Neuropathic Pain

NEUROPATHIC PAIN
Mechanisms, Diagnosis and Treatment

EDITED BY DAVID M. SIMPSON, MD, FAAN

Professor of Neurology
Director, Neuromuscular Division
Director, Clinical Neurophysiology Laboratories
Director, Neuro-AIDS Program
Mount Sinai Medical Center
New York, NY

EDITED BY JUSTIN C. MCARTHUR, MBBS, MPH, FAAN

Professor of Neurology, Pathology, Medicine, and Epidemiology
Director, Department of Neurology
Johns Hopkins University School of Medicine
Neurologist-in-chief
The Johns Hopkins Hospital
Baltimore, MD

EDITED BY ROBERT H. DWORKIN, PHD

Professor of Anesthesiology, Neurology, Oncology, and Psychiatry
Professor, Center for Human Experimental Therapeutics
University of Rochester School of Medicine and Dentistry
Rochester, NY

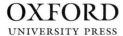
OXFORD
UNIVERSITY PRESS

OXFORD
UNIVERSITY PRESS

Oxford University Press, Inc., publishes works that further
Oxford University's objective of excellence
in research, scholarship, and education.

Oxford   New York
Auckland   Cape Town   Dar es Salaam   Hong Kong   Karachi
Kuala Lumpur   Madrid   Melbourne   Mexico City   Nairobi
New Delhi   Shanghai   Taipei   Toronto

With offices in
Argentina   Austria   Brazil   Chile   Czech Republic   France   Greece
Guatemala   Hungary   Italy   Japan   Poland   Portugal   Singapore
South Korea   Switzerland   Thailand   Turkey   Ukraine   Vietnam

Published by Oxford University Press, Inc.
198 Madison Avenue, New York, New York 10016
www.oup.com

Oxford is a registered trademark of Oxford University Press

Library of Congress Cataloging-in-Publication Data
    Neuropathic pain : mechanisms, diagnosis and treatment / edited by
    David M. Simpson, Justin C. McArthur, Robert H. Dworkin.
        p. ; cm.
    Includes bibliographical references and index.
    ISBN 978–0–19–539470–2 (hardcover : alk. paper)
    I. Simpson, David M.   II. McArthur, Justin C.   III. Dworkin, Robert H.
    [DNLM: 1. Neuralgia. WL 544]

    616.8—dc23
    2011043414

9 8 7 6 5 4 3 2 1
Printed in the United States of America
on acid-free paper

Contents

Foreword

THE IMPACT OF neuropathic pain is well known to those who have experienced it themselves and to the practitioners who specialize in the care of these patients. To many however, the world of neuropathic pain is a secret society. Nearly invisible in all but its most fulminant form, neuropathic pain causes immense suffering accompanied, all too often, by a pervasive sense of alienation as the initiate shuttles from doctor to doctor in search of an answer, if not a cure. The difficulties of neuropathic pain are compounded in that clinical signs are typically subtle, the symptoms may evade description, as Scadding so eloquently noted, and diagnostic tests have only recently become widely available.

It is clear now that there is little to match the pain that arises from neuropathic causes. In their landmark study, Melzack and colleagues demonstrated that neuropathic pain in the form of CRPS exceeded nearly every other cause of pain in the intensity of its effects. So it is that, perhaps more than any other area of medicine, neuropathic pain demands that thoroughgoing scientific knowledge is partnered with the utmost in professional qualities. This volume brings together a wealth of resources to support the experienced practitioner, the inquisitive graduate student, and the devoted medical trainee.

With this book, Drs. Simpson, McArthur, and Dworkin have assembled internationally renowned experts to establish a new cornerstone for future advances. *Neuropathic Pain: Mechanisms, Diagnosis and Treatment* is designed to take the field into the next generation: from the pioneers laboring over first principles to those who will know and understand neuropathic pain as part and parcel of their world of medicine. This is as it should be: as populations around the globe are aging, the incidence of neuropathic pain will continue to climb and hence the need for this work. The capacity to address and effectively treat neuropathic pain is far beyond what any would have dreamed 30 years ago when few but the great specialists held the relevant knowledge in their hands. This book will surely serve to disseminate what is known about neuropathic pain and establish an authoritative foundation for further scientific endeavor and clinical practice.

Beth Murinson

Preface

PERIPHERAL NEUROPATHY IS one of most common neurological disorders in the general population, one which is associated with many diseases. While there are numerous texts on neuromuscular disorders and peripheral neuropathy, relatively few focus on neuropathic pain. During recent decades, there has been a wealth of basic and clinical data expanding our understanding of the mechanisms of neuropathic pain. Unfortunately advances in treatment have lagged behind these pathophysiological findings. This is likely due to a combination of factors, including the limitations in efficacy and safety of existing treatments for neuropathic pain and the methodological challenges of analgesic clinical trials.

This collaborative text is authored by internationally recognized thought leaders in the fields of peripheral neuropathy and neuropathic pain. They include basic scientists, clinicians and clinical researchers, educators, and ethicists. The book is organized into four major sections. The first presents basic mechanisms of peripheral and central neuropathic pain, basic experimental approaches, and the drug discovery pipeline. The second section discusses clinical and diagnostic approaches to neuropathic pain, including recognition of its psychosocial aspects. One chapter presents the strengths and weaknesses of currently employed clinical trial methods, with suggestions for strategies to increase the likelihood that studies will provide a true and valid positive or negative result. The complex ethical and legal issues surrounding pain treatment are also presented, with emphasis on social and economic disparities and the challenges surrounding use of opioid analgesics. The third section is organized around the specific diseases associated with neuropathic pain, illustrating their commonalities and differences. This issue of lumping vs. splitting is particularly timely considering the pathophysiological mechanisms of neuropathic pain of different etiologies and the regulatory approval of agents for these disorders (e.g., diabetic and HIV neuropathy). The last section discusses non-pharmacological treatment approaches and preventive strategies for neuropathic pain. Perhaps the greatest barrier to optimal pain treatment is insufficient education of the health care and lay communities. The final chapter presents strategies to enhance these educational efforts.

We stand on the shoulders of those who preceded us. There are many individuals deserving acknowledgement in providing the teaching and inspiration leading to our entering the daunting field of pain research and management. The editors would like to thank our mentors including Drs. Robert Young, Bhagwan Shahani, Jack Griffin, Guy McKhann, Richard Johnson, Brendan Maher, and Russell Portenoy. We dedicate this book to the memory of Dr. Jack Griffin, whose scholarship, mentorship and kindness touched all that were involved in the field of peripheral neuropathy. We hope that this book will be of interest to students, residents, basic scientists, and both generalists and specialists dealing with patients having neuropathic pain, which includes almost all clinicians.

David M. Simpson, Justin C. McArthur and
Robert H. Dworkin

Contributors

W. David Arnold, MD
Assistant Professor of Neurology
Ohio State University
Columbus, OH

Aditya Bardia, MD, MPH
Medical Oncology Fellow
Johns Hopkins Kimmel Comprehensive Cancer Center
Baltimore, MD

Ralf Baron, Prof. Dr. med.
Head, Division of Neurological Pain Research and
Therapy
Vice Chair, Department of Neurology
Universitätsklinikum Schleswig-Holstein
Kiel, Germany

Andreas Binder
Division of Neurological Pain Research and Therapy
Department of Neurology
Christian-Albrechts-Universität
Kiel, Germany

Tamara B. Bockow
Medical Student
University of Pennsylvania School of Medicine
Philadelphia, PA

Jörgen Boivie, MD, PhD
Department of Neurology
University Hospital
Uppsala, Sweden

Brian Callaghan, MD
Associate Director, Amyotrophic Lateral Sclerosis
(ALS) Clinic
University of Michigan
Ann Arbor, MI

William W. Campbell, MD, MSHA
Professor and Chair
Department of Neurology
Uniformed Services University of Health
Sciences
Bethesda, MD

Craig G. Carroll, DO
Department of Neurology
Naval Medical Center
Portsmouth, VA

Vinay Chaudhry, MD
Professor, Department of Neurology
Johns Hopkins University School of Medicine
Baltimore, MD

Hsinlin T. Cheng, MD, PhD
Assistant Professor
Department of Neurology
University of Michigan
Ann Arbor, MI

Paul J. Christo, MD, MBA
Pain Management Specialist
Johns Hopkins Hospital
Baltimore, MD

Steven P. Cohen, MD
Associate Professor
Department of Anesthesiology/Critical Care
Medicine
Johns Hopkins University School of Medicine
Baltimore, MD

Ross C. Donehower, MD
Professor of Oncology and Medicine
Johns Hopkins University School of Medicine
Director, Division of Medical Oncology
Johns Hopkins Oncology Center
Baltimore, MD

Robert H. Dworkin, PhD
Professor of Anesthesiology, Neurology, Oncology,
and Psychiatry
Professor, Center for Human Experimental
Therapeutics
University of Rochester School of Medicine and
Dentistry
Rochester, NY

Kathryn J. Elliott, MD, JD, MSc
Assistant Professor of Neurology
Mount Sinai School of Medicine
New York, NY

Eva L. Feldman, MD, PhD
Russell N. DeJong Professor of Neurology
University of Michigan
Ann Arbor, MI

Howard L. Fields, MD, PhD
Director of Human Clinical Research,
Gallo Center
Professor of Neurology and Physiology
University of California, San Francisco
San Francisco, CA

Roy Freeman, MD
Professor of Neurology
Harvard Medical School
and
Center for Autonomic and Peripheral
Nerve Disorders
Beth Israel Deaconess Medical Center
Boston, MA

Christopher H. Gibbons MD, MMSc
Assistant Professor of Neurology
Beth Israel Deaconess Medical Center
Boston, MA

Ian Gilron, MD, MSc, FRCPC
Director of Clinical Pain Research
Professor, Anesthesiology & Perioperative Medicine
and Biomedical & Molecular Sciences
Queen's University
Kingston, Ontario, Canada

John W. Griffin, MD[†]
Professor of Neurology
Johns Hopkins University School of Medicine
Baltimore, MD

Scott Haldeman, DC, MD, PhD
Clinical Professor, Department of Neurology
University of California, Irvine
and
Adjunct Professor, Department of Epidemiology
University of California, Los Angeles
and
Research Division
Southern California University of
Health Sciences
Whittier, CA

Per Hansson, MD, DMSci, DDS
Specialist in Neurology and Pain Medicine
Karolinska University Hospital
and
Professor of Clinical Pain Research
Department of Molecular Medicine and Surgery
Karolinska Institutet
Stockholm, Sweden

[†] *Deceased*

R. Norman Harden, MD
Medical Director, Center for Pain Studies
Center for Pain Management
Rehabilitation Institute of Chicago
and
Associate Professor, Physical Medicine and
Rehabilitation
Northwestern University
Chicago, IL

Spencer Heaton, MD
Staff Physician
International Pain Medicine
Desert Pain Institute
Mesa, AZ

Ahmet Höke, MD, PhD
Professor of Neurology and Neuroscience
Director, Neuromuscular Division
Johns Hopkins School of Medicine
Baltimore, MD

Steven H. Horowitz, MD
Department of Neurology
Massachusetts General Hospital
Harvard Medical School
Boston, MA

Mark P. Jensen, PhD
Professor and Vice Chair for Research
Department of Rehabilitation Medicine
University of Washington
Seattle, WA

Christina Jensen-Dahm
Research Assistant
Memory Disorders Research Group
Rigshospitalet
Copenhagen, Denmark

John T. Kissel, MD
Director, Division of Neuromuscular Medicine
Professor of Neurology
Associate Professor of Pediatrics
Ohio State University
Columbus, OH

Michael Lim, MD
Assistant Professor of Neurosurgery
and Oncology
Director of the Metastatic Brain Tumor
Center
Director of Brain Tumor Immunotherapy
Johns Hopkins University School of Medicine
Baltimore, MD

John D. Markman, MD
Associate Professor
Department of Neurosurgery
University of Rochester School of Medicine and
Dentistry
Rochester, NY

John M. Mayer, DC, PhD
Associate Professor and Chiropractor
College of Medicine and School of Physical Therapy
and Rehabilitation Sciences
University of South Florida
Tampa, FL

Justin C. Mcarthur, MBBS, MPH, FAAN
Professor of Neurology, Pathology, Medicine, and
Epidemiology
Director, Department of Neurology
Johns Hopkins University School of Medicine
Neurologist-in-chief
The Johns Hopkins Hospital
Baltimore, MD

Michael R. Moore
Department of Psychology
Willamette University
Salem, OR

Beth B. Murinson, MS, MD, PhD
Associate Professor
Department of Neurology
Johns Hopkins School of Medicine
Baltimore, MD

Trang Nguyen
Department of Neurosurgery
Johns Hopkins School of Medicine
Baltimore, MD

Anne Louise Oaklander, MD, PhD
Associate Professor of Neurology
Massachusetts General Hospital
Harvard Medical School
Boston, MA

Alec B. O'Connor, MD, MPH
Associate Professor of Medicine
University of Rochester School of Medicine and
Dentistry
Rochester, NY

Amanda Peltier, MD, MS
Assistant Professor of Neurology
Vanderbilt Medical Center
Nashville, TN

Karin L. Petersen, MD
Associate Adjunct Professor of Neurology
University of California, San Francisco
San Francisco, CA

Srinivasa N. Raja, MD
Professor
Department of Anesthesiology/Critical Care Medicine
Johns Hopkins University School of Medicine
Baltimore, MD

Pablo F. Recinos, MD
Neurosurgery resident
Department of Neurosurgery
Johns Hopkins Hospital
Baltimore, MD

Gadi Revivo, DO
Center for Pain Management
Rehabilitation Institute of Chicago
Northwestern University
Chicago, IL

Kathryn Richardson, MOTR/L
Center for Pain Management
Rehabilitation Institute of Chicago
Chicago, IL

Tamara S. Ritsema, MP, MMSc, PA-C
Assistant Professor of Health Care Sciences
George Washington University
Washington, DC

Jessica Robinson-Papp, MD
Assistant Professor of Neurology
Mount Sinai Medical Center
New York, NY

Ricardo Horacio Roda, MD, PhD
Clinical Fellow
Department of Neurology
Johns Hopkins School of Medicine
Baltimore, MD

Michael C. Rowbotham, MD
Scientific Director
California Pacific Medical Center Research Institute
San Francisco, CA

Michelle Shufelt, DPT
Center for Pain Management
Rehabilitation Institute of Chicago
Chicago, IL

David M. Simpson, MD, FAAN
Professor of Neurology
Director, Neuromuscular Division
Director, Clinical Neurophysiology
Laboratories
Director-Neuro AIDS Program
Mount Sinai Medical Center
New York, NY

J. Robinson Singleton M.D.
Professor, Neurology
Director, CCTS Clinical Services Core
University of Utah
Salt Lake City, UT

A. Gordon Smith, MD FAAN
Chief of Neuromuscular Medicine
Associate Professor of Neurology and
Pathology
University of Utah School of Medicine
Salt Lake City, UT

Rolf-Detlef Treede, MD
Professor of Neurophysiology
Center for Biomedicine and Medical
Technology Mannheim (CBTM)
Ruprecht-Karls-University of Heidelberg
Mannheim, Germany

Andrew W. Varga, MD, PhD
Department of Neurology
Beth Israel Deaconess Medical Center
Boston, MA

Haleh Van Vliet, MD
University of Rochester School of Medicine
Rochester, NY

Gunnar Wasner, MD
Consultant Neurologist
Division of Neurological Pain Research and
Therapy
Department of Neurology
Christian-Albrechts-Universität
Kiel, Germany

Kayode A. Williams, MD, MBA, FFARCSI
Assistant Professor of Anesthesiology and
Critical Care Medicine
Johns Hopkins University School of Medicine
Baltimore, MD

1

Neuropathic Pain: A Brief Conceptual History

HOWARD L. FIELDS

INTRODUCTION

PAIN IS A familiar part of life for most people and is an expected symptom of many injuries and diseases. Thankfully, over the past century, tremendous progress has been made in our understanding of the neural mechanisms underlying normal pain sensation. Furthermore, as more clinicians have been drawn to pain management, significant improvements in therapy have been achieved. Neuropathic pain, however, remains a significant problem area. Nervous system injury or disease that affects sensory pathways typically impairs normal sensation. However, in some situations, the disease process that impairs normal pain sensation can produce pain and hypersensitivity. For patients with neuropathic pain, the suffering can be severe and have a disturbingly peculiar quality. Because they can be extremely disturbing and resistant to treatment, neuropathic pains are a major challenge to the research and treatment communities. Unfortunately, despite progress in clinical care and improved animal models for research, the mechanisms of neuropathic pain remain enigmatic, even for the most common conditions. Fortunately, the paradoxical combination of impaired pain sensation and ongoing severe pain has drawn the interest and attention of scientists for well over a century and has stimulated both clinical and animal research. This, in turn has led to new ideas and experiments that have broadly informed and advanced the field of pain research. Notable examples of this are the pioneering studies of S. Weir Mitchell and Rene Leriche on causalgia, Henry Head's studies of his own experimentally injured nerve, and Melzack and Wall's Gate Control Hypothesis.[1] More recently, tantalizing glimpses of future progress have accumulated following the seminal work of Gary Bennett to improve animal models of nerve injury pain.[2]

These improved animal models and discoveries in patients have confirmed that some forms of neuropathic pain are caused by increased excitability of small-diameter primary afferent fibers. We are at a point where optimism is justified that the torture of neuropathic pain will be alleviated.

WHAT IS NEUROPATHIC PAIN?

Despite impressive growth in the number of professionals working on this problem, it is surprising that there are still significant areas of controversy about the definition of neuropathic pain. A corollary of this lack of consensus is uncertainty about whether certain clinical syndromes represent a form of neuropathic pain. There are several reasons for this. First and foremost, the neural pathophysiology is unknown, even for the most common painful neuropathic conditions (e.g., painful diabetic polyneuropathy, postherpetic neuralgia, and spinal cord injury). Second, there are several painful conditions that are clearly associated with dysfunction of the nervous system but are not commonly considered to be neuropathic pain (e.g., migraine and cluster headaches, painful epileptic seizures). Third, because large nerve trunks have connective tissue sheaths that are innervated by nociceptors (nervi nervorum), the pain in some neuropathic conditions may be due to inflammatory processes whose activation represents the *normal* function of primary afferent nociceptors. Fourth, some clinical features of neuropathic pain (e.g., allodynia, hyperalgesia) can be produced by activity in normally functioning primary afferent nociceptors and have little specificity either for diagnosis or for understanding the unique pathophysiology of neuropathic pain. Fifth, there are conditions of unknown etiology that share some clinical features with syndromes that are clearly neuropathic (e.g., fibromyalgia). These problems have clouded the very concept of neuropathic pain or, at the very least, have broadened its scope to the point where the value of the concept has declined and in some cases may be confusing rather than informative. Unfortunately, the lumping together of mechanistically diverse conditions has led to less accuracy in diagnosis and has slowed progress in understanding which experimental models correspond to which clinical conditions.

In order to trace the conceptual history of neuropathic pain with clarity, it is essential to define the concept in a way that permits a cogent and accessible story. The simplest approach is to narrow the definition of neuropathic pains to include only those pains that result from abnormal function of neurons. The etiology should be neuropathic if the primary cause is intrinsic to the neuron (e.g., viral damage of primary afferents in herpes zoster, leading either to increased sodium channel function or to deafferentation hypersensitivity of second-order pain transmission neurons). The etiology might be secondary to a condition primarily affecting nonneural tissue (e.g., pathological changes in primary afferents due to nerve compression, infiltration by tumor or by occlusion of a blood vessel that supplies the nerve). The important point is that primary afferent nociceptors normally detect and signal actual or impending damage in a variety of tissues. Their *normal* biological function thus occurs under *pathological conditions* and may involve local metabolic changes that increase their sensitivity. The activity of nociceptors, in turn, causes changes in the central nervous system that lead to further increases in sensitivity. I propose that if the pain is caused by the normal physiological function of the pain afferent pathway, including nociceptive nervi nervorum, it should not be considered neuropathic.

In an individual patient, it may be difficult to determine which are the neuropathic and the nonneuropathic components of the pain. For example, in a patient with an acute herniated intervertebral disc, there may be back and radiating leg pain as well as weakness and sensory loss. This combination of factors is often seen in neuropathic conditions. However, referred pain does not imply a neuropathic mechanism; the pain may be primarily inflammatory and involve the normal function of primary afferent nociceptors that innervate the dura.[3,4] I suggest that we keep an open mind on the issue of whether a particular clinical syndrome is neuropathic until sufficient evidence is amassed to inform the question. Unfortunately, due to real-world pressures to rapidly assess and treat patients, such a thoughtful approach is too often not taken. Consequently, neuropathic pain is frequently misdiagnosed.

EARLY RECOGNITION OF DRAMATIC NEUROPATHIC PAIN SYNDROMES

Distinct Neuropathic Pain Conditions

Some neuropathic pain conditions are so dramatic and distinct in their clinical manifestations that their unique features were widely appreciated for years before anyone knew that their cause had anything to do with the nervous system. Phantom limb pain, herpes zoster, and trigeminal neuralgia are prominent examples of conditions that have been known for millennia and were described in early medical writings. Phantom limb pain is perhaps the most dramatic of these conditions. This is likely due to the mysterious and counterintuitive phenomenon of experiencing pain in an absent extremity. Phantom limb pain has drawn the widespread interest of the public and the artistic community, as well as that of scientists, psychologists, physicians, and the surgeons involved in the amputations. One of the most dramatic descriptions of the condition was provided by Herman Melville in his classic novel *Moby Dick*, published in 1851 (Chapter 108, pp. 432–433):

> Carpenter (speaking to Captain Ahab while fashioning for him a new prosthesis for his amputated leg): "Yes, I have heard something curious on that score, sir; how that a dismasted man never entirely loses the feeling of his old spar, but it will be still pricking him at times. May I humbly ask if it be really so, sir?"
> Captain Ahab: "It is, man....And if I still feel the smart of my crushed leg, though it be now so long dissolved; then, why mayst not thou, carpenter, feel the fiery pains of hell for ever, and without a body? Hah!"

John Hunter, Trigeminal Neuralgia, and the Emerging Concept of Neuropathic Pain

Another example of a unique and dramatic syndrome that has been known for a very long time is trigeminal neuralgia. Despite its rarity, it was recognized and recorded as a clinical entity by early physicians. The first published clinical description was written in 1671 by Johannes Bausch, who suffered from the condition himself (see ref. 5). Later authors provided more accurate and informative clinical descriptions of the condition; however, John Hunter was apparently the first to propose explicitly that pain could arise from injury to nerves. He observed that though the pain often appeared to arise from the teeth, removal of teeth had no effect on the condition. He correctly concluded that this was a different sort of pain. To quote him directly[6]:

> Hence it should appear that the pain in question does not arise from any disease in the part, but it is entirely a nervous affection.

It is clear from this quote that Hunter understood the concept of neuropathic pain, and he may have been the first to publish the idea that it is a distinct clinical phenomenon. Furthermore, although the mechanism of pain in trigeminal neuralgia is still not known, it is likely that it was the first neuropathic pain condition to be correctly understood as such. This eighteenth-century idea was confirmed by the twentieth-century neurosurgeon Walter Dandy, who first reported that many patients with trigeminal neuralgia have a compressive lesion of the root of the trigeminal nerve and experience immediate relief following decompression.[7]

S. Weir Mitchell, the Syndrome of Causalgia, and Sympathetically Maintained Pain

Although the concept of neuropathic pain had been proposed well before he appeared on the scene, no discussion of the history of neuropathic pain would be complete without including the contributions of Silas Weir Mitchell

(1829–1914). Mitchell was an illustrious neurologist, a member of the National Academy of Sciences, and the first president of the American Neurological Society. His unparalleled clinical experience with neuropathic pain was the result of his service as a physician for the Union Army in the American Civil War (1861–1865). At one point, he was responsible for a 400-bed hospital entirely devoted to the care of patients with peripheral nerve injuries. Working nearly a century after John Hunter's first explicit (and correct) publication of the concept of neuropathic pain, Mitchell had the advantage of tremendous advances in medical and biological knowledge of the nervous system. However, it was his vast clinical experience, combined with his extensive knowledge of the normal anatomy and physiology of peripheral nerves, that uniquely qualified him to advance our understanding of neuropathic pain.

Mitchell described a distinct syndrome consisting of burning pain (causalgia) of the upper or lower extremity following traumatic peripheral nerve damage (this is currently referred to as *complex regional pain syndrome type II*). The latency to the onset of the pain was variable, but the intensity of the pain characteristically grew over days to weeks, often as normal strength and sensation were returning. The pain was always most intense in the distal extremity (hand or foot) and often involved the joints. Associated swelling and glossiness of the skin were prominent in most cases. Mitchell also described exquisite hypersensitivity to light touch and exacerbation of the pain by movement or strong emotion. The following is an extract from Mitchell's 1864 (Mitchell SW, Morehouse GR, & Keen WW, *Gunshot Wounds and Other Injuries of Nerves*: Philadelphia: J.B. Lippincott & Co., 1864) book:

> Pain, in the shape of neuralgia like the darting, typical pain of tic douloureux, is a common sequence of nerve wounds. It assumes all kinds of forms, from the burning, which we have yet fully to describe, through the whole catalogue of terms vainly used to convey some idea of variety in torture.... Long after every other trace of the effects of a wound has gone, these neuralgic symptoms are apt to linger, and too many carry with them throughout long years this final reminder of the battle-field.... We have here set apart for distinct consideration that kind of pain which we have before spoken of as burning pain. It is a form of suffering as yet undescribed, and so frequent and terrible as to demand from us the fullest description.... Of the special cause which provokes it we know nothing, except that it has sometimes followed the transfer of pathological changes from a wounded nerve to unwounded nerves, and has then been felt in their distribution.... The part itself is not alone subject to an intense burning sensation, but becomes exquisitely hyperaesthetic, so that a touch or tap of the finger increases the pain. (Chapter 7, pp. 100–103)

EARLY IDEAS ABOUT PATHOPHYSIOLOGY

At the time Mitchell was accumulating his vast store of clinical experience with traumatic nerve injury, he was curious about what made certain lesions painful. He knew that sensory and motor nerves ran in separate pathways and that nerve sheaths had their own separate innervation (nervi nervorum). He was also aware that there was a sympathetic nervous system that controlled blood vessel diameter. The pioneering work of Galvani and Volta in the 1790s had shown that peripheral nerves were electrically sensitive and conducted information to and from the nervous system. By 1852, Helmholtz had measured the conduction velocity of motor axons in the frog and had found a value of about 20 m/s. Despite knowing that peripheral nerves were electrically excitable and conducted information to and from the central nervous system, physiologists did not know how the peripheral nerves worked. Furthermore, although neurologists and physiologists were aware that touch had a different representation than pain and temperature in the central nervous system, Mitchell voiced doubts that there were individual nerve fibers that responded selectively to noxious stimulation. He also expressed doubt that the information in nerves was electrically transmitted because the conduction velocity of nerves as measured by Helmholtz was so much slower than the known speed of electrical pulses in wires.

Mitchell's descriptions of neuralgic conditions are unparalleled, and he clearly understood that direct pathology of the nerve could produce both loss of function and pain. However, he was completely puzzled about the pathophysiology of the pain, and his speculations about how nerves transmit their messages were wide of the mark. In fact, given how little was known at the time about neurophysiology, a basic understanding of the cause of neuralgic pain would have been impossible. It wasn't until the next century that information relevant to causalgia began to trickle in. Perhaps the first clinical breakthrough related to neuropathic pain was the discovery in 1916 by Rene Leriche that stripping the periarterial nerve plexus gave immediate pain relief.[8] Leriche concluded that efferent sympathetic activity in the presence of nerve injury could cause pain. This was confirmed by later workers who found that local anesthesia of the sympathetic efferent outflow to the appropriate limb also gave immediate and complete relief (see ref. 9 for review). The combination of having a dramatically effective intervention, along with the clinical observation that the painful extremity was often very cold and discolored and that the pain relief following sympatholysis correlated with a warmer, drier limb, led to the idea that efferent sympathetic activity could somehow activate pain fibers. This was important because interruption or block of sympathetic efferents normally has no effect on pain sensation. Although there is still some controversy over the nature and ubiquity of sympathetically maintained pain, the idea that sympathetic outflow can generate pain in the distribution of a damaged peripheral nerve is now well established.[10]

From a historical perspective, the discovery of causalgia, its concomitant vegetative signs (e.g., cold, sweaty skin), and, in particular, the later discovery by Leriche that it was relieved by sympathetic blockade were important first steps in understanding one form of neuropathic pain. More important conceptually was the idea that this particular type of pain is mechanistically distinct from somatic pains (i.e., pains resulting from the normal function of primary afferent nociceptors). While

the response of causalgia to sympathetic block suggested that damaged nerve fibers become responsive to efferent sympathetic activity (and this, in a sense, is an explicit, albeit incomplete, explanation of the pain), at the time of Leriche's discovery, the mechanism by which nerve cells transmit information was still unknown. Because of this ignorance, the question of how injury to neurons could cause an increase in their function and how this could lead to pain was still unanswered.

The Discovery of the Action Potential and the First Insights into How Nerve Cells Transmit Information

This situation began to change dramatically following the technical advances that permitted scientists to measure the tiny electrical potentials that are the basis for axonal conduction (i.e., the action potential). The technical breakthrough (ca. 1915–1930) was the invention and improvement of the vacuum tube or thermionic valve. This device provided a method for amplification of the tiny signals generated by single nerve axons up to 5000-fold. The distinguished Cambridge physiologist Edgar Adrian pioneered the use of this method for studying single nerves in the 1920s and shared the Nobel Prize with Charles Sherrington in 1932. Adrian was able to record single action potentials in peripheral axons, elicited by either electrical stimulation or a variety of physiological sensory stimuli, including noxious stimuli. He demonstrated quite dramatically and conclusively that all axons transmit information by means of trains of identical brief electrical pulses. He was, for example, able to show that tactile stimulation produced an increase in firing frequency in a peripheral sensory axon that subsided when the stimulus was terminated (see ref. 11). Furthermore, other axons in other sensory systems generated apparently identical pulses (each pulse was a few hundredths of a volt and lasted for about one-thousandth of a second). Adrian's critical discovery and the insight that followed remain powerful to this day:

Impulses travelling to the brain in the auditory nerve make us hear sounds and impulses of the same kind arranged in much the same way in the optic nerve make us see sights. The mental result must differ because a different part of the brain receives the message and not because the message has a different form.[12]

Although Adrian and others were able to show activity produced by noxious stimuli in single peripheral nerve axons,[13] the ability to record reliably from single unmyelinated axons lay several decades in the future. However, Adrian's discovery that nervous system information is encoded in the temporal sequence of nerve impulses, that is, that the operation of the brain is representational, meant that precise connectivity is required for decoding this information. This principle is the critical conceptual basis for understanding how the nervous system works, and without this discovery a full explanation for pain (or, for that matter, any function of the nervous system) would not be possible. The critical nature of this technical and conceptual advance is affirmed by the dramatic progress in understanding that followed.

Segregation of Function in Peripheral Nerves, Compound Sensation, and the Role of Inhibition in Pain Perception from Henry Head to Melzack and Wall

Based on his careful studies of cutaneous sensation, Henry Head reported that experimental damage to a human cutaneous nerve (his own) produced some curious findings in addition to the expected loss of somatic sensation.[14] He found that there was a transition zone between the region of total sensory loss and the surrounding area of normal sensation. In this transition zone there was a partial loss of sensation but, importantly, stimuli that induced pain in normal skin produced even greater pain when delivered in this transition zone. Thus, he discovered that *partial* nerve damage is associated with *enhanced* pain. Furthermore, he described scattered regions around the transition zone in which light moving tactile stimuli produced significant pain. Based on these and other clinical observations, Head proposed the existence of two cutaneous sensory systems, which he named *epicritic* and *protopathic*. Head further proposed that under most conditions, stimuli

activated both systems and that the epicritic pathway normally inhibited input arriving via the protopathic pathway. Thus, under conditions in which there was predominant damage to the epicritic system, Head proposed that one would see hyperfunction of the protopathic system. Trotter and Davis[15] largely replicated Head's observations using a larger dataset of human experimental nerve injuries and instruments designed to ensure the delivery of identical somatic stimuli in different skin regions.

Over the next two decades, as scientists were able to record ever smaller transient electrical signals, it became clear that peripheral nerves were made up of axons that could be grouped by size and conduction velocity. Joseph Erlanger and Herbert Gasser (who shared the Nobel Prize in 1944 for their work in this area) discovered that each group of axons generated a distinct wave, the compound action potential that could be recorded near the surface of the nerve.[16] They were able to correlate the speed of conduction with the axon diameter and to show that the more slowly conducting axons were more susceptible to local anesthetic infiltration of the peripheral nerve (e.g., see ref. 16). In addition, D.C. Sinclair had shown that applying varying levels of mechanical pressure on a nerve could lead to selective blockade of peripheral axons, with the rapidly conducting larger-diameter myelinated groups the earliest to be blocked (see ref. 17 for review). Using this knowledge and themselves as experimental subjects, William Landau and George Bishop[18] studied the time course of sensory changes following either local anesthetic or pressure block of peripheral nerves. Bishop had already shown that Aδ and C fiber groups could be blocked separately. In this study, Landau and Bishop showed that blockade of Aδ axons produced a loss of pricking pain but preserved deep inflammatory pain. Importantly, they clearly demonstrated that blockade of Aδ fibers resulted in an enhanced subjective experience of pain when using stimuli that produced only moderate pain in normally innervated skin. Along with Head's findings and Trotter and Davies' psychophysical studies of pain following experimental nerve injury, the discovery of an inhibitory interaction between different classes of primary afferent was the impetus for early theories of the pathophysiology of neuropathic pain. This inhibitory interaction, with large fibers inhibiting noxious input from small-diameter primary afferents, was proposed by the clinicians William Livingston[19] and William Noordenbos as contributing factors in neuropathic pain. Noordenbos assumed that it was the predominant loss of large-diameter fibers following acute herpes zoster that led to the phenomenon of summation in patients with postherpetic neuralgia. He observed that the sensation elicited by slowly repeated mechanical stimulation was innocuous at first but built up over time, becoming unbearable, spread spatially, and persisted long after the stimulation had ceased.[20]

THE GATE CONTROL HYPOTHESIS: A TURNING POINT IN THE EVOLUTION OF IDEAS ABOUT PAIN

What Was the Gate Control Hypothesis Trying to Explain?

The publication of the Gate Control Hypothesis in 1965 was a watershed event in the history of pain research, and its publication influenced the course of research and clinical care for several decades.[1] The Gate Control Hypothesis represented a synthesis of clinical, psychophysical, and neurobiological findings and was the first serious attempt to provide a comprehensive theory of pain in the form of a specific, falsifiable neural model. At the time that the Gate Control Hypothesis was proposed, most scientists studying somatosensory function were content with the idea that stimulus intensity was the critical variable governing pain perception. Most believed in the existence of neurons that responded selectively to noxious stimulation and whose activity invariably produced the sensation of pain. That belief was the essence of *specificity theory*. Specificity theory rested on three critical assumptions: (1) There exist specific classes of primary afferent nociceptors whose activity unambiguously signals that a noxious stimulus has been applied in their receptive field. (2) The activity of these neurons is necessary and sufficient to produce the subjective sensation of pain

and no other sensation. (3) Nonnociceptive primary afferents do not normally contribute to pain sensation. Despite the evidence for specificity in somatosensory pain pathways, it is clear (and had been clear since the work of Henry Head) that what an individual normally experiences following a noxious stimulus is a compound sensation. That is, under physiological conditions, noxious stimuli activate several classes of primary afferents (including low-threshold afferents) and activity in more than one type contributes to normal pain sensation. We know this because selective blockade of Aδ fibers blocks pricking pain and changes the quality and timing of what one feels when C fibers are activated. Not only does the quality of the sensation change but, in addition, such blockade enhances the painfulness of a noxious stimulus and produces a state in which ordinarily innocuous stimuli elicit pain. If pain sensation were a simple and reliable consequence of activity in one or more classes of primary afferents, then damage to that afferent should result in a loss of pain sensation, not an enhancement and/or change in quality. Thus, not only is pain a compound sensation, but under normal conditions, a subset of the primary afferents activated by noxious stimuli exerts a net inhibitory influence on the resulting sensation. This was one of the critical observations that Melzack and Wall intended to explain with their new theory. They also wanted to explain why cutting a peripheral nerve usually failed to relieve pain in the innervation territory of that nerve and, finally, they wanted to address Noordenbos' observation that patients with postherpetic neuralgia had a predominant loss of large-diameter peripheral axons and manifested the phenomenon of increasing pain intensity over time with prolonged or repeated stimuli. In addition to the challenges posed by psychophysical studies in subjects with injury or experimental partial blockade of peripheral nerve, Melzack and Wall were aware of the powerful influence of psychological factors on pain perception and they felt, rightfully so, that any general theory of pain must provide a mechanism by which this could occur.

There was a broad understanding, especially among clinicians caring for patients with neuropathic pain, that specificity theory fell short as an explanatory model. Melzack and Wall knew what had to be explained by any valid and comprehensive pain theory. However, given the extensive requirements of a general theory and the primitive state of understanding of central nervous system pain processing at the time, no one really knew how to construct the explanatory neural model. Melzack and Wall proposed that the substantia gelatinosa (SG) was the key. Activity of large-diameter myelinated primary afferents had been shown to depolarize primary afferent terminals in the SG, and this depolarization was associated with presynaptic inhibition. In contrast, Wall had demonstrated that small-diameter primary afferents contacted SG neurons and produced a hyperpolarization of the same terminals. Melzack and Wall proposed that both large- and small-diameter primary afferents converge upon and excite dorsal horn pain transmission cells (they called these *T cells* or *action cells*). In addition, the large-diameter primary afferents excited while the small-diameter afferents inhibited SG interneurons that mediated presynaptic inhibition of the T cells. Thus, small-diameter inputs would remove SG neuron inhibition (i.e., facilitate firing) in T cells. Melzack and Wall guessed that this disinhibition grew gradually with continued small-fiber input and mediated the phenomenon of summation (i.e., the increase in pain over time with continued stimulation). Their model offered an explanation of several of the well-established psychophysical features of pain that could not be explained by specificity theory: (1) how input from large-diameter fibers inhibits input from small-diameter primary afferents (excitation of inhibitory SG cells), (2) summation (progressive disinhibition of T cells), (3) compound sensation (convergence of large- and small-diameter afferents on SG and T cells), and (4) how the sensory quality of large-diameter inputs can switch from innocuous to painful (allodynia or hyperalgesia: shutdown of inhibitory SG neurons by input from small-diameter primary afferents, leaving excitatory input from large-diameter primary afferents to T cells intact).

In addition, their model provided a mechanism, the Central Control Trigger, by which learning and emotional state can influence pain. This Central Control Trigger was involved in an action decision process, modulated by learning and other contextual factors, that could, through descending pathways, inhibit nociceptive transmission at the level of the SG.

A good scientific theory should explain more than previous theories, be more consistent with more observations, and have assumptions and predictions that are testable. Even if it is wrong, a scientific theory is successful if the experiments it suggests lead to new knowledge. The Gate Control Hypothesis passed all these tests. It caught on because it explained the variability of pain using a neural mechanism simple enough to be easily understood, yet detailed enough to be falsified. It made some assumptions, guesses, and predictions, the majority of which have turned out to be wrong. The Gate Control Hypothesis surpassed the other theories because it was more comprehensive, it did not ignore puzzling clinical observations, it included new experimental findings that previous theories did not have to deal with, and it suggested specific experiments. It was a key impetus for modern pain research. What features of the proposal have survived?

The Action System (T Cells)

T cells were vaguely specified by Melzack and Wall. They were referring to a hierarchically organized set of afferent pathways activated by a noxious stimulus and mediating a variety of behaviors usually associated with the subjective experience of pain—for example, escape/withdrawal, orientation, and vocalization. Although no specific pathway was named, pathways from the dorsal horn to the cortex were included; thus, the T cell system would clearly include the spinothalamic tract, which everyone agrees is critical for pain sensation in primates. The key concept for this part of the Gate Control Hypothesis is that T cells have convergent input, have both excitatory and inhibitory input from large-diameter primary afferents, show summation when small-diameter primary afferents are repeatedly activated, and are subject to descending inhibition. These key aspects of the proposal have all, in fact, been confirmed for dorsal horn neurons in cats, primates, and rats. For example, consistent with the model, Price and colleagues[21] showed convincingly in human subjects that with repeated thermal stimulation, noxious pricking first pain progressively declines, while the later throbbing second pain progressively increases. Using the same stimuli in anesthetized primates, they showed that both Aδ (first pain) and C-fiber (second pain) responses progressively decline with repeated stimuli. This finding is consistent with the idea that summation is a central nervous system phenomenon. In fact, shortly after the publication of the Gate Control Hypothesis, Lorne Mendell showed that spinal cord dorsal horn neurons show a progressive increase in activity (wind up) with repeated identical C-fiber stimulation.[22] In 1969, Hillman and Wall[23] showed that lamina 5 neurons in cat dorsal horn receive both excitatory and inhibitory input from low-threshold mechanoreceptors and are primarily excited by more intense mechanical stimulation. Furthermore, Wall, in his classic 1967 paper showing physiological lamination of the dorsal horn,[24] had discovered that lamina 5 neurons with convergent input are subject to powerful descending inhibition. Thus, the concept of the T cell, with convergent input from large and small fibers, summation of sustained or repeated small-fiber input over time, and an inhibitory effect of myelinated input on T-cell responses to input from nonmyelinated primary afferents, appears to be correct.

What about the SG?

This was the most detailed part of the Gate Control Hypothesis and the only part of the mechanism that was based on existing neural data. The SG was known to be packed with interneurons; however, because of their small size, no one had yet recorded from them. Wall had indirect evidence that synapses in the SG controlled the terminals of both large- and small-diameter primary afferents, but he had no direct evidence that primary afferents directly contacted SG cells or that SG cells modulated local primary afferent terminals. The existence of this entire circuit was a guess. Subsequent experiments have shown that it was an inspired guess. Although it is still uncertain whether the proposed connections function in the manner proposed by Melzack and Wall, it is now clear

that there are inhibitory interneurons in the SG and there is indirect evidence that they control T cells. We now know that unmyelinated primary afferents, including identified nociceptors, terminate on both projection neurons and SG interneurons. It is also clear that primary afferent terminals in the SG are subject to modulatory control. However, the involvement of SG neurons in this presynaptic control and the direction of their effect (if any) have not been established. It is also true that myelinated primary afferents can either excite or inhibit T cells. The inhibition requires an interneuron; the excitation may be mono- or polysynaptic. Under pathological circumstances, including inflammation, activation of large-diameter primary afferents, which respond maximally to light mechanical stimuli, produces pain. Since this modality switch can occur without lesions of the nervous system, it is certain that there is an excitatory connection between large-diameter primary afferents that normally respond to innocuous stimuli and at least some second-order neurons that transmit the pain message (*vide infra*).

In the decades following publication of the Gate Control Hypothesis, research into the neural mechanisms underlying pain transmission grew explosively and, as new discoveries accumulated, critical assumptions of the original hypothesis and several of its key assumptions and mechanistic proposals were shown to be wrong. More importantly, new neural mechanisms were discovered that provided a simpler and more accurate explanation for some of the phenomena that the Gate Control Hypothesis attempted to explain. However, although the Gate Control Hypothesis is incomplete and wrong in significant details, it has not yet been replaced by a comprehensive theory. Unfortunately, any future theory that attempts to be comprehensive will have to be much more detailed because it will have much more information to account for. The original Gate Control Hypothesis was simple, comprehensive, and testable. In a sense, Melzack and Wall's signal achievement was to clearly define the questions that pain researchers needed to address and to raise the bar for future explanations by demanding that they be based on specific circuit connections. The publication of the

Gate Control Hypothesis was a milestone that deserves a significant place in the conceptual history of neuropathic pain.

THE MODERN ERA: ALLODYNIA, CENTRAL SENSITIZATION, AND THE MODALITY SWITCH OF INPUT FROM MYELINATED LOW-THRESHOLD MECHANORECEPTORS

One of the most common features of neuropathic pain is the unpleasant sensation produced by innocuous mechanical stimulation of the skin. How this happens in patients with nerve injury is not known; however, elegant psychophysical studies in normal individuals have shown that electrical stimulation of large-diameter myelinated primary afferents can switch from eliciting an innocuous tactile sensation to eliciting pain following activation of nociceptors within the territory of their receptive field.[25] A parallel change in perception is elicited by innocuous moving mechanical stimulation in the same receptive field. This shows that prolonged activation of nociceptors normally leads to allodynia through a change in the central nervous system. This is a very important observation because it proves that activity in nonnociceptive primary afferents can elicit pain. In this case, primary afferent nociceptors are permissive but do not directly cause the perception of pain. This study is also important clinically because it shows that, like summation, allodynia is not an unambiguous diagnostic sign of neuropathic pain. On the other hand, allodynia could be secondary either to a pathological process in the periphery that results in activity in primary afferent nociceptors or to anatomical changes in the spinal cord.

Technical advances in the late 1960s allowed Ed Perl and his colleagues to record reliably from small-diameter primary afferents. They were able to show that distinct subclasses of unmyelinated and small myelinated primary afferents respond selectively to noxious stimuli (i.e., there are primary afferent nociceptors—lots of them).[26,27] Perhaps even more devastating to the Gate Control

Hypothesis, there are distinct classes of C and Aδ fibers that respond selectively and maximally to innocuous touch or temperature change. Furthermore, two important properties of primary afferent nociceptors were completely unknown to Melzack and Wall: sensitization of their peripheral terminals following local tissue damage and their development of spontaneous discharge following damage. These two phenomena are among the likely contributing factors to neuropathic pain. In fact, in 1978, Wall himself acknowledged these issues in an eloquent reframing of the original hypothesis.[28]

THE CURRENT ERA OF NEUROPATHIC PAIN RESEARCH

The Irritable Nociceptor

Severed peripheral nerves form neuromas at their cut ends. Clinicians had known for some time that these neuromas can be exquisitely sensitive to mechanical stimulation. Furthermore, in some cases, local anesthetic infiltration of a neuroma can provide complete, though typically transient, pain relief of pain (e.g., ref. 29). The discovery that a subset of primary afferents are nociceptive and cause pain when selectively activated raised the specific idea that long-term increases in the discharge of such primary afferents following damage to a peripheral nerve could be a significant source of pain. The first experimental evidence for this was provided in 1974 by Pat Wall and Michael Gutnick,[30] who showed that sensory axons innervating an experimental neuroma gave rise to a constant barrage of impulses for up to 5 weeks following nerve injury. Although this observation has been extensively replicated across a variety of peripheral pathologies (e.g., see ref. 31), its interpretation is uncertain because when the primary afferents are cut from their peripheral terminals, they cannot be identified as nociceptors.

Because of this problem, a major advance in neuropathic pain research was required. It came in the form of the explicit use of experimental partial nerve injury. Bennett and Xie[2] were the first to understand and address the problem that complete peripheral nerve transection typically does not elicit a behavioral syndrome that mirrors what is common in patients with neuropathic pain: evidence of discomfort and hyperalgesia in the affected region. To replicate an entrapment neuropathy, which is often painful, Bennett and Xie placed loose ligatures around the common sciatic nerve. They observed hyperalgesia to chemogenic stimulation, allodynia to cold and light mechanical stimulation, and guarding of the affected limb. It is fair to say that the modern era of experimental nerve injury in pain research was catalyzed by this seminal publication. Most scientists currently studying experimental neuropathic pain in animals use some variation of partial nerve injury, and hypersensitivity to cutaneous stimuli is currently the most common measure of pain. One of the great values of the partial nerve injury model is that many of the primary afferents innervating the painful region remain connected to their peripheral transducing terminals. This makes it possible to study individual primary afferents and to determine their conduction velocity and response characteristics (i.e., identify them as nociceptors). Importantly, such studies have shown that nerve injury or inflammation can increase the number of primary afferent nociceptors with spontaneous discharge. This is consistent with the idea that one mechanism of neuropathic pain is the development of spontaneous discharge in primary afferent nociceptors. This in and of itself could lead to hyperalgesia, enhanced summation, and allodynia through physiological mechanisms in the central nervous system. It also implies that to the extent that a neuropathic pain syndrome is due to increased firing of nociceptors, *its central actions will be similar to those of somatic pains without nerve dysfunction.* A corollary of this idea is that such neuropathic pain conditions should respond to centrally acting analgesic drugs that are effective for nonneuropathic pains.

The question of whether an abnormality leading to a selective increase in primary afferent nociceptors can occur in humans was conclusively answered in the affirmative by the clinical discovery of two distinct syndromes characterized by spontaneous episodic pain: erythermalgia and paroxysmal extreme pain disorder.[32] In both conditions, there are point mutations in the gene of a subtype of voltage-gated sodium channels. This channel ($Na_v 1.7$) is highly expressed in primary afferent nociceptors. The pain syndromes associated with mutations in the $Na_v 1.7$ gene cause increases in activation level (reduced threshold) compared to the normal channel, and this results in enhanced firing of primary afferent nociceptors. This extraordinary finding suggests that renewed efforts to study the pathophysiology of neuropathic pain in patients will be a fruitful guide to future understanding.

OVERVIEW

From Hunter's first explicit articulation of the concept of neuropathic pain in 1778 to the present time, we have made great strides in our understanding of the pathophysiology of neuropathic pain. The single most important technical advance that enabled this progress was the ability to record action potentials in single nerve cells. It is this technique that taught us about the different classes of primary afferents and showed us that their interaction (both excitatory and inhibitory) is necessary for the compound sensation we call pain. Ultimately, we learned that changes in the properties and distribution of voltage-gated sodium channels due to pathology in primary afferent nociceptors can be sufficient to cause pain. Furthermore, we learned that a prolonged increase in the activity of unmyelinated primary afferent nociceptors under conditions where large-diameter primary afferents are not active can lead to summation, increased pain, and hyperalgesia to noxious stimuli. In addition, prolonged input from nociceptors can produce a shift in the psychophysical consequence of activity in large-diameter mechanoreceptors such that they produce pain (allodynia) instead of an innocuous tactile sensation. It is likely that this modality switch occurs under both pathological and physiological conditions. These signs are to be expected under pathological conditions, such as entrapment neuropathies that predominantly affect large myelinated primary afferents.

CURRENT SIGNIFICANT CHALLENGES AND OPPORTUNITIES

While it is clear that pathology in the peripheral nervous system can produce cellular, molecular, and anatomical changes in the central nervous system, we have no idea what these central nervous system changes contribute (if anything) to neuropathic pain in patients. Furthermore, we know next to nothing about how injury to the central nervous system can result in pain. There are significant technical barriers to progress in this area. The first is the paucity of reliable direct measures of tonic pain in animals despite the fact that such pain is often the major complaint of patients. In humans, who can tell us what their pain level is, our research tools do not yet have the requisite temporal or spatial resolution to study the relevant central nervous sytem changes. When these technical problems are solved, progress will be rapid. In fact, there is reason to be optimistic that these problems can be addressed. In rodents, there is evidence that pharmaceuticals effective for human neuropathic pain relieve tonic pain in models of neuropathic pain.[33] This is direct evidence that these rodent models have a tonic component. On the human research side, methods have been developed to image ongoing pain, offering hope that central nervous system mechanisms of neuropathic pain can be uncovered.[34] Thus, the study of neuropathic pain not only has a distinguished history but also a promising future.

REFERENCES

1. Melzack R, Wall PD. Pain mechanisms: a new theory. *Science*. 1965;150:971–979.
2. Bennett GJ, Xie YK. A peripheral mononeuropathy in rat that produces disorders of pain sensation like those seen in man. *Pain*. 1988;33:87–107.
3. Bove GM, Light AR. Unmyelinated nociceptors of rat paraspinal tissues. *J Neurophysiol*. 1995;73:1752–1762.
4. Bove GM, Moskowitz MA. Primary afferent neurons innervating guinea pig dura. *J Neurophysiol*. 1997;77:299–308.
5. Eboli P, Stone JL, Aydin S, Slavin KV. Historical characterization of trigeminal neuralgia. *Neurosurgery*. 2009;64:1183–1186; discussion 1186–1187.
6. Hunter J. Nervous pain in the jaw. *The Natural History of the Teeth; Explaining Their Structure, Use, Formation, Growth and Disease, Part II*. 2nd ed. London: J. Johnson; 1778:61–63.
7. Dandy WE. Concerning the cause of trigeminal neuralgia. *Am J Surg*. 1934;24:447–455.
8. Leriche R. De la causalgie envisagee comme une nevrite du sympathique et de son traitement par la denudation et l'excision des plexus nerveux peri-arteriels. *Presse Med*. 1916;24:178–180.
9. Richards RL. Causalgia. A centennial review. *Arch Neurol*. 1967;16:339–350.
10. Baron R, Levine JD, Fields HL. Causalgia and reflex sympathetic dystrophy: does the sympathetic nervous system contribute to the generation of pain? *Muscle Nerve*. 1999;22:678–695.
11. Adrian ED. *The Mechanism of Nervous Action; Electrical Studies of the Neurone*. Oxford: Oxford University Press; 1935.
12. Adrian ED. *The Physical Background of Perception*. Oxford: Clarendon Press; 1947.
13. Zotterman Y. Touch, pain and tickling: an electrophysiological investigation on cutaneous sensory nerves. *J Physiol*. 1939;95:1–28.
14. Head H, Sherren J. The consequences of injury to the peripheral nerves in man. *Brain*. 1905;28:116–138.
15. Trotter W, Davies HM. Experimental studies in the innervation of the skin. *J Physiol*. 1909;38:134–246.
16. Gasser HS. Conduction in nerves in relation to fiber types. *Proc Assn Res Nerv Ment Dis*. 1934;15:35–39.
17. Sinclair DC. *Mechanisms of Cutaneous Sensation*. Oxford: Oxford University Press; 1981.
18. Landau W, Bishop GH. Pain from dermal, periosteal, and fascial endings and from inflammation; electrophysiological study employing differential nerve blocks. *AMA Arch Neurol Psychiatry*. 1953;69:490–504.
19. Livingston WK. *Pain Mechanisms*. New York: Macmillan; 1944.
20. Noordenbos W. *Pain*. Amsterdam: Elsevier; 1959.
21. Price DD, Hu JW, Dubner R, Gracely RH. Peripheral suppression of first pain and central summation of second pain evoked by noxious heat pulses. *Pain*. 1977;3:57–68.
22. Mendell LM. Physiological properties of unmyelinated fiber projection to the spinal cord. *Exp Neurol*. 1966;16:316–332.
23. Hillman P, Wall PD. Inhibitory and excitatory factors influencing the receptive fields

of lamina 5 spinal cord cells. *Exp Brain Res.* 1969;9:284–306.

24. Wall PD. The laminar organization of dorsal horn and effects of descending impulses. *J Physiol.* 1967;188:403–423.

25. Torebjork HE, Lundberg LE, LaMotte RH. Central changes in processing of mechanoreceptive input in capsaicin-induced secondary hyperalgesia in humans. *J Physiol.* 1992;448: 765–780.

26. Bessou P, Perl ER. Response of cutaneous sensory units with unmyelinated fibers to noxious stimuli. *J Neurophysiol.* 1969;32:1025–1043.

27. Burgess PR, Perl ER. Myelinated afferent fibres responding specifically to noxious stimulation of the skin. *J Physiol.* 1967;190:541–562.

28. Wall PD. The gate control theory of pain mechanisms. A re-examination and re-statement. *Brain.* 1978;101:1–18.

29. Chabal C, Jacobson L, Russell LC, Burchiel KJ. Pain response to perineuromal injection of normal saline, epinephrine, and lidocaine in humans. *Pain.* 1992;49:9–12.

30. Wall PD, Gutnick M. Properties of afferent nerve impulses originating from a neuroma. *Nature.* 1974;248:740–743.

31. Fields HL, Rowbotham M, Baron R. Postherpetic neuralgia: irritable nociceptors and deafferentation. *Neurobiol Dis.* 1998;5:209–227.

32. Waxman SG. Nav1.7, its mutations, and the syndromes that they cause. *Neurology.* 2007;69: 505–507.

33. King T, Vera-Portocarrero L, Gutierrez T, Vanderah TW, Dussor G, et al. Unmasking the tonic-aversive state in neuropathic pain. *Nat Neurosci.* 2009;12:1364–1366.

34. Baliki MN, Chialvo DR, Geha PY, Levy RM, Harden RN, et al. Chronic pain and the emotional brain: specific brain activity associated with spontaneous fluctuations of intensity of chronic back pain. *J Neurosci.* 2006;26: 12165–12173.

2

Peripheral and Central Mechanisms of Neuropathic Pain

ROLF-DETLEF TREEDE

INTRODUCTION

NEUROPATHIC PAIN IS defined as "pain caused by a lesion or disease of the somatosensory nervous system" (Table 2-1). Neuropathic pain is a clinical description (and not a diagnosis) which requires a demonstrable lesion or a disease that satisfies established neurological diagnostic criteria. There have been extensive discussions within the International Association for the Study of Pain (IASP) and its Special Interest Group on Neuropathic Pain (NeuPSIG) before this definition was accepted in 2011 (for discussion see Chapter 1 and Refs. [1,2]). Guidelines for the assessment of patients with neuropathic pain are available.[2a,2b] Neuropathic pain is a challenge to health care providers, as it is common, often underdiagnosed, undertreated, and may be associated with suffering, disability, and an impaired quality of life. Standard treatment with conventional analgesics does not typically provide effective relief

of pain, but special treatment regimens have been developed in an evidence-based manner.[3,4] There are also screening tools to detect possible neuropathic pain cases.[5]

In contrast to nociceptive pain, which is caused by physiological activation of peripheral nociceptive nerve terminals by actual or impending tissue damage, chronic neuropathic pain has no beneficial effect. It can arise from damage to the neural pathways at any point from the terminals of the peripheral nociceptors to the cortical neurons in the brain. Neuropathic pain is classified as central (originating from damage of the brain or spinal cord) or peripheral (originating from damage in peripheral nerves, plexus, or roots). Neuropathic pain is also classified on the basis of the character of the insult to the nervous system (e.g., inflammatory, metabolic, vascular, or mechanical). Only a small minority of patients with peripheral nerve injury develop neuropathic pain (5%), whereas in spinal cord injury the percentage is around 50%. It is not

Table 2-1. Definitions

TERM	DEFINITION	COMMENT
Neuropathic pain	Pain caused by a lesion or disease of the somatosensory nervous system.	Neuropathic pain is a clinical description (and not a diagnosis) which requires a demonstrable lesion or a disease that satisfies established neurological diagnostic criteria. The term *lesion* is commonly used when diagnostic investigations (e.g., imaging, neurophysiology, biopsies, lab tests) reveal an abnormality or when there was obvious trauma. The term *disease* is commonly used when the underlying cause of the lesion is known (e.g., stroke, vasculitis, diabetes mellitus, genetic abnormality). *Somatosensory* refers to information about the body per se including visceral organs, rather than information about the external world (e.g., vision, hearing, or olfaction). This definition fits into the nosology of neurological disorders.
Peripheral neuropathic pain	Pain caused by a lesion or disease of the peripheral somatosensory nervous system.	Usage is not identical to that of the term *peripheral neuropathy*. The peripheral somatosensory system includes the peripheral nerve, but also the plexus, DRG and roots (i.e., the entire first neuron of the somatosensory system).
Central neuropathic pain	Pain caused by a lesion or disease of the central somatosensory nervous system.	This term refers to a primary pathology within the central somatosensory system (e.g., injury, stroke, demyelination). It does not refer to secondary neuroplastic changes in the CNS that may result from peripheral neuropathic pain or from nociceptive pain.
Sensitization	Increased responsiveness of nociceptive neurons to their normal input and/or recruitment of a response to normally subthreshold inputs.	Sensitization includes a drop in threshold and an increase in the suprathreshold response. Spontaneous discharges and increases in receptive field size may also occur. This is a neurophysiological term that can only be applied when both input and output of the neural system under study are known (e.g., by controlling the stimulus and measuring the neural event). Clinically, sensitization may only be inferred indirectly from phenomena such as hyperalgesia or allodynia.
Peripheral sensitization	Increased responsiveness and reduced threshold of nociceptive neurons in the periphery to stimulation of their receptive fields.	Peripheral sensitization is often accompanied by spontaneuous activity in nociceptive afferents. This activity has also been interpreted as a drop in heat threshold below body temperature.[6]
Central sensitization	Increased responsiveness of nociceptive neurons in the CNS to their normal or subthreshold afferent input.	This may include increased responsiveness due to dysfunction of endogenous pain control systems.
Hyperalgesia	Increased pain from a stimulus that normally provokes pain.	An augmented response within the somatosensory submodality of nociception and pain. This is a clinical term that does not imply a mechanism. The test stimulus should always be specified, as in "heat hyperalgesia."
Allodynia	Pain due to a stimulus that does not normally provoke pain.	The stimulus leads to an unexpectedly painful response. This is a clinical term that does not imply a mechanism. The test stimulus should always be specified, as in "dynamic mechanical allodynia."

Note: These terms can be found on the IASP website www.iasp-pain.org. For discussion see Loeser and Treede 2008[1] and Treede et al. 2008.[2]

known why the same condition is painful in some patients and painless in others.

CLINICAL PICTURE

Neuropathic pain can be spontaneous (stimulus-independent) or elicited by a stimulus (stimulus-evoked). Spontaneous pain is often described as a constant burning sensation, but it may also include pricking, tingling, or pins and needles, as well as electric shock-like pain.[5] Paresthesias (abnormal but not painful spontaneous sensations) may also occur. Stimulus-evoked pains are elicited by mechanical or thermal stimuli (chemical stimuli are usually not tested). Stimulus-evoked pain may be reduced due to damage to the nociceptive pathways (*hypoalgesia*). *Hyperalgesia* is an increased pain response to a stimulus that activates peripheral nociceptive terminals,[5a] whereas the term *allodynia* has been introduced to describe a pain sensation induced by a stimulus that does not activate nociceptors (such as gentle stroking by a brush) and thus implies a change in central neural processing (Table 2-1). Additionally, there may be other neurological symptoms, signs, and clinical findings (e.g., motor paresis, muscle cramps, autonomic nervous system signs), depending on the site of the lesion.

OVERVIEW OF MECHANISMS

Damage to the somatosensory system leads to negative sensory symptoms (a feeling of numbness) and signs (sensory loss to the somatosensory submodalities touch, proprioception, thermoreception, nociception, or visceroreception). Damaged neurons, however, can also develop spontaneous activity, for example by altered expression of ion channels at the site of axonal damage (neuroma) or in the soma of the damaged neuron (dorsal root ganglion [DRG]). When ectopically generated action potentials are transmitted to the nociceptive network in the brain, this results in a pain sensation that is projected to the receptive field of the damaged neural structure (projected pain; Figure 2.1). Peripheral nerve damage can also lead to secondary changes within the central nervous system, including altered synaptic connectivity and receptive field reorganization. These secondary changes involve local excitatory and inhibitory neurons and

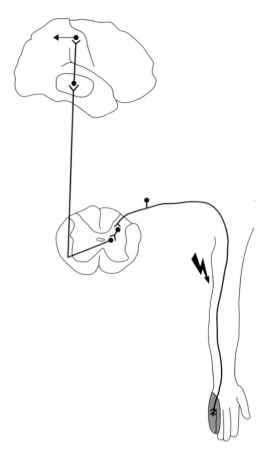

FIGURE 2.1   Projected pain. Damage to a peripheral nerve may lead to generation of action potentials at the site of damage. When these action potentials reach the nociceptive network in the brain, the resulting pain sensation is projected into the peripheral receptive field of the damaged nerve, where this activity would normally originate. Thus, pain in a body part may result from damage to that body part itself or to any site along the neural pathways connecting that body part with the brain.

ascending and descending pathways, as well as microglia and astrocytes.[7,8] When the neural damage is partial, the remaining neural connections may be facilitated due to these secondary changes, leading to positive sensory symptoms (paresthesia and spontaneous pain) and signs (hyperalgesia and allodynia, mostly to mechanical or cold stimuli). In spite of many detailed findings from animal studies, the exact mechanisms of positive sensory signs in patients are as poorly understood as the mechanisms of positive motor signs (spasticity, rigidity, dystonia).

The coexistence of negative and positive sensory phenomena within the same region is prototypical for patients with neuropathic pain.[9] The spatial distribution of these symptoms and signs and the distribution of the projected pain sensation provide information on the neuroanatomical site of neural damage. Current and future therapies for neuropathic pain are directed at ectopic impulse generation (local anesthetics, antiepileptic agents), at central nociceptive signal processing (centrally acting analgesics, modulators of endogenous pain control systems), and at the pathophysiological processes of degeneration, regeneration, and reorganization.[10] In general, systemic neuropathic pain medication has to pass the blood-brain barrier in order to reach its target. Such a barrier is also present in the peripheral nervous system, but the blood-nerve barrier is leaky in the DRG and in peripheral nerve inflammation.

PERIPHERAL MECHANISMS OF NEUROPATHIC PAIN

In peripheral neuropathic pain, the ongoing pain is thought to be due to action potentials that are generated ectopically, that is, not at the normal site near the nerve terminal. According to the injured afferents hypothesis, altered sodium channel expression in injured nerve fibers leads to spontaneous action potential generation either at the site of nerve damage or more rostrally in the DRG.[11] In human neuroma specimens, upregulation of the voltage-gated sodium channels NaV1.3, NaV1.7, and NaV1.8 has been found.[12] There is limited evidence for spontaneous action potential activity from microneurography in humans.[13,14,14a] Observed spontaneous activity was mostly from A fibers, and its origin (peripheral nerve or ganglion) has not been determined.

According to the intact nociceptor hypothesis, intact nociceptors that survive injury and innervate the region subserved by the injured nerve or root are sensitized by the local micromilieu of degenerating nerve fibers and partly denervated target tissue.[8] A key role for uninjured nerve fibers is consistent with the observation that partial rather than complete nerve injury leads to neuropathic pain. After partial nerve injury in the monkey, uninjured C fibers develop spontaneous activity,[15] and in a similar model in the rat, the uninjured nerve fibers are sensitized to mechanical and heat stimuli.[16] This peripheral sensitization to heat may be a result of upregulation of the heat transduction channel TRPV1.[17]

In either case, ectopically generated action potentials are transmitted along the normal neural pathways to the nociceptive network in the brain,[18] ultimately leading to a painful percept. Nociceptive input to the spinal cord dorsal horn may induce use-dependent plasticity in synaptic transmission, a phenomenon readily occurring in all acute pain situations.[19] Thus, ectopic impulse generation and peripheral sensitization may provide the afferent signal to induce central sensitization.

Moreover, afferent nerve fibers sample the local micromilieu by endocytosis and retrograde axonal transport. Injured afferents lose connection with their target tissue and hence are "undertrophed"—for example, for glial cell line-derived neurotrophic factor (GDNF). Denervated target tissue increases expression of growth factors such as nerve growth factor (NGF), leading to "overtrophed" uninjured fibers.[20] An imbalance of growth factors alters gene expression patterns in DRG neurons and thus indirectly affects both afferent encoding and spinal processing.[7,21,22] In addition, axonal transport of neurally generated chemokines such as chemokine (C-C motif) ligand 2 (CCL2) may activate spinal microglia that, in turn, may contribute to central sensitization.[23]

To the extent that analgesic medications act at presynaptic terminals in the spinal cord, expression of the respective receptor molecules by DRG neurons is also relevant, since the central branches of the axons of DRG neurons provide the presynaptic terminals in the spinal dorsal horn. The regulatory $\alpha_2\delta$ subunit of voltage-gated calcium channels (the target of gabapentin and pregabalin) is upregulated in neuropathic pain,[24] whereas μ-opiate receptors are downregulated following nerve injury.[25]

In summary, peripheral nerve damage leads to a complex pattern of altered electrical and chemical signals reaching the spinal cord (Table 2.2). These signals may lead directly to altered pain

Table 2-2. Peripheral Mechanisms of Neuropathic Pain

SIGNAL	PERIPHERAL SOURCE	IMMEDIATE EFFECT	INDIRECT EFFECT
Peripheral sensitization	Uninjured afferents	Hyperalgesia	(Central sensitization)
Ectopic action potentials	Injured or uninjured afferents	Pain	Central sensitization
Trophic factors (GDNF, NGF)	Target tissue, axonal transport via injured or uninjured afferents	Up-/downregulation of genes in DRGneuron	Central sensitization, glia activation
Chemokines (CCL2)	Injured or uninjured afferents	Microglia activation	Central sensitization

perception via normal signal processing in the central nervous system (CNS), but in addition they may also induce changes in central signal processing mechanisms.

NORMAL CENTRAL PROCESSING OF ALTERED PERIPHERAL INPUT

Ectopically generated action potentials are transmitted along the normal neural pathways to the nociceptive network in the brain.[18] This network then interprets these signals as coming from the normal innervation territory of the damaged nerve or root (projected pain). If the peripheral neural signal to a given stimulus is enhanced by peripheral sensitization, CNS neurons will also exhibit an enhanced response to the stimulus without necessarily changing their response properties to their synaptic input.

The reflections of peripheral sensitization in CNS neural activity have been studied for inflammatory pain conditions. Inflammation sensitizes peripheral nociceptive nerve terminals to heat stimuli, and the resulting enhanced peripheral neural responses to heat are faithfully reflected at the thalamic and cortical levels.[26-29] The enhanced responses of thalamic or cortical neurons to peripheral stimulation in arthritic animals[30,31] do not necessarily indicate altered signal processing in thalamus or cortex; instead, these responses may be a reflection of enhanced input from the spinal cord. Likewise, enhanced thalamic and cortical responses to peripheral stimulation in models of peripheral

neuropathic pain may reflect spinal rather than cortical sensitization.[32,33] Enhanced responses of central neurons to peripheral stimulation may simply be a reflection of the enhanced input generated by these stimuli due to peripheral sensitization. Nevertheless, these are important findings indicating that the enhanced input generated in the periphery does reach the brain.

CENTRAL SENSITIZATION

Central sensitization is defined as increased responsiveness of nociceptive neurons in the CNS to their normal or subthreshold afferent input (Table 2.3). Synapses in central nociceptive pathways are subject to activity-dependent plasticity, as shown for the spinal cord[34] and the anterior cingulate gyrus.[35] Spinal dorsal horn neurons that project to the parabrachial nucleus are facilitated by high-frequency input (100 Hz), whereas those projecting to the periaqueductal gray are facilitated by low-frequency input (2 Hz).[36] Some spinal neurons are inhibited by low-frequency input.[37] These phenomena are similar to long-term potentiation (LTP) and long-term depression (LTD) in the hippocampus. The frequency dependence of synaptic plasticity appears to be different between spinal dorsal horn and hippocampus in that some spinal LTP-like processes are induced by relatively low-frequency input, such as the input normally provided by peripheral nociceptive neurons. Moreover, when tested at the behavioral level in humans, both low- and high-frequency

Table 2-3. Central Mechanisms of Neuropathic Pain

EVENT	LOCATION	IMMEDIATE EFFECT
Ectopic action potentials, bursting	Spinal cord or thalamus	Pain
Central sensitization	Spinal cord	Hyperalgesia
Receptive field reorganization	Spinal cord, thalamus, cortex	Hyperalgesia, referred sensations
Loss of inhibition	Brainstem or its descending inputs	Pain and hyperalgesia
Descending facilitation	Brainstem or its ascending inputs	Pain and hyperalgesia

stimulation may induce a hyperalgesia to pin prick in the skin surrounding the stimulation electrode,[38] similar to pinprick hyperalgesia in neuropathic pain.[9] These mechanisms are triggered by primary afferent nociceptive input and are part of the normal plasticity of the nociceptive system. They thus occur after tissue injury as well as after nerve injury.[39] A single bout of conditioning afferent input usually leads to early LTP lasting for up to 24 h, but in some susceptible subjects even this mild input induces late LTP of several days' duration.[40]

Several signal transduction cascades are involved in central sensitization.[41] The presynaptic terminals of nociceptive afferents release glutamate and substance P. Glutamate receptors of the N-methyl-D-aspartate (NMDA)-receptor type and substance P receptors of the neurokinin 1 (NK1)-receptor type are important for the induction of central sensitization.[42] A common denominator of these two signaling pathways is an increase in intracellular calcium. Rapid excitatory neurotransmission usually occurs via glutamate receptors of the α-amino-3-hydroxy-5-methyl-4-isoxazolepropionate (AMPA)-receptor type. AMPA receptors are highly regulated in synaptic plasticity but are normally not calcium-permeable themselves. Recently, it was observed that the spinal dorsal horn contains an unusually high density of calcium-permeable variants of AMPA receptors, which therefore have become an interesting therapeutic target.[43]

The excitability of spinal dorsal horn neurons is controlled by a large network of interneurons, mostly situated in laminae I–III.[44] Many of these interneurons are excitatory and glutamatergic; others are inhibitory and GABAergic (γ-aminobutyric acid) or glycinergic. Thus, excitability of the projection neurons is regulated by several metabotropic (G-protein-coupled) neurotransmitter receptors such as metabotropic glutamate receptors (mGluR) and GABA$_B$.[45] Additional inhibitory control is provided by endogenous opioids and cannabinoids. A loss of inhibitory interneurons has thus been implied in neuropathic pain generation by some authors,[46,47] but others suggest that only the level of activity of inhibitory interneurons may be reduced.[48]

Matters become further complicated by the fact that rapid inhibition via GABA$_A$ or glycin receptors is mediated by increasing the chloride conductance of the membrane, since these receptors are ligand-gated chloride channels. Normal adult CNS neurons maintain a low intracellular chloride concentration by transporting these ions out of the cell via the cotransporter potassium chloride transporter 2 (KCC2); this way, opening of the chloride channel will admit negatively charged ions and lead to hyperpolarization. This mechanism is disrupted in neuropathic pain[49] by a pathway involving microglia activation by adenosine triphosphate (ATP) via the P2X4 receptors, brain-derived neurotrophic factor (BDNF), release and tyrosine kinase receptor B (trkB) receptor activation on dorsal horn neurons.[50] This pathway changes the chloride equilibrium potential in such a way that opening of ligand-gated chloride channels will lead to an outward flux of negatively charged ions and hence depolarization.

DESCENDING CONTROL SYSTEMS

Spinal excitability is modulated by several pathways descending from centers in brainstem, midbrain, diencephalon, and cortex.[51,52] These descending controls may be inhibitory or excitatory. An important switching station is the region of the rostroventral medulla (RVM) that contains many clusters of neurons from which monoaminergic pathways to the spinal cord originate. Activity in RVM is modulated by ascending pathways from the spinal cord and by descending pathways from the periaqueductal gray, parabrachial nucleus, and nucleus tractus solitarii. Descending inhibition is thought to maintain an adequate level of contrast for sensory discrimination. Descending facilitation is thought to contribute to some forms of hyperalgesia, in particular secondary hyperalgesia to pinpricks surrounding a site of tissue injury.

With respect to mechanisms of neuropathic pain, it has been observed that serotonergic pathways are both inhibitory (via 5HT1 receptors) and facilitory (via 5HT3 receptors), whereas noradrenergic pathways are predominantly inhibitory (via α2 adrenoreceptors). Moreover, serotonergic descending facilitation appears to be enhanced following peripheral nerve injury.[53] While neuropathic pain might be due to deficits in descending inhibition, current evidence suggests a more prominent role for enhanced descending facilitation. In addition to noradrenalin and serotonin, other transmitters, such as dopamine, are involved in descending control systems and deficits of these systems may induce clinical signs of neuropathic pain.[54]

ECTOPIC IMPULSE GENERATION WITHIN THE CNS

Denervated neurons tend to become hyperexcitable and may eventually generate spontaneous action potentials without adequate sensory or synaptic input. This phenomenon is well recognized for DRG neurons and probably also applies to neurons in the CNS. Development of or increase in spontaneous activity is one of the hallmarks of central sensitization in spinal neurons.[55] Depending on their tonic drive, spinal neurons can develop endogenous bursting patterns.[45] Bursting activity in the somatosensory thalamus has been observed in patients with neuropathic pain in the course of implantation of stimulating electrodes[56] and is considered a mechanism in neuropathic pain.[57] In animal models of neuropathic pain, there is some evidence that spontaneous activity may be generated within the thalamus itself[33] and that upregulation of the voltage-gated sodium channel NaV1.3 contributes to this spontaneous activity.[58] Changes in electrophysiological properties of CNS neurons allow them to either faithfully transmit, block, or enhance the transfer of nociceptive information to further rostral centers.

Disturbed GABAergic inhibition has been implied in central sensitization in the spinal cord. At the thalamic level, bursting activity has been suggested to be due to an imbalance in lateral inhibition between specific and nonspecific thalamic nuclei via the GABAergic reticular thalamic nucleus, and this concept has recently been formulated as a mathematical model of network activity.[59]

RECEPTIVE FIELD REORGANIZATION

Changes in receptive field size are another hallmark of central sensitization in the spinal cord.[55] Enlarged receptive fields of dorsal horn neurons have also been found in animal models of partial nerve injury,[60] and similar partial lesions induce rapid reorganization of receptive fields of thalamic neurons.[61] In amputation patients, thalamic neurons with receptive fields adjacent to the area of sensory loss occupied a larger part of the thalamic homunculus than was found for the same part of the body in patients without sensory abnormality, that is, patients with movement disorders.[62] This result is consistent with somatotopic reorganization of afferent inputs from the limb that has also been found at the cortical level following limb amputation.[63] Although the extent of cortical reorganization has been found to be correlated with the intensity of phantom limb pain and its treatment,[64] a few caveats apply.

Cortical reorganization in humans has mostly been reported for tactile representation in the primary somatosensory cortex. Hence, it remains to be determined how this change in the tactile homunculus contributes to a painful sensation. An alternative concept has been proposed, namely, that tactile somatotopy is maintained by nociceptive pathways.[65] According to this concept, cortical reorganization would be a consequence, not a cause, of neuropathic pain.

SUMMARY AND CONCLUSIONS

Neuropathic pain arises as a direct consequence of a lesion or a disease affecting the somatosensory system. Damage to the somatosensory system leads primarily to sensory loss (negative sensory signs). As with other neurological conditions, positive signs and symptoms may also occur. These include ongoing pain and hyperalgesia. Ongoing pain is due to ongoing neural activity that may arise at the site of neural damage or more rostrally. Hyperalgesia is due to enhanced excitatory transmission or reduced inhibition or both. Damage to somatosensory pathways in the periphery may induce peripheral sensitization and ectopic impulse generation in the course of degeneration and regeneration at the site of damage, involving interactions of damaged nerve fibers, intact nerve fibers, and Schwann cells. Ectopically generated impulses may be processed along the normal nociceptive pathways, leading to pain perception in the peripheral innervation territory of the damaged structure (projected pain). Excitatory neurotransmission and microglia activation may lead to secondary alterations in central neural processing, including receptive field reorganization and central sensitization. Lesions or diseases of the central somatosensory pathways induce local degeneration and regeneration processes within the CNS leading to central sensitization and spontaneous generation of action potentials. These action potentials may be perceived as projected pain and may induce secondary changes in more rostral CNS structures. Thus, peripheral neuropathic pain invokes both peripheral and central neural mechanisms, whereas central neuropathic pain has to be explained based on CNS mechanisms.

REFERENCES

1. Loeser JD, Treede RD. The Kyoto protocol of IASP Basic Pain Terminology. *Pain*. 2008;137: 473–477.
2. Treede RD, Jensen TS, Campbell JN, Cruccu G, Dostrovsky JO, Griffin JW, Hansson P, Hughes R, Nurmikko T, Serra J.. Redefinition of neuropathic pain and a grading system for clinical use: consensus statement on clinical and research diagnostic criteria. *Neurology*. 2008;70:1630–1635.
2a. Cruccu G, Anand P, Attal N, Garcia-Larrea L, Haanpää M, Jørum E, Serra J, Jensen TS. EFNS guidelines on neuropathic pain assessment. *Eur J Neurol*. 2004;11:153–162.
2b. Haanpää M, Backonja M, Bennett M, Bouhassira D, Cruccu G, Hansson P, Jensen T, Kauppila T, Rice A, Smith BH, Treede R, Baron R. Assessment of neuropathic pain in primary care. *Am J Med*. 2009;122(10 suppl):S13–21.
3. Dworkin RH, O'Connor AB, Backonja M, Farrar JT, Finnerup NB, Jensen TS, Kalso EA, Loeser JD, Miaskowski C, Nurmikko TJ, Portenoy RK, Rice AS, Stacey BR, Treede RD, Turk DC, Wallace MS.. Pharmacologic management of neuropathic pain: evidence-based recommendations. *Pain*. 2007;132:237–51.
4. Attal N, Cruccu G, Baron R, Haanpää M, Hansson P, Jensen TS, Nurmikko T. EFNS guidelines on the pharmacological treatment of neuropathic pain: 2010 revision. *Eur J Neurol*. 2010;17:1113–1123
5. Bennett MI, Attal N, Backonja MM, Baron R, Bouhassira D, Freynhagen R, Scholz J, Tölle TR, Wittchen HU, Jensen TS. Using screening tools to identify neuropathic pain. *Pain*. 2007;127:199–203.
5a. Treede RD, Handwerker HO, Baumgärtner U, Meyer RA, Magerl W. Hyperalgesia and allodynia: taxonomy, assessment, and mechanisms. In: Brune K, Handwerker HO, eds. *Hyperalgesia: Molecular Mechanisms and Clinical Implications*. Seattle: IASP Press; 2004:1–15.
6. Reeh PW, Pethö G. Nociceptor exitation by thermal sensitization—a hypothesis. In: Sandkühler J, Bromm B, Gebhart GF, eds. *Nervous System Plasticity of Chronic Pain*. Progress in Brain Research, Vol. 129. Amsterdam: Elsevier; 2000:39–50.
7. Hökfelt T, Zhang X, Xu X, Wiesenfeld-Hallin Z. Central consequences of periphereal nerve

damage. In: McMahon SB, Koltzenburg M, eds. *Textbook of Pain*. Amsterdam: Elsevier; 2006: 947–959.

8. Campbell JN, Meyer RA. Mechanisms of neuropathic pain. *Neuron*. 2006;52:77–92.

9. Maier C, Baron R, Tölle TR, Binder A, Birbaumer N, Birklein F, Gierthmühlen J, Flor H, Geber C, Huge V, Krumova EK, Landwehrmeyer GB, Magerl W, Maihöfner C, Richter H, Rolke R, Scherens A, Schwarz A, Sommer C, Tronnier V, Uçeyler N, Valet M, Wasner G, Treede RD. Quantitative sensory testing in the German Research Network on Neuropathic Pain (DFNS): somatosensory abnormalities in 1236 patients with different neuropathic pain syndromes. *Pain*. 2010;150:439–450.

10. Campbell JN, Basbaum AI, Dray A, Dubner R, Dworkin RH, Sang CN, eds. *Emerging Strategies for the Treatment of Neuropathic Pain*. Seattle: IASP Press; 2006.

11. Devor M, Wall PD, Catalan N. Systemic lidocaine silences ectopic neuroma and DRG discharge without blocking nerve conduction. *Pain*. 1992;48:261–268.

12. Black JA, Nikolajsen L, Kroner K, Jensen TS, Waxman SG. Multiple sodium channel isoforms and mitogen-activated protein kinases are present in painful human neuromas. *Ann Neurol*. 2008;64:644–653.

13. Campero M, Serra J, Marchettini P, Ochoa JL. Ectopic impulse generation and autoexcitation in single myelinated afferent fibers in patients with peripheral neuropathy and positive sensory symptoms. *Muscle Nerve*. 1998;21:1661–1667.

14. Burchiel KJ, Baumann TK. Pathophysiology of trigeminal neuralgia: new evidence from a trigeminal ganglion intraoperative microneurographic recording— case report. *J Neurosurg*. 2004;101:872–873

14a. Serra J, Bostock H, Solà R, Aleu J, García E, Cokic B, Navarro X, Quiles C. Microneurographic identification of spontaneous activity in C-nociceptors in neuropathic pain states in humans and rats. *Pain* 2012;153(1):42–55.

15. Ali Z, Ringkamp M, Hartke TV, Chien HF, Flavahan NA, Campbell JN, Meyer RA. Uninjured C-fiber nociceptors develop spontaneous activity and alpha adrenergic sensitivity following L6 spinal nerve ligation in the monkey. *J Neurophysiol*. 1999;81:455–466.

16. Shim B, Kim DW, Kim BH, Nam TS, Leem JW, Chung JM. Mechanical and heat sensitization of cutaneous nociceptors in rats with experimental peripheral neuropathy. *Neuroscience*. 2005;132:193–201.

17. Hudson LJ, Bevan S, Wotherspoon G, Gentry C, Fox A, Winter J. VR1 protein expression increases in undamaged DRG neurons after partial nerve injury. *Eur J Neurosci*. 2001;13: 2105–2114.

18. Apkarian AV, Bushnell C, Treede RD, Zubieta J-K. Human brain mechanisms of pain perception and regulation in health and disease. *Eur J Pain*. 2005;9:463–484.

19. Kehlet H, Jensen TS, Woolf CJ. Persistent postsurgical pain: risk factors and prevention. *Lancet*. 2006;367:1618–1625.

20. Griffin JW. The roles of growth factors in painful length-dependent axonal neuropathies. In: Campbell JN, Basbaum AI, Dray A, Dubner R, Dworkin RH, Sang CN, eds. *Emerging Strategies for the Treatment of Neuropathic Pain*. Seattle: IASP Press; 2006:271–290.

21. Boucher TJ, McMahon SB. Neurotrophic factors and neuropathic pain. *Curr Opin Pharmacol*. 2001;1:66–72.

22. Ueda H. Molecular mechanisms of neuropathic pain—phenotypic switch and initiation mechanisms. *Pharmacol Ther*. 2006;109:57–77.

23. Thacker MA, Clark AK, Bishop T, Grist J, Yip PK, Moon LD, Thompson SW, Marchand F, McMahon SB. CCL2 is a key mediator of microglia activation in neuropathic pain states. *Eur J Pain*. 2009;13:263–272.

24. Melrose HL, Kinloch RA, Cox PJ, Field MJ, Collins D, Williams D. [3H] pregabalin binding is increased in ipsilateral dorsal horn following chronic constriction injury. *Neurosci Lett*. 2007;417:187–192

25. Kohno T, Ji RR, Ito N, Allchorne AJ, Befort K, Karchewski LA, Woolf CJ. Peripheral axonal injury results in reduced mu opioid receptor pre- and post-synaptic action in the spinal cord. *Pain*. 2005;117:77–87.

26. Guilbaud G, Benoist JM, Neil A, Kayser V, Gautron M. Neuronal response thresholds to and encoding of thermal stimuli during carrageenin-hyperalgesic-inflammation in the ventro-basal thalamus of the rat. *Exp Brain Res*. 1987;66:421–431.

27. Kenshalo DR, Isensee O. Responses of primate SI cortical neurons to noxious stimuli. *J Neurophysiol*. 1983;50:1479–1496.

28. Kenshalo DR, Chudler EH, Anton F, Dubner R. SI nociceptive neurons participate in the encoding process by which monkeys perceive the intensity of noxious thermal stimulation. *Brain Res*. 1988;454:378–382.

29. Kenshalo DR, Iwata K, Sholas M, Thomas DA. Response properties and organization of

nociceptive neurons in area 1 of monkey primary somatosensory cortex. *J Neurophysiol.* 2000;84:719–729.

30. Dostrovsky JO, Guilbaud G. Nociceptive responses in medial thalamus of the normal and arthritic rat. *Pain.* 1990;40:93–104.

31. Vin-Christian K, Benoist JM, Gautron M, Levante A, Guilbaud G. Further evidence for the involvement of SmI cortical neurons in nociception: modification of their responsiveness over the early stage of a carrageenin-induced inflammation in the rat. *Somatosens Motor Res.* 1992;9:245–261.

32. Guilbaud G, Benoist JM, Gautron M, Willer JC. Primary somatosensory cortex in rats with pain-related behaviours due to a peripheral mononeuropathy after moderate ligation of one sciatic nerve: neuronal responsivity to somatic stimulation. *Exp Brain Res.* 1992;92:227–245.

33. Fischer TZ, Tan AM, Waxman SG. Thalamic neuron hyperexcitability and enlarged receptive fields in the STZ model of diabetic pain. *Brain Res.* 2009;1268:154–161.

34. Randic M, Jiang MC, Cerne R. Long-term potentiation and long-term depression of primary afferent neurotransmission in the rat spinal cord. *J Neurosci.* 1993;13:5228–5241.

35. Zhao TH, Ulzhöfer B, Wu LJ, Xu H, Seeburg PH, Sprengel R, Kuner R, Zhuo M. Roles of the AMPA receptor subunit GluA1 but not GluA2 in synaptic potentiation and activation of ERK in the anterior cingulate cortex. *Mol Pain.* 2009;5:46.

36. Ikeda H, Stark J, Fischer H, Wagner M, Drdla R, Jäger T, Sandkühler J. Synaptic amplifier of inflammatory pain in the spinal dorsal horn. *Science.* 2006;312:1659–1662.

37. Liu XG, Morton CR, Azkue JJ, Zimmermann M, Sandkühler J. Long-term depression of C-fibre-evoked spinal field potentials by stimulation of primary afferent A delta-fibres in the adult rat. *Eur J Neurosci.* 1998;10:3069–3075.

38. Klein T, Magerl W, Hopf HC, Sandkühler J, Treede RD. Perceptual correlates of nociceptive long-term potentiation and long-term depression in humans. *J Neurosci.* 2004;24:964–971.

39. Sandkühler J, Liu X. Induction of long-term potentiation at spinal synapses by noxious stimulation or nerve injury. *Eur J Neurosci.* 1998;10:2476–2480.

40. Pfau D, Klein T, Putzer D, Pogatzki-Zahn E, Treede RD, Magerl W. Analysis of hyperalgesia time courses in humans following painful electrical high-frequency stimulation identifies a possible transition from early to late LTP-like pain plasticity. *Pain.* 2011;152(7):1532–1539.

41. Kuner R. Central mechanisms of pathological pain. *Nat Med.* 2010;16:1258–1266.

42. Liu XG, Sandkühler J. Activation of spinal *N*-methyl-D-aspartate or neurokinin receptors induces long-term potentiation of spinal C-fibre-evoked potentials. *Neuroscience.* 1998;86:1209–1216.

43. Tong CK, MacDermott AB. Both Ca^{2+}-permeable and -impermeable AMPA receptors contribute to primary synaptic drive onto rat dorsal horn neurons. *J Physiol.* 2006;575:133–144.

44. Todd AJ. Neuronal circuitry for pain processing in the dorsal horn. *Nat Rev Neurosci.* 2010;11:823–836.

45. Derjean D, Bertrand S, Le Masson G, Landry M, Morisset V, Nagy F. Dynamic balance of metabotropic inputs causes dorsal horn neurons to switch functional states. *Nat Neurosci.* 2003;6:274–281.

46. Moore KA, Kohno T, Karchewski LA, Scholz J, Baba H, Woolf CJ. Partial peripheral nerve injury promotes a selective loss of GABAergic inhibition in the superficial dorsal horn of the spinal cord. *J Neurosci.* 2002;22:6724–6731.

47. Scholz J, Broom DC, Youn DH, Mills CD, Kohno T, Suter MR, Moore KA, Decosterd I, Coggeshall RE, Woolf CJ. Blocking caspase activity prevents transsynaptic neuronal apoptosis and the loss of inhibition in lamina II of the dorsal horn after peripheral nerve injury. *J Neurosci.* 2005;25:7317–7323.

48. Polgar E, Todd AJ. Tactile allodynia can occur in the spared nerve injury model in the rat without selective loss of GABA or GABA(A) receptors from synapses in laminae I–II of the ipsilateral spinal dorsal horn. *Neuroscience.* 2008;156:193–202.

49. Coull JA, Boudreau D, Bachand K, Prescott SA, Nault F, Sík A, De Koninck P, De Koninck Y. Trans-synaptic shift in anion gradient in spinal lamina I neurons as a mechanism of neuropathic pain. *Nature.* 2003;424:938–942.

50. Coull JA, Beggs S, Boudreau D, Boivin D, Tsuda M, Inoue K, Gravel C, Salter MW, De Koninck Y. BDNF from microglia causes the shift in neuronal anion gradient underlying neuropathic pain. *Nature.* 2005;438:1017–1021.

51. Millan MJ. Descending control of pain. *Prog Neurobiol.* 2002;66:355–474.

52. D'Mello R, Dickenson AH. Spinal cord mechanisms of pain. *Br J Anaesth.* 2008;101:8–16.

53. Suzuki R, Rahman W, Hunt SP, Dickenson AH. Descending facilitatory control of mechanically evoked responses is enhanced in deep dorsal horn neurones following peripheral nerve injury. *Brain Res.* 2004;1019:68–76.

54. Bachmann CG, Rolke R, Scheidt U, Stadelmann C, Sommer M, Pavlakovic G, Happe S, Treede RD, Paulus W. Thermal hypoaesthesia differentiates secondary restless legs syndrome associated with small fibre neuropathy from primary restless legs syndrome. *Brain*. 2010;133:762–770.

55. Latremoliere A, Woolf CJ. Central sensitization: a generator of pain hypersensitivity by central neural plasticity. *J Pain*. 2009;10(9):895–926.

56. Lenz FA, Kwan HC, Dostrovsky JO, Tasker RR. Characteristics of the bursting pattern of action potentials that occurs in the thalamus of patients with central pain. *Brain Res*. 1989;496:357–360.

57. Klit H, Finnerup NB, Jensen TS. Central post-stroke pain: clinical characteristics, pathophysiology, and management. *Lancet Neurol*. 2009;8:857–868.

58. Hains BC, Saab CY, Waxman SG. Changes in electrophysiological properties and sodium channel Nav1.3 expression in thalamic neurons after spinal cord injury. *Brain*. 2005;128:2359–2371

59. Henning Proske J, Jeanmonod D, Verschure PF. A computational model of thalamocortical dysrhythmia. *Eur J Neurosci*. 2011;33(7): 1281–1290.

60. Suzuki R, Kontinen VK, Matthews E, Williams E, Dickenson AH. Enlargement of the receptive field size to low intensity mechanical stimulation in the rat spinal nerve ligation model of neuropathy. *Exp Neurol*. 2000;163:408–413.

61. Brüggemann J, Galhardo V, Apkarian AV. Immediate reorganization of the rat somatosensory thalamus after partial ligation of sciatic nerve. *J Pain*. 2001;2:220–228.

62. Anderson WS, O'Hara S, Lawson HC, Treede RD, Lenz FA. Plasticity of pain-related neuronal activity in the human thalamus. *Prog Brain Res*. 2006;157:353–364.

63. Flor H, Elbert T, Knecht S, Wienbruch C, Pantev C, Birbaumer N, Larbig W, Taub E. Phantom-limb pain as a perceptual correlate of cortical reorganization following arm amputation. *Nature*. 1995;375:482–484.

64. Knecht S, Henningsen H, Elbert T, Flor H, Höhling C, Pantev C, Taub E. Reorganizational and perceptional changes after amputation. *Brain*. 1996;119:1213–1219.

65. Pettit MJ, Schwark HD. Capsaicin-induced rapid receptive field reorganization in cuneate neurons. *J Neurophysiol*. 1996;75:1117–1125.

3

Experimental Approaches to Neuropathic Pain

RICARDO HORACIO RODA AND AHMET HÖKE

DEFINITIONS OF NEUROPATHIC PAIN SYMPTOMS IN HUMANS AND CORRESPONDING ANIMAL MODELS

NEUROPATHIC PAIN IS a generic term used to characterize a range of symptoms described by patients. Those that suffer from this syndrome can experience inappropriate reactions to both noxious and nonnoxious stimuli, as well as spontaneous pain that is not generated or precipitated by any external stimuli. *Allodynia* refers to a painful response to an otherwise nonnoxious stimulus. The nature of the stimuli can be mechanical (such as simple touch), thermal (to a mild cold or warm temperature), or chemical (to irritants including capsaicin). *Hyperalgesia*, on the other hand, refers to an exaggerated response to a mildly noxious stimulus. Both the latency to pain and its intensity are altered.

Mechanical and thermal modalities are used to elicit hyperalgesic and allodynic reactions in animal models of neuropathy. Mechanical hyperalgesia can be demonstrated by applying precise amounts of force with an analgesiometer, a pressure instrument with a ball tip, whereas thermal hyperalgesia is elicited by directing a controllable heat source to the paws of rats. Examples of nonnoxious mechanical sensory inputs that became allodynic in neuropathy include pressure with serially graded von Frey filaments or camel hairbrushes. Normally tolerable water temperatures or the cold sensation of evaporating acetone on the skin also become nontolerable.

Anatomically, the pathophysiology of neuropathic pain involves peripheral injury as well as central processing alterations in the spinal cord or brain. In this manner, toxic neuropathies such as chemotherapy and diabetes injure the peripheral nerves, but at least some of their effects are mediated by reorganization of spinal synapses. In a more direct manner, spinal cord injury leads to symptoms of both allodynia and hyperalgesia.

Several methods have been developed to study allodynia, hyperalgesia, and spontaneous pain in animals, especially rats. Using different methods and different anatomical locations for the initial injury (peripheral nerve, spinal nerve, and spinal cord), animal behavior and reactions to stimuli have been studied. This chapter will review these animal models and their utility in evaluating the efficacy of drugs for neuropathic pain. We will also compare and contrast these models to the human condition.

PERIPHERAL NERVOUS SYSTEM MODELS

Traumatic Models

A relatively large number of animal models have been developed to study peripheral nerve biology following complete nerve transection and injury. However, the relevance of these models to the larger human neuropathic pain population is limited because most of the symptoms experienced by patients suffering from neuropathic pain arise from incomplete nerve injuries. These include traumatic injuries that do not completely transect the nerve or partial ongoing metabolic insults such as those from diabetes. The initial injury triggers a response that must interpreted by the whole neuraxis as noxious, and at least part of this signal needs to be relayed through spared nerve fibers. Therefore, attempts to mimic neuropathic pain in most animal models have sought to create injury in some fibers while sparing others.

CHRONIC CONSTRICTION INJURY

In the chronic constriction and injury (CCI) model, this goal is achieved by placing loosely held sutures around the common sciatic nerve (Figure 3.1).[1] This leads to Wallerian degeneration of some of the afferent and efferent fibers while sparing most of the afferent fibers. A few days following surgery to place the sutures, rats display behavioral responses characteristic of neuropathic pain. These behavioral responses include mechanical, thermal, and chemical hyperalgesia as well

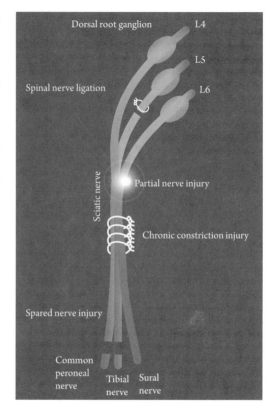

FIGURE 3.1 Animal models of neuropathic pain.

Source: Reprinted with permission from Niederberger E, Kühlein H, Geisslinger G. Update on the pathobiology of neuropathic pain. *Expert Rev Proteomics.* 2008;5(6):799–818. Copyright Expert Reviews Ltd.

as thermal allodynia and spontaneous pain behaviors. In rats after CCI, mechanical hyperalgesia is often measured using an analgesiometer. This device applies a known pressure to an animal's paw using a conical stylus with a hemispherical tip, which is applied to the dorsum of the paw while the animal is held in place. The amount of pressure required to induce paw withdrawal is then recorded. Commercially available apparatuses are available to carry out this test. Thermal hyperalgesia is measured using a radiant heat source aimed at the paw on the surgical side; the time to hind paw withdrawal-reflex after heat application is measured and compared to that on the nonoperated side. Thermal hyperalgesia is then inferred by a quicker withdrawal time. After CCI, using this method, hyperalgesia is noted to last for a few months, followed by limb hypoalgesia. In an analogous manner, application of a noxious chemical (e.g., mustard oil or formalin) to the operated paw can be used to model hyperalgesia. The chemical is applied to both hind paws, and then the cumulative duration of hind paw withdrawal is compared to that of the nonoperated control side. Finally, in the CCI model, mechanical hyperalgesia is often measured using von Frey filaments of increasing rigidity. The animals are placed in a wire cage and an operator applies the von Frey filaments until a paw withdrawal is noted. Both the latency of withdrawal and the filament rigidity at which consistent withdrawal takes place are used to measure hyperalgesia from a nonnoxious mechanical stimulus.

In addition to various measures of hyperalgesia, thermal allodynia can also be measured in CCI models of neuropathic pain. In this test, rats are placed on a cooled or warmed plate set to a temperature known to be nonnoxious to control animals. Their behavior and time to withdrawal of the paw are then recorded. The cumulative duration and frequencies of hind paw withdrawals are noted. Should withdrawal occur, an allodynia-like response is scored. In CCI animals, spontaneous pain can also be scored by observing the rat's behavior. Failure to gain weight, suppression of appetite, and guarding of the paw are commonly used measures to evaluate spontaneous pain. Despite their usefulness, in contrast to the induced hyperalgesia behaviors, these assays have more variability and are therefore less often used in preclinical studies.

The main advantage of the CCI model is its ability to reproduce the essential elements of neuropathic pain, especially hyperalgesia. Also, an ideal control is present with the sham-operated paw. Unfortunately, most of the measured variables depend in one way or another on a paw-withdrawal reflex. Not every rat in which ligatures are placed develops neuropathic symptoms, which leads to variability in the number of responder animals per experiment. Another advantage of the model is its flexibility. In addition to in vivo electrophysiological studies, one can carry out ex vivo electrophysiological studies with controlled molecular or pharmacological interventions. For example, neuronal discharges in cultured spinal cord slices occurring during central sensitization can be measured,[2] and tetrodotoxin-resistant (TTXr) sodium channel blockage experiments using small RNA molecules can be carried out.[3] An experimental variation of the CCI model resorts to the use of a polyethylene cuff instead of ligatures, with similar results.[4]

The primary rationale for developing models such as CCI has been to test potential therapies for neuropathic pain. To this end, the CCI model has been an invaluable platform for drug testing. Tricyclic antidepressants (TCAs) are often used to manage neuropathic symptoms in humans. Their effectiveness has been demonstrated in the rat CCI model. In one of the earliest work, Ardid and Guilbaud showed that various TCAs, including clomipramine, amitriptyline, and desipramine, reduce mechanical hyperalgesia in a naloxone-reversible manner.[5] Others have shown that in the CCI model, amitriptyline reduces symptoms of thermal and mechanical hyperalgesia.[6,7] In the study by Bomholt et al., duloxetine (a serotonin-norepinephrine reuptake inhibitor) was found to have a treatment profile similar to that of amitriptyline; however, citalopram (a selective serotonin reuptake inhibitor) was successful in ameliorating thermal hyperalgesia but not mechanical hypersensitivity. Human studies have corroborated these animal data. Antidepressants have been shown to be effective in treating diabetic,[8] human immunodeficiency virus (HIV),[9] and postherpetic neuropathies.[10] Gabapentin, an antagonist of α2δ calcium ion channels, which was initially approved as an antiepileptic, is effective in treating CCI-induced hyperalgesia,[11] an observation paralleled by human clinical trials.[12] Carbamazepine reduces hyperalgesia and allodynia from chronic constriction injury.[7] This is a result validated in human trials as well.[13]

Other unusual pharmacological approaches to the treatment of neuropathy, such as the use of tramadol,[7] midazolam,[14] methotrexate,[15] and anandamide uptake inhibitors,[16] have been reported to be useful in CCI-induced neuropathic pain. Experimentally, this system has been used extensively in drug development to test new agents such as biologics like anti-TrkA[17] antibodies and the glial modulatory drug AV411[18] and will likely remain as one of the important models in the development of symptomatic therapies for neuropathic pain.

SEGMENTAL SPINAL NERVE LIGATION

The segmental spinal nerve ligation (SNL) model is another extensively used model of neuropathic pain (Figure 3.1).[19] It differs from CCI in that ligation is done at a specific spinal level (usually L5 and L6 together or L5 by itself) as opposed to the whole sciatic nerve or a part of the nerve.[1,20] Experimentally, this system was found to reproduce the neuropathic findings seen in CCI. Thermal hyperalgesia and mechanical allodynia appeared within 5 days of surgery.[19] Interestingly, signs of allodynia developed on the corresponding spinal level on the contralateral side. These "mirror image" changes are also seen in other partial nerve injury models. In addition to these induced neuropathic pain behaviors, rats undergoing SNL exhibit behavior suggestive of spontaneous pain such as licking or pulling the nails with their teeth on the operated paws.

A specific neuropathic pain syndrome that SNL mimics is *causalgia*, which refers to a constellation of symptoms of burning pain, hyperalgesia, and allodynia that is occasionally seen after partial nerve injury. It is partially driven by sympathetic overactivity and responds to treatment by early sympathectomy. Mirroring the human response, sympathectomy appears to relieve some of the neuropathic symptoms in rats with SNL.[21] Furthermore, the response to sympathectomy provides a built-in positive control for efficacy trials with new medications or interventions. Other advantages of the model include a stereotyped surgery that allows for easy standardization and sparing of unaffected spinal levels that permit mechanistic studies on central sensitization. Finally, the SNL model has been translated to primates.[22] A tight SNL at the L7 level in the primate *Macaca fascicularis* results in mechanical allodynia and thermal allodynia to heat (using a thermal probe) and cold (using acetone drops on the paw and cold baths).

In preclinical studies, the SNL model has been used to test a number of strategies for the treatment of neuropathic pain. Both carbamazepine and gabapentin were shown to be effective in reducing mechanical allodynia and cold hyperalgesia.[23] Other antiepilectics, including felbamate and lamictal, have also been tested.[24] Intraperitoneal and intrathecal pregabalin were shown to reduce tactile and cold allodynia. In human trials, pregabalin has been shown to be effective in treating diabetic neuropathy[25] but not HIV neuropathy.[26]

The underlying physiology in neuropathic pain has also been probed using the SNL system. Among other things, it has shed some light on the role of the redistribution of Na(V)1.8 channels in uninjured axons[27] and has allowed for genetic studies of double knockdowns of Na(V)1.8 and Na(V)1.7 channels[28] as well as studies of the contribution of Na(V)1.3 channels in the development of neuropathic pain.[29]

The usefulness of SNL as a drug screen is evidenced by reports on the effectiveness of cannabinoids such as AM1241,[30] MDA-7,[31] and WIN55,212-2,[32] and other pharmacologics such as adenosine kinase inhibitors (ABT-702),[33] glial modulatory drugs (AV411),[18] gabapentin,[34] minocycline,[35] snail-derived conantokin-G ligand MVIIA,[36] and the TRPA-1 antagonists HC-030031[37] as well as dexamethasone[38] and sildenafil[39] in relieving neuropathic pain. Most of these studies, however, await validation and confirmation in clinical trials.

PARTIAL NERVE LIGATION

In an attempt to recreate causalgia in partial nerve injury, Seltzer and colleagues modified the CCI model by inducing a partial nerve injury (Figure 3.1).[20] They exposed the sciatic nerve and introduced a tight ligature in such a manner that the dorsal one-third to one-half of the nerve thickness was trapped in the ligature. This system induced rapid onset of neuropathic behaviors in rats. The authors reported mechanical hyperalgesia, as measured by a single pinprick with a sharply pointed plastic rod, and mechanical allodynia with von Frey filaments. In addition, animals exhibited heat hyperalgesia (paw withdrawal to pulses of infrared heat from a laser) and cold allodynia as measured by the duration of paw flicks when rats were placed on a cold plate at 5°C. Animals with partial nerve ligation also developed signs of spontaneous pain (guarding of the operated side) but did not display autotomy.

Similar to the CCI and SNL models, partial nerve ligation has been utilized to test the efficacy of several analgesics. Gabapentin was found to be helpful in decreasing mechanical and thermal allodynia.[40] In another report, oxcarbazepine and carbamazepine did not influence mechanical hyperalgesia or tactile allodynia, whereas gabapentin reduced tactile allodynia.[41] The TCA amitriptyline prevented thermal hyperalgesia if given after the injury was performed on the animal.[42]

SPARED NERVE INJURY

In order to create a reliable and reproducible system of neuropathic pain while also sparing any collateral damage that may take place during surgery, Woolf and colleagues developed a spared nerve injury (SNI) model of neuropathic pain.[43] The sciatic nerve is exposed and the common peroneal and tibial nerves are sectioned, leaving the sural nerve intact. In this initial study, a subset of mice had the nerves crushed as opposed to ligated; these animals developed transient neuropathic pain. The following neuropathic features were noted: (1) mechanical allodynia as measured by von Frey filaments of increasing force; (2) mechanical hyperalgesia, as noted by pinprick withdrawal time; (3) cold allodynia, tested with a drop of acetone on the paw; and (4) heat hyperalgesia, tested using the Hargreaves method with a Hugo Basile apparatus. Symptoms were noted to evolve rapidly after surgery. Sensory changes occurred in the distribution of the sural and saphenous nerves as well, but no mirror changes on the contralateral side were evident. Pharmacological testing of the SNI model has demonstrated that neuropathic pain is relieved by amitriptyline,[44] gabapentin,[45,46] and opioids[47] but not by venlafaxine.[48] As noted previously, many of these medications have proven successful to varying degrees in treating human neuropathies.

Models of Pain Due to Metabolic and Toxic Neuropathies

DIABETIC NEUROPATHY

Neuropathic pain is a common feature of diabetic neuropathy. In order to study the pathogenesis and test treatment strategies, several rat models of diabetic neuropathy have been developed. Additional details can be found in Chapter 11. These models include chemically induced diabetes (using the beta cell toxic compounds alloxan and streptozotocin) and genetic models of type 1 (biobreeding Worcester [BB/W]) and type 2 diabetes (Zucker diabetic rats), as well as prediabetic rats fed a high-fat diet that develop neuropathy.

Injection of the pancreatic B-cell toxic compound streptozotocin or alloxan leads to rapid induction of hyperglycemia in rodents. Hypothetically, it mimics the onset of type 1 diabetes, as well as the onset of neuropathic symptoms. This system has been particularly useful in studying diabetic rats in a normal genetic background. Rodents tested in this manner have been evaluated for thermal hyperalgesia using the tail flick test[49,50] and the hot plate method[49,51]; mechanical hyperalgesia using the Randall-Sellito method[49,52,53]; mechanical allodynia using von Frey filaments[54]; and chemical allodynia using formalin injection to the paw.[49,51,54,55]

There are two well-known commercially available lines that develop insulin-dependent diabetes (BB/W) and hyperglycemia (Zucker). Both rats have been shown to develop behaviors consistent with neuropathy. These rats display thermal hyperalgesia in the tail flick test,[50] as well as the paw withdrawal method described by Hargreaves.[56–59] In addition, they develop mechanical allodynia as measured using von Frey filaments.[56]

As interest in impaired glucose tolerance and peripheral neuropathy has increased, a prediabetic model of peripheral neuropathy has been developed.[60] In this model, rats are fed a high-fat diet and develop features that mimic alimentary obesity, including high insulin and free fatty acids levels as well as hyperglycemia. The advantage of this model is that studies are carried out in a normal genetic background. Behavioral characteristics displayed by these mice include mechanical allodynia and thermal hyperalgesia.

Several analgesics, including pregabalin, TCAs, diclofenac, and morphine, have been evaluated in diabetic rat models. Animal results suggest that TCAs are effective in managing diabetic neuropathic pain.[58,59,61,62] Several reports have arrived at the same conclusion with human subjects.[8,63–66] Morphine has also been shown to have a short-term effect in diabetic rats.[61] As a correlation, opioids also provide some relief from the pain of diabetic neuropathy in humans.[67,68]

CHEMOTHERAPY-INDUCED PERIPHERAL NEUROPATHY

Peripheral neuropathy is a common side effect of many chemotherapy regimens, often limiting the use of higher, more effective doses of cancer drugs. The extent of chemotherapy-induced peripheral neuropathy is often dose-dependent, and the fiber type involved varies with the drug. Neuropathic pain is a common feature for most of these drugs, but is especially seen with cisplatin, vincristine, and paclitaxel.[69] Most animal models used to study chemotherapy-induced painful neuropathies use similar outcome measures. The desired drug (cisplatin, paclitaxel, or vincristine) is applied to rats in different dosing regimens and to a final total cumulative dose.[70] A limiting factor in these studies is the systemic effects of chemotherapy on the rats. At higher cumulative doses, motor deficits and failure to thrive are noted in the animals.[71]

Studies of vincristine neurotoxicity were initially carried out in rats after injection of the drug into the tail vein.[72] Daily intravenous injections of up to 200 µg/kg for 2 weeks resulted in mechanical hyperalgesia (using the Randall Selitto paw-withdrawal test), mechanical allodynia (using von Frey filaments), and thermal allodynia (the Hargreaves method). Additionally, rotarod testing demonstrated that at a dose of 200 µg/kg there was an effect on motor performance, emphasizing the importance of finding an appropriate dosing regimen to obtain a sensory deficit without motor abnormalities. Due to the high incidence of systemic side effects, Weng et al. modified this method using intraperitoneal delivery.[73] Mechanical and thermal allodynia without motor deficits were seen with this alternative delivery route.

Similar to other neuropathic pain models, vincristine neuropathy models have been used to evaluate the efficacy of various medications. For example, the antidepressant venlafaxine was shown to be effective in reducing hyperalgesia in a rat model of vincristine neuropathy.

In addition, the C-fiber evoked flexor reflex, which is used to analyze central pain processing in rats, was also depressed.[74] Gabapentin was found to improve both cold and mechanical allodynia thresholds in rats with paclitaxel and vincristine neuropathy.[75] Surprisingly, a randomized, controlled trial of gabapentin failed to show any effect on chemotherapy-induced neuropathy in humans.[76] Nonetheless, some evidence suggests that it might be useful as an adjuvant to opioids.[77] The antiepileptic drug topiramate demonstrated relief of mechanical allodynia and hyperalgesia in a rat model of vincristine-induced neuropathy.[78] In clinical trials, topiramate has also been reported to relieve neuropathic pain in humans.[79]

Initial studies looking into neurophysiological and structural changes in paclitaxel-induced neuropathy in rats were conducted by several research groups. Behavioral changes and the nature of the deficits observed in rats, interestingly, were found to be dependent on the method of paclitaxel administration. Campana et al. demonstrated thermal hypoalgesia after intraperitoneal administration of paclitaxel (1.2 mg/kg/day) given five times per week for 3 weeks or given every third day for 10 days.[80] Authier et al. demonstrated that with a single 32 mg/kg intraperitoneal dose of paclitaxel, mechanical hyperalgesia became evident in rats; however, on a more prolonged dosing regimen of five weekly doses of 16 mg/kg, thermal hypoalgesia developed as well.[81] In spite of this, they were unable to demonstrate any type of allodynia with either dosing regimen. Others also showed behavioral differences based on their dosing regimen.[82] Polomano et al. were able to model the neuropathy induced by paclitaxel by dosing rats intraperitoneally on four alternate days (days 1, 3, 5, and 7) with doses of 0.5, 1.0, and 2.0 mg/kg.[83] Abnormal heat hyperalgesia, mechanical allodynia, and cold allodynia in the hind paws were noted.

There has been extensive drug screening using this system, with mixed results when they were applied to humans. For example, the antiepileptics ethosuximide and topiramate were shown to relieve the mechanical allodynia of paclitaxel in rats.[78,84] Other anticonvulsants, such as oxcarbazepine[78] and carbamazepine,[85] have not been successful in doing so. Additional animal studies have demonstrated the anti-nociceptive effects of magnesium, venlafaxine, gabapentin, and clomipramine.[85] In spite of a remarkable case report of successful treatment with venlafaxine,[79] human trials have been less successful in replicating these outcomes.[86]

Cisplatin-induced neuropathy models have been developed and show typical features of neuropathic pain.[87] More recently, however, attention has been directed at developing reliable animal models of oxaliplatin-induced peripheral neuropathy because of widespread use of oxaliplatin in colon cancer and its unique presentation of cold allodynia in patients. In one of the earlier models, neuropathy induced by repeated injections of oxaliplatin resulted in cold hyperalgesia and allodynia, as well as mechanical allodynia.[85] A study directly comparing the early stages of oxaliplatin- and cisplatin-induced neuropathy replicated the clinical features with differential responses to thermal stimuli.[88] In animals, magnesium and venlafaxine produced an antinociceptive effect, but gabapentin, clomipramine, and lidocaine only improved allodynia.[85] These findings in the animal model mirror a clinical report indicating that a combination of venlafaxine and topiramate successfully relieved pain in a patient with oxaliplatin neuropathy.[79]

SPINAL CORD INJURY AND NEUROPATHIC PAIN

Neuropathic pain is a common feature of chronic spinal cord injury and affects the quality of life of many patients.[89,90] Spinal cord injury is a heterogeneous disorder with multiple mechanisms of injury. Mirroring this clinical observation, animal models designed to induce central neuropathic pain from spinal cord injury include spinal cord ischemia, spinal cord hemisection, and spinal contusion models.

In the spinal cord ischemia model, to achieve ischemia at a specific level of the spinal cord in rats, a photo-reactive chemical is injected at a particular spinal level and the area is irradiated with a laser beam. This leads to an intravascular photochemical reaction, vessel occlusion, and ischemia. Using this system, Hao et al. were able to demonstrate mechanical allodynia to light touch by stroking the skin and the threshold of vocalization to various ratings of von Frey filaments.[91] A drawback of this model is that spinal cord injury may be extensive if the laser irritation is too prolonged. Histological analysis is required to demonstrate that there is no damage to dorsal roots or dorsal columns, excluding a peripheral cause for the central pain. This spinal cord ischemic injury model has been used to determine the effectiveness of tocainide, morphine, baclofen, muscinol, clinidine, carbamezepine, pentobarbital, and guanethidine in treating pain.[91] Using the ischemic model of spinal cord injury, Erichsen et al. were able to demonstrate that codeine is particularly effective in reducing neuropathic pain behavior in rats, validating the usefulness of the model.[47]

In order to better mimic the traumatic spinal cord injury, a spinal cord contusion injury model has been developed by carefully monitoring weight drops on animals.[92,93] The system consists of an impactor that can be raised to specific heights and then dropped onto an open spinal cord while the rat in held in place in a stereotaxic instrument. This produces a relatively reproducible stereotyped response and has been shown to produce mechanical as well as thermal allodynia in rat models.[94] This model has been used to evaluate the underlying mechanisms of central pain; among many other studies, expression levels of the sodium channel Na(V)1.3 mRNA, which has been implicated in peripheral mechanisms of neuropathic pain, were shown to be unregulated in spinal cord contusion.[95] Using this setup, after moderate contusion injury, intraperitoneal gabapentin was shown to improve mechanical and thermal allodynia in adult rats.[94] Human trials have validated the use of gabapentin in human spinal cord injury patients as well.[96,97]

Another model of central pain due to spinal cord injury has utilized Brown-Sequard-like spinal hemisection. Both mechanical and thermal allodynia were observed in animals with hemisected spinal cords at the thoracic level utilizing paw withdrawal as well as behavioral endpoints.[98,99] Thermal allodynia was examined in an experimental setup in which each paw was individually heated by 1°C steps, and behaviors such as head turning and guarding of the paw or brisk paw withdrawal with a lick were scored.[98,99]

A common theme in these studies has been evaluation of the role of neuron-glia interactions in the generation and persistence of neuropathic pain behavior after spinal cord injury.[100] In animal models of spinal cord injury, there is hyperexcitibility of the dorsal horn neurons below the injury level[101] and chronic activation of microglia diffusely.[102,103] These observations are similar to what has been reported after peripheral nerve injury with activation of microglia in the spinal cord and hyperexcitibility of dorsal horn neurons.[104,105] The relevance of microglial activation in neuropathic pain has been shown by studies in which selective inhibition of microglial activation resulted in restoration of morphological, electrophysiological, and behavioral changes.[106,107]

VISCERAL PAIN MODELS

Visceral pain in various forms afflicts a significant number of patients and account for a large percentage of patients with chronic pain.[108,109] Animal models have been developed for pelvic pain due to endometriosis,[110] interstitial cystitis,[111] and prostatitis.[112] Most of the studies on neuropathic pain due to visceral syndromes have been done with models of interstitial cystitis. In one of the more commonly used versions, interstitial cystitis and pelvic pain are induced by intraperitoneal administration of cyclophosphamide.[113,114] An anticancer agent, cyclophosphamide is metabolized into acrolein in the kidney, which accumulates in the bladder. Acrolein is an irritant to the bladder and results in inflammation and visceral pain. Cyclophosphamide-treated rats developed behavior typical of spontaneous pain within 15–30 minutes of administration of the drug.[113] The pain behavior was scored using an arbitrary scale based on respiratory rate, posture, and eye opening in freely moving rats. The presence of neuropathic pain was validated in this model because morphine was able to reverse the spontaneous pain behavior. Others have developed a similar model in the mouse[115] and have validated its utility with morphine, keteroloc, and duloxetine.[116] Interestingly, the antiepileptic drug gabapentin had no benefit in this model, and clinical experience seems to mirror this observation.[117]

Another model of interstitial cystitis involved administration of pseudorabies virus into the abductor caudalis dorsalis muscle of female mice.[118] The presence of neurogenic pain was evaluated using von Frey hair stimulation of the pelvic region. In this model there was intense mast cell-mediated inflammation of the bladder suggesting a direct relationship between neurogenic pain and bladder inflammation. Furthermore, this model was used to evaluate the crosstalk between the bladder and other abdominal organs; lidocaine administration into the colon was sufficient to block bladder pain.[119] Recently, the same model was used to demonstrate the therapeutic efficacy of neurokinin 1 receptor and histamine receptor antagonists.[120] In the same model, gabapentin had no therapeutic effect. The relationship between other pelvic organs and the bladder has been studied in other models of interstitial cystitis as well. For example, intrarectal delivery of a colonic irritant, trinitrobenzenesulfonic acid, results in sensitization of bladder afferents to bladder distention or intravesical capsaicin.[121,122] Taken together, the results of these studies suggest that there is crosstalk between the genitourinary and gastrointestinal innervation that results in an augmented neuropathic pain syndrome.

CONCLUSIONS

Multiple animal models have been developed for various conditions with neuropathic pain to study mechanisms of disease and test the therapeutic utility of potential drug candidates. Despite their utility, animal models do not provide complete mechanistic insight into neuropathic pain or predict therapeutic efficacy in patients. The reasons for these observations are likely to be many. One potential pitfall is that chronic neuropathic pain is a complicated illness with both peripheral and central mechanisms, and nonprimate models may lack the complexity of the interactions between the central and peripheral nervous systems. The models may be able to replicate only a single aspect of the neuropathic pain, and drugs developed on the basis of such mechanistic insights may be able to provide only partial relief. Furthermore, a given patient with chronic neuropathic pain may experience different types of pain with different mechanisms that evolve over time. This observation may necessitate combination therapies to tackle different mechanisms of chronic pain. Animal models that replicate such complexities will be required to test drug therapies, not only singly but also in combination.

REFERENCES

1. Bennett GJ, Xie YK. A peripheral mononeuropathy in rat that produces disorders of pain sensation like those seen in man. *Pain.* 1988;33(1):87–107.
2. Balasubramanyan S, Stemkowski PL, Stebbing MJ, Smith PA. Sciatic chronic constriction injury produces cell-type-specific changes in the electrophysiological properties of rat substantia gelatinosa neurons. *J Neurophysiol.* 2006;96(2):579–590.
3. Dong XW, Goregoaker S, Engler H, et al. Small interfering RNA-mediated selective knockdown of NaV1.8 tetrodotoxin-resistant sodium channel reverses mechanical allodynia in neuropathic rats. *Neuroscience.* 2007;146(2):812–821.
4. Mosconi T, Kruger L. Fixed-diameter polyethylene cuffs applied to the rat sciatic nerve induce a painful neuropathy: ultrastructural morphometric analysis of axonal alterations. *Pain.* 1996;64(1):37–57.
5. Ardid D, Guilbaud G. Antinociceptive effects of acute and "chronic" injections of tricyclic antidepressant drugs in a new model of mononeuropathy in rats. *Pain.* 1992;49(2):279–287.
6. Bomholt SF, Mikkelsen JD, Blackburn-Munro G. Antinociceptive effects of the antidepressants amitriptyline, duloxetine, mirtazapine and citalopram in animal models of acute, persistent and neuropathic pain. *Neuropharmacology.* 2005;48(2):252–263.
7. De Vry J, Kuhl E, Franken-Kunkel P, Eckel G. Pharmacological characterization of the chronic constriction injury model of neuropathic pain. *Eur J Pharmacol.* 2004;491(2–3):137–148.
8. Max MB, Lynch SA, Muir J, Shoaf SE, Smoller B, Dubner R. Effects of desipramine, amitriptyline, and fluoxetine on pain in diabetic neuropathy. *N Engl J Med.* 1992;326(19):1250–1256.
9. Kieburtz K, Simpson D, Yiannoutsos C, et al. A randomized trial of amitriptyline and mexiletine for painful neuropathy in HIV infection. AIDS Clinical Trial Group 242 Protocol Team. *Neurology.* 1998;51(6):1682–1688.
10. Max MB, Schafer SC, Culnane M, Smoller B, Dubner R, Gracely RH. Amitriptyline, but not lorazepam, relieves postherpetic neuralgia. *Neurology.* 1988;38(9):1427–1432.
11. Pradhan AAA, Yu XH, Laird JMA. Modality of hyperalgesia tested, not type of nerve damage, predicts pharmacological sensitivity in rat models of neuropathic pain. *Eur J Pain* (*London*). 2009;14(5):503–509.
12. Serpell MG. Gabapentin in neuropathic pain syndromes: a randomised, double-blind, placebo-controlled trial. *Pain.* 2002;99(3):557–566.
13. Wiffen PJ, McQuay HJ, Moore RA. Carbamazepine for acute and chronic pain. *Cochrane Database of Systematic Reviews* (*Online*). 2005(3):CD005451–CD005451.
14. Shih A, Miletic V, Miletic G, Smith LJ. Midazolam administration reverses thermal hyperalgesia and prevents gamma-aminobutyric acid transporter loss in a rodent model of neuropathic pain. *Anesth Anal.* 2008;106(4):1296–1302; table of contents,1296–1302.
15. Scholz J, Abele A, Marian C, et al. Low-dose methotrexate reduces peripheral nerve injury-evoked spinal microglial activation and neuropathic pain behavior in rats. *Pain.* 2008;138(1):130–142.
16. Costa B, Siniscalco D, Trovato AE, et al. AM404, an inhibitor of anandamide uptake, prevents pain behaviour and modulates cytokine and apoptotic pathways in a rat model of neuropathic pain. *Br J Pharmacol.* 2006;148(7):1022–1032.
17. Ugolini G, Marinelli S, Covaceuszach S, Cattaneo A, Pavone F. The function neutralizing anti-TrkA antibody MNAC13 reduces inflammatory and neuropathic pain. *Proc Natl Acad Sci USA.* 2007;104(8):2985–2990.
18. Ledeboer A, Liu T, Shumilla JA, et al. The glial modulatory drug AV411 attenuates mechanical allodynia in rat models of neuropathic pain. *Neuron Glia Biol.* 2006;2(4):279–291.
19. Kim SH, Chung JM. An experimental model for peripheral neuropathy produced by segmental spinal nerve ligation in the rat. *Pain.* 1992;50(3):355–363.
20. Seltzer Z, Dubner R, Shir Y. A novel behavioral model of neuropathic pain disorders produced in rats by partial sciatic nerve injury. *Pain.* 1990;43(2):205–218.
21. Kim SH, Chung JM. Sympathectomy alleviates mechanical allodynia in an experimental animal model for neuropathy in the rat. *Neurosci Lett.* 1991;134(1):131–134.
22. Carlton SM, Lekan HA, Kim SH, Chung JM. Behavioral manifestations of an experimental model for peripheral neuropathy produced

by spinal nerve ligation in the primate. *Pain.* 1994;56(2):155–166.

23. Chapman V, Suzuki R, Chamarette HL, Rygh LJ, Dickenson AH. Effects of systemic carbamazepine and gabapentin on spinal neuronal responses in spinal nerve ligated rats. *Pain.* 1998;75(2–3):261–272.

24. Hunter JC, Gogas KR, Hedley LR, et al. The effect of novel anti-epileptic drugs in rat experimental models of acute and chronic pain. *Eur J Pharmacol.* 1997;324(2–3):153–160.

25. Arezzo JC, Rosenstock J, Lamoreaux L, Pauer L. Efficacy and safety of pregabalin 600 mg/d for treating painful diabetic peripheral neuropathy: a double-blind placebo-controlled trial. *BMC Neurol.* 2008;8:33–46.

26. Simpson DM, Schifitto G, Clifford DB, et al. Pregabalin for painful HIV neuropathy: a randomized, double-blind, placebo-controlled trial. *Neurology.* 74(5):413–420.

27. Gold MS, Weinreich D, Kim C-S, et al. Redistribution of Na(V)1.8 in uninjured axons enables neuropathic pain. *J Neurosci.* 2003;23(1):158–166.

28. Nassar MA, Levato A, Stirling LC, Wood JN. Neuropathic pain develops normally in mice lacking both Na(v)1.7 and Na(v)1.8. *Mol Pain.* 2005;1:24–33.

29. Nassar MA, Baker MD, Levato A, et al. Nerve injury induces robust allodynia and ectopic discharges in Nav1.3 null mutant mice. *Mol Pain.* 2006;2:33–43.

30. Ibrahim MM, Deng H, Zvonok A, et al. Activation of CB2 cannabinoid receptors by AM1241 inhibits experimental neuropathic pain: pain inhibition by receptors not present in the CNS. *Proc Natl Acad Sci USA.* 2003;100(18):10529–10533.

31. Naguib M, Diaz P, Xu JJ, et al. MDA7: a novel selective agonist for CB2 receptors that prevents allodynia in rat neuropathic pain models. *Br J Pharmacol.* 2008;155(7):1104–1116.

32. Bridges D, Ahmad K, Rice AS. The synthetic cannabinoid WIN55,212–2 attenuates hyperalgesia and allodynia in a rat model of neuropathic pain. *Br J Pharmacol.* 2001;133(4):586–594.

33. Suzuki R, Stanfa LC, Kowaluk EA, Williams M, Jarvis MF, Dickenson AH. The effect of ABT-702, a novel adenosine kinase inhibitor, on the responses of spinal neurones following carrageenan inflammation and peripheral nerve injury. *Br J Pharmacol.* 2001;132(7):1615–1623.

34. Hahm TS, Ahn HJ, Bae C-D, et al. Protective effects of gabapentin on allodynia and alpha 2 delta 1-subunit of voltage-dependent calcium channel in spinal nerve-ligated rats. *J Korean Med Sci.* 2009;24(1):146–151.

35. Guasti L, Richardson D, Jhaveri M, et al. Minocycline treatment inhibits microglial activation and alters spinal levels of endocannabinoids in a rat model of neuropathic pain. *Mol Pain.* 2009;5:35–45.

36. Hama A, Sagen J. Antinociceptive effects of the marine snail peptides conantokin-G and conotoxin MVIIA alone and in combination in rat models of pain. *Neuropharmacology.* 2009;56(2):556–563.

37. Eid SR, Crown ED, Moore EL, et al. HC-030031, a TRPA1 selective antagonist, attenuates inflammatory- and neuropathy-induced mechanical hypersensitivity. *Mol Pain.* 2008;4:48–58.

38. Beaudry F, Girard C, Vachon P. Early dexamethasone treatment after implantation of a sciatic-nerve cuff decreases the concentration of substance P in the lumbar spinal cord of rats with neuropathic pain. *Can J Veterinary Res = Rev Can Recherche Vétérinaire.* 2007;71(2):90–97.

39. Huang LJ, Yoon MH, Choi JI, Kim WM, Lee HG, Kim YO. Effect of sildenafil on neuropathic pain and hemodynamics in rats. *Yonsei Med J.* 2010;51(1):82–87.

40. Castañé A, Célérier E, Martín M, et al. Development and expression of neuropathic pain in CB1 knockout mice. *Neuropharmacology.* 2006;50(1):111–122.

41. Fox A, Gentry C, Patel S, Kesingland A, Bevan S. Comparative activity of the anti-convulsants oxcarbazepine, carbamazepine, lamotrigine and gabapentin in a model of neuropathic pain in the rat and guinea-pig. *Pain.* 2003;105(1–2):355–362.

42. McCarson KE, Ralya A, Reisman SA, Enna SJ. Amitriptyline prevents thermal hyperalgesia and modifications in rat spinal cord GABA(B) receptor expression and function in an animal model of neuropathic pain. *Biochem Pharmacol.* 2005;71(1–2):196–202.

43. Decosterd I, Woolf CJ. Spared nerve injury: an animal model of persistent peripheral neuropathic pain. *Pain.* 2000;87(2):149–158.

44. Arsenault A, Sawynok J. Perisurgical amitriptyline produces a preventive effect on afferent hypersensitivity following spared nerve injury. *Pain.* 2009;146(3):308–314.

45. Erichsen HK, Blackburn-Munro G. Pharmacological characterisation of the spared nerve injury model of neuropathic pain. *Pain.* 2002;98(1–2):151–161.

46. Rode F, Jensen DG, Blackburn-Munro G, Bjerrum OJ. Centrally-mediated antinociceptive actions of GABA(A) receptor agonists in the rat spared nerve injury model of neuropathic pain. *Eur J Pharmacol.* 2005;516(2):131–138.

47. Erichsen HK, Hao J-X, Xu X-J, Blackburn-Munro G. Comparative actions of the opioid analgesics morphine, methadone and codeine in rat models of peripheral and central neuropathic pain. *Pain.* 2005;116(3):347–358.

48. Rode F, Broløs T, Blackburn-Munro G, Bjerrum OJ. Venlafaxine compromises the antinociceptive actions of gabapentin in rat models of neuropathic and persistent pain. *Psychopharmacology.* 2006;187(3):364–375.

49. Courteix C, Eschalier A, Lavarenne J. Streptozocin-induced diabetic rats: behavioural evidence for a model of chronic pain. *Pain.* 1993;53(1):81–88.

50. Lee JH, McCarty R. Glycemic control of pain threshold in diabetic and control rats. *Physiol Behav.* 1990;47(2):225–230.

51. Calcutt NA, Malmberg AB, Yamamoto T, Yaksh TL. Tolrestat treatment prevents modification of the formalin test model of prolonged pain in hyperglycemic rats. *Pain.* 1994;58(3):413–420.

52. Ahlgren SC, Levine JD. Mechanical hyperalgesia in streptozotocin-diabetic rats. *Neuroscience.* 1993;52(4):1049–1055.

53. Malcangio M, Tomlinson DR. A pharmacologic analysis of mechanical hyperalgesia in streptozotocin/diabetic rats. *Pain.* 1998;76(1–2):151–157.

54. Calcutt NA, Jorge MC, Yaksh TL, Chaplan SR. Tactile allodynia and formalin hyperalgesia in streptozotocin-diabetic rats: effects of insulin, aldose reductase inhibition and lidocaine. *Pain.* 1996;68(2–3):293–299.

55. Malmberg AB, Yaksh TL, Calcutt NA. Antinociceptive effects of the GM1 ganglioside derivative AGF 44 on the formalin test in normal and streptozotocin-diabetic rats. *Neurosci Lett.* 1993;161(1):45–48.

56. Brussee V, Guo G, Dong Y, et al. Distal degenerative sensory neuropathy in a long-term type 2 diabetes rat model. *Diabetes.* 2008;57(6):1664–1673.

57. Kamiya H, Murakawa Y, Zhang W, Sima AAF. Unmyelinated fiber sensory neuropathy differs in type 1 and type 2 diabetes. *Diabetes/Metab Res Rev.* 2005;21(5):448–458.

58. Oltman CL, Davidson EP, Coppey LJ, Kleinschmidt TL, Yorek MA. Treatment of Zucker diabetic fatty rats with AVE7688 improves vascular and neural dysfunction. *Diabetes, Obesity Metab.* 2009;11(3):223–233.

59. Stevens MJ, Zhang W, Li F, Sima AAF. C-peptide corrects endoneurial blood flow but not oxidative stress in type 1 BB/Wor rats. *Am J Physiol Endocrinol Metab.* 2004;287(3):E497–E505.

60. Obrosova IG, Ilnytska O, Lyzogubov VV, et al. High-fat diet–induced neuropathy of pre-diabetes and obesity. *Diabetes.* 2007;56(10):2598–2608.

61. Courteix C, Bardin M, Chantelauze C, Lavarenne J, Eschalier A. Study of the sensitivity of the diabetes-induced pain model in rats to a range of analgesics. *Pain.* 1994;57(2):153–160.

62. Yamamoto H, Shimoshige Y, Yamaji T, Murai N, Aoki T, Matsuoka N. Pharmacological characterization of standard analgesics on mechanical allodynia in streptozotocin-induced diabetic rats. *Neuropharmacology.* 2009;57(4):403–408.

63. Kvinesdal B, Molin J, Frøland A, Gram LF. Imipramine treatment of painful diabetic neuropathy. *JAMA.* 1984;251(13):1727–1730.

64. Max MB, Culnane M, Schafer SC, et al. Amitriptyline relieves diabetic neuropathy pain in patients with normal or depressed mood. *Neurology.* 1987;37(4):589–596.

65. Max MB, Kishore-Kumar R, Schafer SC, et al. Efficacy of desipramine in painful diabetic neuropathy: a placebo-controlled trial. *Pain.* 1991;45(1):3–9.

66. McQuay HJ, Tramèr M, Nye BA, Carroll D, Wiffen PJ, Moore RA. A systematic review of antidepressants in neuropathic pain. *Pain.* 1996;68(2–3):217–227.

67. Gimbel JS, Richards P, Portenoy RK. Controlled-release oxycodone for pain in diabetic neuropathy: a randomized controlled trial. *Neurology.* 2003;60(6):927–934.

68. Watson CPN, Moulin D, Watt-Watson J, Gordon A, Eisenhoffer J. Controlled-release oxycodone relieves neuropathic pain: a randomized controlled trial in painful diabetic neuropathy. *Pain.* 2003;105(1–2):71–78.

69. Quasthoff S, Hartung HP. Chemotherapy-induced peripheral neuropathy. *J Neurol.* 2002;249(1):9–17.

70. Authier N, Balayssac D, Marchand F, et al. Animal models of chemotherapy-evoked painful peripheral neuropathies. *Neurotherapeutics.* 2009;6(4):620–629.

71. Golden JP, Johnson EM. Models of chemotherapy drug-induced peripheral neuropathy. *Drug Discovery Today: Dis Models.* 2004;1(2):186–191.

72. Aley KO, Reichling DB, Levine JD. Vincristine hyperalgesia in the rat: a model of painful vincristine neuropathy in humans. *Neuroscience.* 1996;73(1):259–265.

73. Weng HR, Cordella JV, Dougherty PM. Changes in sensory processing in the spinal dorsal horn accompany vincristine-induced hyperalgesia and allodynia. *Pain.* 2003;103(1–2):131–138.

74. Marchand F, Alloui A, Pelissier T, et al. Evidence for an antihyperalgesic effect of venlafaxine in vincristine-induced neuropathy in rat. *Brain Res.* 2003;980(1):117–120.

75. Xiao W, Boroujerdi A, Bennett GJ, Luo ZD. Chemotherapy-evoked painful peripheral neuropathy: analgesic effects of gabapentin and effects on expression of the alpha-2-delta type-1 calcium channel subunit. *Neuroscience.* 2007;144(2):714–720.

76. Caraceni A, Zecca E, Bonezzi C, et al. Gabapentin for neuropathic cancer pain: a randomized controlled trial from the Gabapentin Cancer Pain Study Group. *J Clin Oncol.* 2004;22(14):2909–2917.

77. Rao RD, Michalak JC, Sloan JA, et al. Efficacy of gabapentin in the management of chemotherapy-induced peripheral neuropathy: a phase 3 randomized, double-blind, placebo-controlled, crossover trial (N00C3). *Cancer.* 2007;110(9):2110–2118.

78. Xiao W, Naso L, Bennett GJ. Experimental studies of potential analgesics for the treatment of chemotherapy-evoked painful peripheral neuropathies. *Pain Med (Malden, Mass.).* 2008;9(5):505–517.

79. Durand J-P, Alexandre J, Guillevin L, Goldwasser F. Clinical activity of venlafaxine and topiramate against oxaliplatin-induced disabling permanent neuropathy. *Anti-Cancer Drugs.* 2005;16(5):587–591.

80. Campana WM, Eskeland N, Calcutt NA, Misasi R, Myers RR, O'Brien JS. Prosaptide prevents paclitaxel neurotoxicity. *Neurotoxicology.* 1998;19(2):237–244.

81. Authier N, Gillet JP, Fialip J, Eschalier A, Coudore F. Description of a short-term Taxol-induced nociceptive neuropathy in rats. *Brain Res.* 2000;887(2):239–249.

82. Dina OA, Chen X, Reichling D, Levine JD. Role of protein kinase Cepsilon and protein kinase A in a model of paclitaxel-induced painful peripheral neuropathy in the rat. *Neuroscience.* 2001;108(3):507–515.

83. Polomano RC, Mannes AJ, Clark US, Bennett GJ. A painful peripheral neuropathy in the rat produced by the chemotherapeutic drug, paclitaxel. *Pain.* 2001;94(3):293–304.

84. Flatters SJL, Bennett GJ. Ethosuximide reverses paclitaxel-and vincristine-induced painful peripheral neuropathy. *Pain.* 2004;109(1–2):150–161.

85. Ling B, Authier N, Balayssac D, Eschalier A, Coudore F. Behavioral and pharmacological description of oxaliplatin-induced painful neuropathy in rat. *Pain.* 2007;128(3):225–234.

86. Mielke S, Sparreboom A, Mross K. Peripheral neuropathy: a persisting challenge in paclitaxel-based regimes. *Eur J Cancer (Oxford, England: 1990).* 2006;42(1):24–30.

87. Tredici G, Tredici S, Fabbrica D, Minoia C, Cavaletti G. Experimental cisplatin neuronopathy in rats and the effect of retinoic acid administration. *J Neuro-Oncol.* 1998;36(1):31–40.

88. Ta LE, Low PA, Windebank AJ. Mice with cisplatin and oxaliplatin-induced painful neuropathy develop distinct early responses to thermal stimuli. *Mol. Pain.* 2009;5:9.

89. Calmels P, Mick G, Perrouin-Verbe B, Ventura M. Neuropathic pain in spinal cord injury: identification, classification, evaluation. *Ann Phys Rehabil Med.* 2009;52(2):83–102.

90. Cardenas DD, Felix ER. Pain after spinal cord injury: a review of classification, treatment approaches, and treatment assessment. *PM&R.* 2009;1(12):1077–1090.

91. Hao JX, Xu XJ, Aldskogius H, Seiger A, Wiesenfeld-Hallin Z. Allodynia-like effects in rat after ischaemic spinal cord injury photochemically induced by laser irradiation. *Pain.* 1991;45(2):175–185.

92. Gruner JA. A monitored contusion model of spinal cord injury in the rat. *J Neurotrauma.* 1992;9(2):123–128.

93. Scheff SW, Rabchevsky AG, Fugaccia I, Main JA, Lumpp JE. Experimental modeling of spinal cord injury: characterization of a force-defined injury device. *J Neurotrauma.* 2003;20(2):179–193.

94. Hulsebosch CE, Xu GY, Perez-Polo JR, Westlund KN, Taylor CP, McAdoo DJ. Rodent model of chronic central pain after spinal cord contusion injury and effects of gabapentin. *J Neurotrauma.* 2000;17(12):1205–1217.

95. Hains BC, Klein JP, Saab CY, Craner MJ, Black JA, Waxman SG. Upregulation of sodium channel Nav1.3 and functional involvement in neuronal hyperexcitability associated with central neuropathic pain after spinal cord injury. *J Neurosci.* 2003;23(26):8881–8892.

96. Levendoglu F, Ogün CO, Ozerbil O, Ogün TC, Ugurlu H. Gabapentin is a first line drug for the treatment of neuropathic pain in spinal cord injury. *Spine.* 2004;29(7):743–751.

97. Tai Q, Kirshblum S, Chen B, Millis S, Johnston M, DeLisa JA. Gabapentin in the treatment of neuropathic pain after spinal cord injury: a prospective, randomized, double-blind, crossover trial. *J Spinal Cord Med.* 2002;25(2):100–105.

98. Christensen MD, Everhart AW, Pickelman JT, Hulsebosch CE. Mechanical and thermal allodynia in chronic central pain following spinal cord injury. *Pain.* 1996;68(1):97–107.

99. Christensen MD, Hulsebosch CE. Chronic central pain after spinal cord injury. *J Neurotrauma.* 1997;14(8):517–537.

100. Hulsebosch CE, Hains BC, Crown ED, Carlton SM. Mechanisms of chronic central neuropathic pain after spinal cord injury. *Brain Res Rev.* 2009;60(1):202–213.

101. Hao JX, Xu XJ, Yu YX, Seiger A, Wiesenfeld-Hallin Z. Transient spinal cord ischemia induces temporary hypersensitivity of dorsal horn wide dynamic range neurons to myelinated, but not unmyelinated, fiber input. *J Neurophysiol.* 1992;68(2):384–391.

102. Hains BC, Klein JP, Saab CY, Craner MJ, Black JA, Waxman SG. Upregulation of sodium channel Nav1.3 and functional involvement in neuronal hyperexcitability associated with central neuropathic pain after spinal cord injury. *J Neurosci.* 2003;23(26):8881–8892.

103. Sroga JM, Jones TB, Kigerl KA, McGaughy VM, Popovich PG. Rats and mice exhibit distinct inflammatory reactions after spinal cord injury. *J Comp Neurol.* 2003;462(2):223–240.

104. Coyle DE. Partial peripheral nerve injury leads to activation of astroglia and microglia which parallels the development of allodynic behavior. *Glia.* 1998;23(1):75–83.

105. Fu KY, Light AR, Matsushima GK, Maixner W. Microglial reactions after subcutaneous formalin injection into the rat hind paw. *Brain Res.* 1999;825(1–2):59–67.

106. Hains BC, Waxman SG. Activated microglia contribute to the maintenance of chronic pain after spinal cord injury. *J Neurosci.* 2006;26(16):4308–4317.

107. Zhao P, Waxman SG, Hains BC. Modulation of thalamic nociceptive processing after spinal cord injury through remote activation of thalamic microglia by cysteine cysteine chemokine ligand 21. *J Neurosci.* 2007;27(33):8893–8902.

108. Wesselmann U, Czakanski PP. Pelvic pain: a chronic visceral pain syndrome. *Curr Pain Headache Rep.* 2001;5(1):13–19.

109. Wesselmann U, Burnett AL, Heinberg LJ. The urogenital and rectal pain syndromes. *Pain.* 1997;73(3):269–294.

110. Story L, Kennedy S. Animal studies in endometriosis: a review. *ILAR J.* 2004;45(2):132–138.

111. Wesselmann U. Interstitial cystitis: a chronic visceral pain syndrome. *Urology.* 2001;57 (6 suppl 1):32–39.

112. Vykhovanets EV, Resnick MI, MacLennan GT, Gupta S. Experimental rodent models of prostatitis: limitations and potential. *Prostate Cancer Prostatic Dis.* 2007;10(1):15–29.

113. Boucher M, Meen M, Codron JP, Coudore F, Kemeny JL, Eschalier A. Cyclophosphamide-induced cystitis in freely-moving conscious rats: behavioral approach to a new model of visceral pain. *J Urol.* 2000;164(1):203–208.

114. Lanteri-Minet M, Bon K, de Pommery J, Michiels JF, Menetrey D. Cyclophosphamide cystitis as a model of visceral pain in rats: model elaboration and spinal structures involved as revealed by the expression of c-Fos and Krox-24 proteins. *Exp Brain Res.* 1995;105(2):220–232.

115. Bon K, Lichtensteiger CA, Wilson SG, Mogil JS. Characterization of cyclophosphamide cystitis, a model of visceral and referred pain, in the mouse: species and strain differences. *J Urol.* 2003;170(3):1008–1012.

116. Wantuch C, Piesla M, Leventhal L. Pharmacological validation of a model of cystitis pain in the mouse. *Neurosci Lett.* 2007;421(3):250–252.

117. Phatak S, Foster HE Jr. The management of interstitial cystitis: an update. *Nat Clin Pract Urol.* 2006;3(1):45–53.

118. Chen MC, Keshavan P, Gregory GD, Klumpp DJ. RANTES mediates TNF-dependent lamina propria mast cell accumulation and barrier dysfunction in neurogenic cystitis. *Am J Physiol Renal Physiol.* 2007;292(5):F1372–F1379.

119. Rudick CN, Chen MC, Mongiu AK, Klumpp DJ. Organ cross talk modulates pelvic pain. *Am J Physiol Regul Integr Comp Physiol.* 2007;293(3):R1191–R1198.

120. Rudick CN, Schaeffer AJ, Klumpp DJ. Pharmacologic attenuation of pelvic pain in a murine model of interstitial cystitis. *BMC Urol.* 2009;9:16–24.

121. Ustinova EE, Gutkin DW, Pezzone MA. Sensitization of pelvic nerve afferents and mast cell infiltration in the urinary bladder following chronic colonic irritation is mediated by neuropeptides. *Am J Physiol Renal Physiol.* 2007;292(1):F123–F130.

122. Winnard KP, Dmitrieva N, Berkley KJ. Cross-organ interactions between reproductive, gastrointestinal, and urinary tracts: modulation by estrous stage and involvement of the hypogastric nerve. *Am J Physiol Regul Integr Comp Physiol.* 2006;291(6):R1592–R1601.

4

Drug Discovery for Neuropathic Pain

IAN GILRON

INTRODUCTION

NEUROPATHIC PAIN PREVALENCE estimates have been recently reported to be as high as 8% of the general population.[1,2] In the United States alone, chronic pain has been estimated to cost over US$150 billion annually in health care, disability, and other related costs,[3] with over US$40 billion attributable to neuropathic pain. Current management of neuropathic pain involves a carefully considered, multimodal and multidisciplinary strategy, which may incorporate both pharmacological and nonpharmacological therapies.[4] Subsequent to early clinical observations—over 40 years ago—suggesting a role for antidepressants,[5] anticonvulsants[6] and, more recently, opioids,[7] multiple clinical trials have confirmed the efficacy of these "old" classes of drugs, which are currently among the most commonly used agents for neuropathic pain.[8] More recently, however, the development of various preclinical models[9] and subsequent elucidation of multiple molecular mechanisms[10] have

pointed to several novel therapeutic candidates[11,12] (see Table 4.1), thus reinforcing the rationale for a coordinated translational approach to new drug discovery for neuropathic pain. The observation that at least 50 new molecular entities have reached clinical stages of development emphasizes the high level of both scientific and commercial interest in neuropathic pain.[12] Thus, the purpose of this chapter is to provide a brief introduction to the progression of investigative efforts aimed at identifying and developing new molecular entities for the treatment of neuropathic pain. The design and conduct of phase 3 pivotal "registration" trials is not discussed but has been recently reviewed in detail elsewhere (e.g., see Chapter 9 of this volume and ref. 13).

GENERAL OVERVIEW OF DRUG DEVELOPMENT

As succinctly summarized by the U.S. Food and Drug Administration (FDA) in 2004,[14,15] the

Table 4-1. Emerging Drugs in Neuropathic Pain Circa 2007

DRUG	ORIGINATOR COMPANY	ACTION	INDICATION	CLINICAL TRIAL PHASE	COMMENTS
CLUTAMATE ANTAGONISTS					
AZD-9272	AstraZeneca	Metabotropic glutamate, receptor-1 modulator	Neuropathic pain	Phase I	
Brivaracetam	UCB	Levitiracetam analogue, anticonvulsant	Neuropathic pain	Phase II	
CNS-5161	CeNeS	NMDA antagonist	Neuropathic pain	Phase II	
CHF-3381	Chiesi	NMDA antagonist, MAO inhibitor	Neuropathic pain	Phase II	
Dextromethorphan-quinidine combination	Avanir	NMDA antagonist and cytochrome P450 inhibitor	Painful diabetic neuropathy	Phase III	Combined formulation
EAA-090	Wyeth	NMDA antagonist	Painful diabetic neuropathy	Phase II	
NS-1209	NeuroSearch	AMPA antagonist	Neuropathic pain	Phase I	
RGH-896	Gedeon Richter	NMDA antagonist ("2B" selective)	Neuropathic pain	Phase II	
CYTOKINE INHIBITORS					
AV-411 (ibudilast)	Avigen	Cytokine inhibitor, glial attenuator, IL-1β and IL-6 inhibitor	Diabetic neuropathy	Phase II	
Lenalidomide (CC-5013)	Celgene	Thalidomide derivative	Complex regional pain syndrome	Phase II	
Thalidomide	Celgene	TNF antagonist	Complex regional pain syndrome, arachnoiditis	Phase II	
VANILLOID-RECEPTOR AGONISTS					
ALGRX-4975 (capsaicin, injectable)	Corgentech	Vanilloid-receptor agonist	Neuropathic pain	Phase II	Injectable

(*continued*)

Table 4-1. (continued)

DRUG	ORIGINATOR COMPANY	ACTION	INDICATION	CLINICAL TRIAL PHASE	COMMENTS
NGX-4010 (capsaicin, dermal patch)	NeurogesX	Vanilloid-receptor agonist	Neuropathic pain	Phase III	Topical formulation
Resiniferatoxin	Afferon	Vanilloid-receptor agonist	Neuropathic pain	Phase II	
WL-1001	Winston Laboratories	Vanilloid-receptor agonist	Postherpetic neuralgia	Phase II	
CATECHOLAMINE MODULATORS					
AGN-199981	Allergan	α_{2b}-Adrenergic agonist	Neuropathic pain	Phase II	
Bicifadine	Dov Pharmaceutical	Serotonin-noradrenaline reuptake inhibitor, glutamate antagonist	Neuropathic pain	Phase II	
Desvenlafaxine SR	Wyeth	Serotonin-noradrenaline reuptake inhibitor	Painful diabetic neuropathy	Phase III	
Radaxafine HCl	GlaxoSmithKline	Noradrenaline-dopamine reuptake inhibitor	Neuropathic pain	Phase I	
(S,S)- reboxetine	Pfizer	Selective noradrenaline reuptake inhibitor	Postherpetic neuralgia	Phase II	
ION-CHANNEL BLOCKERS					
Gabapentin ER	Depomed	Calcium-channel ($\alpha_2\delta$ subunit) antagonist	Postherpetic neuralgia	Phase II	ER
Ralfinamide	Newron	Sodium-channel blocker N-type calcium-channel blocker	Neuropathic pain	Phase II	
SPI-860	Scion Pharmaceuticals	N-type calcium-channel antagonist (Cav2.2) Nav1.8 channel antagonist	Neuropathic pain	Phase I	

ANTICONVULSANT DRUGS					
Lacosamide (SPM-927)	Schwarz Pharma	Amino acid anticonvulsant	Neuropathic pain	Phase III	
Lamotrigine, once daily	GlaxoSmithKline	Anticonvulsant	Neuropathic pain	Phase III	
Valrocemide	Teva Pharmaceuticals	Valproate-like anticonvulsant	Neuropathic pain	Phase II	
OPIOID AGONISTS					
Oravescent fentanyl	Cephalon	Opioid	Neuropathic pain	Phase III	Effervescent buccal formulation
Tramadol ER	TheraQuest Biosciences	μ-Opioid agonist and serotonin-noradrenaline re-uptake inhibitor	Neuropathic pain Postherpetic neuralgia	Phase III	Controlled release
CANNABINOID AGONISTS					
KDS-2000	Kadmus Pharmaceuticals	Topical cannabinoid agonist	Postherpetic neuralgia	Phase II	
IP-751	Manhattan Pharmaceuticals	Cannabinoid derivative TNF antagonist, lipoxygenase inhibitor, interleukin antagonist	Neuropathic pain	Phase II	
COX INHIBITORS					
GSK-644784	GlaxoSmithKline	COX-2 inhibitor	Neuropathic pain	Phase II	
GW-406381	GlaxoSmithKline	COX-2 inhibitor	Neuropathic pain	Phase III	
ACETYLCHOLINE MODULATORS					
ABT-894	Abbott Laboratories	Nicotinic agonist	Neuropathic pain	Phase 1	
ACV-1	Metabolic Pharmaceuticals	Nicotinic antagonist	Neuropathic pain	Phase 1	

(*continued*)

Table 4-1. (continued)

DRUG	ORIGINATOR COMPANY	ACTION	INDICATION	CLINICAL TRIAL PHASE	COMMENTS
ADENOSINE AGONISTS					
GW-493838	GlaxoSmithKline	Adenosine agonist	Neuropathic pain	Phase II	
T-62	King Pharmaceuticals	Adenosine agonist	Neuropathic pain	Phase I	
OTHER DRUGS					
Amitriptyline plus ketamine	EpiCept Pharmaceuticals	Tricyclic antidepressant plus NMDA antagonist	Neuropathic pain	Phase III	Combined topical
Cizolirtine	Esteve Laboratories	CGRP/substance P release inhibitor	Neuropathic pain	Phase II	
DA-5018	Dong-A	Neurokinin-1 receptor antagonist	Diabetic neuropathy, postherpetic neuralgia	Phase II	
GPI-16072	MGI Pharma	N-acetylated α-linked acidic, dipeptidase inhibitor	Neuropathic pain	Phase I	
M-40403	ActivBiotics	Superoxide dismutase mimetic	Neuropathic pain	Phase II	
MK-0686	Merck	Undisclosed	Postherpetic neuralgia	Phase II	
MK-0759	Merck	Undisclosed	Postherpetic neuralgia	Phase II	
PD-217,014	Pfizer	Undisclosed	Postherpetic neuralgia	Phase II	
Prosaptide	Savient Pharmaceuticals	Neurotrophic factor	HIV neuropathy	Phase II	
QR-333	Quigley Pharma	Topical flavonoid	Diabetic neuropathy	Phase II	Topical formulation
Sildenafil	Pfizer	Phosphodiesterase inhibitor	Painful diabetic neuropathy	Phase II	
TRO-19622	Trophos	Novel class, cholesterol-like molecule	Neuropathic pain	Phase I	

CGRP: calcitonin gene-related peptide; ER: extended release; MAO: monoamine oxidase; SR: sustained release; IL-2: interleukin-2; TNF: tumour necrosis factor; COX-2: cyclooxygenase-2.

Source: Gilron I, Coderre TJ. Emerging drugs in neuropathic pain. *Expert Opin Emerg Drugs.* 2007;12(1):113–126. Copyright © 2007, Informa Healthcare. Reproduced with permission of Informa Healthcare.

"critical path" of drug development begins with the processes aimed at identifying new therapeutic targets through to preclinical and then clinical drug development and culminates in regulatory approval and market launch (Figure 4-1). As one might imagine, this is an exceedingly complex as well as time- and resource-intensive series of processes requiring close interplay between the fields of science, health care, government regulation, and business. The design and conduct of studies of new molecular entities is generally initiated by the sponsor (i.e., the drug manufacturer or academic investigator) but is closely regulated and supervised by government regulators (e.g., the FDA and the European Medicines Agency). Administrative processes regarding government regulation of drug development activities (e.g., investigational new drug [IND] application; new drug application [NDA]) obviously vary from one country to another and are discussed in detail elsewhere (http://www.fda.gov; http://www.emea.europa.eu; ref. 16).

Discovery of novel therapeutic agents may be achieved through various strategies, including (1) novel target design or modification based on previous knowledge of the target or receptor structure, (2) high-throughput screening of large libraries of chemical or biological entities for the desired activity, (3) synthesis of novel biological agents based on previous knowledge about putative genetic mechanisms, (4) repositioning of a known drug for a new therapeutic use (e.g., gabapentin), and (5) combining known drugs for additive or synergistic effects.[17] As Figure 4.1 illustrates, preclinical evaluation of candidate molecules involves (1) demonstration of the desired therapeutic efficacy using available assays of drug effect (e.g., allodynia in the rat nerve constriction injury model),[18] (2) safety testing for organ toxicities, mutagenicity, and teratogenicity in nonhuman species,[19] and (3) development of synthetic approaches that could ultimately lead to mass production of the molecular entity of interest. Preclinical safety evaluation of a new molecular entity

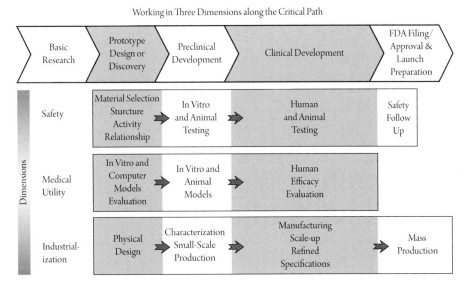

FIGURE 4.1 The critical path of drug development.

Source: From Woodcock J, Woosley R. The FDA critical path initiative and its influence on new drug development. *Annu Rev Med.* 2008;59:1–12.

most often continues even as early clinical development commences.

In the absence of any no-go signals from preclinical safety or efficacy results obtained until that point, clinical development starts with phase 1 "first-in-human" studies. Phase 1 studies are generally small (e.g., 20–50 subjects per trial) and are conducted with an emphasis on safety in order to determine the maximal tolerated dose of an agent and to measure and document observed toxicities.[17] While commonly conducted with healthy volunteers,[20] phase 1 trials may involve patients suffering from the target condition if considerable toxicities are anticipated (e.g., cancer chemotherapy) and may also involve the application of experimental conditions (e.g., human intradermal capsaicin-induced pain) in order to confirm that the range of doses studied in phase 1 is associated with relevant target engagement.[21] Following reassuring safety outcomes from phase 1, a subsequent program of somewhat larger phase 2 trials continues to evaluate safety, now conducted in patients with the target condition (e.g., diabetic neuropathy), but with the proof-of-concept goal of demonstrating treatment efficacy against the disease of interest.[22] Given convincing evidence of safety and efficacy from this set of early phase trials, the next definitive step of drug development involves the design, regulation, and completion of substantially larger (e.g., 250–1000 patients) phase 3 "pivotal" trials that provide data that support the regulatory decision to either approve or reject an application to market the new product.[17] Subsequent to drug licensing approval and market launch, phase 4 or postmarketing trials, sponsored by the manufacturer or by independent academic investigators, can serve to evaluate product safety in much larger populations (e.g., 2000–10,000) and/or to study the new product for indications or in clinical situations beyond those indicated in the approved labeling.[23]

PRECLINICAL IDENTIFICATION AND EFFICACY EVALUATION OF INVESTIGATIONAL DRUGS

Preclinical research is clearly a critical component of drug discovery and involves strategies of pharmacological target identification, preclinical proof-of-concept development, and drug safety and toxicology evaluations, all of which must integrate dynamically with evolving early human research programs.[24]

Identification of novel targets for the treatment of neuropathic pain relies heavily upon investigative efforts to better understand the underlying biological mechanisms of this set of disorders (e.g., see Chapters 1 and 2 of this volume). However, it is also important to recognize the potential of translational research involving preclinical development of new chemical entities that belong to drug classes with known clinical efficacy for human neuropathic pain (e.g., novel opioids, antidepressants, anticonvulsants). Together with these two important sources of information guiding future identification of therapeutic targets, novel technologies such as high-throughput candidate screening serve to facilitate concurrent evaluation of multiple candidate drugs. As some illustrative examples, identification of the role of the purinergic P2X$_7$ receptor (P2X$_7$R) and the transient receptor potential vanilloid 1 receptor (TRPV1) in neuropathic pain modulation followed by high-throughput screening has led to the evaluation of several promising P2X$_7$ receptor antagonists[25] and TRPV1 receptor antagonists[26] for the treatment of neuropathic pain. With the development and refinement of whole genome sequencing and analysis,[27] genomic research has provided another important source of potential neuropathic pain treatment targets. For example, evaluation of altered gene expression in dorsal root ganglia of neuropathic animals has served, in one study, to further support a putative role of the sodium channel alpha subunit *Scn11a* and the cool receptor *Trpm8*[28] and, in another study, to identify 39 genes not previously known to play a role in the induction and/or maintenance of neuropathic pain.[29]

In vivo preclinical efficacy evaluations of candidate drugs for neuropathic pain have generally involved the development and implementation of animal models that seek to emulate this group of clinical disorders. Previously developed models have involved mechanical, thermal, and inflammatory injuries to peripheral nerves (which generally produce mononeuropathies) as well as the creation of infectious, metabolic, and toxic conditions (which generally produce polyneuropathies) that result in behavioral manifestations of neuropathic pain in the experimental animal such as hyperalgesia and allodynia.[9] Table 4.2 and Figure 4.2 provide nonexhaustive lists of several animal models that have been used for the evaluation of potential neuropathic pain therapeutics. Table 4.3 describes results from experiments of various drugs tested in the chronic constriction injury and spinal nerve ligation models.[30]

EARLY HUMAN STUDIES

Phase 1 Trials

Although classically thought of as dose-ranging, drug safety evaluations in healthy volunteers,[17] first-in-human phase 1 drug trials have evolved somewhat in their diversity with respect to methodology and research objectives. Broadly speaking, these trials are meant to evaluate pharmacokinetics (PK) and adverse effect profiles in order to better guide subsequent proof-of-concept efficacy trials. However, several innovations to this concept have been introduced. For example, the need to generate PK and tolerability data, which would be clinically relevant, has led to the introduction of surrogate biomarkers of treatment effect (e.g., suppression of capsaicin-induced allodynia) so as to demonstrate target engagement within the studied dose range.[21] Also, the FDA's release of a regulatory guidance[48] on exploratory treatment INDs has led to the concept of small-scale, low-dose "phase 0" trials in which presumably subtherapeutic doses of a new molecular entity are evaluated for their intended biological effects in order to guide more expeditiously subsequent development efforts.[49]

Clearly, the methodology, outcome measures, and focus of any phase 1 trial will be dictated by the clinical setting of the target indication and, more importantly, by preclinical

Table 4-2. Examples of Preclinical Models of Neuropathic Pain

MODEL	DESCRIPTION	REF.
Rat sciatic nerve section	Unilateral section of the nerve and encapsulation of its cut end in a polyethylene tube	Wall et al.[31]
Chronic constriction injury	Unilateral application of four loosely tied chromic gut sutures at the mid-thigh level of the sciatic nerve	Bennett et al.[32]
Partial sciatic nerve ligation	Unilateral ligation of the sciatic nerve at the high-thigh level with one-third to one-half the thickness of the sciatic nerve trapped in the ligature.	Seltzer et al.[33]
Spinal nerve (L5/L6) ligation	Unilateral tight ligation of L5 and L6 spinal nerves just distal to their dorsal root ganglia	Kim and Chung[34]
Spared nerve ligation	Axotomy and ligation of tibial and common peroneal nerves (leaving the sural nerve intact)	Decosterd and Woolf[35]
Sciatic cyroneurolysis	Unilateral freezing of the proximal sciatic nerve with a −60°C cryoprobe	DeLeo et al.[36]
Sciatic inflammatory neuritis	Injection of zymosan from yeast cells around the sciatic nerve	Chacur et al.[37]
Postherpetic neuralgia model	Establishment of a chronic varicella-zoster viral infection	Fleetwood-Walker et al.[38]
Diabetic neuropathy model	Induction of diabetes following injection of streptozocin in the rat	Wuarin-Bierman et al.[39]
Cancer chemotherapy-induced neuropathy	Daily administration of vincristine to the rat for 2 weeks	Aley et al.[40]

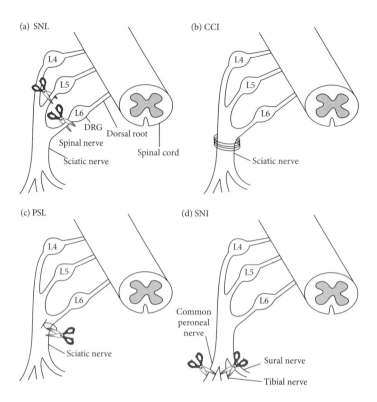

FIGURE 4.2   Animal models of neuropathetic pain. CCl, chronic constriction injury; DRG, dorsal root ganglion; PSL, partial scistic nerve ligation; SNL, spinal nerve ligation.

information obtained to date about the anticipated effects and toxicities of the investigational drug. Although the majority of early human studies conducted by pharmaceutical manufacturers remain unpublished, a few recent publications have described some approaches to phase 1 trials in the development of potential analgesic therapies. One dose-ranging, placebo- and alfentanil-controlled study evaluated the safety and PK of the ultra-short-acting opioid, remifentanil (GI87084B) in 48 healthy volunteers in an intensively monitored setting with pulse oximetry, continuous electrocardiography, end-tidal CO_2 monitoring, and radial artery monitoring.[50] In this design, subjects were treated with intravenous study drug infusions (given over 60 s) of placebo ($n = 7$), alfentanil ($n = 4$ per dose group at 8, 16, and 32 µg/kg, respectively), and remifentanil ($n = 4$–5 per dose group at 0.0625, 0.125, 0.25, 0.5, 1.0,

1.5, and 2.0 µg/kg, respectively). This study demonstrated that, for statistically significant and dose-dependent respiratory depression (measured by increases in arterial PCO_2 and decreases in arterial PO_2), remifentanil was approximately 23 times more potent than alfentanil. Relatively frequent adverse effects with remifentanil, particularly at higher doses, included a sensation of warmth and somnolence/dizziness, as well as speech and visual disturbances. Comparisons of PK with alfentanil suggested that remifentanil had a smaller volume of distribution (0.39 vs. 0.52 L/kg for alfentanil) and an extremely short elimination half-life (9.5 vs. 58 minutes for alfentanil). The $t_{1/2}$ keo (half-time for equilibration between plasma and the effect compartment) was calculated as 1.3 minutes for remifentanil.[50] An added feature of this study was the concurrent measurement of mechanical pain thresholds using an experimental

Table 4-3. Effects of Analgesic Compounds in the Chronic Constriction Injury (CCI) and Spinal Nerve Ligation (SNL) Models of Neuropathic Pain[a]

COMPOUND	ROUTE	TIME (MIN)	MODEL	STIMULATION	EFFECTS	REFERENCE
Morphine (Sigma)	i.v.	10	CCI	Randall	60% at 0.1 mg/kg 80% at 0.3 mg/kg 100% at 0.6 mg/kg	Attal et al.[41]
	s.c.	30	CCI	von Frey	0% at 1 mg/kg 50% at 3 mg/kg	Gonzalez et al.[42]
	i.t.	60	SNL	von Frey	35% at 30 µg/kg	Ossipov et al.[43]
Gabapentin (Sigma)	p.o.	60	CCI	Randall	0% at 20 mg/kg 75% at 100 mg/kg 100% at 300 mg/kg	Boyce et al.[44]
	i.p.	60	CCI	Cold	0% at 30 mg/kg 57% at 100 mg/kg 78% at 300 mg/kg	Hunter et al.[45]
	i.p.	60	SNL	von Frey	0% at 30 mg/kg 60% at 100 mg/kg 60%at 300 mg/kg	Hunter et al.[45]
Lamotrigine (Lamicital; Wellcome)	p.o.	60	CCI	Randall	5% at 3 mg/kg 40% at 10 mg/kg 100% at 20 mg/kg	Boyce et al.[44]
	s.c.	60	CCI	Cold	0% at 10 mg/kg 50% at 30 mg/kg 70% at 100 mg/kg	Hunter et al.[45]
	s.c.	60	SNL	von Frey	0% at 10 mg/kg 0% at 30 mg/kg 0% at 100 mg/kg	Hunter et al.[45]
MK-801 (Tocris)	i.p.	60	CCI	Randall	4% at 0.07 mg/kg 45% at 0.2 mg/kg 100% at 0.7 mg/kg	Boyce et al.[44]
Amitriptyline (Sigma)	i.p.	60	SNL	von Frey	0% at 1.5 mg/kg 0% at 5 mg/kg 0% at 10 mg/kg	Esser and Sawynok[46]
	i.p.	60	SNL	Thermal	50% at 1 mg/kg 75% at 3 mg/kg 100% at 10 mg/kg	Esser and Sawynok[46]
Desipramine (RBI)	s.c.	60	SNL	von Frey	0% at 1 mg/kg 0% at 30 mg/kg 0% at 100 mg/kg	Jett et al.[47]
	s.c.	60	SNL	Pinprick	0% at 1 mg/kg 25% at 30 mg/kg 75% at 100 mg/kg	Jett et al.[47]

[a]Results are expressed as percent effects. Compounds were injected by various routes of administration— intraperitoneal (i.p.), oral (p.o.), intrathecal (i.t.), intravenous (i.v.), and subcutaneous (s.c.)—and their effects were evaluated on various pain outcomes described in Support Protocols 1 (thermal), 2 (Randall and pinprick), 3 (von Frey), and 4 (cold).

Source: From Bennett GJ, Chung JM, Honore M, Seltzer Z. Models of neuropathic pain in the rat. Curr Protoc Neurosci 2003. Chapter 9: Unit 9.14. This material is reproduced with permission of Current Protocols and John Wiley & Sons, Inc.

pressure-transduced, spring-loaded rod applied to each subject's tibia and sternum. According to measured pain thresholds, both remifentanil and alfentanil demonstrated statistically significant dose-dependent analgesia, and the estimated potency of remifentanil was approximately 22 times that of alfentanil. These careful preliminary drug safety evaluations contributed to the ultimate development of remifentanil that is now used widely as an intraoperative analgesic agent.[51]

Another report demonstrated the safety of a novel AMPA (α-amino-3-hydroxy-5-methyl-4-isoxazole-proprionic acid)/kainate antagonist, LY293558, in 25 healthy human volunteers.[52] A preliminary ascending dose study ranging from 0.01 to possibly as high as 2.0 mg/kg indicated cumulative dose-dependent side effects including headache, sedation, and visual symptoms (blurry vision and transient peripheral "white clouds") that generally occurred between 15 and 60 minutes after the drug infusion. Intensive visual evaluations (with visual evoked potentials and electroretinography) ruled out any long-term sequelae of these brief visual symptoms, and the median maximal tolerated dose based on tolerability of these adverse effects was estimated at 1.3 mg/kg.[52] Similar to the phase 1 study of remifentanil discussed above, this study expanded beyond routine safety evaluations to also measure the effects of LY293558 on brief nociceptive stimuli (electrical and thermal detection and pain thresholds) in normal skin and on spontaneous pain, brush allodynia, and pinprick hyperalgesia in skin sensitized by intradermal capsaicin injection. Although LY293558 had no effect on brief nociception in normal skin, it did reduce capsaicin-induced spontaneous pain as well as brush allodynia. These early careful investigations were instrumental in facilitating subsequent clinical evaluation of LY293558 for postoperative[53] and acute migraine[54] pain.

A more recently published phase 1 trial described the safety and PK of CNS 5161, a novel N-methyl-D-aspartate (NMDA) receptor antagonist.[55] In this placebo-controlled, double-blind, randomized trial, CNS 5161 was administered as a single intravenous infusion to 24 of 32 healthy human volunteers (doses ranged from 30 to 2000 μg). Relatively frequent dose-related side effects that were self-limited and mild in severity included paresthesias, lightheadedness, drowsiness, and headache. A transient dose-dependent rise in both diastolic and systolic blood pressure was observed, but all subjects returned to their normal hemodynamics within 24 hours of drug infusion. Reported PK parameters included a volume of distribution of 296 L, a clearance of 106 L/h, and an elimination half-life of 2.95 h. The reasonable safety profile generated by this phase 1 trial led to a subsequent clinical trial of CNS 5161 in patients with neuropathic pain; however, that trial was abandoned after two patients entering the 750 μg dose group developed sustained systolic hypertension.[56]

Preclinical Human Pain Models

Although some examples suggest that drug treatment responses in certain types of experimental pain do not always predict efficacy in clinical pain conditions,[57] preclinical human pain models provide an early and efficient opportunity to corroborate—in humans—prior laboratory animal observations of antinociceptive activity (e.g., see ref. 52). Also, as mentioned above, evaluating the effects of novel agents on measures of human experimental pain stimuli may provide a clinically relevant context for the early evaluation of PK and drug safety. Over the past 20 years or so, investigators have developed several preclinical human pain models that are safe, that do not cause long-term tissue injury, and that activate different nociceptive and antinociceptive pathways.[58–60] Tables 4.4A and 4.4B include nonexhaustive lists of preclinical human pain models together with examples of the drug treatment response for each. One important broad distinction among these models should be made between brief noxious stimuli transmitted via normal nociceptive pathways and the experimental induction of brief peripheral and/or central sensitization leading to hyperalgesia and/or allodynia and/or spontaneous pain.[59] More detailed consideration of each experimental model may allow for matching between its putative operant pain mechanism (e.g., inflammation, glutamate

Table 4-4A. Experimental Pain Models Involving Brief Nociceptive Pain

STIMULUS/MODEL	DESCRIPTION	EXAMPLES
Direct heat to skin	Application of a contact thermode, usually to the subject's volar forearm, over an increasing range of temperatures to measure heat detection, pain detection, pain tolerance thresholds, and pain intensity/unpleasantness	Intravenous morphine >0.06 mg/kg decreases sensory and affective visual analog scores[61] Oral gabapentin 1200 mg: no effect[62]
Laser heat to skin	Brief application of argon- or CO_2-laser stimulation of subject's skin to measure pain and laser-evoked potentials	High-dose alfentanil reduces argon laser-induced pain[63]
Cold to skin (e.g., cold pressor test)	Immersion of subject's hand in a temperature-controlled water bath at approximately 1°C to measure pain, time to pain detection, and time to pain tolerance	Oral morphine 0.5 mg/kg decreases cold pain, increases detection and tolerance thresholds[64]
Electrical skin stimulation	Transcutaneous electrical stimulation of the skin below the patella with a silver electrode in 1 mA increasing increments at a frequency of 2 Hz	Morphine, but not THC, increased the electrical pain detection threshold[65]
Interdigital web pinching	A pressure stimulus of 10 N applied to the interdigital web space between the second and third fingers with a 0.28 cm^2 circular probe	Static pressure pain intensity reduced by oral ibuprofen
Intramuscular hypertonic saline	0.5 mL of hypertonic saline (5%) infused through a 27 gauge, 20 mm needle into the middle portion of the right anterior tibial muscle over 20 s	Pain induced by intramuscular hypertonic saline reduced by both alfentanil and morphine[66]
Electrical tooth pulp stimulation	Application of a silver electrode to the dried tooth surface to deliver 1 s trains of electrical stimuli in 1 μA incremental steps	Pain induced by electrical tooth pulp stimulation reduced by intravenous fentanyl but not diazepam[67]
Ischemic pain	Subjects repeatedly and isotonically lift a 3 kg weight following application of a tourniquet to the upper arm that is inflated to a pressure of 100 mmHg above the subject's systolic blood pressure	Ischemic pain reduced by intravenous adenosine, ketamine, and morphine[68]
Esophageal distention	A 14 French, 45 mm long latex balloon inserted with its center 10 cm above the lower esophageal sphincter is inflated with air at a rate of 170 mL/s	Pain induced by esophageal distention reduced by oral imipramine[69]
Sural nerve stimulation (nociceptive reflex)	Constant current rectangular pulse electrical stimulation of the sural nerve along its retromalleolar path as five pulses delivered at 200 Hz or—for temporal summation—that stimulus burst repeated five times at a frequency of 3 Hz	Pain tolerance threshold to single sural nerve stimulation reduced in poor metabolizers of tramadol[70]
Nasal mucosa stimulation with CO_2	Carbon dioxide gas (at 55%–66%) is administered in one nostril over a stimulus duration of 250 ms	Pain induced by intranasal CO_2 reduced by oral imipramine but not tramadol[71]

Table 4-4B. Experimental Pain Models Involving Peripheral and/or Central Sensitization

STIMULUS/MODEL	DESCRIPTION	EXAMPLES
Experimental burn injury	6 min skin application of a 25 x 50 mm thermode at 47°C to the medial surface of the calf resulting in a first-degree burn injury with erythema lasting for less than 1 day with no visible edema or blister	Neither ketamine nor morphine reduced the heat pain detection threshold in the area of the burn; ketamine, but not morphine, reduced the surrounding area of pinprick hyperalgesia and brush allodynia and also reduced temporal summation pain[72]
Continuous electrical skin stimulation	A stainless steel needle is inserted intracutaneously in the central volar forearm and continuous electrical stimuli ranging from 30 to 70 mA are delivered at a frequency of 5 Hz	Intravenous ketamine and alfentanil, but not lidocaine, reduced electrically evoked pain as well as surrounding pinprick hyperalgesia and tactile allodynia[73]
Ultraviolet (UVB) radiation	The lateral thigh is exposed to a 5 cm diameter circular area of calibrated source of UVB light radiation to produce a mild sunburn injury	Intravenous remifentanil, but not oral gabapentin, reduced UVB-induced secondary hyperalgesia[57]
Freeze lesion	A 290 g, 15 mm diameter copper cylinder is cooled to –28°C and applied to the anterior thigh for 10 s to induce a small area of skin inflammation	Intravenous remifentanil reduced hyperalgesia to blunt stimuli in the area of the freeze lesion[74]
Topical capsaicin	Capsaicin, dissolved in ethanol and mixed with a moisturizing cream to a final concentration of 1%, is applied to the skin on the dorsolateral aspect of the foot over a 2.5 cm diameter area for 1 h	Topical capsaicin-induced hyperalgesia suppressed by intravenous ketamine[75]
Heat-capsaicin sensitization	Forearm skin is sensitized by heating the skin with a thermode to 45°C for 5 min and then covering the area with 0.075% capsaicin cream	Heat-capsaicin sensitization suppressed by oral gabapentin[62]
Intradermal capsaicin	250 µg capsaicin in a 10 mg/mL solution is injected intradermally into the volar forearm	Capsaicin-induced pain and brush allodynia reduced by intravenous infusion of the AMPA/kainiate antagonist, LY293558[52]
Esophageal hydrochloric acid infusion	Hydrochloric acid (0.15 mol/L) is infused with an infusion pump into the lower esophagus, 3 cm above the lower esophageal sphincter, at 8 mL/min for 30 min	Intravenous ketamine prevented acid-induced esophageal hypersensitivity[76]

Note: Each model described above may vary across different studies with respect to specific methodology; each description refers to only one example of that particular model.

receptor activation, TRPV1 receptor activation, or visceral distention) and the target condition of interest (e.g., osteoarthritis, diabetic neuropathy, postherpetic neuralgia, or irritable bowel syndrome). Following application of the relevant noxious stimulus, study measures may include the effect of the study intervention on pain intensity, pain unpleasantness, peristimulus skin surface area of allodynia or hyperalgesia, or surface electroencephalographic evoked potentials.

Outcome Measures and Surrogate Biomarkers in Phase 1 Trials

Often, in contrast with phase 1 trials, phase 2 to 4 clinical trials generally need to be based upon the most clinically relevant outcomes, such as overall pain experience, physical and emotional function, and treatment tolerability.[77,78] However, it should be emphasized that more focused attention on pharmacodynamics in phase 1 trials may be facilitated by a variety of semiobjective evaluative approaches including quantitative sensory testing (QST),[58] laser-evoked potentials,[79] and functional brain imaging[80] that may serve to confirm drug-specific target engagement and also elucidate pain mechanisms that may best respond to the study treatment (e.g., antihyperalgesia, antiallodynia). For example, QST evidence that the AMPA/kainate antagonist, LY293558, has no effect on thermal nociception in normal skin (unlike opioids)—but significantly reduces pain and areas of allodynia following intradermal capsaicin injection—serves to describe more precisely the antinociceptive effects and potential clinical applications of this drug.[52] As another example, the measurement of laser-evoked potentials, when studied in normal versus ultraviolet B-irradiated skin, may serve to distinguish between diverse pharmacological mechanisms such as those of opioids versus nonsteroidal anti-inflammatory drugs.[79] Finally, the use of functional magnetic resonance imaging (fMRI) may similarly provide another surrogate marker of drug action. In a previous study, gabapentin was shown to significantly reduce mechanical punctate stimulation-induced activation of the brainstem and insular cortex and also to reduce deactivation in the occipital, temporal, and frontal cortices. However, these drug effects were only observed during capsaicin-induced sensitization and not in normal skin.[81] Despite these robust findings using fMRI evaluation, it is interesting to note that the trends for pain intensity reduction with gabapentin treatment of capsaicin-induced sensitization actually failed to reach statistical significance, further supporting the role of such surrogate markers in smaller early phase studies.

CLINICAL PROOF-OF-CONCEPT STUDIES

Phase 2 or proof-of-concept clinical trials generally involve study sizes of 100–200 patients with the target condition of interest.[17] This is the first exploratory opportunity to evaluate the clinical efficacy of the study drug for its intended use and, most importantly, to predict the ultimate success of this drug in large-scale pivotal phase 3 licensing trials. Given that over 60% of new drugs fail in phase 2, this is clearly a stage of development associated with intense focus and attention.[82] Although beyond the scope of this chapter, it must be emphasized that statistical considerations for phase 2 trials are absolutely critical given that the outcomes of these trials may lead to two misguided decisions: (1) to abandon a drug that might have ultimately succeeded or (2) to proceed to a series of very costly phase 3 trials that ultimately fail to achieve regulatory approval due to efficacy or safety limitations.[83] Challenges in designing phase 2 trials include (1) selecting the appropriate target population (e.g., the one most likely to succeed, such as diabetic neuropathy, versus a larger target market such as low back pain), (2) determining the drug dosage range (e.g., the lowest effective dose versus the maximal tolerated dose), (3) inclusion of placebo and/or active comparators, and (4) several methodological issues including primary outcome and analysis, sample size, and criteria for a meaningful effect (e.g., any statistically significant pain reduction versus at least 30% pain reduction).

Given the importance of a placebo comparator in phase 3 trials of novel analgesic drugs, placebo considerations are also central to the design of phase 2 trials. In the setting of neuropathic pain treatment, responses to placebo are known to vary widely,[84,85] and this clearly has an important impact on trial outcomes. For example, in one painful diabetic neuropathy trial, 300 mg of pregabalin demonstrated statistical superiority over placebo,[86] whereas the same dose in another trial failed to do so,[87] partially due to a more pronounced placebo response in the latter investigation. One strategy to improve the apparent precision of such trials involves the exclusion of placebo responders (e.g., >30% pain reduction during a placebo run-in period),[88] although this may overestimate drug efficacy compared to subsequent phase 3 trials that may not employ this strategy. On the other hand, the use of an active placebo (i.e., a drug with no analgesic effects that mimics the side effects of the study drug) to improve the quality of blinding[89–92] may provide a more realistic estimation of drug efficacy and guide the earlier abandonment of ultimately unsuccessful candidates. In addition to placebo comparators, the inclusion of a positive control or "*active comparator*" (i.e., a drug with known efficacy for the target condition) may prove quite valuable in early drug development. Whereas a placebo comparator provides a measure of assay sensitivity (i.e., trial methods can detect study drug efficacy), an active comparator may confirm assay sensitivity (e.g., in the event of no significant difference between placebo and the study drug) and also demonstrate "upside" assay sensitivity (i.e., trial methods can detect additional efficacy above the positive control).[93] In addition to validating the trial methodology used, inclusion of an active comparator adds clinical relevance to early phase 2 trial results.

Although several PK-pharmacodynamic questions may have been answered in earlier phase 1 trials, it may also be useful and important to incorporate PK measures in phase 2 trials given a variety of issues associated with the target condition as opposed to healthy volunteers (e.g., genetic variations in drug metabolism, use of concomitant medications, hepatic/renal dysfunction). The potential value of concurrent PK evaluations can be illustrated by a neuropathic pain trial that compared imipramine to paroxetine.[94] Results from this study suggested that both drugs are superior to placebo for pain and other outcomes and, further,

that imipramine was significantly more efficacious than paroxetine. However, in this trial, paroxetine was administered to all patients at a fixed dose of 40 mg/day, whereas imipramine was individually titrated in order to reach plasma drug levels of 400 to 600 nmol/L. Thus, titrating imipramine to optimal plasma levels could, in part, explain the superior efficacy observed with this drug.[94] Thus, this example further illustrates the importance of careful attention to PK early in drug development.

Several innovative alternatives to a classical double-blind, parallel, placebo-controlled trial may serve to more efficiently rule in or rule out a potential drug candidate in phase 2. As we continue to learn more about the heterogeneity of disease mechanisms in neuropathic pain,[95] it is important to recognize that promising new therapies may be of value only to a subset of individuals with the target condition. This is illustrated by the example of a diabetic neuropathy trial that showed that although only 30% of patients responded to treatment with transdermal clonidine in the first phase of that trial (i.e., a negative trial if average responses from all patients are considered), treatment efficacy in this subset was subsequently confirmed by second-phase, repeated drug-placebo crossover.[96] Further recognition of the need to identify the treatment response in subsets of target populations has led to the evolution of various *enriched enrollment* designs such as the enriched enrollment, randomized withdrawal design.[97–100] Other methodological innovations in development include two-stage designs whereby an interim analysis of the first-stage results guide the decision either to stop for futility or to progress to later-phase trials.[101] Also, sequential *response-adaptive* designs whereby statistical power is enhanced by skewing participant allocation to the better treatment group have been proposed for use in neuropathic pain trials.[102,103]

CONCLUSION

Evidence of current treatment patterns suggests that pharmacotherapy is an important and widely used component of multimodal, multidisciplinary neuropathic pain management. Despite this, treatment success with current drugs for neuropathic pain is often hindered by incomplete efficacy and treatment-limiting toxicities emphasizing the need for improved therapies. The past several decades have seen an explosion of knowledge about the biological mechanisms underlying neuropathic pain that has led to the expanded preclinical development of novel therapeutic candidates. In contrast to the large number of promising agents identified in preclinical investigations, however, surprisingly few new drugs have become available to humans suffering from neuropathic pain. Recent recognition of these apparent disappointments has inspired a reappraisal of current preclinical pain models. Such reflections have emphasized the need for model refinements that incorporate the diverse biopsychosocial elements of human pain such as sex, genotype, and social communication[104] and have demonstrated that preclinical drug evaluations must be conducted with more rigor, methodological uniformity, and transparent reporting[105] with the expectation of future improvements in predictive value. As in other health-related therapeutic areas, drug discovery for neuropathic pain requires an intensely focused, interactive, multidisciplinary and translational approach in order to effectively foster the development of new promising therapies for those who continue to suffer in pain.

REFERENCES

1. Bouhassira D, Lantéri-Minet M, Attal N, Laurent B, Touboul C. Prevalence of chronic pain with neuropathic characteristics in the general population. *Pain*. 2008;136:380–387.
2. Torrance N, Smith BH, Bennett MI, Lee AJ. The epidemiology of chronic pain of predominantly neuropathic origin. Results from a general population survey. *J Pain*. 2006;7:281–289.
3. Turk DC. Clinical effectiveness and cost-effectiveness of treatments for patients with chronic pain. *Clin J Pain*. 2002;18:355–365.
4. Gilron I, Watson CP, Cahill CM, Moulin DE. Neuropathic pain: a practical guide for the clinician. *CMAJ*. 2006;175(3):265–275.
5. Woodforde JM, Dwyer B, McEwen BW, De Wilde FW, Bleasel K, Connelley TJ, Ho CY. Treatment of post-herpetic neuralgia. *Med J Aust*. 1965;2(21):869–872.
6. Graham JG, Zilkha KJ. Treatment of trigeminal neuralgia with carbamazepine: a follow-up study. *Br Med J*. 1966;1(5481):210–211.
7. Rowbotham MC, Reisner-Keller LA, Fields HL. Both intravenous lidocaine and morphine reduce the pain of postherpetic neuralgia. *Neurology*. 1991;41(7):1024–1028.
8. Finnerup NB, Otto M, McQuay HJ, Jensen TS, Sindrup SH. Algorithm for neuropathic pain treatment: an evidence based proposal. *Pain*. 2005;118(3):289–305.
9. Wang LX, Wang ZJ. Animal and cellular models of chronic pain. *Adv Drug Deliv Rev*. 2003;55(8):949–965.
10. Campbell JN, Meyer RA. Mechanisms of neuropathic pain. Neuron. 2006;52(1):77–92.
11. Dray A. Neuropathic pain: emerging treatments. *Br J Anaesth*. 2008;101(1):48–58.
12. Gilron I, Coderre TJ. Emerging drugs in neuropathic pain. *Expert Opin Emerg Drugs*. 2007;12(1):113–126.
13. Dworkin RH, Turk DC, Peirce-Sandner S, Baron R, Bellamy N, Burke LB, Chappell A, Chartier K, Cleeland CS, Costello A, Cowan P, Dimitrova R, Ellenberg S, Farrar JT, French JA, Gilron I, Hertz S, Jadad AR, Jay GW, Kalliomäki J, Katz NP, Kerns RD, Manning DC, McDermott MP, McGrath PJ, Narayana A, Porter L, Quessy S, Rappaport BA, Rauschkolb C, Reeve BB, Rhodes T, Sampaio C, Simpson DM, Stauffer JW, Stucki G, Tobias J, White RE, Witter J. Research design considerations for confirmatory chronic pain clinical trials: IMMPACT recommendations. *Pain*. 2010;149(2):177–193.
14. FDA. 2004: http://www.fda.gov/ScienceResearch/SpecialTopics/CriticalPathInitiative/default.htm.
15. Woodcock J, Woosley R. The FDA critical path initiative and its influence on new drug development. *Annu Rev Med*. 2008;59:1–12.
16. Holbein ME. Understanding FDA regulatory requirements for investigational new drug applications for sponsor-investigators. *J Invest Med*. 2009;57(6):688–694.
17. Berkowitz BA. Development and regulation of drugs. In: Katzung BG, ed. *Basic and Clinical Pharmacology*. 11th ed. New York: McGraw-Hill; 2009:67–75.
18. Negus SS, Vanderah TW, Brandt MR, Bilsky EJ, Becerra L, Borsook D. Preclinical assessment of candidate analgesic drugs: recent advances and future challenges. *J Pharmacol Exp Ther*. 2006;319(2):507–514.
19. Lord PG, Nie A, McMillian M. Application of genomics in preclinical drug safety evaluation. *Basic Clin Pharmacol Toxicol*. 2006;98(6):537–546.
20. Redfern WS, Wakefield ID, Prior H, Pollard CE, Hammond TG, Valentin JP. Safety

pharmacology—a progressive approach. *Fundam Clin Pharmacol*. 2002;16(3):161–173.

21. Chizh BA, Sang CN. Use of sensory methods for detecting target engagement in clinical trials of new analgesics. *Neurotherapeutics*. 2009;6(4):749–754.

22. Miller R, Ewy W, Corrigan BW, Ouellet D, Hermann D, Kowalski KG, Lockwood P, Koup JR, Donevan S, El-Kattan A, Li CS, Werth JL, Feltner DE, Lalonde RL. How modeling and simulation have enhanced decision making in new drug development. *J Pharmacokinet Pharmacodyn*. 2005;32(2):185–197.

23. Griessinger N, Sittl R, Likar R. Transdermal buprenorphine in clinical practice—a post-marketing surveillance study in 13,179 patients. *Curr Med Res Opin*. 2005;21(8):1147–1156.

24. Olejniczak K, Gunzel P, Bass R. Preclinical testing strategies. *Drug Inf J*. 2001;35:321–336.

25. Romagnoli R, Baraldi PG, Cruz-Lopez O, Lopez-Cara C, Preti D, Borea PA, Gessi S. The P2X7 receptor as a therapeutic target. *Expert Opin Ther Targets*. 2008;12(5):647–661

26. Culshaw AJ, Bevan S, Christiansen M, Copp P, Davis A, Davis C, Dyson A, Dziadulewicz EK, Edwards L, Eggelte H, Fox A, Gentry C, Groarke A, Hallett A, Hart TW, Hughes GA, Knights S, Kotsonis P, Lee W, Lyothier I, McBryde A, McIntyre P, Paloumbis G, Panesar M, Patel S, Seiler MP, Yaqoob M, Zimmermann K. Identification and biological characterization of 6-aryl-7-isopropylquinazolinones as novel TRPV1 antagonists that are effective in models of chronic pain. *J Med Chem*. 2006;49(2):471–474.

27. Walker SJ, Worst TJ, Freeman WM, Vrana KE. Functional genomic analysis in pain research using hybridization arrays. *Methods Mol Med*. 2004;99:239–253.

28. Persson AK, Gebauer M, Jordan S, Metz-Weidmann C, Schulte AM, Schneider HC, Ding-Pfennigdorff D, Thun J, Xu XJ, Wiesenfeld-Hallin Z, Darvasi A, Fried K, Devor M. Correlational analysis for identifying genes whose regulation contributes to chronic neuropathic pain. *Mol Pain*. 2009;5:7.

29. Maratou K, Wallace VC, Hasnie FS, Okuse K, Hosseini R, Jina N, Blackbeard J, Pheby T, Orengo C, Dickenson AH, McMahon SB, Rice AS. Comparison of dorsal root ganglion gene expression in rat models of traumatic and HIV-associated neuropathic pain. *Eur J Pain*. 2009;13(4):387–398.

30. Bennett GJ, Chung JM, Honore M, Seltzer Z. Models of neuropathic pain in the rat. *Curr Protoc Neurosci*. 2003;chap 9:unit 9.14.

31. Wall PD, Devor M, Inbal R, Scadding JW, Schonfeld D, Seltzer Z, Tomkiewicz MM. Autotomy following peripheral nerve lesions: experimental anaesthesia dolorosa. *Pain*. 1979;7(2):103–111.

32. Bennett GJ, Xie YK. A peripheral mononeuropathy in rat that produces disorders of pain sensation like those seen in man. *Pain*. 1988;33(1):87–107.

33. Seltzer Z, Dubner R, Shir Y. A novel behavioral model of neuropathic pain disorders produced in rats by partial sciatic nerve injury. *Pain*. 1990;43(2):205–218.

34. Kim SH, Chung JM. An experimental model for peripheral neuropathy produced by segmental spinal nerve ligation in the rat. *Pain*. 1992;50(3):355–363.

35. Decosterd I, Woolf CJ. Spared nerve injury: an animal model of persistent peripheral neuropathic pain. *Pain*. 2000;87(2):149–158.

36. DeLeo JA, Coombs DW, Willenbring S, Colburn RW, Fromm C, Wagner R, Twitchell BB. Characterization of a neuropathic pain model: sciatic cryoneurolysis in the rat. *Pain*. 1994;56(1):9–16.

37. Chacur M, Milligan ED, Gazda LS, Armstrong C, Wang H, Tracey KJ, Maier SF, Watkins LR. A new model of sciatic inflammatory neuritis (SIN): induction of unilateral and bilateral mechanical allodynia following acute unilateral peri-sciatic immune activation in rats. *Pain*. 2001;94(3):231–244.

38. Fleetwood-Walker SM, Quinn JP, Wallace C, Blackburn-Munro G, Kelly BG, Fiskerstrand CE, Nash AA, Dalziel RG. Behavioural changes in the rat following infection with varicella-zoster virus. *J Gen Virol*. 1999;80(pt 9): 2433–2436.

39. Wuarin-Bierman L, Zahnd GR, Kaufmann F, Burcklen L, Adler J. Hyperalgesia in spontaneous and experimental animal models of diabetic neuropathy. *Diabetologia*. 1987;30(8):653–658.

40. Aley KO, Reichling DB, Levine JD. Vincristine hyperalgesia in the rat: a model of painful vincristine neuropathy in humans. *Neuroscience*. 1996;73(1):259–265.

41. Attal N, Chen YL, Kayser V, Guilbaud G. Behavioural evidence that systemic morphine may modulate a phasic pain-related behaviour in a rat model of mononeuropathy. *Pain*. 1991;47:65–70.

42. Gonzalez MI, Field MJ, Hughes J, Singh L. Evaluation of selective NK1 receptor antagonist CI-1021 in animal models of inflammatory and neuropathic pain. *J Pharmacol Exp Ther*. 2000;294:444–450.

43. Ossipov MH, Lopez Y, Nichols ML, Bian D, Porreca F. The loss of antinociceptive efficacy of spinal morphine in rats with nerve ligation is prevented by reducing spinal afferent drive. *Neurosci Lett*. 1995;199:87–90.

44. Boyce S, Wyatt A, Webb JK, O'Donnell R, Mason G, Rigby M, Sirinathsinghji D, Hill RG, Rupniak NMJ. Selective NMDA NR2B antagonists induce antinociception without motor dysfunction: correlation with restricted localization of NR2B subunit in dorsal horn. *Neuropharmacology*. 1999;38:611–623.

45. Hunter JC, Gogas KR, Hedley LR, Jacobson LO, Kassotakis L, Thompson J, Fontana DJ. The effects of novel anti-epileptic drugs in rat experimental models of acute and chronic pain. *Eur J Pharmacol*. 1997;324:153–160.

46. Esser MJ, Sawynok J. Acute amitriptyline in a rat model of neuropathic pain: differential symptom and route effects. *Pain*. 1999;80: 643–653.

47. Jett MF, McGuirk J, Waligora D, Hunter JC. The effects of mexiletine, desipramine and fluox-etine in rat models involving centralsensitiza-tion. *Pain*. 1997;69:161–169.

48. FDA 2006: http://www.fda.gov/downloads/Drugs/GuidanceComplianceRegulatoryInfor-mation/Guidances/UCM078933.pdf.

49. Kummar S, Rubinstein L, Kinders R, Parchment RE, Gutierrez ME, Murgo AJ, Ji J, Mroczkowski B, Pickeral OK, Simpson M, Hollingshead M, Yang SX, Helman L, Wiltrout R, Collins J, Tomaszewski JE, Doroshow JH. Phase 0 clinical trials: conceptions and misconceptions. *Cancer J*. 2008;14(3):133–137.

50. Glass PS, Hardman D, Kamiyama Y, Quill TJ, Marton G, Donn KH, Grosse CM, Hermann D. Preliminary pharmacokinetics and phar-macodynamics of an ultra-short-acting opi-oid: remifentanil (GI87084B). *Anesth Analg*. 1993;77(5):1031–1040.

51. Komatsu R, Turan AM, Orhan-Sungur M, McGuire J, Radke OC, Apfel CC. Remifentanil for general anaesthesia: a systematic review. *Anaesthesia*. 2007;62(12):1266–1280.

52. Sang CN, Hostetter MP, Gracely RH, Chappell AS, Schoepp DD, Lee G, Whitcup S, Caruso R, Max MB. AMPA/kainate antagonist LY293558 reduces capsaicin-evoked hyperalgesia but not pain in normal skin in humans. *Anesthesiology*. 1998;89(5):1060–1067.

53. Gilron I, Max MB, Lee G, Booher SL, Sang CN, Chappell AS, Dionne RA. Effects of the 2-amino-3-hydroxy-5-methyl-4-isoxazole-proprionic acid/kainate antagonist LY293558 on spontaneous and evoked postoperative pain. *Clin Pharmacol Ther*. 2000;68(3):320–327.

54. Sang CN, Ramadan NM, Wallihan RG, Chappell AS, Freitag FG, Smith TR, Silberstein SD, John-son KW, Phebus LA, Bleakman D, Ornstein PL, Arnold B, Tepper SJ, Vandenhende F. LY293558, a novel AMPA/GluR5 antagonist, is efficacious and well-tolerated in acute migraine. *Cephalal-gia*. 2004;24(7):596–602.

55. Walters MR, Bradford AP, Fischer J, Lees KR. Early clinical experience with the novel NMDA receptor antagonist CNS 5161. *Br J Clin Pharma-col*. 2002;53(3):305–311.

56. Forst T, Smith T, Schütte K, Marcus P, Pfützner A, CNS 5161 Study Group. Dose escalating safety study of CNS 5161 HCl, a new neuronal glutamate receptor antagonist (NMDA) for the treatment of neuropathic pain. *Br J Clin Pharma-col*. 2007;64(1):75–82.

57. Gustorff B, Hoechtl K, Sycha T, Felouzis E, Lehr S, Kress HG. The effects of remifenta-nil and gabapentin on hyperalgesia in a new extended inflammatory skin pain model in healthy volunteers. *Anesth Analg*. 2004;98(2): 401–407.

58. Arendt-Nielsen L, Yarnitsky D. Experimental and clinical applications of quantitative sensory testing applied to skin, muscles and viscera. *J Pain*. 2009;10(6):556–572.

59. Staahl C, Olesen AE, Andresen T, Arendt-Nielsen L, Drewes AM. Assessing analgesic actions of opioids by experimental pain models in healthy volunteers—an updated review. *Br J Clin Phar-macol*. 2009;68(2):149–168.

60. Staahl C, Olesen AE, Andresen T, Arendt-Nielsen L, Drewes AM. Assessing efficacy of non-opioid analgesics in experimental pain models in healthy volunteers: an updated review. *Br J Clin Pharmacol*. 2009;68(3):322–341.

61. Price DD, Von der Gruen A, Miller J, Rafii A, Price C. A psychophysical analysis of morphine analgesia. *Pain*. 1985;22(3):261–269.

62. Dirks J, Petersen KL, Rowbotham MC, Dahl JB. Gabapentin suppresses cutaneous hyperalgesia following heat-capsaicin sensitization. *Anesthe-siology*. 2002;97(1):102–107.

63. Petersen-Felix S, Arendt-Nielsen L, Bak P, Fischer M, Zbinden AM. Psychophysical and electrophysiological responses to experimen-tal pain may be influenced by sedation: com-parison of the effects of a hypnotic (propofol) and an analgesic (alfentanil). *Br J Anaesth*. 1996;77(2):165–171.

64. Pud D, Yarnitsky D, Sprecher E, Rogowski Z, Adler R, Eisenberg E. Can personality traits

and gender predict the response to morphine? An experimental cold pain study. *Eur J Pain*. 2006;10(2):103–112.

65. Naef M, Curatolo M, Petersen-Felix S, Arendt-Nielsen L, Zbinden A, Brenneisen R. The analgesic effect of oral delta-9-tetrahydrocannabinol (THC), morphine, and a THC-morphine combination in healthy subjects under experimental pain conditions. *Pain*. 2003;105(1–2):79–88.

66. Schulte H, Segerdahl M, Graven-Nielsen T, Grass S. Reduction of human experimental muscle pain by alfentanil and morphine. *Eur J Pain*. 2006;10(8):733–741.

67. Gracely RH, Dubner R, McGrath PA. Fentanyl reduces the intensity of painful tooth pulp sensations: controlling for detection of active drugs. *Anesth Analg*. 1982;61(9):751–755.

68. Segerdahl M, Ekblom A, Sollevi A. The influence of adenosine, ketamine, and morphine on experimentally induced ischemic pain in healthy volunteers. *Anesth Analg*. 1994;79(4):787–791.

69. Peghini PL, Katz PO, Castell DO. Imipramine decreases oesophageal pain perception in human male volunteers. *Gut*. 1998;42(6):807–813.

70. Enggaard TP, Poulsen L, Arendt-Nielsen L, Brøsen K, Ossig J, Sindrup SH. The analgesic effect of tramadol after intravenous injection in healthy volunteers in relation to CYP2D6. *Anesth Analg*. 2006;102(1):146–150.

71. Hummel T, Hummel C, Friedel I, Pauli E, Kobal G. A comparison of the antinociceptive effects of imipramine, tramadol and anpirtoline. *Br J Clin Pharmacol*. 1994;37(4):325–333.

72. Warncke T, Stubhaug A, Jørum E. Ketamine, an NMDA receptor antagonist, suppresses spatial and temporal properties of burn-induced secondary hyperalgesia in man: a double-blind, cross-over comparison with morphine and placebo. *Pain*. 1997;72(1–2):99–106.

73. Koppert W, Dern SK, Sittl R, Albrecht S, Schüttler J, Schmelz M. A new model of electrically evoked pain and hyperalgesia in human skin: the effects of intravenous alfentanil, S(+)-ketamine, and lidocaine. *Anesthesiology*. 2001;95(2):395–402.

74. Lötsch J, Angst MS. The mu-opioid agonist remifentanil attenuates hyperalgesia evoked by blunt and punctuated stimuli with different potency: a pharmacological evaluation of the freeze lesion in humans. *Pain*. 2003;102(1–2):151–161.

75. Andersen OK, Felsby S, Nicolaisen L, Bjerring P, Jensen TS, Arendt-Nielsen L. The effect of Ketamine on stimulation of primary and secondary hyperalgesic areas induced by capsaicin—a double-blind, placebo-controlled, human experimental study. *Pain*. 1996;66(1):51–62.

76. Willert RP, Woolf CJ, Hobson AR, Delaney C, Thompson DG, Aziz Q. The development and maintenance of human visceral pain hypersensitivity is dependent on the *N*-methyl-D-aspartate receptor. *Gastroenterology*. 2004;126(3):683–692.

77. Turk DC, Dworkin RH, Allen RR, Bellamy N, Brandenburg N, Carr DB, Cleeland C, Dionne R, Farrar JT, Galer BS, Hewitt DJ, Jadad AR, Katz NP, Kramer LD, Manning DC, McCormick CG, McDermott MP, McGrath P, Quessy S, Rappaport BA, Robinson JP, Royal MA, Simon L, Stauffer JW, Stein W, Tollett J, Witter J. Core outcome domains for chronic pain clinical trials: IMMPACT recommendations. *Pain*. 2003;106(3):337–345.

78. Dworkin RH, Turk DC, Farrar JT, Haythornthwaite JA, Jensen MP, Katz NP, Kerns RD, Stucki G, Allen RR, Bellamy N, Carr DB, Chandler J, Cowan P, Dionne R, Galer BS, Hertz S, Jadad AR, Kramer LD, Manning DC, Martin S, McCormick CG, McDermott MP, McGrath P, Quessy S, Rappaport BA, Robbins W, Robinson JP, Rothman M, Royal MA, Simon L, Stauffer JW, Stein W, Tollett J, Wernicke J, Witter J, IMMPACT. Core outcome measures for chronic pain clinical trials: IMMPACT recommendations. *Pain*. 2005;113(1–2):9–19.

79. Chizh BA, Priestley T, Rowbotham M, Schaffler K. Predicting therapeutic efficacy—experimental pain in human subjects. *Brain Res Rev*. 2009;60(1):243–254.

80. Wise RG, Tracey I. The role of fMRI in drug discovery. *J Magn Reson Imaging*. 2006;23:862–876.

81. Iannetti GD, Zambreanu L, Wise RG, Buchanan TJ, Huggins JP, Smart TS, Vennart W, Tracey I. Pharmacological modulation of pain-related brain activity during normal and central sensitization states in humans. *Proc Natl Acad Sci USA*. 2005;102(50):18195–18200.

82. Kola I, Landis J. Can the pharmaceutical industry reduce attrition rates? *Nat Rev Drug Discov*. 2004;3(8):711–715.

83. Chen C, Beckman RA. Optimal cost-effective designs of Phase II proof of concept trials and associated go-no go decisions. *J Biopharm Stat*. 2009;19(3):424–436.

84. Quessy SN, Rowbotham MC. Placebo response in neuropathic pain trials. *Pain*. 2008;138(3):479–483.

85. Wasan AD, Kaptchuk TJ, Davar G, Jamison RN. The association between psychopathology and placebo analgesia in patients with discogenic low back pain. *Pain Med*. 2006;7(3):217–228.

86. Rosenstock J, Tuchman M, LaMoreaux L, Sharma U. Pregabalin for the treatment of painful diabetic peripheral neuropathy: a double-blind, placebo-controlled trial. *Pain*. 2004;110(3):628–638.

87. Tölle T, Freynhagen R, Versavel M, Trostmann U, Young JP Jr. Pregabalin for relief of neuropathic pain associated with diabetic neuropathy: a randomized, double-blind study. *Eur J Pain*. 2008;12(2):203–213.

88. Ziegler D, Ametov A, Barinov A, Dyck PJ, Gurieva I, Low PA, Munzel U, Yakhno N, Raz I, Novosadova M, Maus J, Samigullin R. Oral treatment with alpha-lipoic acid improves symptomatic diabetic polyneuropathy: the SYDNEY 2 trial. *Diabetes Care*. 2006;29(11):2365–2370.

89. Max MB, Schafer SC, Culnane M, Smoller B, Dubner R, Gracely RH. Amitriptyline, but not lorazepam, relieves postherpetic neuralgia. *Neurology*. 1988;38(9):1427–1432.

90. Dellemijn PL, Vanneste JA. Randomised double-blind active-placebo-controlled crossover trial of intravenous fentanyl in neuropathic pain. *Lancet*. 1997;349(9054):753–758.

91. Gilron I, Booher SL, Rowan MS, Smoller MS, Max MB. A randomized, controlled trial of high-dose dextromethorphan in facial neuralgias. *Neurology*. 2000;55(7):964–971.

92. Gilron I, Bailey JM, Tu D, Holden RR, Weaver DF, Houlden RL. Morphine, gabapentin, or their combination for neuropathic pain. *N Engl J Med*. 2005;352(13):1324–1334.

93. Max MB, Portenoy RK, Laska EM, eds. *Advances in Pain Research and Therapy: The Design of Analgesic Clinical Trials*. Vol. 18. New York: Raven Press;1991.

94. Sindrup SH, Gram LF, Brøsen K, Eshøj O, Mogensen EF. The selective serotonin reuptake inhibitor paroxetine is effective in the treatment of diabetic neuropathy symptoms. *Pain*. 1990;42(2):135–144.

95. Baron R, Tölle TR, Gockel U, Brosz M, Freynhagen R. A cross-sectional cohort survey in 2100 patients with painful diabetic neuropathy and postherpetic neuralgia: differences in demographic data and sensory symptoms. *Pain*. 2009;146(1–2):34–40.

96. Byas-Smith MG, Max MB, Muir J, Kingman A. Transdermal clonidine compared to placebo in painful diabetic neuropathy using a two-stage "enriched enrollment" design. *Pain*. 1995;60(3):267–274.

97. McQuay HJ, Derry S, Moore RA, Poulain P, Legout V. Enriched enrolment with randomized withdrawal (EERW): time for a new look at clinical trial design in chronic pain. *Pain*. 2008;135(3):217–220.

98. Crofford LJ, Mease PJ, Simpson SL, Young JP Jr, Martin SA, Haig GM, Sharma U. Fibromyalgia relapse evaluation and efficacy for durability of meaningful relief (FREEDOM): a 6-month, double-blind, placebo-controlled trial with pregabalin. *Pain*. 2008;136(3): 419–431.

99. Katz N. Enriched enrollment randomized withdrawal trial designs of analgesics: focus on methodology. *Clin J Pain*. 2009;25(9):797–807.

100. Gilron I, Wajsbrot D, Therrien F, Lemay J. A randomized, placebo-controlled trial of pregabalin for the treatment of peripheral neuropathic pain. Presented at the meeting of the Canadian Pain Society, Quebec, Canada, May 2009.

101. Whitehead J, Valdés-Márquez E, Lissmats A. A simple two-stage design for quantitative responses with application to a study in diabetic neuropathic pain. *Pharm Stat*. 2009;8(2):125–135.

102. Zhang L, Rosenberger WF. Response-adaptive randomization for clinical trials with continuous outcomes. *Biometrics*. 2006;62(2):562–569.

103. Biswas A, Bhattachary R, Zhang L. Optimal response-adaptive designs for continuous responses in phase III trials. *Biomed J*. 2007;49(6):928–940.

104. Mogil JS. Animal models of pain: progress and challenges. *Nat Rev Neurosci*. 2009;10(4): 283–294.

105. Rice AS, Cimino-Brown D, Eisenach JC, Kontinen VK, Lacroix-Fralish ML, Machin I; Preclinical Pain Consortium, Mogil JS, Stöhr T. Animal models and the prediction of efficacy in clinical trials of analgesic drugs: a critical appraisal and call for uniform reporting standards. *Pain*. 2008;139(2):243–247.

5

Definitions, Anatomical Localization, and Signs and Symptoms of Neuropathic Pain

GUNNAR WASNER, ANDREAS BINDER, AND RALF BARON

DEFINITION OF NEUROPATHIC PAIN

ACCORDING TO RECENT estimates, 19% of all adults suffer from chronic pain and 40% of all visits to a general practitioner are due to chronic pain. Chronic pain represents a severe burden for many patients, with significant impairments of daily life and the quality of life, and is challenging for the treating physician in terms of both diagnosis and management. Chronic pain conditions can be primarily divided into two categories: *nociceptive* pain occurs as a consequence of tissue disease or damage, while the sensory nervous system is unimpaired and thus functionally intact, (e.g., osteoarthritis), whereas *neuropathic* pain arises when the afferent nervous system itself is diseased or damaged[1] (e.g., postherpetic neuralgia). Furthermore, other chronic pain disorders should be taken into account in the diagnosis, such as pain associated with psychoses, somatoform pain disorders, or pain *sine materia* (diagnosed by

exclusion), for all of which there is no evidence for any nociceptive and neuropathic processes.

Neuropathic pain syndromes are defined as *pain arising as a direct consequence of a lesion or disease affecting the somatosensory system.* The term *disease* refers to identifiable disease processes such as inflammatory conditions, auto-immune conditions, or channelopathies, while the term *lesion* refers to macro- or microscopically identifiable damage. The restriction to the somatosensory system is important, because diseases and lesions of other parts of the nervous system may cause nociceptive pain. For example, lesions or diseases of the motor system may lead to spasticity or rigidity and thus may indirectly cause nociceptive muscle pain. The latter pain conditions are now excluded from the condition of neuropathic pain. If possible, neuropathic pain should be classified as being of peripheral or central origin in terms of the location of the lesion or disease process (Table 5.1).

Table 5-1. Disease-/Anatomy-Based Classification of Painful Peripheral Neuropathies

FOCAL, MULTIFOCAL
    Phantom pain, stump pain, nerve transection pain (partial or complete)
    Neuroma (posttraumatic or postoperative)
    Posttraumatic neuralgia
    Entrapment syndromes
    Mastectomy
    Postthoracotomy
    Morton's neuralgia
    Painful scars
    Herpes zoster and postherpetic neuralgia
    Diabetic mononeuropathy, diabetic amyotrophy
    Ischemic neuropathy
    Borreliosis
    Connective tissue disease (vasculitis)
    Neuralgic amyotrophy
    Peripheral nerve tumors
    Radiation plexopathy
    Plexus neuritis (idiopathic or hereditary)
    Trigeminal or glossopharyngeal neuralgia
    Vascular compression syndromes
GENERALIZED (POLYNEUROPATHIES)
    Metabolic or Nutritional
        Diabetic, often "burning feet syndrome"
        Alcoholic
        Amyloid
        Hypothyroidism
        Beriberi, pellagra
    Drugs
        Antiretrovirals, cisplatin, disulfiram, ethambutol, isoniazid, nitrofurantoin, thalidomide, thiouracil, vincristine, chloramphenicol, metronidazole, taxoids, gold
    Toxins
        Acrylamide, arsenic, clioquinol, dinitrophenol, ethylene oxide, pentachlorophenol, thallium
    Hereditary
        Amyloid neuropathy
        Fabry's disease
        Charcot-Marie-Tooth disease type 5, type 2B
        Hereditary sensory and autonomic neuropathy (HSAN) type 1, type 1B
    Malignant
        Carcinomatous (paraneoplastic), myeloma
    Infective or Postinfective, Immune
        Acute or inflammatory polyradiculoneuropathy (Guillain-Barré syndrome), borreliosis, human immunodeficiency virus

(continued)

Table 5-1. (continued)

Other Polyneuropathies
  Erythromelalgia
  Idiopathic small-fiber neuropathy
  Trench foot (cold injury)
CENTRAL PAIN SYNDROMES
  Vascular Lesions in the Brain (Especially in the Brainstem and Thalamus) and Spinal Cord
    Infarct
    Hemorrhage
    Vascular malformation
  Multiple Sclerosis
  Traumatic Spinal Cord Injury Including Iatrogenic Cordotomy
  Traumatic Brain Injury
  Syringomyelia and Syringobulbia
  Tumors
  Abscesses
  Inflammatory Diseases Other Than Multiple Sclerosis; Myelitis Caused by Viruses, Syphilis
  Epilepsy
  Parkinson's Disease
MIXED-PAIN SYNDROMES
  Chronic low back pain with radiculopathy
  Cancer pain with malignant plexus invasion
  Complex regional pain syndromes

Source: Adapted from Baron R. Mechanisms of disease: neuropathic pain—a clinical perspective. *Nat Clin Pract Neurol.* 2006;2:95–106.

ANATOMICAL LOCALIZATION OF NEUROPATHIC PAIN

In clinical practice, neuropathic pain is frequently classified according to the underlying etiology of the disorder and the anatomical location of the specific lesion.[2] Hence, the majority of patients with painful lesions in the nervous system can be allocated to one of the following two classes[3] (Table 5.1): neuropathic pain after the development of peripheral nerve lesions or neuropathic pain after the development of lesions in the central nervous system.

Neuropathic Pain After Development of Peripheral Nerve Lesions

Painful peripheral neuropathies may be caused by trauma or ischemia or may result from inflammatory, toxic, metabolic, or degenerative processes; they may also have hereditary causes. For the differential diagnosis of possible underlying causes, the anatomical distribution pattern of the affected nerves is of great importance and leads to a grouping of painful peripheral neuropathies:

• Symmetrical generalized polyneuropathies are diseases affecting many nerves simultaneously.
• Asymmetrical neuropathies have a focal or multifocal distribution or are the result of processes affecting the brachial or lumbosacral plexuses.

Neuropathic Pain After Development of Lesions in the Central Nervous System

All lesions causing central pain affect the somatosensory pathways. They may be located at any level of the neuraxis. Thus, lesions at the first synapse in the dorsal horn of the spinal cord or trigeminal nuclei, along the ascending pathways through the spinal cord and brainstem, in the thalamus, in the subcortical white matter, and in the cerebral cortex have all been reported.[4] The most common are cerebrovascular lesions, multiple sclerosis (MS) lesions, and traumatic spinal cord injuries (SCI). In these diseases the incidence of neuropathic pain is approximately 8%, 28%, and 40%, respectively.[5] In stroke the pain is most frequently a hemipain (75%). In MS it affects one or both sides, more often in the legs (87%) than in the upper extremities (31%). Trigeminal neuralgia, caused by a lesion in the brainstem, occurs in 5% of all MS patients.

SENSORY SIGNS AND SYMPTOMS OF NEUROPATHIC PAIN

The characteristic symptoms and signs of neuropathic pain make it distinct from other chronic pain syndromes in which the nervous system remains unaltered, that is, nociceptive pain. Thus, an important aim of the clinical examination and the recording of patients´ history is correctly categorizing the type and quality of pain. In addition to identifying nociceptive or neuropathic types, other chronic pain disorders should be ruled out. For example, both nociceptive and neuropathic processes may contribute to an overall clinical picture of *mixed pain*, as in chronic low back pain with pathology of the spine, vertebral discs. and nerve root.[6,7]

Pain associated with nerve injury has a number of clinical characteristics[3] (Table 5.2). If a peripheral nerve with a cutaneous branch or a central somatosensory pathway is involved, almost always an area of abnormal sensation can be identified and the patient's maximum pain is coexistent with or lies within an area of sensory deficit. This is a key diagnostic feature for pain of neuropathic origin. This sensory deficit may, for instance, involve a reduced perception of noxious and thermal stimuli, which in turn may indicate damage to small-diameter afferent fibers or to the spinothalamic tract.

In addition to these negative somatosensory signs (deficit in function), patients with neuropathic conditions also frequently present with positive somatosensory signs (enhanced perception). Paresthesias (ant crawling sensation, tingling) are not painful, but they are uncomfortable. Painful positive signs may be *spontaneous* (not stimulus-induced), such as ongoing pain and spontaneous shooting, electric shock-like sensations, or may occur as *evoked* types of pain (stimulus-induced pain, hypersensitivity) characterized by several sensory abnormalities, either adjacent to or within skin areas of sensory deficit. Frequently, patients report mechanical hypersensitivity and/or hypersensitivity to heat and cold. Two types of hypersensitivity can be distinguished:

- *Allodynia* is defined as pain in response to a stimulus that does not normally provoke pain. For instance, with mechanical allodynia, even very gentle mechanical stimuli such as slight bending of hairs may evoke severe pain.
- *Hyperalgesia* is defined as increased pain sensitivity in response to a painful stimulus.

Another evoked type of pain is *summation*, which occurs as progressive aggravation of pain in response to slowly repeated stimulation with mildly painful stimuli—for example, pinprick. Some patients with nerve injury have a nearly pure hypersensitive syndrome in which no sensory deficit is demonstrable.[8]

For the diagnosis of neuropathic pain conditions, the quality of the reported sensations should also be taken into account; neuropathic pain is frequently experienced as burning and/or shooting pain with unusual tingling, crawling, or electric shock-like sensations (dysesthesias).

None of the characteristics described above is always present in patients with neuropathic pain or absolutely diagnostic of neuropathic pain. However, if these sensory signs and symptoms occur, the diagnosis of neuropathic pain is likely.

CLINICAL ASSESSMENT OF SENSORY SIGNS (BEDSIDE TESTS)

A precise clinical evaluation requires a standardized method for the assessment of patients.

Table 5-2. Definition and Assessment of Negative and Positive Sensory Symptoms and Signs in Neuropathic Pain

	SYMPTOM/SIGN	DEFINITION	ASSESSMENT (BEDSIDE EXAMINATION)	EXPECTED PATHOLOGICAL RESPONSE
Negative signs and symptoms	Hypoesthesia	Reduced sensation to nonpainful stimuli	Touch skin with painter's brush, cotton swab, or gauze	Reduced perception, numbness
	Pall-hypoesthesia	Reduced sensation to vibration	Apply tuning fork on bone or joint	Reduced perception threshold
	Hypoalgesia	Reduced sensation to painful stimuli	Prick skin with single pin stimulus	Reduced perception, numbness
	Therm-hypoesthesia	Reduced sensation to cold/warm stimuli	Contact skin with objects at 10°C (metal roller, glass with water, coolants like acetone) Contact skin with objects at 45°C (metal roller, glass with water)	Reduced perception
Spontaneous sensations/pain	Paraesthesia	Nonpainful ongoing sensation (ant crawling)	Grade intensity (0–10) Area in cm^2	—
	Paroxysmal pain	Shooting electric shock-like attacks for several seconds	Number per time Grade intensity (0–10) Threshold for evocation	—
	Superficial pain	Painful ongoing sensation, often of a burning quality	Grade intensity (0–10) Area in cm^2	—

Evoked pain			
Mechanical dynamic allodynia	Normally nonpainful light moving stimuli on skin evoke pain	Stroke skin with painter's brush, cotton swab, or gauze	Sharp burning superficial pain Present in the primary affected zone but spreads beyond it into unaffected skin areas (secondary zone)
Mechanical static allodynia	Normally nonpainful gentle static pressure stimuli on skin evoke pain	Apply manual gentle mechanical pressure to the skin	Dull pain Present in the area of affected (damaged or sensitized) primary afferent nerve endings (primary zone)
Mechanical punctate, pinprick hyperalgesia	Normally stinging but nonpainful stimuli evoke pain	Manually prick the skin with a safety pin, sharp stick, or stiff von Frey hair	Sharp superficial pain Present in the primary affected zone but spreads beyond it into unaffected skin areas (secondary zone)
Temporal summation	Repetitive application of identical single noxious stimuli is perceived as increasing pain sensation (windup-like pain)	Prick the skin with a safety pin at intervals <3s for 30 s	Sharp superficial pain of increasing intensity
Cold allodynia	Normally nonpainful cold stimuli evoke pain	Contact skin with objects at 20°C (metal roller, glass with water, coolants like acetone) Control: contact skin with objects of skin temperature	Painful, often burning temperature sensation Present in the area of affected (damaged or sensitized) primary afferent nerve endings (primary zone)
Heat allodynia	Normally non painful heat stimuli evoke pain	Contact skin with objects at 40°C (metal roller, glass with water) Control: contact skin with objects at skin temperature	Painful burning temperature sensation Present in the area of affected (damaged or sensitized) primary afferent nerve endings (primary zone)
Mechanical deep somatic allodynia	Normally nonpainful pressure on deep somatic tissues evokes pain	Apply manual light pressure to joints or muscles	Deep pain at joints or muscles

Source: Adapted from Baron R. Mechanisms of disease: neuropathic pain—a clinical perspective. *Nat Clin Pract Neurol.* 2006;2:95–106.

The sensory bedside examination should include testing the following: touch, pinprick, pressure, cold, heat, vibration, and temporal summation[9,10] (see the definition in Table 5.2). In order to assess loss (negative sensory signs) or gain (positive sensory signs) of somatosensory function, the individual responses can be divided into normal, decreased, or increased function. For stimulus-evoked (positive) pain types, hyperalgesic or allodynic responses are distinguished, and the dynamic or static character of the stimulus should be taken into account.[11]

The following assessment tools are suggested (see also Table 5.2):

• Touch can be assessed by gently applying a cotton swab or a soft brush to the skin.
• Pinprick sensation is tested with sharp pinprick stimuli—for example, using a safety pin or a stiff von Frey hair.
• Gentle pressure on muscle and joints is applied in order to identify deep pain.
• Cold and heat sensation is measured using thermal stimuli—for example, metal objects kept at 20 or 45°C or a glass of water with a corresponding temperature; for the assessment of cold sensation, acetone spray might also be used.
• Vibration is assessed with a tuning fork (128 Hz) placed at strategic points (interphalangeal joints, etc.).
• Temporal summation (windup-like pain), the clinical equivalent of increasing neuronal activity following repetitive noxious C-fiber stimulation of more than 0.3 Hz, can be assessed using mechanical and thermal stimuli—for example, pinprick with a safety pin at intervals of <3 s for 30 s.

If a patient presents with allodynia or hyperalgesia, these can be quantified by measuring the intensity and area. Currently, it is generally agreed that assessments should be carried out in the area of maximum pain while using the contralateral body side as a control, if possible. It must be borne in mind, however, that a mirror site may not necessarily represent a true control site, since after the development of a unilateral nerve or root lesion, contralateral segmental changes cannot be excluded.

Of note, the areas of distribution of abnormal sensations need to be taken into account. In neuropathic conditions, primary and secondary areas are distinguished; the primary area corresponds to the tissue supplied by damaged nerves, whereas the secondary area lies outside this innervation territory. Mechanical hypersensitivity often expands into the secondary area.

SCREENING TOOLS TO DISTINGUISH NEUROPATHIC PAIN FROM OTHER CHRONIC PAIN STATES

Modern research into the mechanisms of neuropathic pain clearly revealed that nerve lesions lead to dramatic changes in the peripheral and central nervous systems, making neuropathic pain distinct from other chronic pain types in which the nociceptive system is intact. Furthermore, neuropathic pain states require different therapeutic approaches, such as the use of anticonvulsants and antidepressants, which are not effective in nociceptive pain. To make the situation even more complex, many chronic pain states are characterized by a combination of both pain types. The best examples of so-called mixed pain syndromes are chronic radicular back pain, tumor pain, and complex regional pain syndrome. For the clinician, it is therefore of the utmost importance to have valid screening tools that differentiate neuropathic pain from nociceptive pain or estimate the neuropathic pain component in mixed pain syndromes. The easiest approach would be to use somatosensory symptoms assessed by questionnaires or history questions or simple signs testable at the bedside that are characteristic for neuropathic pain. A summary of all available screening tools is published elsewhere.[12]

A clinician-administered 10-item questionnaire (**DN4**) consists of sensory descriptors (7 items) as well as signs related to the bedside sensory examination (3 items).[9] The sensory descriptors address the quality of the pain (burning, painful cold, electric shocks) and associated symptoms (tingling, pins and needles, numbness, itching). The clinical examination consists of the assessment of hypoesthesia to touch and prick and allodynia to brush. This questionnaire was validated in 160 patients presenting with pain of nociceptive and neuropathic origin and showed that 86.0% of patients were correctly identified (sensitivity 82.9%, specificity 89.9%).

Another approach to distinguish neuropathic from nonneuropathic pain uses a patient-based questionnaire with nine questions without the need of examinations by the physician (**PainDETECT**).[13] The questionnaire uses slightly different sensory descriptors (seven items: burning pain, tingling or prickling [electricity], sensitivity to touch [clothes, blanket], pain caused by light pressure [e.g., with a finger], shooting pain or electric shock-like pain, occasional painful cold or heat [e.g., in a bathtub], and numbness), the question of whether the pain is spatially radiating, and a question addressing the individual pain pattern. This questionnaire was validated in 392 patients with pain of either predominantly neuropathic origin ($n = 167$, e.g., postherpetic neuralgia, painful polyneuropathies, nerve trauma) or predominantly nociceptive origin ($n = 225$, e.g., osteoarthritis, mechanical low back pain, inflammatory arthropathies). Patients were diagnosed according to the results of two independent pain specialists who determined the predominant pain type (neuropathic versus nociceptive) on the basis of of clinical experience as well as neurological examination, electrophysiological methods, or imaging techniques. This questionnaire showed a correct classification rate of 82.5% (sensitivity 80.8%, specificity 84.7%).

However, a recent study raised several caveats on the approach using screening tools.[11] This study looked prospectively at symptoms and signs in 214 patients with suspected chronic neuropathic pain that were a priori classified by pain experts as having so-called definite, possible, or unlikely neuropathic pain. Pain symptoms and descriptors were recorded, and sensory tests including pinprick stimulation, examination for cold-evoked pain by an acetone drop, and brush-evoked pain were carried out to determine if symptoms and signs cluster differently in groups of patients with increasing evidence of neuropathic pain. Several symptoms (touch- or cold-provoked pain) and signs (brush-evoked allodynia) were more prominent in patients with definite or possible neuropathic pain. However, there was considerable overlap with the clinical presentation of patients with unlikely neuropathic pain. Even worse, the pain descriptors used could not distinguish between the three clinical categories.

ASSESSMENT SCALES FOR NEUROPATHIC PAIN SIGNS AND SYMPTOMS IN LONGITUDINAL STUDIES

Most clinical trials in neuropathic pain only use the pain intensity measured on a rating scale as a primary endpoint. It is very likely that therapies influence the different aspects of pain quality differently. Thus, the different symptoms, like hyperalgesia and allodynia, should be assessed independently and the change in these symptoms should also be documented during therapy. Several assessment tools have been proposed for the use in clinical trials.

The **Neuropathic Pain Scale (NPS)**[14] was the first pain quality assessment tool specifically devoted to neuropathic pain assessment. It includes 10 pain quality items rated on 0–10 numerical scales and a temporal assessment of pain. In the NPS each item is rated separately, but in further studies, various composite scores using selected items were proposed, although these changes have not been formally validated.[15] The NPS has been used in several neuropathic pain trials,[15–18] some of them reporting better sensitivity of some descriptors compared to others in response to treatments such as gabapentin, cannabinoids, or opioids.[16,18,19] The main limitation of the NPS is that it lacks several common pain qualities, particularly those associated with the paroxysmal dimension of neuropathic pain.

The **Pain Quality Assessment Scale (PQAS)** has been developed to assess pain qualities that are present with both neuropathic and nonneuropathic pain conditions.[18] Three pain quality factors were identified representing paroxysmal pain, superficial pain, and deep pain.[20] However, the three-factor division may be too broad to capture specific dimensions of neuropathic pain. To date, no data exist regarding the use of this scale in blinded neuropathic pain trials.

The **Neuropathic Pain Symptom Inventory (NPSI)** contains 10 descriptors representing five distinct dimensions—burning pain, deep pain, paroxysmal pain, evoked pain, paresthesia/dysesthesia—and 2 temporal items designed to assess pain duration and the number of pain paroxysms.[9] The NPSI has been validated in patients with definite neuropathic pain of peripheral or central origin.[9,21] In a clinical trial, it was found that several neuropathic pain dimensions were particularly sensitive to the treatment effect.[22] Importantly, the factorial structure of the NPSI makes it suitable to capture different aspects of neuropathic pain that likely have distinct underlying pathophysiological mechanisms.[21,23] For example, it has recently been found that the various NPSI pain qualities of neuropathic pain were correlated to neurophysiological data in patients with carpal tunnel syndrome. Paroxysmal pain was associated with impairment of nonnociceptive A-β fibers, as indicated by nerve conduction velocity, while spontaneous ongoing pain was related to damage of nociceptive fibers, as indicated by laser-evoked potential amplitudes.[23]

The **SF-MPQ-2**[24] is a revised and expanded version of the Short Form McGill Questionnaire that was recently developed to measure the symptoms of both neuropathic and nonneuropathic pain. It contains seven new items specifically related to neuropathic pain, and the scoring of each symptom is based on 0–10 numerical scales. The sensitivity to change was confirmed in a double-blind trial of diabetic neuropathic pain. A factor analysis identified four subscales: continuous pain, intermittent pain, predominantly neuropathic pain, and an affective descriptor. The validation study of the SFMPQ-2, however, was mainly based on a very large Internet survey with several limitation (i.e. the representativeness of the sample was not controlled, and participants were asked to self-report their pain conditions). Thus, further studies are necessary to confirm the psychometric properties of the SFMPQ-2 in properly diagnosed groups of patients with neuropathic or mixed pain syndromes.

STANDARDIZED PROTOCOLS TO ASSESS SENSORY SIGNS QUANTITATIVELY

Quantitative sensory testing (QST) is a sophisticated neurophysiological technique for the assessment of both the nociceptive and non-nociceptive afferent systems in the periphery and the central nervous system. Standardized mechanical and thermal stimuli are applied (e.g., graded von Frey hairs, several pinprick stimuli, pressure algometers, quantitative thermotesting), and they assess both loss of function (minus signs) and gain of function (positive signs). Sensory symptoms such as allodynia or hyperalgesia can be quantified by measuring intensity, threshold for elicitation, duration, and area.

The standardized protocol for QST that was recently proposed by the nationwide German Network on Neuropathic Pain (DFNS)[25] analyzes the precise somatosensory phenotype of neuropathic pain patients via 13 parameters of sensory testing procedures (Figure 5-1). Initially, an age- and gender-matched database for absolute and relative QST reference data was established in a nationwide multicenter trial for healthy human subjects that allows for the evaluation of pathological ranges of plus or minus signs in patients. Currently, this database comprises complete sensory profiles of 180 healthy volunteers and more than 2000 neuropathic pain patients with a variety of indications; the data on the healthy volunteers were analyzed for influence of body side and region, age, and gender. The QST allows for an assessment of the following parameters: thermal detection and pain thresholds (including a test for the presence of paradoxical heat sensations), mechanical detection thresholds to von Frey filaments and a tuning fork (64 Hz), mechanical pain thresholds to pinprick stimuli and blunt pressure, stimulus/response functions for pinprick and dynamic mechanical allodynia (pain to light touch), and repetitive pinprick stimulation for the determination of pain summation (windup ratio). On the basis of reference data for most variables, this DFNS protocol can detect pathological values of positive and negative signs. In an analysis of 1236 neuropathic pain patients with pain of various

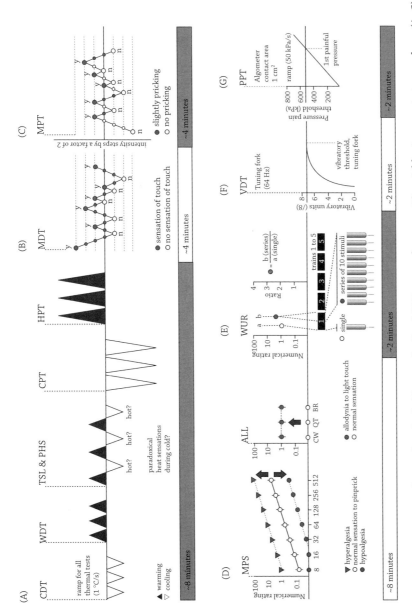

FIGURE 5.1. QST—a battery of sensory tests: figure of methods. The standardized QST protocol assesses 13 variables in seven test procedures (A–G). All procedures are presented, including a time frame for testing over one area. (A) Thermal testing (CDT, cold detection threshold; WDT, warm detection threshold; TSL, thermal sensory limen for alternating warm and cold stimuli; PHS, number of paradoxical heat sensations during the TSL procedure; CPT, cold pain threshold; HPT, heat pain threshold); this comprises detection and pain thresholds for cold, warm, or hot stimuli (C- and A-δ fiber mediated). (B) (MDT, mechanical detection threshold); this tests for A-β fiber function using von Frey filaments. (C) (MPT, mechanical pain sensitivity) for pinprick stimuli and dynamic mechanical allodynia (ALL) for dynamic mechanical allodynia; this again assesses A-δ-mediated sensitivity to sharp stimuli (pinprick) and also A-β fiber-mediated sensitivity to stroking light touch (CW, cotton wisp; QT, cotton wool tip; BR, brush). (E) (WUR, windup ratio); this compares the verbal ratings within five trains of a single pinprick stimulus (a) with a series (b) of 10 repetitive pinprick stimuli to calculate WUR as the ratio b/a. (F) (VDT, vibration detection threshold); this tests again for A-β fiber function using a Rydel-Seiffer 64 Hz tuning fork. (G) (PPT, pressure pain threshold); this is the only test for deep pain sensitivity, probably mediated by muscle C- and A-δ fibers.

Source: After Rolke R, Baron R, Maier C, et al. Quantitative sensory testing in the German Research Network on Neuropathic Pain (DFNS): standardized protocol and reference values. *Pain.* 2006;123:231–243. This figure has been reproduced with permission of the International Association for the Study of Pain (IASP®). The figure may not be reproduced for any other purpose without permission.

etiologies, the precise frequency of somatosensory abnormalities in the affected skin areas was determined. Table 5.3 shows an example of these data for two neuropathic conditions. These data are of the utmost importance for the design of clinical trials in which compounds that are known to target specific sensory signs are tested.[26]

This approach of addressing individual sensory signs, however, has one potential limitation: according to animal research, one single sign can probably not be linked to exactly one underlying pathophysiological mechanism. On the contrary, it is likely that several entirely different underlying pathophysiological mechanisms may cause one specific sign. Thus, rather than looking at just a single parameter, a particular pathophysiological mechanism may be predicted more precisely by a specific constellation of sensory signs, that is, a profile of signs consisting of a combination of negative and positive sensory phenomena.

For example, standardized QST methods, as described above, can clearly differentiate between various phenotypic subtypes of postherpetic neuralgia patients, each with distinct sensory symptom constellations.[25] The profile of patient 1 in Figure 5.2 shows a predominant gain of sensory function with heat pain hyperalgesia (HPT), pinprick mechanical hyperalgesia (MPS), dynamic mechanical allodynia (ALL), and static hyperalgesia to blunt pressure (PPT). In terms of pathophysiological mechanisms, this profile points to a combination of peripheral and central sensitization. In contrast, the QST profile of patient 2 shows a predominant loss of sensory function, with cold (CDT) and warm detection thresholds (WDT), thermal sensory limen (TSL), heat pain thresholds (HPT), tactile detection thresholds (MDT), and mechanical pain thresholds to pinprick stimuli (MPT) all lying below the normal range and thus reflecting a loss of function. This profile points to a combined small- and large-fiber sensory deafferentation. Despite these very different profiles and thus different pain-generating mechanisms, both patients suffered from spontaneous burning pain of similar intensity.

Table 5-3 Frequency of Pathological Values in Percent (Gain and Loss) for Complex Regional Pain Syndromes (CRPS) and Polyneuropathies (PNP)

	GAIN		LOSS	
	CRPS	PNP	CRPS	PNP
	N = 403	N = 343	N = 403	N = 343
CDT	2.7	0.3	32.5	40.2
WDT	2.5	0.9	26.6	18.4
TSL	2.7	0.6	26.9	36.7
CPT	30.5	1.5	5.2	—
HPT	40.1	7.0	7.7	5.0
PPT	66.3	5.0	3.3	13.2
MPT	28.7	11.1	10.0	21.9
MPS	46.6	8.5	6.2	5.0
WUR	13.1	6.9	2.7	0.4
MDT	9.5	0.3	35.2	39.8
VDT	1.5	—	35.4	45.9
PHS	9.4	37.3	—	—
DMA	24.1	12.0	—	—

Thirteen variables of QST are shown. Thermal testing: CDT, cold detection threshold; WDT, warm detection threshold; TSL, thermal sensory limen for alternating warm and cold stimuli; PHS, number of paradoxical heat sensations during the TSL procedure; CPT, cold pain threshold; HPT, heat pain threshold; MDT, mechanical detection threshold; MPT, mechanical pain threshold; MPS, mechanical pain sensitivity; WUR, windup ratio; VDT, vibration detection threshold; PPT, pressure pain threshold; DMA, dynamic mechanical allodynia.

#Source: From Maier C, Baron R, Tölle TR, Binder A. Quantitative sensory testing in the German Research Network on Neuropathic Pain (DFNS): Somatosensory abnormalities in 1236 patients with different neuropathic pain syndromes. Pain. 2010;150:439–450.

ASSESSMENT TOOLS TO DEFINE SUBGROUPS OF PATIENTS WITH SPECIFIC SENSORY SYMPTOM PROFILES

For exact QST profiling as described above, 13 somatosensory tests are conducted; in total, these take more than 1 h of the physician´s and the patient´s time. For practical reasons, this approach can therefore be used only in research settings and in fairly small proof-of-concept trials. Large clinical phase III trials require different comprehensible assessment strategies. Furthermore, since pain is a subjective

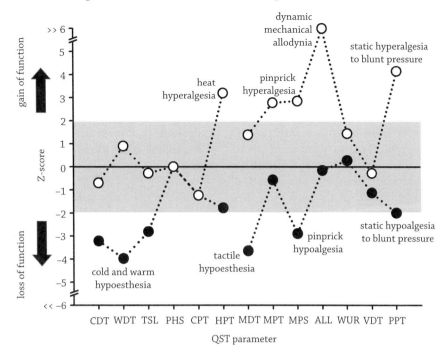

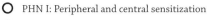

FIGURE 5.2. Z-score sensory profiles of two patients suffering from postherpetic neuralgia (PHN). **Patient PHN I** (open circles) shows the QST profile of a 70-year-old woman suffering from PHN for 8 years. Ongoing pain was 80 on a 0–100 numerical rating scale. The profile shows a predominant gain of sensory function in terms of heat pain hyperalgesia (HPT), pinprick mechanical hyperalgesia (MPS), dynamic mechanical allodynia (ALL), and static hyperalgesia to blunt pressure (PPT) outside the 95% confidence interval of the distribution of healthy subjects (gray zone). This profile is consistent with a combination of peripheral and central sensitization. **Patient PHN II** (filled circles) shows the QST profile of a 71-year-old woman with pain for 8 months. Ongoing pain was 70 on a 0–100 numerical rating scale. The profile shows predominant loss of sensory function. Note the cold (CDT) and warm detection thresholds (WDT), thermal sensory limen (TSL), heat pain thresholds (HPT), tactile detection thresholds (MDT), and mechanical pain thresholds to pinprick stimuli (MPT) outside the normal range, as indicated by the gray zone. This profile is consistent with a combined small- and large-fiber sensory deafferentation. Z-score: number of standard deviations between patient data and the group-specific mean value.

Source: After Rolke R, Baron R, Maier C, et al. Quantitative sensory testing in the German Research Network on Neuropathic Pain (DFNS): standardized protocol and reference values. *Pain*. 2006;123:231–243. This figure has been reproduced with permission of the International Association for the Study of Pain (IASP®). The figure may not be reproduced for any other purpose without permission.

phenomenon, it is still not clear whether QST parameters (e.g., a pain perception threshold to a small thermal stimulus) are able to give a real picture of the patients' subjective experience and whether these parameters are thus clinically relevant, as perceived by the patients themselves.[27,28] Alternatively, patient-reported outcomes (PROs), which collect health-related data directly from the patients,[29] may be able to capture subtle differences in individual somatosensory characteristics.

Symptom Questionnaires

A cross-sectional cohort survey recently confirmed that PROs can indeed be used to classify neuropathic pain on the basis of the patients' perceived sensory neuropathic symptoms. In this survey, among others, the painDETECT questionnaire (see above) was used to analyze 498 patients with postherpetic neuralgia and 1623 patients with painful diabetic polyneuropathy.[30] In order to identify relevant subgroups of patients with a characteristic symptom profile in this cohort, a hierarchical cluster analysis was performed. The clusters correspond to the patterns of questionnaire scores, thereby revealing the typical pathological structure of each group. Using this approach, five distinct clusters (subgroups) of patients were detected, each showing a characteristic sensory profile, that is, a typical constellation and combination of neuropathic symptoms (Figure 5.3). These five sensory profiles show notable differences concerning the expression of symptoms. In postherpetic neuralgia (PHN) and diabetic painful neuropathy (DPN), for example, all subgroups and their respective sensory profiles occur in relevant numbers in both conditions but their frequencies differ; thus, it is tempting to speculate about the underlying pathophysiological mechanisms potentially operating in these phenotypic subgroups. Three examples are discussed in detail:

Subgroup 1 occurs nearly three times more frequently in PHN compared to DPN. The predominant features in this subgroup are moderate to severe spontaneous burning pain in combination with mild to moderate dynamic mechanical allodynia (the latter being more intense in PHN than in DPN). Numbness occurred very rarely, which indicates intact cutaneous innervation without any signs of degeneration. This profile might indicate preserved but irritable nociceptors with secondary sensitization of central nociceptive neurons. Interestingly, the sensory perceptions of this group of patients closely resemble the constellation of sensory signs previously described with QST for a subset of patients (see Figure 5.2). Pharmacological compounds that modulate neuronal sensitization might be favorable for this particular group.

Subgroup 2 is characterized by clinically relevant pain attacks. These patients might be particularly suitable for clinical trials with drugs that

are expected to reduce ectopic neuronal firing in nociceptors, such as sodium channel blockers.

Subgroup 4 patients experience a combination of substantial dynamic mechanical allodynia and deep somatic hyperalgesia. Predominant involvement of afferents innervating deep somatic structures may explain this profile, and cutaneous allodynia might be caused by convergent afferent input of deep somatic and skin nerves on central nociceptive neurons. Again, compounds that interfere with central sensitization could be more successful for this group of patients.

The predominant features of subgroup 5 patients are considerable burning pain, paresthesias, and numbness but a lack of clinically relevant dynamic mechanical allodynia, thermal hyperalgesia, or pain attacks. This profile points to severe deafferentation of the affected skin, and a length-dependent denervation of afferent neurons (which occurs more often in diabetic neuropathy) might be a good explanation for these findings. Patients in this subgroup might be the most suitable candidates for clinical trials with drugs that are expected to have an effect on spontaneous afferent sensations rather than on evoked pain types. Again, this constellation of sensory signs has previously been described with QST, as shown for patient 2 in Figure 5.2.

The sensory profile of subgroup 3 patients (a large subgroup of patients who comprised one-third of the entire cohort) came somewhat as a surprise since the values for all parameters were concentrated mainly around the zero line, implying moderate perception of all parameters. There are several potential explanations for this finding: Some patients may, of course, perceive all neuropathic symptoms with similar frequency and intensity; it is, however, unlikely, both from clinical experience and quantitative sensory testing studies, that this applies to such a large group of patients (30%). Another explanation for this type of profile might be a psychological phenomenon in which several patients have a tendency to score all questions in a similar or identical manner, possibly because they are unable to discriminate between the different sensory abnormalities and therefore give the same score to all questions. Whatever the explanation for this finding is, these patients

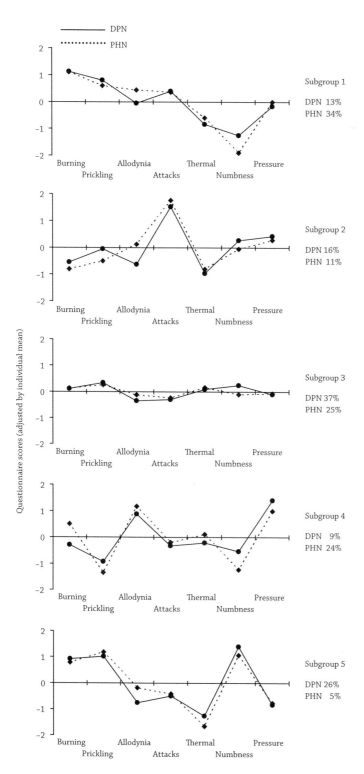

FIGURE 5.3. Subgrouping of patients according to sensory profiles using patient-reported outcomes. To identify relevant subgroups of patients characterized by a characteristic symptom constellation, a hierarchical cluster analysis was performed. The clusters are represented by the patterns of questionnaire scores (adjusted individual mean; see below), thus showing the typical pathological structure of the respective groups. Using this approach, five clusters (subgroups) with distinct symptom profiles could be detected. Sensory profiles show remarkable differences in the expression of the symptoms.[30] %, frequency of occurrence; DPN, diabetic painful neuropathy; PHN, postherpetic neuralgia. Adjusted individual mean: in order to eliminate interindividual differences in the general perception of sensory stimuli (differences in individual pain perception thresholds), a score was calculated in which the given 0–5 score of each question was subtracted by the mean of all values marked in the seven questions. In this individual score, values above 0 indicate a sensation that is more intense than the individual mean pain perception; values below 0 indicate a sensation that is less intense than the individual mean pain perception.

Source: Baron R, Tölle TR, Gockel U, Brosz M, Freynhagen R. A cross-sectional cohort survey in 2100 patients with painful diabetic neuropathy and postherpetic neuralgia: Differences in demographic data and sensory symptoms. Pain. 2009 Nov;146(1–2):34–40. Epub 2009 Jul 9.

should probably be excluded from clinical trials in which the effect of a compound on specific symptoms is evaluated.

Interview in Combination with the Bedside Examination

A recent study used a combination of structured interview and standardized bedside examination for the assessment of pain-related symptoms and signs in 130 patients with peripheral neuropathic pain (painful diabetic polyneuropathy, PHN, or radicular back pain) and in 57 patients with nonneuropathic (axial) low back pain.[31] The interview consisted of 16 questions with a total of 46 items concerning pain localization, pain quality, evoked pains, and additional sensory qualities such as dysesthesia and numbness. The physical examination included 23 bedside tests providing information about 39 items covering trophic and autonomic cutaneous signs, evoked pains, and sensory deficits. Readily available tools such as von Frey filaments, the eraser end of a pencil, a safety pin, and so on were used to test for tactile stimulation, blunt pressure, vibration, pinprick, temperature, position, and passive movement, among other factors. This approach enabled the researcher to distinguish six subgroups of patients with neuropathic pain and two subgroups of patients with nonneuropathic pain. In this study, the physical examination was shown to be more sensitive for the distinction of pain subtypes than the symptoms assessed by the interview.

RATIONALE FOR A NEW CLASSIFICATION OF NEUROPATHIC PAIN BASED ON SIGNS AND SYMPTOMS

The traditional and initial clinical approach to patients presenting with pain has basically always been an examination and classification of the patient on the basis of the topography of the lesion and the underlying pathology. If the underlying disorder causing the *symptom* of pain has been properly diagnosed, disease-modifying or even disease-curing therapies may be initiated. In many disorders associated with pain (e.g., bacterial meningitis, neuroborreliosis,

osteoarthritis, cancer, rheumatoid arthritis, ischemic heart disease, stroke), the symptom, that is, the pain, rapidly disappears after the relevant therapy has been administered.

This approach is certainly valid, and knowledge of the underlying pathology is essential; however, what happens if the symptom itself becomes a disease? In many patients, pain persists despite treatment of the underlying disease and becomes a chronic problem. In other patients, the underlying disease such as diabetes, cancer, or vasculitis is known but cannot be cured, and again, the patient is left with chronic pain.

Clinical experience and rather discouraging systematic research related to therapy in chronic pain have shown that a strategy directed at examining, classifying, and treating pain on the basis of anatomy or underlying disease is often of no or little help to the patients.[32] This has become very clear in some recent randomized clinical trials performed in PDN. In these trials the study medication failed to demonstrate efficacy, although the compound showed encouraging results in preclinical and early clinical studies.[17] Do these negative results really indicate lack of efficacy or is it more likely that specific characteristics of the patient population, the selected etiology, or the defined primary outcome have obscured a positive response[33]?

Observations like this have raised the question of whether an entirely different approach of analyzing pain on the basis of underlying mechanisms might be appropriate for the examination and classification of patients in order to obtain more favorable treatment results. The increasing knowledge of the mechanisms causing chronic pain together with the discovery of new molecular targets for modifying pain has supported the demand for alternative ways to treat pain. Since new treatments are being developed on the basis of the biological mechanisms that underlie pain, Woolf and other authors[3,34] have emphasized the need for a treatment approach directed at mechanism(s) rather than at diseases. One area that desperately requires a new treatment approach like this one is neuropathic pain.

Although it is fairly difficult to study mechanisms of pain generation in human patients, the expression of sensory abnormalities, that is, the somatosensory phenotype, points to some pathophysiological dysfunctions in afferent processing, and it is likely that specific pathophysiological mechanisms are associated with characteristic signs or sign constellations of hypo- and hypersensitivity to mechanical and thermal stimuli.

Various combinations of symptoms and sensory abnormalities may occur, with some patients suffering from spontaneous pain, dysesthesias, and electric shock-like pain, whereas in others the affected body area is hypersensitive to temperature or touch.[3] Therefore, a feasible way forward might be to classify and subgroup patients with neuropathic pain on the basis of their somatosensory phenotype. It is highly likely that subgroups of patients with different sign and symptom constellations—that is, different somatosensory phenotypes—will also respond differently to treatment. This, in turn, suggests that patients participating in clinical trials should be stratified on the basis of this new classification scheme; that is, rather than being subgrouped on the basis of their underlying etiology, patients should be subgrouped on the basis of their phenotypic profile. This approach may not only reduce the pathophysiological heterogeneity within the groups being investigated, it may also increase the power to detect a positive treatment result.

Even though a subtype classification based on afferent profiles is very attractive, there are some limitations, and it needs to be stressed that it will not be possible to allocate all patients to a particular subgroup. Thus, the suggested subgroup allocation needs to be seen as a statistical approximation of a best fit. Furthermore, in some patients, many heterogeneous patterns of sensory dysfunction can be detected in adjacent cutaneous areas.[35] Accordingly, various investigations, such as detailed testing of sensory function, chemical stimulation with capsaicin, and assessment of epidermal innervation density in patients with PHN, have clearly shown areas of relative preservation of sensory functions in close proximity to areas of impaired thermal sensation, both within the affected dermatome.[36] It also needs to be emphasized that sensory profiles may vary considerably over the time course of the disease. This might be in line with the observation that some patients respond very well to treatment early in the course of the disease and subsequently become more and more refractory along with the development of chronicity.

Another limitation in the predictive value of QST measurements for therapy was recently revealed by two independent studies on topically applied lidocaine. Topical lidocaine is assumed to act on ectopic discharges in hyperactive nociceptive fibers; thus, it was hypothesized that it might be particularly beneficial for patients with sensitized peripheral nociceptors rather than for patients with a loss of dermal nociceptors. Contrary to this hypothesis, however, no association between skin biopsies (epidermal and subepidermal innervation) or QST and the response to lidocaine was found in painful neuropathies.[37] Furthermore, PHN patients responded well to lidocaine even if the skin was completely deprived of nociceptors.[38] This disappointing finding once again emphasizes that the entire scenario of the individual somatosensory perception, and thus the whole variety of sensory abnormalities, requires precise analysis and might be more appropriate both for the investigation of the underlying mechanisms and as a potential predictor of treatment success.

Bearing these limitations in mind, a classification of patients based on the sensory profile within the most painful skin area allows for detection of the predominant individual sensory profile and the most likely underlying pain-generating mechanism.

CONCLUSION

The approach of classifying and subgrouping patients with neuropathic pain on the basis of symptoms or signs facilitates the stratification of patients in clinical trials based on sensory profiles and thus potential underlying mechanisms. Results of questionnaires or QST analyses can be used to calculate a priori to which subgroup one particular patient belongs with the highest probability. The future benefits of such a selection process will be twofold: (1) In clinical proof-of-concept trials, the study population can be enriched prospectively on the basis of a priori defined entry criteria. This enrichment with patients who potentially require a specific treatment will increase the likelihood of positive trial outcomes. (2) In clinical practice, it will be possible to establish an individualized therapy, that is, to identify the right patients who require a specific treatment option.

ACKNOWLEDGMENTS

Supported by the German Ministry of Research and Education, the German Research Network on Neuropathic Pain (BMBF, 1EM01/04), the National Health and Medical Research Council of Australia (NHMRC), the Ministry for Science and Education of Schleswig-Holstein, the EFIC-Grünenthal-Grant (EGG), the IMI "Europain" collaboration and industry members of this are: Astra Zeneca, Pfizer, Esteve, UCB-Pharma, Sanofi Aventis, Grünenthal, Eli Lilly, Neuroscience Technologies and Boehringer Ingelheim. This research was made possible by the support of Pfizer and Grünenthal GmbH. We would like to thank Birgit Brett for linguistic revision.

REFERENCES

1. Treede RD, Jensen TS, Campbell JN, et al. Neuropathic pain. Redefinition and a grading system for clinical and research purposes. *Neurology*. 2008;70:1630–1635.
2. Jensen TS, Baron R. Translation of symptoms and signs into mechanisms in neuropathic pain. *Pain*. 2003; 102:1–8.
3. Baron R. Mechanisms of disease: neuropathic pain—a clinical perspective. *Nat Clin Pract Neurol*. 2006;2:95–106.
4. Leijon G, Boivie J, Johansson I. Central post-stroke pain—neurological symptoms and pain characteristics. *Pain*. 1989;36:13–25.
5. Siddall PJ, McClelland JM, Rutkowski SB, Cousins MJ. A longitudinal study of the prevalence and characteristics of pain in the first 5 years following spinal cord injury. *Pain*. 2003;103:249–257.
6. Baron R, Binder A. How neuropathic is sciatica? The mixed pain concept. *Orthopäde*. 2004;33:568–575.
7. Freynhagen R, Rolke R, Baron R, et al. Pseudoradicular and radicular low-back pain—a disease continuum rather than different entities? Answers from quantitative sensory testing. *Pain*. 2008;135:65–74.
8. Fields HL, Rowbotham M, Baron R. Postherpetic neuralgia: irritable nociceptors and deafferentation. *Neurobiol Dis*. 1998;5:209–227.
9. Bouhassira D, Attal N, Fermanian J, et al. Development and validation of the Neuropathic Pain Symptom Inventory. *Pain*. 2004;108:248–257.
10. Cruccu G, Anand P, Attal N, et al. EFNS guidelines on neuropathic pain assessment. *Eur J Neurol*. 2004;11:153–162.
11. Rasmussen PV, Sindrup SH, Jensen TS, Bach FW. Symptoms and signs in patients with suspected neuropathic pain. *Pain*. 2004;110:461–469.
12. Bennett MI, Attal N, Backonja MM, et al. Using screening tools to identify neuropathic pain. *Pain*. 2007;127:199–203.
13. Freynhagen R, Tölle TR, Baron R. painDETECT—ein Palmtop-basiertes Verfahren für Versorgungsforschung, Qualitätsmanagement und Screening bei chronischen Schmerzen. *Akt Neurol*. 2005; 34:P641.
14. Galer BS, Jensen MP. Development and preliminary validation of a pain measure specific to neuropathic pain: the Neuropathic Pain Scale. *Neurology*. 1997;48:332–338.
15. Galer BS, Jensen MP, Ma T, Davies PS, Rowbotham MC. The lidocaine patch 5% effectively treats all neuropathic pain qualities: results of a randomized, double-blind, vehicle-controlled, 3-week efficacy study with use of the neuropathic pain scale. *Clin J Pain*. 2002;18:297–301.
16. Levendoglu F, Ogun CO, Ozerbil O, Ogun TC, Ugurlu H. Gabapentin is a first line drug for the treatment of neuropathic pain in spinal cord injury. *Spine (Phila, Pa, 1976)*. 2004;29:743–751.
17. Vinik AI, Tuchman M, Safirstein B, et al. Lamotrigine for treatment of pain associated with diabetic neuropathy: results of two randomized, double-blind, placebo-controlled studies. *Pain*. 2007;128:169–179.
18. Jensen MP, Gammaitoni AR, Olaleye DO, Oleka N, Nalamachu SR, Galer BS. The Pain Quality Assessment Scale: assessment of pain quality in carpal tunnel syndrome. *J Pain*. 2006;7:823–832.
19. Rog DJ, Nurmikko TJ, Friede T, Young CA. Randomized, controlled trial of cannabis-based medicine in central pain in multiple sclerosis. *Neurology*. 2005;65:812–819.
20. Victor TW, Jensen MP, Gammaitoni AR, Gould EM, White RE, Galer BS. The dimensions of pain quality: factor analysis of the Pain Quality Assessment Scale. *Clin J Pain*. 2008;24:550–555.
21. Attal N, Fermanian C, Fermanian J, Lanteri-Minet M, Alchaar H, Bouhassira D. Neuropathic pain: are there distinct subtypes depending on the aetiology or anatomical lesion? *Pain*. 2008;138:343–353.

22. Ranoux D, Attal N, Morain F, Bouhassira D. Botulinum toxin type A induces direct analgesic effects in chronic neuropathic pain. *Ann Neurol*. 2008;64:274–283.

23. Truini A, Padua L, Biasiotta A, et al. Differential involvement of A-delta and A-beta fibres in neuropathic pain related to carpal tunnel syndrome. *Pain*. 2009;145:105–109.

24. Dworkin RH, Turk DC, Revicki DA, et al. Development and initial validation of an expanded and revised version of the Short-Form McGill Pain Questionnaire (SF-MPQ-2). *Pain*. 2009;144:35–42.

25. Rolke R, Baron R, Maier C, et al. Quantitative sensory testing in the German Research Network on Neuropathic Pain (DFNS): standardized protocol and reference values. *Pain*. 2006;123:231–243.

26. Maier C., Baron R, Tölle TR, et al. Quantitative sensory testing in the German Research Network on Neuropathic Pain (DFNS): somatosensory abnormalities in 1236 patients with different neuropathic pain syndromes. *Pain*. 2010;150:439–450.

27. McDermott AM, Toelle TR, Rowbotham DJ, Schaefer CP, Dukes EM. The burden of neuropathic pain: results from a cross-sectional survey. *Eur J Pain*. 2006;10:127–135.

28. Davies M, Brophy S, Williams R, Taylor A. The prevalence, severity, and impact of painful diabetic peripheral neuropathy in type 2 diabetes. *Diabetes Care*. 2006;29:1518–1522.

29. Acquadro C, Berzon R, Dubois D, et al. Incorporating the patient's perspective into drug development and communication: an ad hoc task force report of the Patient-Reported Outcomes (PRO) Harmonization Group meeting at the Food and Drug Administration, February 16, 2001. *Value Health*. 2003;6:522–531.

30. Baron R, Tölle TR, Gockel U, Brosz M, Freynhagen R. A cross sectional cohort survey in 2100 patients with painful diabetic neuropathy and postherpetic neuralgia: differences in demographic data and sensory symptoms. *Pain*. 2009; 146:34–40.

31. Scholz J, Mannion RJ, Hord DE, et al. A novel tool for the assessment of pain: validation in low back pain. *PLoS Med*. 2009;6:e1000047.

32. Dworkin RH, O'Connor AB, Backonja M, et al. Pharmacologic management of neuropathic pain: evidence-based recommendations. *Pain*. 2007; 132:237–251.

33. Katz J, Finnerup NB, Dworkin RH. Clinical trial outcome in neuropathic pain: relationship to study characteristics. *Neurology*. 2008;70:263–272.

34. Woolf CJ, Bennett GJ, Doherty M, et al. Towards a mechanism-based classification of pain? *Pain*. 1998;77:227–229.

35. Pappagallo M, Oaklander AL, Quatrano-Piacentini AL, Clark MR, Raja SN. Heterogeneous patterns of sensory dysfunction in postherpetic neuralgia suggest multiple pathophysiologic mechanisms. *Anesthesiology*. 2000;92:691–698.

36. Petersen KL, Fields HL, Brennum J, Sandroni P, Rowbotham MC. Capsaicin evoked pain and allodynia in post-herpetic neuralgia. *Pain*. 2000; 88:125–133.

37. Herrmann DN, Pannoni V, Barbano RL, Pennella-Vaughan J, Dworkin RH. Skin biopsy and quantitative sensory testing do not predict response to lidocaine patch in painful neuropathies. *Muscle Nerve*. 2006;33:42–48.

38. Wasner G, Kleinert A, Binder A, Schattschneider J, Baron R. Postherpetic neuralgia: topical lidocaine is effective in nociceptor-deprived skin. *J Neurol*. 2005;252:677–686.

6

Diagnostic Testing

Nerve Conduction Studies, Quantitative Sensory Testing, Autonomic Testing, Skin/Nerve Biopsy, and Pain Scales

ANDREW W. VARGA AND CHRISTOPHER H. GIBBONS

NEUROPATHIC PAIN IS not a disease or a diagnosis, but rather a complex physiological manifestation caused by an injury to the peripheral or central nervous system. A significant and ongoing debate currently rages about the utility of diagnostic localization in patients with neuropathic pain, particularly when the pain has become chronic and has a mixed nociceptive and neuropathic picture.[1-4] However, it is clear that diagnosis of a treatable underlying disorder is still critical to the prevention and management of many neuropathic pain conditions, requiring the use of many available tools to confirm or deny a specific diagnosis.

Two general categories of investigation can be considered when attempting to identify a source of neuronal damage: tests that measure neurological function or neurological structure. Measures of neurological function range from simple physical examinations and pain assessment questionnaires to complex neurophysiological assessments of nerve fiber subtypes through nerve conduction studies, autonomic testing, or quantitative sensory testing. Measures of neurological structure can be directly investigated by pathological examination of nerve fiber tissue through sural nerve biopsy or cutaneous skin biopsy. Anatomical details of nerve fibers can be monitored through a variety of imaging modalities, but they will not be addressed in this chapter.

A variety of methods exist to study neural structure and function, and each technique has its own strengths and limitations. The relevance of an abnormal test result must be considered in the context of the patient's underlying neuropathic condition to avoid attributing the pain to an unrelated test result. In this chapter, we will provide a brief overview of the various diagnostic tests that may be considered in the evaluation of a patient with neuropathic pain.

NERVE CONDUCTION STUDIES

Overview

Nerve conduction studies play an extensive role in the evaluation of peripheral nerve function.[5–7] The basic principle of nerve conduction studies is that a supramaximal electrical stimulation can initiate a neural impulse that propagates along a sensory, motor, or mixed nerve fiber. There are differences between the results of these two techniques: sensory conductions measure the velocity of the transmission along the sensory nerve by stimulating at one site and recording over the same nerve at another site, while motor conductions stimulate along the nerve but record over a muscle.

Sensory nerves are stimulated and recorded over the nerve fiber itself, resulting in a sensory nerve action potential (SNAP). The SNAP amplitude is a relative measure of the number of axons that conduct between stimulation and recording sites. Reductions in SNAP amplitude suggest a pathological process affecting the number of axons.[8] Sensory distal latencies measure the time elapsed between the stimulation of a nerve and the arrival of an action potential at the recording site. When stimulating at a proximal and a distal site of a nerve, the conduction velocity can be measured by dividing the distance by the difference in distal latencies. Conduction velocities provide a relative measure of axonal myelination; reductions below normative values with intact sensory amplitudes suggest a problem primarily affecting the myelin sheathing and not the axon itself.[8]

Unlike sensory nerves, motor nerves are stimulated over the nerve while the potential is recorded over the muscle itself. The compound muscle action potential (CMAP) represents the sum of the synchronous electrical activity of the activated muscle fibers under the recording electrode. Similar to the SNAP, the CMAP amplitude is an approximate measure of the number of conducting axons. The CMAP recording electrode is placed directly over the belly of the muscle while a reference electrode is placed over the tendon of the same muscle. Motor distal latencies therefore include the time necessary for transmission across the neuromuscular junction and spread along the muscle membrane in addition to propagation along the nerve fiber.[9] Motor conduction velocities are also calculated by dividing the distance between two stimulating sites by the difference in distal latencies.

Diagnostic Utility

Nerve conduction studies aid in localizing damage to specific regions of the peripheral nervous system. Impairments to sensory nerve conduction indicate damage to a specific nerve; if the conduction study is normal, this indicates that a lesion is proximal to the dorsal root ganglia. Motor nerve conduction studies determine if weakness is due to damage to the peripheral nerve or some other component of the motor unit. The ability to differentiate between peripheral neuropathy, radiculopathy, and mononeuropathies, or between sensory and motor selective damage, can narrow a differential diagnosis dramatically. Nerve conduction studies can also determine if neuropathic damage is primarily demyelinating (reduced conduction velocity) or axonal (reduced amplitude) and can also localize the region of damage. An example of the direct utility of nerve conduction studies is the patient that presents with burning pain in the feet and has clear evidence of an entrapment of the posterior tibial nerve at the tarsal tunnel; surgical decompression could relieve the neuropathic symptoms.[10] In contrast, if the same patient did not have evidence of damage to the posterior tibial nerve, and instead had normal nerve conduction studies, a diagnosis of small-fiber neuropathy could be considered with entirely different treatments.[11]

Strengths

Nerve conduction studies have been extensively evaluated across a range of normal and disease-related conditions with comprehensive data on sensitivity and specificity.[12,13] Nerve conduction studies have been utilized in clinical trials investigating neuropathy, both in response to disease modification and for relief of neuropathic pain.[14,15] Manufacturers of electromyographic (EMG) equipment follow standard guidelines for production, so results can be interpreted and compared using different types of equipment across studies and institutions. Because of this standardization, nerve conductions studies can provide diagnostic certainty leading to direct treatment and clinical response in a variety of disparate medical conditions such as distal polyneuropathy, acute and chronic demyelinating neuropathies, neuromuscular junction defects, and focal entrapment syndromes.[12,16]

Weaknesses

Although nerve conductions studies can be very powerful tools in the assessment of peripheral nerve fiber function, they only investigate the largest and most rapidly conducting myelinated nerve fibers. Small myelinated and unmyelinated nociceptive fibers, frequently implicated in many neuropathic pain syndromes, cannot be measured using these techniques.[17] Many patients with severe neuropathic pain from diseases such as distal small-fiber neuropathy, amyloidosis, complex regional pain syndrome, or focal dermatomal injuries from herpes zoster may have completely normal nerve conduction studies.[11,18,19]

QUANTITATIVE SENSORY TESTING

Overview

Quantitative sensory testing (QST) is a standardized, quantifiable method to assess many aspects of physical sensation, such as vibration and thermal and pain perception thresholds.[20] The QST is rooted in the neurological sensory exam, where monofilament sensation testing, vibratory testing with a tuning fork, and pain sensation testing with a pin have been guiding principles. Quantitative sensory testing is considered a psychophysical test in which stimulation is applied to a subject and the subject must indicate when a response is detected.[21,22] A number of QST testing paradigms exist; two of the most commonly used are the method of limits and the method of levels.

The *method of limits* starts with a stimulus that is below the threshold of detection and

gradually increases in intensity until a subject detects the sensation[23,24] (Figure 6-1). For example, thermal stimuli might start at a neutral (undetectable) temperature (32°C) and gradually increase for warm detection or gradually decrease for cold detection. The subject would indicate at what temperature he or she felt an initial sensation. After several trials, most subjects can provide a reliable and reproducible result. The same approach can be used for painful stimuli, in which the subject responds to a gradually increasing (or decreasing) temperature indicating the heat-pain and cold-pain thresholds, respectively. This testing paradigm is highly dependent on the ability of the subject to detect and respond to the stimuli, so mental status and physical ability to respond may alter the results.[22]

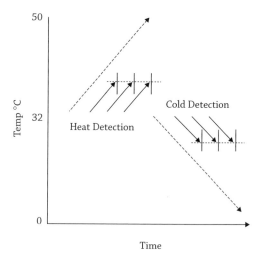

FIGURE 6.1 Quantitative sensory testing—method of limits. This figure demonstrates a sample testing paradigm for detection of heat and cold detection thresholds. In this example, a sample stimulus gradually changes in intensity. If the patient does not respond to the stimulus, it will continue until a maximal (or minimal) threshold is reached, shown as the initial long-dash line. However, if the patient responds to a stimulus (the vertical line stopping the stimulus), an average of the results is taken and recorded as the sensory detection threshold (shown as the dotted lines). This example reveals a hypothetical, and perfect, patient response. More variability to the response is the norm, requiring more careful analysis of the results to determine validity.

The *method of levels* incorporates applied stimuli of standard intensity and duration. The subject indicates if a response was detected by a "yes" or "no" (Figure 6-2).[23,24] The stimulation is increased or decreased accordingly, depending on the patient's response. This paradigm can be conducted with thermal, thermal pain, or vibratory detection thresholds. This *forced-choice* approach reduces confounding variables such as reaction time but dramatically increases the duration of testing.[25] A number of additional complexities can be inserted into the testing paradigm that can increase sensitivity and specificity, but at the cost of additional testing time.[26]

Diagnostic Utility

Quantitative sensory testing can identify regions of cutaneous abnormality to aid in the diagnosis of peripheral neuropathy or mononeuropathies. The strongest evidence for the use of QST comes

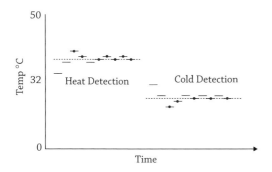

FIGURE 6.2 Quantitative sensory testing—method of levels. This figure demonstrates a sample paradigm for detection of heat and cold thresholds using a method of levels. An unchanging stimulus of a certain temperature is provided, and the subject responds whether he or she feels it (shown by the line with a circle) or not (the straight line). This methods uses a *four, two, one stepping paradigm* in which the initial changes are larger (four steps) until a detection is noted; then the distance between steps decreases (two steps apart) until a threshold is determined by single steps (the dotted line) for both heat and cold detection thresholds. This example reveals a clear patient response; a more variable response prolong the number of steps, increases the duration of testing, and may reduce the validity of the result.

from studies of diabetic peripheral neuropathy, in which many clinical trials have utilized QST in a longitudinal fashion to study changes in peripheral nerve function.[27-29] Quantitative sensory testing can also detect neuropathies severe enough to put subjects at risk for ulceration or neurogenic arthropathy.[30] Quantitative sensory testing may also play a role in the diagnosis of toxic neuropathies, small-fiber neuropathies, and entrapment neuropathies.[21,31-34]

Strengths

Quantitative sensory testing can measure responses from large myelinated nerve fibers, lightly myelinated nerve fibers, and even unmyelinated nerve fibers.[21] This method has been widely published across clinical trials and is widely accepted as a research tool.[23,35,36] The topographical distribution of sensory loss seen in QST can identify specific patterns of nerve injury, such as a length-dependent neuropathy or focal mononeuropathy. Quantitative sensory testing is easily repeated and can be used to monitor disease progression in cases of diabetic or other neuropathies. In addition, QST can monitor nerve recovery after injury.[30,33] Unlike nerve conduction studies, which can only investigate peripheral nerve fibers, QST can identify sensory loss from damage anywhere along the neural axis, including the central nervous system.[37-40]

Weaknesses

Quantitative sensory testing has been studied in a variety of clinical scenarios over many years, yet it has never achieved the same widespread use as nerve conduction studies and is therefore not as widely available. Manufacturers of QST equipment do not provide identical stimuli or testing techniques; thus, results cannot be interpreted across studies using different equipment or testing paradigms.[41] In addition, the psychophysical nature of the test leads to variability due to differences in medication effects, personal bias, and testing environments.[22] After a certain period of time, most subjects will begin to lose focus. Further testing only reduces testing reliability, so the examiner must be cognizant of testing fatigue.

AUTONOMIC TESTING

Overview

Tests of autonomic function can assess the parasympathetic, sympathetic adrenergic, and sympathetic cholinergic portions of the autonomic nervous system (ANS). Due to the widespread distribution of autonomic innervation, there are a large variety of organ- specific tests that can assess autonomic function (genitourinary, gastrointestinal, ophthalmic, pulmonary, etc.). This chapter will discuss the most common autonomic tests and those most relevant to the investigation of diseases resulting in neuropathic pain.

Tests of cardiovascular function monitor both the sympathetic and parasympathetic branches of the ANS and can examine the integrity of the ANS from the atria and ventricles to the peripheral vascular system. In most cases, both the sympathetic and parasympathetic components of these tests can be derived simultaneously using continuous, noninvasive, beat-to-beat blood pressure monitoring with continuous electrocardiographic (ECG) recording. Tests of cardiovascular parasympathetic function include the heart rate response to deep breathing, the heart rate response to a Valsalva maneuver, and the heart rate response to standing (Figures 6-3 and 6-4). Heart rate variability declines with age and with diseases that damage the ANS, such as diabetes, human immunodeficiency virus (HIV) and amyloidosis.[42–46] Age- and sex-based normative data are available, values below which suggest damage to the parasympathetic nervous system.[47,48] Tests of sympathetic adrenergic function include the blood pressure response to the Valsalva maneuver, the tilt table test, the standing test, and the

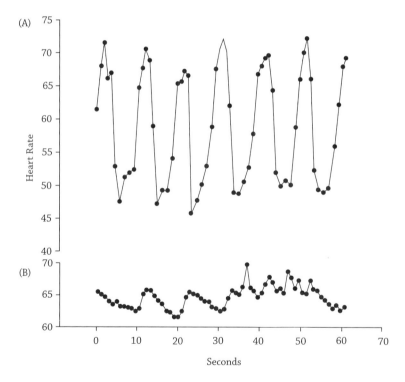

FIGURE 6.3 The heart rate variation in response to deep breathing. The natural variation in heart rate (the sinus arrhythmia) is exaggerated in response to slow, deep breaths. Increasing age and damage to the autonomic nervous system can reduce the normal variability and suggest dysfunction of the parasympathetic nervous system. In (A), a young, healthy individual is breathing at a rate of six breaths per minute and has a variation in heart rate of more than 20 beats, which is normal. A patient with peripheral autonomic neuropathy (B) has reduced heart rate variability, with a variation of less than five beats, which is abnormal.

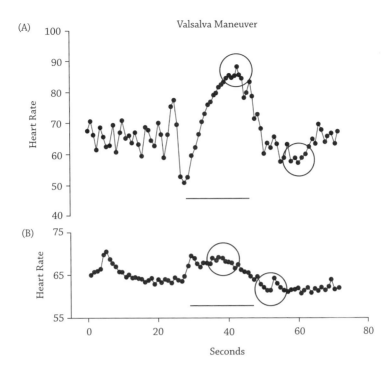

FIGURE 6.4 The heart rate response to a Valsalva maneuver. As an individual exhales against resistance (the solid black line from 30–45 seconds above the x-axis), there is a significant change in the heart rate, a measure of parasympathetic function. In (A), a normal individual has a large change in heart rate, with a Valsalva ratio of 1.6 (the circles denote maximum and minimum values). A patient with peripheral autonomic neuropathy (the same one from Figure 6.3) has a reduced heart rate response, with a ratio of only 1.1.

cold pressor test.[49] Orthostatic hypotension is diagnosed as a fall in systolic blood pressure of ≥20 mmHg or in diastolic blood pressure of ≥10 mmHg within 3 min of upright tilt or standing.[49a] [position paper 1996] The Valsalva maneuver and the cold pressor test are useful adjunctive studies for the overall assessment of autonomic function, but individually they have lower sensitivity and specificity than the tilt or standing test for diagnosing sympathetic adrenergic dysfunction.[50]

Tests of sudomotor autonomic function are often referred to as *sweat tests*. Sudomotor nerves extend throughout the skin, are closely integrated with thermal regulation, and play a critical role in heat dissipation. Tests of sudomotor function may include the quantitative sudomotor axon reflex test (QSART) or the thermoregulatory sweat test (TST). Although a number of additional tests of sudomotor function exist, such as the silicone impression

technique,[51,52] quantitative direct and indirect reflex testing,[53] and the sweat-spot test, they are not as widely utilized. Both the QSART and the TST study sweat production, the QSART through a humidity detection capsule that is placed on the skin and the TST through an indicator dye that changes color in the presence of moisture (sweat). With QSART, production of sweat is stimulated by acetyl-choline iontophoresis, causing a local axon reflex-mediated sweat production. This is measured by the local change in humidity in the capsule (Figure 6-5).

In contrast, a TST places the subject in a heated chamber to raise the core body temperature by approximately 1–1.5°C, causing sweat production over the entire body. An indicator dye is applied over the subject's entire body and changes color where sweat is produced, creating a topographical map of sweat production[54] (Figure 6-6). The major difference between

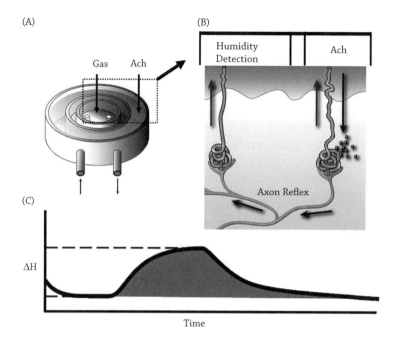

FIGURE 6.5   Quantitative sudomotor axon reflex testing (QSART). A capsule that contains three concentric chambers (A) is placed over the skin. The outermost circle is filled with acetylcholine (or another charged substance) and is iontophoresed into the skin to stimulate sweating. The middle capsule acts as a vapor barrier to prevent seepage of the acetylcholine into the innermost chamber, where changes in humidity are monitored. The acetylcholine causes direct sweating (B) in sweat glands under that portion of the capsule, but also causes axon reflex sweating in more distal sweat glands where sweat detection is measured. The output (C) is measured as a change in humidity (ΔH) over time and can be quantified by maximal changes or area under the curve analysis.

these techniques is that QSART measures postganglionic sweat production (i.e., it evaluates local sudomotor nerve fiber integrity in the region of testing), while the TST measures both pre- and postganglionic sweat production simultaneously (but is unable to localize the site of the lesion).

Diagnostic Utility

Tests of cardiovascular autonomic function may detect early signs of a length-dependent neuropathy and may support other tests of peripheral nerve function. Studies have demonstrated abnormal autonomic tests in patients with painful neuropathy[55]; however, the overall diagnostic utility of cardiovascular autonomic function testing in patients with neuropathic pain is not clear. The measured endpoints are not themselves directly implicated in most neuropathic pain conditions.

Tests of sudomotor function have a much greater historical role in the evaluation of neuropathic pain in diseases such as complex regional pain syndrome, where localized sudomotor and vasomotor dysfunction is easily detected. Quantitative sudomotor axon reflex testing is used to detect a difference in sudomotor function between opposite limbs or in a length-dependent fashion against which established normative values are compared.[52,56] The TST is a topographic measure of sudomotor function that can identify length-dependent neuropathies, specific radiculopathies, or injuries to specific nerves (Figure 6-6).[52,57]

Strengths

Autonomic function testing has well-established normative values and a long history of clinical testing across a number of specific diseases. Autonomic testing may also provide the earliest

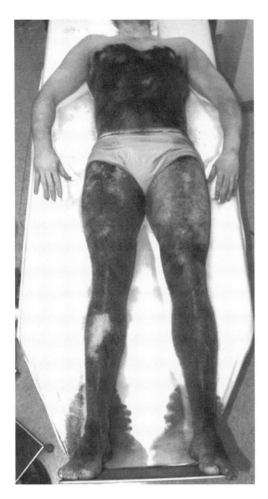

underlying nerve injury when the cause of neuropathic pain is unknown.

Weaknesses

Despite its clinical utility in many diseases that result in autonomic neuropathies, cardiovascular autonomic testing is still unlikely to play a major role in the diagnosis of neuropathic pain states. Autonomic testing, although relatively easy to perform, is available at only a few generalized testing centers. Sudomotor function testing carries more direct clinical diagnostic utility in neuropathic pain states but, unfortunately, is even less widely available than cardiovascular autonomic testing. Many tests of sudomotor function can be performed without specialized testing equipment, but few physicians have the time to take advantage of such opportunities. Most autonomic tests are lengthy to administer, with generally poor reimbursement by insurers.

SKIN AND NERVE BIOPSY

Overview

Pathological evaluation of nerve fiber structure has historically been the only means to diagnose certain types of rare neuropathies, such as amyloidosis, sarcoidosis, and vasculitis. The most common site of nerve biopsy is the sural nerve. The superficial peroneal nerve is also occasionally used, particularly when a simultaneous muscle biopsy is required.[59] The nerve biopsy has slowly gone out of favor as other tests of nerve fiber structure and function have become more widely utilized and more easily accessible. There are few remaining disorders in which sural nerve biopsy is essential for diagnosis, but the diagnosis of demyelinating and multiple mononeuropathies can be aided by the use of nerve biopsy.[60] Unfortunately, for the procedure to have any diagnostic utility, nerve biopsies must be performed at centers with experience in processing the tissue.

A more recent addition to the armamentarium of the neurologist has been the development of skin biopsy as a means to directly assess the cutaneous nociceptive C fibers.[18] Although not universally available, skin biopsy has achieved widespread use for both clinical

FIGURE 6.6   Thermoregulatory sweat test (TST). An individual is placed in a chamber where the core temperature is increased by 1.5°C, causing diffuse sweat production to cool the body. An indicator dye (in this case alizarin red) is placed over the individual and turns purple in the presence of sweat. In a normal response, the entire body would be covered completely. In this example, the subject has had a thoracic sympathectomy and so does not sweat above T4. The subject also had an injury to the right lateral cutaneous nerve of the calf (a branch of the peroneal nerve) during knee surgery several years ago that was previously unknown but is clearly evident in the territory of absent sweating.

neurophysiological evidence of a distal small-fiber neuropathy.[58] The combination of cardiovascular autonomic and sudomotor function testing can identify many patients with subtle nerve fiber damage, thus providing support for a diagnosis of

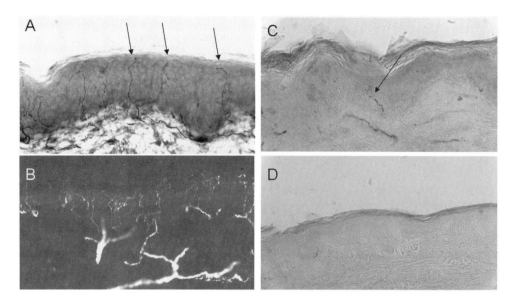

FIGURE 6.7   Cutaneous innervation by skin biopsy. Nerve fibers (shown with arrows), stained with the pan-axonal marker PGP 9.5, can be seen extending from the dermal to the epidermal layers by light microscopy (A) and confocal microscopy (B). The fibers are often more easily identified by confocal imaging due to a reduction in background staining, thereby improving the visual contrast. However, the dermal-epidermal junction is more difficult to identify without the use of additional stains (such as collagen or basement membrane proteins). A patient with a distal small-fiber neuropathy and reduced nerve fiber density is seen, with a single nerve fiber remaining in the epidermal layer (shown with the arrow in C). A patient with a severe reduction in both dermal and epidermal nerve fibers can be seen in (D).

and research purposes.[61,62] In most cases, a standard 3 mm dermatological punch biopsy specimen is obtained and the tissue is stained with the pan-axonal marker protein gene product 9.5 (PGP 9.5)[63] (Figure 6-7). This minimally invasive technique is now more popular than sural nerve biopsy with both patients and physicians. Epidermal nociceptive C fibers can be quantified using standard counting techniques and compared to age-based normative values.[64] Abnormalities are seen in a length-dependent fashion in many peripheral neuropathies, but reduced nerve fiber counts are also seen with focal abnormalities due to mononeuropathies, radiculopathy, and other peripheral nerve injuries.[65]

Diagnostic Utility

Nerve biopsies has provided very useful diagnostic discrimination, as well as altered management, in 60% of 50 consecutive patients referred for nerve biopsy.[60] The most common

diseases aided by biopsy include vasculitis, amyloidosis, sarcoidosis, and leprosy. The diagnostic utility of nerve biopsies extends to a large number of other diseases, including anti-myelin associated glycoprotein (anti-MAG) neuropathy, chronic inflammatory demyelinating polyradiculoneuropathy, small-fiber neuropathies, hereditary neuropathies, giant axonal neuropathy, and neoplastic infiltration, but the relatively high rate of adverse outcomes and the increasing value of noninvasive testing warrant cautious use of this investigatory tool.[66]

Skin biopsy can quantify the number of nociceptive C fibers seen in a given tissue section and can therefore diagnosis a length-dependent neuropathy, a focal neuropathy, or other damage to small unmyelinated nerve fibers. Abnormal findings can be seen in acquired or systemic diseases that result in neuropathy, such as diabetes, HIV, sarcoidosis, celiac disease, Sjogren syndrome, and other neuropathies affecting small nerve fibers.[67-71] The true utility of the skin biopsy technique is the ability to quantify the number of unmyelinated C fibers in a given sample. The results can be compared against standard values to document the presence or absence of neuropathy, as well as to document disease progression or remission in the same subject.[72–74] Skin biopsy is often helpful in conditions of painful small-fiber neuropathy, in which other functional and structural tests may yield normal results.

Strengths

Although not frequently utilized, nerve biopsy is still the most definitive means to diagnose certain types of rare neuropathy, such as amyloidosis, vasculitis, and sarcoidosis (particularly when other tissues or organ systems are not affected). In many cases, no other test is available to confirm these diagnoses. If necessary, a biopsy can be repeated on the opposite limb to identify ongoing disease or the response to therapy. In general, a nerve biopsy is recommended only in patients with symptoms that are very distressing to the patient, or are progressively worsening, and when the diagnosis cannot be made through less invasive means.

Skin biopsy is a simple, minimally invasive technique to quantify the number of epidermal nerve fibers. Standardized methodologies have been agreed upon and normative values published by a number of different testing centers.[75,76] Tests can document a length-dependent neuropathy or focal damage in diseases such as complex regional pain syndrome.[77,78] Morphological abnormalities, such as nerve fiber swellings, can further augment the utility of skin biopsies by suggesting ongoing axonal damage to nerve fibers.[79,80] Finally, skin biopsies are becoming more widely utilized to investigate structural changes to other parts of the nervous system, such as autonomic nerve fibers, although these preliminary data need further validation.[81,82]

Weaknesses

Nerve biopsy can provide a great deal of information on the health of the peripheral nervous system, but it is invasive and results in a permanent sensory deficit that may be painful to many patients.[59,60] Few centers have the experience to properly perform the biopsy and analyze the tissue, thus limiting the access to this procedure. In addition, the number of different tissue preparations and stains necessary for making a diagnosis can be broad, labor-intensive and time-consuming.

Skin biopsy can determine that a neuropathy exists but, unlike nerve biopsies, it cannot identify the reason for the neuropathy.[65,83] For example, skin biopsy cannot reliably differentiate vasculitic, demyelinating, or amyloid neuropathies. Some patients with painful symptoms suggestive of small-fiber neuropathy may have normal skin biopsies. This may be due to ongoing small nerve fiber damage that has not yet reduced nerve fiber density to a level below the normal range, or it may be due to functional impairments of nociceptive C fibers that have not resulted in measurable structural damage.

PAIN SCORES

Pain is a complex physiological phenomenon that crosses physiological, emotional, and social boundaries. Though there has been a push to treat pain as an additional vital sign, quantifying pain has been fraught with difficulty. While mechanisms to quantify pain exist, including quantitative sensory testing, skin biopsy, imaging, and nerve conduction studies, these are impractical to perform on a routine basis and do not likely capture many subjective pain qualities.

On the surface, it seems rather straightforward to attempt to qualify pain with simple verbal assessments—though even these can be divided into purely qualitative adjectival descriptors and pseudoquantitative numerical estimates. Still, such scales tend to focus primarily on the intensity of pain and fail to capture other important components, such as affective aspects of pain (i.e., how much pain is bothersome), temporal changes, effects of medicines, interference with daily activities, pain location, association with specific disease entities, or pain descriptors that might suggest differing underlying neurophysiological mechanisms. Literally hundreds of pain scales have been created with staggering variability and specificity. There is even a pain scale that specifically evaluates the relative pain caused by different hymenopteran stings (the Schmidt Sting Pain Index) with elaborate descriptions.[84]

Like any measurement tool, pain scales are only useful if they satisfy certain criteria, primarily validity, responsiveness, and reliability. *Validity* refers to the appropriateness of a scale for a specific end and asks whether the scale is measuring the intended outcome. This type of validity typically falls under the more specific category *content validity*. Researchers care most about two other types of validity, namely, *criterion validity*, which assesses a scale's ability to detect changes with treatment or predict important outcomes,[85] and *construct validity*, which evaluates a scale's ability to recapitulate the findings of scales that measure the same pain dimension. Although construct validity has some utility, it is one aspect that has been criticized, since the comparator may be flawed in its own right, and differences can be exaggerated if the comparator is measuring blended dimensions of pain. *Responsiveness* examines the ability of a scale to manifest clinically important changes over time in regard to treatment or natural history. Although responsiveness is in fact a component of criterion validity,[86] it tends to be examined as a separate category due to its importance in clinical trials. *Reliability* refers to the ability of a scale to yield reproducible results, both within an individual patient and across patients. Reliability can be confounded by a number of variables, including the setting, the interaction with the test administrator, motivational factors, and emotional state.[85] Scales that make a great effort to satisfy these criteria can become increasingly complex and need to be balanced with the factor of participant burden—both for the administrator and for the test recipient.

PAIN SCORES—INTENSITY SCALES

Overview

Perhaps the most obvious component of pain and the aspect for which the earliest scales were developed is pain intensity. Numerical rating scales (NRS), visual analog scales (VAS), and verbal rating scales (VRS) represent the most common measures of pain intensity.[87] Numerical rating scales consist of a range of numbers, typically 0 through 10 (although many variants exist). Examinees are told that 0 represents "no pain" and 10 "the worst imaginable pain" and then are asked to state, write, or circle the number that best indicates either their pain at the moment or their average level of pain over the past 24 hours. Visual analog scales typically contain a horizontal line, the ends of which are labeled with pain descriptors similar to those in the numerical rating scales (e.g., "no pain" at one end and "the worst imaginable pain" at the other). Examinees are then asked to intersect the line at the point that represents their estimate of the pain. Visual analog scales consist of a list of adjectival descriptors of pain, typically consisting of four to eight words describing increasing pain intensity. Patients are asked which word best describes their pain intensity, and a post hoc numerical value is assigned to each adjective. Interestingly, rescue analgesics themselves have been used to construct pain scales based on the class used, the amount used, and the time until used.[88] However, these data can be obscured by patients taking multiple rescue medications, physicians' and patients' attitudes toward the use of rescue medications, patients' concurrent use of nonpharmacological means to alleviate pain, and patients' use of analgesic medicines for alternative reasons. An overview of these pain scales is shown in Table 6.1.

Diagnostic Utility

Numerical scales reflect relative pain gradations; thus, changes in the pain score may reflect uncertain levels of significant pain reduction. In order to avoid the challenges of interpreting relative changes to pain scores in the absence of clinical outcomes, Farrar et al. defined a clinically relevant change in pain as one not requiring a rescue dose during the titration phase of clinical trials examining pain relief for breakthrough cancer pain.[89] They found that an absolute change of 2 points on a 0–10 numerical rating scale or a 33% change on a 0–100 percentage scale represented the change most balanced in sensitivity and specificity for detecting meaningful pain reduction.[89] This was later corroborated in a study in which an average change of 1.8

Table 6-1. Pain Scores—Intensity Scales

SCALE NAME	BRIEF DESCRIPTION	PAIN DIMENSION	STRENGTHS	WEAKNESSES
Numerical rating scale (NRS)	A simple numerical scale, typically from 0 to 10	Any, though typically intensity	Simplicity of administration	Patients treat scale nonlinearly
Visual analogue scale (VAS)	A numerical scale with a visual analog, such as horizontal or vertical lines or faces	Any, though typically intensity	Also relatively simple	Can confuse the elderly or sedated
Verbal rating scale (VRS)	A purely adjectival descriptive scale to which rankings are added post hoc	Any, though typically intensity	Allows for more concrete expression	Gradations can be arbitrary
Faces Pain Scale	Combination of numerical ands visual analog scale showing faces of increasing distress	Any, though typically intensity	Widely used in children and correlates with other NRS	Less reliable in young children; the optimal number of faces is unclear; underrates pain in adult men
Face, leg, arm, cry, and consolability (FLACC)	Measure of pain in children by observation	Intensity	Allows for pain rating in children who may not otherwise verbalize pain well	Observer bias; requires an interaction to rate consolability
Children's Hospital Eastern Ontario Pain Scale (CHEOPS)	Measure of pain in children by observation	Intensity	Allows for pain rating in children who may not otherwise verbalize pain well; test based solely on observation.	Observer bias

points on a 0–10 scale or 36% on a 0–100 scale represented a "meaningful change" in a cohort of patients who were asked retrospectively to rate such changes in pain.[90]

Assessing pain intensity can be challenging in both children and cognitively impaired older adults. The Faces Pain Scale represents a combination of an NRS and a VAS—in this case, one in which the visual analogues are faces depicting increasing distress. This scale has been employed widely in children and correlates well with other scales including an NRS.[91] Interestingly, two of the more commonly used scales in children are not self-report scales, but rather observational scales. FLACC is an acronym for face, leg, arm, cry, and consolability in which an observer rates

each of these categories on a 0- to 2-point scale, for a maximum total of 10.[92] CHEOPS similarly evaluates six categories (cry, facial, verbal, torso, wound touching, and legs), with a minimum score of 4 and a maximum score of 13.[93] Notably, other objective observational measures, such as respiratory rate and heart rate, correlate only loosely with pain intensity, perhaps because of their nonspecificity.[94]

Strengths

All three types of scales (numerical, visual, verbal) demonstrate good validity, reliability, and responsiveness, and all three scales correlate well with each other at least in terms of the directionality, if not the magnitude, of responses, the NRS appear to have the fewest complicating factors. The basic three scales are all very simple to administer and require little time and effort. The Faces Pain Scale is a useful adaptation that is helpful in the assessment of pain intensity in children.

Weaknesses

Visual analog scales tend to be less preferred by patients. Difficulty completing VAS has been demonstrated in patients with advanced age or with high opioid intake.[95,96] Verbal rating scales tend to be highly influenced by the adjectives used, their connotations, and their nonlinear nature (i.e., the difference between "very mild" and "mild" being the same as that between "mild" and "moderate"). A study comparing NRS and VRS in palliative care patients, in which the VRS contained six items labeled "none," "very mild," "mild," "moderate," "severe," and "very severe," demonstrated that although there was strong directional correlation, the "mild" descriptor corresponded to an 11-point NRS score of anywhere between 2 and 6 and a "moderate" descriptor of anywhere between 3 and 7 at baseline.[97] There has also been some question about the use of the Faces Pain Scale, especially in very young children, as to how finely they discriminate levels of pain and what the optimal number of faces should be.[98] This scale has also been validated in adults. However, at least one study demonstrated an underrating of pain in men due to a bias against choosing the strongest level of pain because of the presence of tears on the face.[99] Cognitively impaired older adults may also have difficulty rating their pain. In a comparison between a 5-item VRS, a 7-item faces scale, a 21-point horizontal box scale, and two vertical 21-point scales measuring pain intensity and unpleasantness, respectively, the 21-point horizontal box scale emerged as best in regard to psychometrics and validity.[100]

PAIN SCORES—TEMPORAL SCALES

Overview

Even the best scale of pain intensity suffers from its temporal limitations, as pain intensity is rarely static. If the pain is not constant, the frequency of pain episodes can be an important contributor to an individual's overall pain. When interventions are used, pharmacological or otherwise, the latency to relief as well as overall relief duration are therefore important factors.

Diagnostic Utility

One of the most frequently used scales that attempts to address this issue is the Brief Pain Inventory (BPI), in which four numerical scales, ranging from 0 to 10 and covering instantaneous pain intensity and worst, least, and average pain over a specified time, are averaged into a single score.[101] Other common scales attempting to measure temporal aspects include four- or five-item VRS in which individuals are asked to judge the frequency of their pain from "never" to "always." An overview of the BPI is shown in Table 6.2.

Strengths

The BPI has been shown to be highly internally consistent and has been validated across many cultures.[85] A reduction in the temporal frequency of pain can be as powerful a predictor of successful treatment as a reduction in the intensity of the pain.

Weaknesses

The temporal qualities of pain are strongly subject to recall bias. Attempts to solve the recall problem have utilized regular monitoring of pain through portable devices, but this substantially increases the time, complexity, and cost of the pain assessment. Although not utilized in routine clinical practice, this type of study is now entering use in clinical treatment trials of pain.

PAIN SCORES—AFFECTIVE SCALES

Overview

In addition to pain intensity, there are sensory components (e.g., burning, itching) and affective

Table 6-2. Pain Scores—Temporal and Affective Scales

SCALE NAME	BRIEF DESCRIPTION	PAIN DIMENSION	STRENGTHS	WEAKNESSES
Brief Pain Inventory (BPI)	Asks patients to estimate the worst, least, and average pain over a specified duration	Temporal	Acknowledges the nonstatic nature of pain	Recall bias
McGill Pain Questionnaire (MPQ)	Addresses four categories of pain using 78 verbal pain descriptors divided into 20 categories	Sensory, affective, evaluative, and miscellaneous	Affective component can be empirically distinguished from pain intensity	Cumbersome to administer
Short form McGill Pain Questionnaire (SF-MPQ)	Addresses two categories of pain using 15 pain descriptors	Sensory and affective pain	Easier to administer than the MPQ; broad experience in clinical trials of neuropathic pain	
Short form McGill Pain Questionnaire 2 (SF-MPQ-2)	Adds 7 questions to the SF-MPQ designed to evaluate neuropathic pain and uses an expanded 0–10 numerical rating scale for all questions	Sensory, affective, and neuropathic pain	Addresses a broad variety of pain components; responsive to changes in pain character and intensity	Not designed to differentiate neuropathic from nonneuropathic pain

descriptors (unpleasant, depressing) that contribute to an individual's overall pain. Studies have shown that the affective component can be empirically distinguished from the pain intensity.[95]

Diagnostic Utility

The scale used most often to address the affective component to pain is the McGill Pain Questionnaire (MPQ) and its subsidiary, the Short-Form MPQ (SF-MPQ).[102,103] The McGill Pain Questionnaire addresses four categories of pain: sensory, affective, evaluative, and miscellaneous. This scale uses 78 verbal pain descriptors divided into 20 categories as well as a total pain severity rating. The SF-MPQ addresses 15 sensory and affective verbal pain descriptors and calculates a total score as well as sensory and affective subset scores. More recently, the SF-MPQ-2 was devised in an effort to incorporate the affective component of pain with descriptors designed to address neuropathic pain.[104]

This scale contains seven additional questions (for a total of 22), asking patients to evaluate the feelings dull, electric shock, cold-freezing, pain caused by light touch, itching, tingling or pins and needles, and numbness. The authors are careful to point out that their wording was specifically chosen to consider nonpainful dysesthesias or paresthesias, which may differentiate the SF-MPQ-2 from other scales of neuropathic pain (see the section below on neuropathic pain). Additionally, in an effort to provide increased responsiveness, all 22 questions use an expanded 0–10 NRS compared to the prior 4-point rating scale. An overview of these affective scales is shown in Table 6.2.

Strengths

Because of its relative brevity, the SF-MPQ is easier to administer than the MPQ and has been shown to be reliable, well validated, and responsive.[95] The SF-MPQ also includes a pain intensity scale and a VAS in addition to the affective and sensory components. The SF-MPQ, because of its ease of administration, has been widely utilized in clinical trials and has been very successful in identifying the response to treatment.[105-107]

Weaknesses

The MPQ is lengthy and generally cumbersome to administer, but most of the drawbacks have been resolved using the aforementioned short form.

PAIN SCORES—INTERFERENCE SCALES

Overview

Pain interference is a concept that addresses the extent to which an individual's pain affects his or her quality of life across different domains. Rather than addressing how severe the pain is (pain intensity), interference measures how much the pain affects an individual's ability to participate in a specific task or perform an activity of daily living such as sleeping or walking.

Diagnostic Utility

The pain scale used most commonly to address interference is the Brief Pain Inventory Pain Interference Scale, which consists of seven 0–10 numerical scales. Individuals are asked to rate their pain's interference with general activities, mood, walking ability, work, interpersonal relations, sleep, and life enjoyment.[101] While this scale addresses pain interference alone, there are two commonly used scales that combine pain intensity and pain interference. The Bodily Pain Scale of the Medical Outcomes Study 36 Item Short Form (SF-36) measures various quality-of-life dimensions including ratings of general health, physical function, physical and emotional role limits, social function, mental health, bodily pain, and energy/vitality.[108] With regard specifically to cancer pain, the European Organization for Research and Treatment of Cancer Quality of Life Questionnaire for Cancer (EORTC QLQ-C30) assesses six quality-of-life domains and seven symptom domains including two 4-point verbal rating scales assessing

pain intensity and interference.[109] An overview of interference scales is shown in Table 6.3.

Strengths

The Brief Pain Inventory Pain Interference Scale is a simple, rapidly administered test and a reliable means to quantify the degree of interference that pain causes in daily life. The SF-36 and the EORTC QLQ-C30 both have good internal consistency and reliability despite containing a component of pain intensity.

Weaknesses

Both the SF-36 and the EORTC QLQ-C30 correlate only loosely correlate with measures of strict pain intensity, supporting the notion that pain interference is a distinct pain dimension.[85] This suggests that an additional scale of pain intensity is required in most cases.

NEUROPATHIC PAIN

Overview

Neuropathic pain is thought to differ from nociceptive pain (both somatic and visceral) in that the underlying pathophysiology and treatment methods likely differ. There has been a recent redefinition of neuropathic pain to refer to pain arising as a consequence of a lesion or disease affecting the somatosensory system.[110] Because of the imprecision in identifying neuropathic pain, due partly to the lack of specific diagnostic tools, an algorithm was created to help categorize the probability of neuropathic pain as unlikely, possible, probable, and definite. The algorithm was based on criteria examining whether the pain distribution is anatomically plausible, whether the history suggests a relevant lesion or disease, whether negative or positive sensory signs exist confined to the innervation territory, and whether other diagnostic testing exists to confirm a lesion or disease explaining the neuropathic pain.[110]

Diagnostic Utility

One of the earliest scales to address neuropathic pain was called, appropriately, the

Table 6-3. Pain Scores—Interference Scales

SCALE NAME	BRIEF DESCRIPTION	PAIN DIMENSION	STRENGTHS	WEAKNESSES
Brief Pain Inventory Pain Interference Scale	Seven 0–10 NRS asking individuals to rate their pain's interference with general activity, mood, walking ability, work, interpersonal relations, sleep, and life enjoyment	Interference	Addresses interference only	Cumbersome to administer
Medical Outcomes Study 36 Item Short Form (SF-36)	Measures various quality-of-life dimensions including ratings of general health, physical function, physical and emotional role limits, social function, mental health, bodily pain, and energy/vitality	Interference	Nondisease specific and most commonly used of the generic measures of health-related quality of life	Blends interference and intensity
European Organization for Research and Treatment of Cancer Quality of Life Questionnaire for Cancer (EORTC QLQ-C30)	Assesses six quality-of-life domains and seven symptom domains including two 4-point VRS assessing pain intensity and interference	Interference	Specific for cancer pain	Blends interference and intensity

Neuropathic Pain Scale (NPS).[111] The NPS consists of 10 questions, 6 of which address the qualities sharp, hot, cold, dull, itchy, and sensitivity to light touch or clothing on 0–10 scales. Four of these items (sharp, cold, itchy, and sensitivity) were derived from patients' descriptions of pain in postherpetic neuralgia and were thought to differentiate postherpetic neuralgia from diabetic neuropathy or complex regional pain syndrome. Similarly, the Neuropathic Pain Symptom Inventory (NPSI) evaluates symptoms of neuropathic pain, including the descriptors burning, squeezing, pressure, electric shocks, stabbing, pins and needles, and tingling, and includes three questions regarding allodynia from either brushing, pressure, or cold.[112] While both of these scales address symptoms of neuropathic pain and were shown to be responsive to pain treatments, they were not specifically designed to differentiate neuropathic from nonneuropathic pain.

Attempts were made to help distinguish neuropathic from nociceptive pain, some by interview alone and other combining interview with physical tests.[113] The Neuropathic Pain Questionnaire (NPQ) and the Neuropathic Pain Screening Questionnaire (ID Pain scale) contain 12 and 6 interview questions, respectively, designed to elucidate neuropathic pain.[114,115] Of the 12 questions in the NPQ, 10 relate to sensory responses and 2 describe affective components (how unpleasant and how overwhelming the pain seems). The ID Pain scale gives 1 point to positive responses for pins/needles pain, electric shock or shooting pain, hot or burning pain, numbness, and pain evoked by light touch (allodynia) and subtracts 1 point for pain limited to joints. The Neuropathic Pain Detection Questionnaire (PainDETECT) is a scale designed to identify neuropathic pain specifically in low back pain.[116] It includes seven weighted sensory symptoms, one question regarding radiation,

Table 6-4. Neuropathic Pain Scales

SCALE NAME	BRIEF DESCRIPTION	PAIN DIMENSION	STRENGTHS	WEAKNESSES
Neuropathic Pain Scale (NPS)	10 questions, 6 of which address neuropathic pain	Neuropathic pain	One of the first scales to address neuropathic pain	Not specifically designed to differentiate neuropathic from nonneuropathic pain
Neuropathic Pain System Inventory (NPSI)	12 questions, 10 of which address neuropathic pain, including 3 addressing allodynia	Neuropathic pain	Relative ease of administration	Not specifically designed to differentiate neuropathic from nonneuropathic pain
Neuropathic Pain Questionnaire (NPQ)	12 interview questions designed to elucidate neuropathic pain	Neuropathic pain	Relative ease of administration	Less sensitive and specific than scales incorporating physical tests
Neuropathic Pain Screening Questionnaire (ID Pain)	6 interview questions designed to elucidate neuropathic pain	Neuropathic pain	Relative ease of administration	Less sensitive and specific than scales incorporating physical tests
Neuropathic Pain Detection Questionnaire (PainDETECT)	9 interview questions designed to identify neuropathic pain specifically in low back pain	Neuropathic pain	Designed to identify neuropathic pain specifically in low back pain	Unclear utility for other types
Leeds Assessment of Neuropathic Signs and Symptoms (LANSS)	Combines 5 sensory interview questions (prickling/tingling, sudden/electric shock, hot/burning, skin changes, skin hypersensitivity) with two physical tests (brush allodynia and raised pinprick threshold)	Neuropathic pain	Adding physical tests improves sensitivity and specificity	More burdensome to administer
Douleur Neuropathique en 4 Questions (DN4)	Similar to LANSS, with 2 additional interview questions about cold or freezing pain as well as itching and one additional physical test concerning the raised threshold to soft touch	Neuropathic pain	Adding physical tests improves sensitivity and specificity	More burdensome to administer
Standardized Evaluation of Pain (StEP)	Heavier emphasis on tests: 6 questions and 10 tests that allowed the best discrimination between neuropathic and nonneuropathic pain	Neuropathic pain	Novel approach to identify the most useful interview questions and tests, achieving the highest sensitivity and specificity thus far	Validated only in low back pain

and one regarding the temporal quality of the pain. As discussed under affective pain scales, the SF-MPQ has been recently updated to include seven questions addressing different components of neuropathic pain (SF-MPQ-2, Table 6.2).[104]

Three other scales have been developed that combine interview questions and physical tests. The addition of physical tests compared to interview questions alone generally resulted in higher diagnostic accuracy for neuropathic pain. The earliest of these was the Leeds Assessment of Neuropathic Signs and Symptoms (LANSS), which combined five sensory interview questions (concerning prickling/tingling, sudden/electric shock, hot/burning, skin changes, and skin hypersensitivity) with two physical tests (brush allodynia and raised pinprick threshold).[117] The Douleur Neuropathique en 4 Questions (DN4) was similar, with differences including two additional interview questions about cold or freezing pain as well as itching and one additional physical test concerning the raised threshold to soft touch.[118] The most recent addition to these tests is the Standardized Evaluation of Pain (StEP).[4] This study began with a set of 16 interview questions and 23 bedside tests applied to a population of patients with various types of neuropathic or nonneuropathic pain. The authors then used classification tree analysis to determine the subset of questions and tests that allowed the best discrimination between neuropathic and nonneuropathic pain and validated this subset in a population of patients with low back pain. The result was a reduced set of six questions and 10 tests. An overview of these neuropathic pain scales is shown in Table 6.4.

Strengths

Many of the neuropathic pain tests are relatively simple to administer (NPQ, IDPain). These assessments have extended the use of questionnaires from the routine assessments of a particular domain of pain into the categories of diagnostic testing. The StEP back pain assessment method has achieved greater than 90% sensitivity and specificity for identifying neuropathic versus nociceptive pain through its emphasis on the importance of physical tests over interview questions.

Weaknesses

The newer protocols require more sophisticated clinical assessments combining examination findings with responses to questions and are therefore more complicated to administer. In addition, not all assessment tools are in universal agreement. For example, in the StEP protocol, the interview question for burning pain and the physical sign for brush allodynia actually reduced the score for neuropathic pain, at least in regard to radicular low back pain. This was in contrast to the findings in the LANSS and DN4 protocols, in which burning pain and brush allodynia increased the score for neuropathic pain. Additional studies incorporating these new guidelines are required to determine the ultimate utility of these new protocols.

REFERENCES

1. Finnerup NB, Sindrup SH, Jensen TS. Chronic neuropathic pain: mechanisms, drug targets and measurement. *Fundam Clin Pharmacol.* 2007;21(2):129–136.
2. Woolf CJ. Pain: moving from symptom control toward mechanism-specific pharmacologic management. *Ann Intern Med.* 2004;140(6): 441–451.
3. Costigan M, Scholz J, Woolf CJ. Neuropathic pain: a maladaptive response of the nervous system to damage. *Annu Rev Neurosci.* 2009;32:1–32.
4. Scholz J, Mannion RJ, Hord DE, et al. A novel tool for the assessment of pain: validation in low back pain. *PLoS Med.* 2009;6(4):e1000047.
5. Chopra JS, Hurwitz LJ. A comparative study of peripheral nerve conduction in diabetes and non-diabetic chronic occlusive peripheral vascular disease. *Brain.* 1969;92:83–96.
6. Vrethem M, Boivie J, Arnqvist H, Holmgren H, Lindstrom T. Painful polyneuropathy in patients with and without diabetes: clinical, neurophysiologic, and quantitative sensory characteristics. *Clin J Pain.* 2002;18(2):122–127.
7. Dyck PJ, Kratz KM, Lehman KA, et al. The Rochester Diabetic Neuropathy Study: design, criteria for types of neuropathy, selection bias, and reproducibility of neuropathic tests. *Neurology.* 1991;41:799–807.

8. Dyck PJ. Invited review: limitations in predicting pathologic abnormality of nerves from the EMG examination. *Muscle Nerve.* 1990;13(5): 371–375.

9. Bril V, Ellison R, Ngo M, Bergstrom B, Raynard D, Gin H. Electrophysiological monitoring in clinical trials. Roche Neuropathy Study Group [see comments]. *Muscle Nerve.* 1998;21(11):1368–1373.

10. Franson J, Baravarian B. Tarsal tunnel syndrome: a compression neuropathy involving four distinct tunnels. *Clin Podiatr Med Surg.* 2006;23(3):597–609.

11. Lacomis D. Small-fiber neuropathy. *Muscle Nerve.* 2002;26(2):173–188.

12. Bird SJ, Brown MJ, Spino C, Watling S, Foyt HL. Value of repeated measures of nerve conduction and quantitative sensory testing in a diabetic neuropathy trial. *Muscle Nerve.* 2006;34(2): 214–224.

13. Cornblath DR, Chaudhry V, Carter K, et al. Total neuropathy score: validation and reliability study. *Neurology.* 1999;53(8):1660–1664.

14. Freeman R, McIntosh KA, Vijapurkar U, Thienel U. Topiramate and physiologic measures of nerve function in polyneuropathy. *Acta Neurol Scand.* 2007;115(4):222–231.

15. Misawa S, Kuwabara S, Kanai K, et al. Aldose reductase inhibition alters nodal Na^+ currents and nerve conduction in human diabetics. *Neurology.* 2006;66(10):1545–1549.

16. Kincaid JC, Price KL, Jimenez MC, Skljarevski V. Correlation of vibratory quantitative sensory testing and nerve conduction studies in patients with diabetes. *Muscle Nerve.* 2007;36(6): 821–827.

17. Mori K, Iijima M, Koike H, et al. The wide spectrum of clinical manifestations in Sjogren's syndrome-associated neuropathy. *Brain.* 2005;128(pt 11):2518–2534.

18. Polydefkis M, Hauer P, Griffin JW, McArthur JC. Skin biopsy as a tool to assess distal small fiber innervation in diabetic neuropathy. *Diabetes Technol Ther.* 2001;3(1):23–28.

19. England JD, Gronseth GS, Franklin G, et al. Evaluation of distal symmetric polyneuropathy: the role of autonomic testing, nerve biopsy, and skin biopsy (an evidence-based review). *Muscle Nerve.* 2009;39(1):106–115.

20. Zaslansky R, Yarnitsky D. Clinical applications of quantitative sensory testing (QST). *J Neurol Sci.* 1998;153(2):215–238.

21. Magda P, Latov N, Renard MV, Sander HW. Quantitative sensory testing: high sensitivity in small fiber neuropathy with normal NCS/EMG. *J Peripher Nerv Syst.* 2002;7(4):225–228.

22. Freeman R, Chase KP, Risk MR. Quantitative sensory testing cannot differentiate simulated sensory loss from sensory neuropathy. *Neurology.* 2003;60(3):465–470.

23. Rolke R, Baron R, Maier C, et al. Quantitative sensory testing in the German Research Network on Neuropathic Pain (DFNS): standardized protocol and reference values. *Pain.* 2006;123(3):231–243.

24. Bennett MI, Attal N, Backonja MM, et al. Using screening tools to identify neuropathic pain. *Pain.* 2007;127(3):199–203.

25. Dyck PJ, Zimmerman IR, Johnson DM, et al. A standard test of heat-pain responses using CASE IV. *J Neurol Sci.* 1996;136(1–2):54–63.

26. Backonja MM, Walk D, Edwards RR, et al. Quantitative sensory testing in measurement of neuropathic pain phenomena and other sensory abnormalities. *Clin J Pain.* 2009;25(7):641–647.

27. Smith AG, Ramachandran P, Tripp S, Singleton JR. Epidermal nerve innervation in impaired glucose tolerance and diabetes-associated neuropathy. *Neurology.* 2001;57(9):1701–1704.

28. Ametov AS, Barinov A, Dyck PJ, et al. The sensory symptoms of diabetic polyneuropathy are improved with alpha-lipoic acid: the SYDNEY trial. *Diabetes Care.* 2003;26(3):770–776.

29. Brown MJ, Bird SJ, Watling S, et al. Natural progression of diabetic peripheral neuropathy in the Zenarestat study population. *Diabetes Care.* 2004;27(5):1153–1159.

30. Freeman R, Stewart JD. *Quantitative Sensory Testing.* Rochester, MN: American Academy of Electrodiagnostic Medicine; 1996.

31. Jamal GA, Hansen S, Weir AI, Ballantyne JP. The neurophysiologic investigation of small fiber neuropathies. *Muscle Nerve.* 1987;10(6):537–545.

32. Chaudhry V, Rowinsky EK, Sartorius SE, Donehower RC, Cornblath DR. Peripheral neuropathy from taxol and cisplatin combination chemotherapy: clinical and electrophysiological studies. *Ann Neurol.* 1994;35(3):304–311.

33. Shy ME, Frohman EM, So YT, et al. Quantitative sensory testing: report of the Therapeutics and Technology Assessment Subcommittee of the American Academy of Neurology. *Neurology.* 2003;60(6):898–904.

34. Bleecker ML. Vibration perception thresholds in entrapment and toxic neuropathies. *J Occup Med.* 1986;28(10):991–994.

35. Chaudhry V, Eisenberger MA, Sinibaldi VJ, Sheikh K, Griffin JW, Cornblath DR. A prospective study of suramin-induced peripheral neuropathy. *Brain.* 1996;119(pt 6):2039–2052.

36. Forsyth PA, Balmaceda C, Peterson K, Seidman AD, Brasher P, DeAngelis LM. Prospective study

of paclitaxel-induced peripheral neuropathy with quantitative sensory testing. *J Neuro-Oncol.* 1997;35(1):47–53.

37. MacGowan DJ, Janal MN, Clark WC, et al. Central poststroke pain and Wallenberg's lateral medullary infarction: frequency, character, and determinants in 63 patients [see comments]. *Neurology.* 1997;49(1):120–125.

38. Krassioukov A, Wolfe DL, Hsieh JT, Hayes KC, Durham CE. Quantitative sensory testing in patients with incomplete spinal cord injury. *Arch Phys Med Rehabil.* 1999;80(10):1258–1263.

39. Birklein F, Riedl B, Sieweke N, Weber M, Neundorfer B. Neurological findings in complex regional pain syndromes—analysis of 145 cases. *Acta Neurol Scand.* 2000;101(4):262–269.

40. Boivie J. Central pain and the role of quantitative sensory testing (QST) in research and diagnosis. *Eur J Pain.* 2003;7(4):339–343.

41. Maser RE, Laudadio C, Lenhard MJ, DeCherney GS. A cross-sectional study comparing two quantitative sensory testing devices in individuals with diabetes. *Diabetes Care.* 1997;20(2):179–181.

42. Maser RE, Lenhard MJ. Cardiovascular autonomic neuropathy due to diabetes mellitus: clinical manifestations, consequences, and treatment. *J Clin Endocrinol Metab.* 2005;90(10):5896–5903.

43. Suarez GA, Clark VM, Norell JE, et al. Sudden cardiac death in diabetes mellitus: risk factors in the Rochester diabetic neuropathy study. *J Neurol Neurosurg Psychiatry.* 2005;76(2):240–245.

44. Vinik AI, Ziegler D. Diabetic cardiovascular autonomic neuropathy. *Circulation.* 2007;115(3): 387–397.

45. Neild PJ, Amadi A, Ponikowski P, Coats AJ, Gazzard BG. Cardiac autonomic dysfunction in AIDS is not secondary to heart failure. *Int J Cardiol.* 2000;74(2–3):133–137.

46. Freeman R. Autonomic peripheral neuropathy. *Lancet.* 2005;365(9466):1259–1270.

47. Ziegler D, Laux G, Dannehl K, et al. Assessment of cardiovascular autonomic function: age related normal ranges and reproducibility of spectral analysis, vector analysis, and standard tests of heart rate variation and blood pressure responses. *Diabetic Med.* 1992;9:166–175.

48. Low PA, Denq JC, Opfer-Gehrking TL, Dyck PJ, O'Brien PC, Slezak JM. Effect of age and gender on sudomotor and cardiovagal function and blood pressure response to tilt in normal subjects. *Muscle Nerve.* 1997;20(12):1561–1568.

49. Low PA. Testing the autonomic nervous system. *Semin Neurol.* 2003;23(4):407–421.

49a. Freeman R, Wieling W, Axelrod FB, Benditt DG, Benarroch E, Biaggioni I, Cheshire WP, Chelimsky T, Cortelli P, Gibbons CH, Goldstein DS, Hainsworth R, Hilz MJ, Jacob G, Kaufmann H, Jordan J, Lipsitz LA, Levine BD, Low PA, Mathias C, Raj SR, Robertson D, Sandroni P, Schatz I, Schondorff R, Stewart JM, van Dijk JG. Consensus statement on the definition of orthostatic hypotension, neurally mediated syncope and the postural tachycardia syndrome. *Clin Auton Res.* 2011;21(2): 69–72.

50. Freeman R. Assessment of cardiovascular autonomic function. *Clin Neurophysiol.* 2006;117(4): 716–730.

51. Vilches JJ, Navarro X. New silicones for the evaluation of sudomotor function with the impression mold technique. *Clin Auton Res.* 2002;12(1):20–23.

52. Illigens BM, Gibbons CH. Sweat testing to evaluate autonomic function. *Clin Auton Res.* 2009;19(2):79–87.

53. Gibbons CH, Illigens BM, Centi J, Freeman R. QDIRT: quantitative direct and indirect test of sudomotor function. *Neurology.* 2008;70(24):2299–2304.

54. Fealey RD, Low PA, Thomas JE. Thermoregulatory sweating abnormalities in diabetes mellitus. *Mayo Clin Proc.* 1989;64(6):617–628.

55. Novak V, Freimer ML, Kissel JT, et al. Autonomic impairment in painful neuropathy. *Neurology.* 2001;56(7):861–868.

56. Low PA, Caskey PE, Tuck RR, Fealey RD, Dyck PJ. Quantitative sudomotor axon reflex test in normal and neuropathic subjects. *Ann Neurol.* 1983;14:573–580.

57. Fealey RD, Low PA, Thomas JE. Thermoregulatory sweating abnormalities in diabetes mellitus. *Mayo Clin Proc.* 1989;64(6):617–628.

58. Low VA, Sandroni P, Fealey RD, Low PA. Detection of small-fiber neuropathy by sudomotor testing. *Muscle Nerve.* 2006;34(1):57–61.

59. Theriault M, Dort J, Sutherland G, Zochodne DW. A prospective quantitative study of sensory deficits after whole sural nerve biopsies in diabetic and nondiabetic patients. Surgical approach and the role of collateral sprouting. *Neurology.* 1998;50(2):480–484.

60. Gabriel CM, Howard R, Kinsella N, et al. Prospective study of the usefulness of sural nerve biopsy. *J Neurol Neurosurg Psychiatry.* 2000;69(4):442–446.

61. Lauria G. Recent developments in the management of peripheral neuropathy using skin biopsy. *Rev Neurol (Paris).* 2007;163(12): 1266–1270.

62. Lauria G, Lombardi R, Camozzi F, Devigili G. Skin biopsy for the diagnosis of peripheral neuropathy. *Histopathology.* 2009;54(3):273–285.

63. Kennedy WR, Wendelschafer-Crabb G. The innervation of human epidermis [see comments]. *J Neurol Sci.* 1993;115(2):184–190.

64. Lauria G, Holland N, Hauer P, Cornblath DR, Griffin JW, McArthur JC. Epidermal innervation: changes with aging, topographic location, and in sensory neuropathy. *J Neurol Sci.* 1999;164(2):172–178.

65. Sommer C, Lauria G. Skin biopsy in the management of peripheral neuropathy. *Lancet Neurol.* 2007;6(7):632–642.

66. Vallat JM, Vital A, Magy L, Martin-Negrier ML, Vital C. An update on nerve biopsy. *J Neuropathol Exp Neurol.* 2009;68(8):833–844.

67. Scott LJ, Griffin JW, Luciano C, et al. Quantitative analysis of epidermal innervation in Fabry disease. *Neurology.* 1999;52(6):1249–1254.

68. Nolano M, Provitera V, Crisci C, et al. Small fibers involvement in Friedreich's ataxia. *Ann Neurol.* 2001;50(1):17–25.

69. Chai J, Herrmann DN, Stanton M, Barbano RL, Logigian EL. Painful small-fiber neuropathy in Sjogren syndrome. *Neurology.* 2005;65(6):925–927.

70. Pardo CA, McArthur JC, Griffin JW. HIV neuropathy: insights in the pathology of HIV peripheral nerve disease. *J Peripher Nerv Syst.* 2001;6(1):21–27.

71. Polydefkis M, Hauer P, Sheth S, Sirdofsky M, Griffin JW, McArthur JC. The time course of epidermal nerve fibre regeneration: studies in normal controls and in people with diabetes, with and without neuropathy. *Brain.* 2004;127(pt 7):1606–1615.

72. Holland NR, Stocks A, Hauer P, Cornblath DR, Griffin JW, McArthur JC. Intraepidermal nerve fiber density in patients with painful sensory neuropathy. *Neurology.* 1997;48(3):708–711.

73. Lauria G, McArthur JC, Hauer PE, Griffin JW, Cornblath DR. Neuropathological alterations in diabetic truncal neuropathy: evaluation by skin biopsy. *J Neurol Neurosurg Psychiatry.* 1998;65(5):762–766.

74. Polydefkis M, Hauer P, Sheth S, Sirdofsky M, Griffin JW, McArthur JC. The time course of epidermal nerve fibre regeneration: studies in normal controls and in people with diabetes, with and without neuropathy. *Brain.* 2004;127(pt 7):1606–1615.

75. McArthur JC, Stocks EA, Hauer P, Cornblath DR, Griffin JW. Epidermal nerve fiber density: normative reference range and diagnostic efficiency [see comments]. *Arch Neurol.* 1998;55(12):1513–1520.

76. Lauria G, Sghirlanzoni A, Lombardi R, Pareyson D. Epidermal nerve fiber density in sensory ganglionopathies: clinical and neurophysiologic correlations. *Muscle Nerve.* 2001;24(8):1034–1039.

77. Oaklander AL, Romans K, Horasek S, Stocks A, Hauer P, Meyer RA. Unilateral postherpetic neuralgia is associated with bilateral sensory neuron damage. *Ann Neurol.* 1998;44(5):789–795.

78. Oaklander AL, Rissmiller JG, Gelman LB, Zheng L, Chang Y, Gott R. Evidence of focal small-fiber axonal degeneration in complex regional pain syndrome-I (reflex sympathetic dystrophy). *Pain.* 2006;120(3):235–243.

79. Lauria G, Morbin M, Lombardi R, et al. Axonal swellings predict the degeneration of epidermal nerve fibers in painful neuropathies. *Neurology.* 2003;61(5):631–636.

80. Gibbons CH, Griffin JW, Polydefkis M, et al. The utility of skin biopsy for prediction of progression in suspected small fiber neuropathy. *Neurology.* 2006;66(2):256–258.

81. Gibbons CH, Illigens BM, Wang N, Freeman R. Quantification of sweat gland innervation: a clinical-pathologic correlation. *Neurology.* 2009;72(17):1479–1486.

82. Dabby R, Vaknine H, Gilad R, Djaldetti R, Sadeh M. Evaluation of cutaneous autonomic innervation in idiopathic sensory small-fiber neuropathy. *J Peripher Nerv Syst.* 2007;12(2):98–101.

83. Lauria G, Devigili G. Skin biopsy as a diagnostic tool in peripheral neuropathy. *Nat Clin Pract Neurol.* 2007;3(10):546–557.

84. Schmidt JO, Blum MS, Overal WL. Comparative enzymology of venoms from stinging Hymenoptera. *Toxicon.* 1986;24(9):907–921.

85. Jensen MP. The validity and reliability of pain measures in adults with cancer. *J Pain.* 2003;4(1):2–21.

86. Hays RD, Hadorn D. Responsiveness to change: an aspect of validity, not a separate dimension. *Qual Life Res.* 1992;1(1):73–75.

87. Kremer E, Atkinson JH, Ignelzi RJ. Measurement of pain: patient preference does not confound pain measurement. *Pain.* 1981;10(2):241–248.

88. Silverman DG, O'Connor TZ, Brull SJ. Integrated assessment of pain scores and rescue morphine use during studies of analgesic efficacy. *Anesth Analg.* 1993;77(1):168–170.

89. Farrar JT, Portenoy RK, Berlin JA, Kinman JL, Strom BL. Defining the clinically important difference in pain outcome measures. *Pain.* 2000;88(3):287–294.

90. Hanley MA, Jensen MP, Ehde DM, et al. Clinically significant change in pain intensity ratings in persons with spinal cord injury or amputation. *Clin J Pain.* 2006;22(1):25–31.

91. von Baeyer CL, Spagrud LJ, McCormick JC, Choo E, Neville K, Connelly MA. Three new datasets supporting use of the Numerical Rating Scale (NRS-11) for children's self-reports of pain intensity. *Pain.* 2009;143(3):223–227.

92. Merkel SI, Voepel-Lewis T, Shayevitz JR, Malviya S. The FLACC: a behavioral scale for scoring postoperative pain in young children. *Pediatr Nurs.* 1997;23(3):293–297.

93. Lyon F, Dawson D. Oucher or CHEOPS for pain assessment in children. *Emerg Med J.* 2003;20(5):470.

94. von Baeyer CL, Spagrud LJ. Systematic review of observational (behavioral) measures of pain for children and adolescents aged 3 to 18 years. *Pain.* 2007;127(1–2):140–150.

95. Dworkin RH, Turk DC, Farrar JT, et al. Core outcome measures for chronic pain clinical trials: IMMPACT recommendations. *Pain.* 2005;113(1–2):9–19.

96. Jensen MP, Dworkin RH, Gammaitoni AR, Olaleye DO, Oleka N, Galer BS. Assessment of pain quality in chronic neuropathic and nociceptive pain clinical trials with the Neuropathic Pain Scale. *J Pain.* 2005;6(2):98–106.

97. Ripamonti CI, Brunelli C. Comparison between numerical rating scale and six-level verbal rating scale in cancer patients with pain: a preliminary report. *Support Care Cancer.* 2009;17(11):1433–1434.

98. Decruynaere C, Thonnard JL, Plaghki L. How many response levels do children distinguish on faces scales for pain assessment? *Eur J Pain.* 2009;13(6):641–648.

99. Ramer L, Richardson JL, Cohen MZ, Bedney C, Danley KL, Judge EA. Multimeasure pain assessment in an ethnically diverse group of patients with cancer. *J Transcult Nurs.* 1999;10(2):94–101.

100. Chibnall JT, Tait RC. Pain assessment in cognitively impaired and unimpaired older adults: a comparison of four scales. *Pain.* 2001;92(1–2):173–186.

101. Cleeland CS, Ryan KM. Pain assessment: global use of the Brief Pain Inventory. *Ann Acad Med Singapore.* 1994;23(2):129–138.

102. Melzack R. The McGill Pain Questionnaire: major properties and scoring methods. *Pain.* 1975;1(3):277–299.

103. Melzack R. The short-form McGill Pain Questionnaire. *Pain.* 1987;30(2):191–197.

104. Dworkin RH, Turk DC, Revicki DA, et al. Development and initial validation of an expanded and revised version of the Short-form McGill Pain Questionnaire (SF-MPQ-2). *Pain.* 2009;144(1–2):35–42.

105. Rice AS, Maton S. Gabapentin in postherpetic neuralgia: a randomised, double blind, placebo controlled study. *Pain.* 2001;94(2):215–224.

106. Kochar DK, Jain N, Agarwal RP, Srivastava T, Agarwal P, Gupta S. Sodium valproate in the management of painful neuropathy in type 2 diabetes—a randomized placebo controlled study. *Acta Neurol Scand.* 2002;106(5):248–252.

107. Rosenstock J, Tuchman M, LaMoreaux L, Sharma U. Pregabalin for the treatment of painful diabetic peripheral neuropathy: a double-blind, placebo-controlled trial. *Pain.* 2004;110(3):628–638.

108. Ware JE Jr., Sherbourne CD. The MOS 36-item short-form health survey (SF-36). I. Conceptual framework and item selection. *Med Care.* 1992;30(6):473–483.

109. Park KU. Assessment of change of quality of life in terminally ill patients under cancer pain management using the EORTC Core Quality of Life Questionnaire (QLQ-C30) in a Korean sample. *Oncology.* 2008;74(suppl 1):7–12.

110. Treede RD, Jensen TS, Campbell JN, et al. Neuropathic pain: redefinition and a grading system for clinical and research purposes. *Neurology.* 2008;70(18):1630–1635.

111. Galer BS, Jensen MP. Development and preliminary validation of a pain measure specific to neuropathic pain: the Neuropathic Pain Scale. *Neurology.* 1997;48(2):332–338.

112. Bouhassira D, Attal N, Fermanian J, et al. Development and validation of the Neuropathic Pain Symptom Inventory. *Pain.* 2004;108(3):248–257.

113. Cruccu G, Truini A. Tools for assessing neuropathic pain. *PLoS Med.* 2009;6(4):e1000045.

114. Krause SJ, Backonja MM. Development of a neuropathic pain questionnaire. *Clin J Pain.* 2003;19(5):306–314.

115. Portenoy R. Development and testing of a neuropathic pain screening questionnaire: ID Pain. *Curr Med Res Opin.* 2006;22(8):1555–1565.

116. Freynhagen R, Baron R, Gockel U, Tolle TR. painDETECT: a new screening questionnaire to identify neuropathic components in patients with back pain. *Curr Med Res Opin.* 2006;22(10):1911–1920.

117. Bennett M. The LANSS Pain Scale: the Leeds assessment of neuropathic symptoms and signs. *Pain.* 2001;92(1–2):147–157.

118. Bouhassira D, Attal N, Alchaar H, et al. Comparison of pain syndromes associated with nervous or somatic lesions and development of a new neuropathic pain diagnostic questionnaire (DN4). *Pain.* 2005;114(1–2):29–36.

7

Psychosocial Aspects of Neuropathic Pain

MARK P. JENSEN, MICHAEL R. MOORE, AND TAMARA B. BOCKOW

PSYCHOSOCIAL FACTORS, SUCH as patients' beliefs or attributions, coping responses, and social support, are key components of biopsychosocial models of chronic pain.[1] However, the majority of studies that support the importance of psychosocial factors in chronic pain have focused on musculoskeletal pain problems, such as low back pain and headaches. Only recently have researchers begun to examine the importance of psychosocial factors in neuropathic pain conditions, such as those associated with surgery (e.g., postsurgical neuropathic pain following amputation), herpes zoster (postherpetic neuralgia), diabetes (painful diabetic neuropathy), and central neuropathic pain conditions (e.g., poststroke pain, pain in individuals with spinal cord injury [SCI] and multiple sclerosis [MS]).

The purpose of this chapter is to evaluate the role that psychosocial factors may play in adjustment to and management of neuropathic pain. It begins with a brief overview and description of the psychosocial factors that have been identified as important in nonneuropathic pain conditions. We then review the findings from recent correlational and treatment outcome research that has examined the association of these factors and both pain severity and pain interference in individuals with neuropathic pain. This is followed by a summary of the findings from studies that have investigated the effects of psychosocial interventions on pain severity and functioning in patients with neuropathic pain. The chapter ends with a brief discussion of the research and clinical implications of the findings from this body of research.

PSYCHOSOCIAL FACTORS AND CHRONIC PAIN

Psychosocial factors refer to both (1) psychological factors that lie within the person and (2) social factors in the person's immediate social environment. The psychological factors most often examined as they relate to pain severity and pain interference are (1) coping, (2) beliefs/attributions, and (3) catastrophizing responses. The social factors most often examined are (1) environmental responses (usually from the spouse or family, but also from health care providers) to patients' pain behaviors and (2) general or global social support.

PSYCHOLOGICAL FACTORS

Coping

Coping responses can be defined as efforts to manage stressful events. The goal of pain-coping responses is to decrease the severity of pain and/or the negative effects of pain on functioning. The pain-coping literature has classified coping responses into two basic categories: (1) adaptive coping (coping responses generally thought to contribute to positive outcomes, also sometimes referred to as *active coping* and *wellness-coping* responses) and (2) maladaptive coping (coping responses generally thought to contribute to long-term negative outcomes,

also referred to as *passive coping*, *pain-focused coping*, or *pain control* strategies).[2]

Research, which in the past was performed mostly in patient populations with musculoskeletal or nociceptive pain conditions, supports both (1) the importance of pain-coping responses as predictors of patient functioning and (2) a pattern of associations indicating that the use of adaptive coping responses tends to be positively associated with measures of patient adjustment and negatively with measures of dysfunction, and that the use of maladaptive coping responses shows the opposite pattern. The coping responses that have been shown to be most closely linked to patient functioning are listed in Table 7.1.[3–14] Findings from one of the few prospective longitudinal studies (determining whether coping activity at one point in time predicts subsequent adjustment) in this area has shown that guarding and asking for assistance, both hypothesized to be maladaptive, predict subsequent work status, with infrequent use of these strategies associated with higher levels of return to work.[15]

Table 7-1. Pain-Coping Strategies Associated with Measures of Patient Functioning in Samples of Individuals with Chronic Pain

COPING RESPONSE	DESCRIPTION
	ADAPTIVE PAIN-COPING RESPONSES
Task persistence	Continuing with a valued activity regardless of pain level
Seeking social support	Asking for emotional support from friends and family members (predictive of positive psychological functioning)
Coping self-statements	Saying reassuring things to oneself (predictive of positive psychological functioning)
Pacing	Engaging in valued activities in a slow but steady (i.e., non-pain-contingent) manner
Self-hypnosis	Using a cue to achieve a relaxed state and increased perceived comfort
	MALADAPTIVE COPING RESPONSES
Guarding	Avoiding the use of a body part or holding it still or in an unusual position to reduce pain
Resting	Electing to reduce activity and/or rest when experiencing pain
Asking for assistance	Asking for help with a chore from a friend or family member when experiencing pain

Beliefs and Attributions

Pain-related beliefs and attributions reflect a patient's understanding of the causes of pain and its meaning. Like coping responses, pain beliefs have been classified as adaptive or maladaptive, depending on how they are hypothesized to affect patient functioning. The beliefs that have been shown to predict patient functioning in nonneuropathic pain conditions are listed in Table 7.2.[9,14,16-19]

Catastrophizing

Pain-related catastrophizing is the tendency to focus on pain and the negative effects it has on one's life. It is listed as a factor separate from coping and beliefs because it can be viewed either as a set of negative beliefs and attributions[20] or as a type of coping response that one uses to elicit support from others.[21] Examples of pain-related catastrophizing responses, pulled from one of the most commonly used measures of this construct, include "I keep thinking about how badly I want the pain to stop," "I can't seem to keep it out of my mind," and "I wonder whether something serious may happen."[22]

Catastrophizing thoughts in response to pain have been shown to be among the psychosocial factors most consistently linked to higher levels of pain and both psychological and physical dysfunction in populations of individuals with chronic pain.[18,23,24] Moreover, longitudinal research indicates that catastrophizing at one point in time prospectively predicts the subsequent development or worsening of depressive symptoms, consistent not only with a causal role of catastrophizing in the development of depressive symptoms, but also with the conclusion that catastrophizing is distinct from depression.[25]

SOCIAL FACTORS

Pain-Contingent Social Responses

In the late 1960s, Wilbert Fordyce and colleagues thought that it might be useful to make pain behaviors a primary treatment target in the treatment of chronic pain.[26] Fordyce noted that the only way people communicate to others how they are doing is through their behaviors. He classified the behaviors most important to chronic pain into two types: (1) pain behaviors such as guarding, complaining of pain, and resting that can communicate pain to others (many of which also fall under the category of maladaptive coping) and (2) well behaviors such as regular exercise and participation in valued activities.[27]

Fordyce also noted that operant theory hypothesizes that all behavior, including pain and wellness behavior, is influenced by the environmental responses to that behavior; when

Table 7-2. Pain-Related Beliefs Associated with Measures of Patient Functioning in Samples of Individuals with Chronic Pain

COPING RESPONSE	DESCRIPTION
ADAPTIVE PAIN-RELATED BELIEF	
Perceived control	The belief that one has the skills or resources to control pain or its negative effects on one's life
MALADAPTIVE PAIN-RELATED BELIEFS	
Disability	The belief that one is necessarily disabled by pain
Harm	The belief that pain is a signal that physical damage is occurring
Medication	The belief that pain-contingent analgesics are appropriate for chronic pain management

behavior is followed by reinforcers, there is an increase in the frequency of the behavior, and when punishers or the lack of reinforcers follow behavior, there is a decrease in the frequency of the behavior. Based on this operant model of pain, he hypothesized that a treatment program that systematically ignores pain behavior and reinforces well behavior would benefit patients. This model is at the foundation of many chronic pain treatment programs, and research supports the efficacy of such programs.[28,29] Moreover, research from a number of studies indicates that solicitous responses (i.e., pain-contingent positive responses that are thought to be reinforcing, such as affection and attention, as well as offers to take over chores and responsibilities) are positively associated with measures of pain intensity and disability, consistent with an operant model of pain.[30,31]

Social Support

Although *pain-contingent* positive responses from the environment are thought to contribute to greater patient dysfunction, *nonpain-contingent* positive responses (i.e., consistent with general or global support) are hypothesized to buffer the negative impact of stress and contribute to positive functioning—in particular, positive psychological functioning. Research supports these hypothesized associations in samples of individuals with chronic pain.[32,33] Based on these findings, clinicians commonly encourage family members of patients with chronic pain to provide ongoing emotional support and affection (positive global support) while encouraging (reinforcing) patient well behaviors such as active engagement in activities and to avoid the encouragement or reinforcement of pain behaviors (i.e., solicitous responses) such as rest and inactivity.

EVIDENCE REGARDING THE CORRELATES OF PSYCHOSOCIAL FACTORS IN NEUROPATHIC PAIN CONDITIONS

In the previous section, we described the psychosocial factors that have been most often shown to be associated with functioning in patients with nonneuropathic pain conditions.

In this section, we summarize the evidence regarding the importance of these factors as they are associated (or not) with key outcomes or functioning domains in patients with neuropathic pain.

Prior to presenting the results of this review, however, some words of caution are needed regarding the interpretation of findings from these (largely) correlational study designs. An important strength of correlational studies, whether they estimate the associations between variables at a single point in time (e.g., cross-sectional correlational designs) or the associations between variables over time (e.g., prospective prediction designs), is that they can be completed relatively easily. They only require that an investigator administer measures of psychosocial factors and measures of pain and patient functioning to study participants at one or more points in time; no intervention or treatment is required. Because of the ease of performing correlational studies, there tends to be many more such studies than true experiments, which are much more time-consuming and difficult to perform. At the same time, however, given that correlational studies do not involve systematic manipulation(s) of psychosocial factors, causality cannot be concluded from the findings of these studies.

To illustrate this very important point, let us say that there is a pain-coping strategy that results in (causes) significant pain reduction that lasts for several hours every time it is used. For this reason, patients may use this coping strategy more often when their average pain levels are higher than when their pain levels are lower; it would not be necessary to use the coping response when pain levels are very low. A correlational study would therefore demonstrate a strong positive association between the use of this (effective) coping response and pain intensity, such that more use of the coping response is linked to higher levels of pain. This does not mean, however, that the coping response *caused* higher pain levels; in fact, in this example, just the opposite is true. Moreover, because pain can contribute to disability, sleep problems, and distress, more frequent use of this coping response might also be shown to be significantly associated with disability, sleep problems, and psychological dysfunction.

Therefore, positive associations between a coping response, or other psychosocial factors, and measures of patient dysfunction could potentially be due to the fact that the coping response is an adaptive and helpful one.

As another example, there may be another coping response that contributes to increases in pain and disability; inactivity and pain-contingent rest, for example, are thought by many clinicians to have this effect.[27] In this case, more use of the coping response would be associated positively with measures of pain intensity and dysfunction. So, the same finding—a positive correlation between a psychosocial factor and measures of pain and disability—could result from the fact that the psychosocial factor effectively reduces pain and disability or causes an increase in pain and disability.

As a third example, it is possible, even likely, that functioning domains themselves influence both pain-related psychosocial factors and other functioning domains. Depression, for example, may contribute to general inactivity and use of passive pain-coping responses while also contributing to lower levels of activity and disability. Thus, significant associations between passive coping responses and measures of disability could be observed because a third variable, in this case depression, influences both; significant associations can be found between variables even if or when they have little causal impact on each other.

In short, strong and consistent associations between psychosocial factors (such as beliefs, coping, catastrophizing, and social factors) and measures of important outcome or functioning domains can tell us that psychosocial factors *might* play some role in patient functioning, but we are unable to draw conclusions from the findings of correlational studies regarding (1) whether the psychosocial factors being examined are necessarily helpful (adaptive) or not helpful (maladaptive) and (2) whether the psychosocial factors actually influence adjustment or just predict (or reflect) adjustment. Still, correlational studies are useful for telling us if, at a minimum, psychosocial factors are linked to important outcome variables, given the fact that a lack of association can be used as evidence against their importance (i.e., an association is a necessary but not sufficient condition

for causality). These studies can also tell us which psychosocial factors are most likely to be important, and therefore the ones that should be targeted in future (experimental) studies that can then be used to determine if causal associations among variables actually do exist.

COPING

We were able to identify 18 studies that examined the associations between measures of coping and adjustment in samples of patients with neuropathic pain conditions.[34–51] Significant associations between coping responses and patient adjustment were found in all but one of these studies (Hanley and colleagues[38] did not find a significant association between the use of resting as a coping strategy and subsequent changes in pain intensity, depression, and pain interference, in a longitudinal prospective prediction study examining patients with postamputation pain), although a very large variety of measures of coping (and of adjustment) were assessed in these studies.

More use of *increasing activities* as a way to cope with pain was associated with better psychological functioning in a sample of patients with multiple sclerosis,[35] although it also predicted subsequent *increases* in pain interference in a sample of patients with postherpetic neuralgia.[40] More use of *rest* as a way to cope with pain was found to be associated with (1) higher levels of pain intensity in patients with acquired amputation and MS,[42,49] (2) more pain interference in patients with acquired amputation, SCI, and MS,[42,45,49] and (3) lower levels of psychological functioning in patients with MS.[49] More use of *coping self-statements* (i.e., repeating reassuring thoughts to oneself) was linked to better psychological functioning in a sample of patients with SCI[45] and to higher levels of activity in a sample of patients with postherpetic neuralgia.[40] However, these coping self-statements were also associated with higher levels of pain interference in a sample of patients with MS and pain.[49]

Greater use of *praying and hoping* was shown to be significantly associated with more pain interference in a sample of patients with postherpetic neuralgia[40] and less pain severity in a sample of patients with acquired amputation,[41] but praying and hoping was also associated with higher levels of physical dysfunction in that same sample of patients with an amputation.[41] The coping strategy of *task persistence* was shown to be associated with less pain interference in samples of patients with SCI and pain[45,49] and also with higher levels of psychological functioning and less pain in a sample of patients with neuropathic pain associated with human immunodeficiency virus (HIV) infection.[44] A number of additional pain-coping responses have been examined in these studies, although they were examined in only one study each. Many of these responses were found to be associated with different measures of patient functioning in samples of patients with neuropathic pain (e.g., asking for assistance[45] and use of guarding[49] were shown to be associated with more pain interference in patients with SCI).

BELIEFS AND ATTRIBUTIONS

Pain-related beliefs have been studied less often than pain-related coping in samples of patients with neuropathic pain conditions; we identified only 10 studies.[34,35,39,41,45,49,51–54] The belief domain studied most often in this research is *perceived control*, including perceived control over pain or its impact, as well as perceived control over life. The findings from these studies are quite consistent across neuropathic pain populations; when significant effects are found, a greater sense of control is associated with less disability, less pain intensity, and greater life satisfaction and well-being in patients with SCI,[45,51,53,54] MS,[49,51] and acquired amputation.[41,53]

Other pain-related beliefs found to be associated with measures of patient functioning include (1) a sense of oneself as necessarily disabled by pain (associated with less psychological functioning and more pain interference in an SCI sample[45] and with more pain intensity, more pain interference, and less psychological functioning in an MS sample[49]); (2) a belief that pain is an indication of physical damage (associated with more pain interference in an SCI sample[45]); and (3) a sense of helplessness about pain (associated with more disability and depression and less perceived well-being in an SCI sample[51]).

In addition, pain-related beliefs have been shown to prospectively predict changes in patient functioning over time. For example, higher levels of pain-related fear of movement assessed before surgery were shown to prospectively predict disability and pain intensity both 6 weeks and 6 months after the surgery in a sample of patients with lumbosacral radicular pain. Specifically, belief (1) in personal control over pain, (2) that one is necessarily disabled by pain, and (3) that pain is a sign of physical harm, assessed at one point in time, all prospectively predicted subsequent changes in psychological functioning.[34] Higher control beliefs, lower disability beliefs, and fewer harm beliefs predicted improvements in function.[34]

CATASTROPHIZING

The strong and consistent association between catastrophizing cognitions and measures of patient functioning demonstrated in the non-neuropathic chronic pain literature is replicated in samples of patients with neuropathic pain. We identified 17 studies that examined these relationships.[35,37–42,48–51,55–60] Frequency of catastrophizing was consistently shown to be associated with higher levels of pain interference, pain intensity, depression, and disability in samples of patients with MS,[35,49] HIV-related neuropathic pain,[37,55] SCI,[45,48,51,56,58,59] postherpetic neuralgia,[40] acquired amputation,[41,42,60] and other mixed neuropathies.[57]

Moreover, longitudinal studies have found that the level of pain-related catastrophizing assessed at one point in time prospectively predicts subsequent changes in measures of patient functioning, and additional longitudinal studies have shown that *changes* in catastrophizing from an initial assessment to a follow-up assessment point are associated with *changes* in patient functioning. For example, Hanley and colleagues assessed the frequency of catastrophizing cognitions 1 month after an amputation, and found that those patients reporting *more* initial catastrophizing demonstrated the most *improvement* in depression (to the 12-month and 24-month follow-up points) and in pain interference (to the 24-month follow-up point).[38] They speculated that those patients who were catastrophizing more in the first few weeks following amputation had more room to improve (i.e., they could show greater decreases in catastrophizing than those who began treatment with lower levels of catastrophizing, and they could show greater decreases in the functioning domains that might be influenced by catastrophizing than those who were catastrophizing less). This idea is consistent with the finding that 1-month to 6-month post-amputation decreases in catastrophizing are associated with decreases in pain interference and improvement in psychological functioning over these same time periods.[39] Another study, reporting a similar result, found that higher levels of pain-related catastrophizing 1 month after an amputation predicted more improvement in depression from this time point to 6 months after the amputation.[42]

SOCIAL FACTORS

Nine studies were identified that examined the associations between measures of social factors (including global social support as well as pain-contingent solicitous, and negative/punishing responses from significant others) and measures of functioning in samples of individuals with neuropathic pain, although all but one of these studied patients with a history of amputation or SCI.[38,42,47,49,54,61–63] The results of four cross-sectional studies looking at global social support had very consistent findings. All four (one studying patients with SCI, two studying patients with acquired amputation, and one studying patients with MS and pain) found positive associations between perceived global social support and measures of psychological functioning (i.e., less depression, higher ratings of global quality of life, more life satisfaction).[49,61–63] Two additional studies found more social support to be associated with less pain interference.[49,63]

The findings from two studies looking at the correlates of negative significant-other (mostly spouse) responses to patient pain behaviors in patients with SCI were also consistent; in both studies, more negative responses were found to be associated with worse outcomes—specifically, more depression, pain interference, and pain severity.[47,62] On the other hand, of the three studies examining the correlates of solicitous

responses (which would be predicted to contribute to greater disability if they are reinforcing, according to operant models) in patients with SCI, two found more solicitous responses to be associated with poorer functioning (more affective pain severity[56] and more pain interference[62]) and one found a positive association between solicitous responses and functioning (more life satisfaction[54]).

Three studies examined the ability of measures of global social support and solicitous significant-other responses to predict outcome measures in longitudinal designs in persons with acquired amputations. In these studies, initial assessments of social support were consistently associated with subsequent improvement (in pain interference,[38,42] in depression,[42] and in mobility and occupational functioning[63]). On the other hand, and consistent with operant models, higher initial levels of solicitous responses were associated with subsequent increases in pain interference[38,42] and depression.[42]

SUMMARY OF RESEARCH ON THE ASSOCIATIONS BETWEEN PSYCHOSOCIAL FACTORS AND FUNCTIONING

As a group, the studies examining the associations between psychosocial factors (coping, beliefs, catastrophizing, and social factors) and measures of physical and psychological functioning in patients with different neuropathic pain conditions demonstrate that psychosocial factors are often linked to measures of key patient quality-of-life domains. Keeping in mind the caveat that correlation cannot be used as evidence for causality, the findings are still consistent with psychosocial models of pain and suggest the possibility, but do not prove that, (1) how patients cope with neuropathic pain, (2) what patients think about their pain, (3) whether or not they catastrophize when they experience pain, and (4) how others respond to the patient when he or she experiences pain could all potentially play a role in the patient's ultimate quality of life.

In terms of the strongest and most consistent associations found, the findings suggest that pain-contingent rest and task persistence may be the coping responses most closely linked to patient outcomes in these populations. Beliefs that appear to be most predictive of patient functioning include those reflecting a sense of control over pain and its effects, as well as beliefs regarding the meaning of pain (i.e., whether or not pain reflects a threat to one's physical well-being and whether or not one is necessarily disabled by pain). Consistent with the literature on patient populations presenting with pain as a primary complaint, catastrophizing cognitions are consistently and strongly related to many negative outcomes (in cross-sectional studies). A few longitudinal studies found that high levels of catastrophizing can predict subsequent improvement in functioning (related to the possibility that such individuals may have more room for improvement in catastrophizing than individuals who report fewer catastrophizing cognitions). Finally, the findings regarding social support appear consistent; patients reporting higher levels of global social support generally report higher levels of functioning in cross-sectional studies, and they report more improvement in functioning in longitudinal studies. Solicitous responses, on the other hand, appear to be associated with more physical disability (although such responses may be linked to higher levels of life satisfaction in some patient populations) in cross-sectional studies, and they seem to predict subsequent decreases in functioning (more pain interference and depression) in longitudinal studies.

EVIDENCE REGARDING THE EFFICACY OF PSYCHOSOCIAL TREATMENTS IN INDIVIDUALS WITH NEUROPATHIC PAIN CONDITIONS

The evidence reviewed above demonstrates that coping, beliefs, catastrophizing, and social factors are all associated with the severity and impact of neuropathic pain. However, this evidence does not support the conclusion that psychosocial factors necessarily impact or influence neuropathic pain and its effects on an individual's quality of life; these correlational results could also be found if patient functioning has an impact on these psychosocial variables.

Evidence for causality will need to come from true experiments in which a psychosocial factor (e.g., catastrophizing cognitions) is systematically altered in one group of individuals and not in another, and then this manipulation is shown to affect pain or another functioning variable in the experimental group but not in the control group.

Controlled trials of psychosocial interventions provide one model for testing causal hypotheses. In such studies, patients are assigned to receive a treatment that is designed to alter one or more psychosocial factors versus a treatment that is designed to control for time and therapist attention but is not thought to alter the targeted factor(s). If the treatment condition shows a larger effect on an outcome variable, such as pain intensity, relative to the control condition, this could be used as evidence that psychosocial variables influence patient outcomes. Moreover, when significant treatment benefits for a psychosocial intervention are found, this provides empirical support for offering that treatment to patients with neuropathic pain as a way to improve their quality of life.

Treatment outcome research of psychosocial interventions for neuropathic pain is in its infancy; we were able to identify only five controlled studies that examined the effects of treatments designed to alter psychosocial variables in samples of patients with neuropathic pain. These published studies include three controlled trials examining the effects of cognitive-behavioral therapy for pain management in persons with mixed disabilities (including patients with acquired amputation, cerebral palsy, MS, and SCI,[64] patients with SCI,[65] and patients with HIV-related peripheral neuropathic pain[55]) and two controlled trials of self-hypnosis training for pain management in patients with neuropathic pain (one including patients with SCI[66] and another including patients with MS[67]).

Cognitive-Behavior Therapy (CBT)

A cognitive-behavioral approach is consistent with biopsychosocial models of pain and is based on the assumptions that (1) psychological and physical functioning are maximized when people replace maladaptive ways of thinking, feeling, and responding with adaptive ones and (2) treatment of complex problems, such as chronic pain and its interference with functioning, should address thoughts, feelings, and behaviors and not one to the exclusion of others.[68] Most CBT interventions, then, include teaching patients strategies for altering thoughts and feelings, as well as teaching and encouraging adaptive pain-coping responses. As mentioned previously, there is evidence from controlled trials that CBT interventions can result in improvements in pain severity, pain-coping responses, pain-related beliefs, behavioral expressions of pain, and social role functioning in patients with nonneuropathic pain conditions.[28,29]

Three controlled trials have examined the efficacy of CBT for the treatment of neuropathic pain. In the first of these, Evans and colleagues randomly assigned 61 patients with HIV-related peripheral neuropathic pain to receive six 1-h sessions of CBT or supportive psychotherapy.[55] The authors of this study did not specify the contents of their CBT intervention, although they did mention that the therapists were graduate psychology students who attended weekly supervision meetings to ensure the fidelity of the treatment program. Of the 61 patients who began treatment, 28 dropped out, with more dropping out of the CBT condition (16) than the supportive psychotherapy condition (12), with most of the dropouts (61%) attending only the first session. However, among those who completed the treatment, significant pre- to posttreatment decreases in pain intensity were reported (in both treatment groups). Participants in the CBT group, however, reported substantial and statistically significant decreases in pain interference and psychological distress, while those in the supportive psychotherapy condition showed fewer gains in these domains that were not statistically significant.

In a second study, 18 individuals with acquired amputation ($n = 4$), SCI ($n = 10$), cerebral palsy ($n = 2$) and MS ($n = 2$) participated in eight 90-minute sessions of either cognitive restructuring ($n = 13$) or an education control condition ($n = 5$).[64] The cognitive intervention had a primary goal of decreasing maladaptive cognitions, and taught participants to identify these cognitions and use a variety of

strategies (thought-stopping, logical evaluation of thought content, development and repetition of reassuring self-statements) to replace them with reassuring ones. The education control intervention was designed to be interesting and informative but to not specifically alter beliefs, feelings, or coping responses. Participants rated both interventions positively, but those in the cognitive restructuring condition reported greater pre- to posttreatment decreases in pain intensity than those in the education control condition.

In a third study, 27 patients with SCI and chronic pain participated in a comprehensive pain management program consisting of 20 sessions over 10 weeks that included (1) education in pain physiology and pharmacology; (2) CBT sessions that included training in mindfulness, attention-diverting coping strategies, cognitive restructuring, social skills training, activity pacing, goal setting, and meetings with a role model; (3) training in relaxation techniques, stretching, and light exercise; and (4) bodily awareness training.[65] Twelve patients with SCI-related neuropathic pain were identified from clinic participants and matched to the first 12 participants in the treatment group; 11 of these agreed to participate in an outcomes data collection group (i.e., they made up a standard care condition). The participants in the pain management program reported significant pretreatment to 12-month follow-up decreases in anxiety and depression and an improvement in sleep quality. Significant differences from pretreatment to 12-month follow-up between the treatment and control participants emerged for depression and a measure of "sense of coherence," which was designed to assess successful coping with stressors, with the participants in the pain management program showing greater improvement than the control participants on both measures.

Self-Hypnosis Training

Hypnosis for pain management has a long history, but only recently have controlled trials been performed in various chronic pain conditions, with the findings from these studies supporting its efficacy across a wide range of conditions.[69,70] Two controlled studies have studied the efficacy of hypnosis in samples of patients with neuropathic pain.

In the first of these studies, 22 patients with MS and chronic pain were recruited into a quasi-experimental trial—quasi-experimental because 8 of the 22 were assigned to received 10 sessions of hypnosis treatment, while only a subset of 14 were randomly assigned to receive 10 sessions of either hypnosis or a relaxation training control treatment.[67] Self-hypnosis training consisted of teaching participants to enter a relaxed (trance) state and then respond to suggestions for comfort and pain relief as well as suggestions for not being bothered or upset by pain. The treatment sessions were recorded, and participants were encouraged to practice self-hypnosis at home during treatment as well as after treatment ended by listening to the audio recording and also by practicing on their own without the recording. Participants in the hypnosis condition reported greater pre- to posttreatment decreases in average daily pain intensity and pain interference (that was maintained to a 3-month follow-up assessment) than participants in the relaxation training condition.

In a second similar study, 37 adults with SCI and chronic pain (17 of whom had neuropathic pain and 20 of whom had musculoskeletal pain) were randomly assigned to received 10 sessions of either self-hypnosis training or electromyographic (EMG) biofeedback relaxation training.[66] Participants in both treatment conditions reported substantial, but similar, decrease in pain intensity from before to after the treatment sessions. However, the participants who received self-hypnosis training, but not those who received relaxation training, reported statistically significant reductions in daily average pain from pre- to posttreatment, which were maintained at 3-month follow-up. Interestingly, when the possible effects of pain type (neuropathic vs. nonneuropathic) on outcome were examined, significant treatment effects were found for those with neuropathic pain but not for those with nonneuropathic pain. Given the exploratory nature of the secondary analyses related to pain type, their replication is needed before concluding that hypnosis is more helpful for neuropathic pain problems than for nonneuropathic ones. But if replicated, such

findings might be related to the recent finding that some chronic pain can produce long-lasting changes in the cortex; changes that can then make a person more susceptible to interpret sensations as pain.[71,72] It is possible that neuropathic pain conditions may be more likely than nonneuropathic conditions to produce central (cortical) changes that contribute to the experience of pain, and pain due to central changes could potentially be more responsive to the effects of hypnotic treatments than pain caused by ongoing nociception. This admittedly speculative idea is consistent (1) with findings that persons with amputations may be particularly responsive to hypnotic interventions[73] and (2) with the knowledge that amputation produces significant central cortical changes.[74,75] In any case, the findings suggest that individuals with severe neuropathic pain might benefit from self-hypnosis training in order to reduce their perceived pain intensity.

CLINICAL IMPLICATIONS

Clearly, biomedical factors play an important, if not a central, role in the severity of neuropathic pain. By definition, neuropathic pain involves injury or disruption of the central or peripheral nervous system, and the presence of such an injury is clearly a biological factor. However, the evidence linking psychosocial factors to the severity and impact of neuropathic pain, as well as the preliminary studies indicating that treatments targeting psychosocial factors can reduce pain and pain interference, strongly suggest that psychosocial factors should be considered when assessing a patient's neuropathic pain. Moreover, the evidence indicates that patients with neuropathic pain should not necessarily be offered or provided *only* with biomedical treatments. In fact, the preliminary evidence, reviewed above, suggests that many patients with neuropathic pain can benefit specifically from CBT and self-hypnosis training.

The evidence may be used to provide clinicians with a preliminary empirical guide for developing a CBT intervention that may have the maximum efficacy for patients with neuropathic pain. First, and consistent with the model underlying CBT,[68] the evidence suggests that such an intervention should target coping, beliefs, catastrophizing cognitions, *and* social factors. A treatment that targets only one of these factors may be less effective than one that addresses each factor that has been linked to patient outcomes. Regarding the specific domains to target within each of these psychosocial factors, the evidence suggests that reasonable treatment goals in individuals with neuropathic pain would be to (1) decrease the use of rest and increase the use of task persistence as a way to cope with pain; (2) teach coping responses that provide the patient with an increased sense of control over pain (with self-hypnosis strategies probably being more effective than relaxation strategies)[66,67]; (3) teach cognitive restructuring strategies that would allow patients to transform catastrophizing cognitions into reassuring ones and to alter the meaning of pain from an indication of harm or a significant threat to a problem that is manageable and controllable[64]; and (4) facilitate social interventions, including couples counseling when indicated, to (a) increase the availability and overall quality of social support and (b) decrease the frequency of solicitous and punishing significant-other responses.

In the meantime, the field would also benefit from additional research that tests the efficacy of psychosocial interventions in various groups of patients with neuropathic pain; the available studies, while promising, have limitations (e.g., use of quasi-experimental designs versus true experimental designs, relatively small sample sizes) that need to be addressed in future studies in order to better understand the outcome domains that are most strongly affected by psychosocial treatments and also to understand the neuropathic pain populations that are most likely to benefit from these treatments. In the meantime, however, there is now adequate evidence for recommending that patients with neuropathic pain be offered psychosocial interventions if they express an interest in such therapy. Doing anything less puts these individuals at risk for suffering more than is necessary.

REFERENCES

1. Gatchel RJ, Turk DC. *Psychosocial Factors in Pain: Critical Perspectives.* New York: Guilford Press; 1999.

2. Jensen MP, Turner JA, Romano JM, Nielson WR. *Chronic Pain Coping Inventory: Professional Manual.* Lutz, FL: Psychological Assessment Resources; 2008.

3. Ersek M, Turner JA, Kemp CA. Use of the chronic pain coping inventory to assess older adults' pain coping strategies. *J Pain.* 2006;7:833–842.

4. Garcia-Campayo J, Pascual A, Alda M, et al. Coping with fibromyalgia: usefulness of the Chronic Pain Coping Inventory-42. *Pain.* 2007;132(suppl 1): S68–S76.

5. Jensen MP, Turner JA, Romano JM. Changes in beliefs, catastrophizing, and coping are associated with improvement in multidisciplinary pain treatment. *J Consult Clin Psychol.* 2001;69:655–662.

6. Jensen MP, Keefe FJ, Lefebvre JC, et al. One- and two-item measures of pain beliefs and coping strategies. *Pain.* 2003;104, 453–469.

7. Jensen MP, Turner JA, Romano JM. Changes after multidisciplinary pain treatment in patient pain beliefs and coping are associated with concurrent changes in patient functioning. *Pain.* 2007;131:38–47

8. Jensen MP, Patterson DR. Hypnotic treatment of chronic pain. *J Behav Med.* 2006;29:95–124

9. Nielson WR, Jensen MP. Relationship between changes in coping and treatment outcome in patients with fibromyalgia syndrome. *Pain.* 2004;109:233–241.

10. Nielson WR, Jensen MP, Hill ML. An activity pacing scale for the chronic pain coping inventory: development in a sample of patients with fibromyalgia syndrome. *Pain.* 2001;89: 111–115.

11. Romano JM, Jensen MP, Turner JA. The Chronic Pain Coping Inventory-42: reliability and validity. *Pain.* 2003;104:65–73.

12. Tan G, Jensen MP, Robinson-Whelen S, et al. Coping with chronic pain: a comparison of two measures. *Pain.* 2001;90:127–133

13. Tan G, Nguyen Q, Anderson KO, et al. Further validation of the chronic pain coping inventory. *J Pain.* 2005;6:29–40.

14. Turner JA, Jensen MP, Romano JM. Do beliefs, coping, and catastrophizing independently predict functioning in patients with chronic pain? *Pain.* 2000;85:115–125.

15. Truchon M, Côté D. Predictive validity of the Chronic Pain Coping Inventory in subacute low back pain. *Pain.* 2005;116:205–212.

16. Jensen MP, Turner JA, Romano JM. Correlates of improvement in multidisciplinary treatment of chronic pain. *J Consult Clin Psychol.* 1994;62:172–179.

17. Jensen MP, Keefe FJ, Lefebvre JC, et al. One- and two-item measures of pain beliefs and coping strategies. *Pain*. 2003;104:453–469.

18. Jensen MP, Karoly P. Control beliefs, coping efforts, and adjustment to chronic pain. *J Consult Clin Psychol*. 1991;59:431–438.

19. Tait RC, Chibnall JT. Development of a brief version of the Survey of Pain Attitudes. *Pain*. 1997;70:229–235.

20. Jensen MP, Turner JA, Romano JM, et al. Coping with chronic pain: a critical review of the literature. *Pain*. 1991;47:249–283.

21. Sullivan M, Thorn B, Haythornthwaite J, et al. Theoretical perspectives on the relation between catastrophizing and pain. *Clin J Pain*. 2001;17:52–64.

22. Sullivan MJL, Bishop SR, Pivik J. The Pain Catastrophizing Scale: development and validation. *Psychol Assess*. 1995;7:524–532.

23. Boothby J, Thorn BE, Stroud MW, at al. Coping with pain. In: Turk DC, Gatchel RJ, eds. *Psychosocial Factors in Pain: Critical Perspectives*. New York: Guilford Press; 1999:343–359.

24. Keefe FJ, Rumble ME, Scipio CD, et al. Psychological aspects of persistent pain: current state of the science. *J Pain*. 2004;5:195–211.

25. Keefe FJ, Caldwell DS, Williams DA, et al. Pain coping skills training in the management of osteoarthritic knee pain: II. Follow-up results. *Behav Ther*. 1990;21:435–447.

26. Fordyce WE, Fowler RS, DeLateur B. An application of behavior modification technique to a problem of chronic pain. *Behav Res Ther*. 1968;6:105–107.

27. Fordyce WE. *Behavioral Methods for Chronic Pain and Illness*. St. Louis, MO: Mosby Year Book; 1976.

28. Morley S, Eccleston C, Williams A. Systematic review and meta-analysis of randomized controlled trials of cognitive behaviour therapy and behaviour therapy for chronic pain in adults, excluding headache. *Pain*. 1999;80:1–13.

29. van Tulder MW, Ostelo R, Vlaeyen JW, et al. Behavioral treatment for chronic low back pain: a systematic review within the framework of the Cochrane Back Review Group. *Spine*. 2001;26:270–281.

30. Romano JM, Turner JA, Jensen MP, et al. Chronic pain patient-spouse behavioral interactions predict patient disability. *Pain*. 1995;63:353–360.

31. Schwartz L, Jensen MP, Romano JM. The development and psychometric evaluation of an instrument to assess spouse responses to pain and well behavior in patients with chronic pain: the Spouse Response Inventory. *J Pain*. 2005;6:243–252.

32. Kerns RD, Rosenberg R, Otis JD. Self-appraised problem solving and pain-relevant social support as predictors of the experience of chronic pain. *Ann Behav Med*. 2002;24:100–105.

33. López-Martínez AE, Esteve-Zarazaga R, Ramírez-Maestre C. Perceived social support and coping responses are independent variables explaining pain adjustment among chronic pain patients. *J Pain*. 2008;9:373–379.

34. den Boer JJ, Oostendorp RA, Beems T, et al. Continued disability and pain after lumbar disc surgery: the role of cognitive-behavioral factors. *Pain*. 2006;123:45–52.

35. Douglas C, Wollin JA, Windsor C. Biopsychosocial correlates of adjustment to pain among people with multiple sclerosis. *Clin J Pain*. 2008;24:559–567.

36. Gallagher P, MacLachlan M. Psychological adjustment and coping in adults with prosthetic limbs. *Behav Med*. 1999;25:117–124.

37. Griswold GA, Evans S, Spielman L, et al. Coping strategies of HIV patients with peripheral neuropathy. *AIDS Care*. 2005;17:711–720.

38. Hanley MA, Jensen MP, Ehde DM, et al. Psychosocial predictors of long-term adjustment to lower-limb amputation and phantom limb pain. *Disabil Rehabil*. 2004;26:882–893.

39. Hanley MA, Raichle K, Jensen MP, et al. Pain castastrophizing and beliefs predict changes in pain interference and psychological functioning in persons with spinal cord injury. *J Pain*. 2008;9:863–871.

40. Haythornthwaite JA, Clark MR, Pappagallo M, et al. Pain coping strategies play a role in the persistence of pain in post-herpetic neuralgia. *Pain*. 2003;106:453–460.

41. Hill A, Niven CA, Knussen C. The role of coping in adjustment to phantom limb pain. *Pain*. 1995;62:79–86.

42. Jensen MP, Ehde DM, Hoffman AJ, et al. Cognitions, coping and social environment predict adjustment to phantom limb pain. *Pain*. 2002;95:133–142.

43. Kennedy P, Lowe R, Grey N, et al. Traumatic spinal cord injury and psychological impact: a cross-sectional analysis of coping strategies. *Br J Clin Psychol*. 1995;34:627–639.

44. Kowal J, Overduin LY, Balfour L, et al. The role of psychological and behavioral variables in quality of life and the experience of bodily pain among persons living with HIV. *J Pain Symptom Manage*. 2008;36:247–258.

45. Molton IR, Stoelb BL, Jensen MP, et al. Psychosocial factors and adjustment to chronic pain in

spinal cord injury: replication and cross-validation. *J Rehabil Res Dev.* 2009;46:31–42.

46. Persson LC, Lilja A. Pain, coping, emotional state and physical function in patients with chronic radicular neck pain. A comparison between patients treated with surgery, physiotherapy or neck collar—a blinded, prospective randomized study. *Disabil Rehabil.* 2001;23:325–335.

47. Summers JD, Rapoff MA, Varghese G, et al. Psychosocial factors in chronic spinal cord injury pain. *Pain.* 1991;47:183–189.

48. Turner JA, Jensen MP, Warms CA, et al. Catastrophizing is associated with pain intensity, psychological distress, and pain-related disability among individuals with chronic pain after spinal cord injury. *Pain.* 2002;98:127–134.

49. Osborne TL, Jensen MP, Ehde DM, et al. Psychosocial factors associated with pain intensity, pain-related interference, and psychological functioning in persons with multiple sclerosis and pain. *Pain.* 2007;127:52–62.

50. Richardson C, Glenn S, Horgan M, et al. A prospective study of factors associated with the presence of phantom limb pain six months after major lower limb amputation in patients with peripheral vascular disease. *J Pain.* 2007;8:793–801; erratum: 8:998.

51. Wollaars MM, Post MW, van Asbeck FW, et al. Spinal cord injury pain: the influence of psychologic factors and impact on quality of life. *Clin J Pain.* 2007;23:383–391.

52. Katz J, McDermott MP, Cooper EM, et al. Psychosocial risk factors for postherpetic neuralgia: a prospective study of patients with herpes zoster. *J Pain.* 2005;6:782–790.

53. Rudy TE, Lieber SJ, Boston JR, et al. Psychosocial predictors of physical performance in disabled individuals with chronic pain. *Clin J Pain.* 2003;19:18–30.

54. Widerström-Noga EG, Cruz-Almeida Y, Martinez-Arizala A, et al. Internal consistency, stability, and validity of the spinal cord injury version of the multidimensional pain inventory. *Arch Phys Med Rehabil.* 2006;87:516–523.

55. Evans S, Fishman B, Spielman L, et al. Randomized trial of cognitive behavior therapy versus supportive psychotherapy for HIV-related peripheral neuropathic pain. *Psychosomatics.* 2003;44:44–50.

56. Giardino ND, Jensen MP, Turner JA, et al. Social environment moderates the association between catastrophizing and pain among persons with spinal cord injury. *Pain.* 2003;106:19–25.

57. Sullivan MJ, Lynch ME, Clark AJ. Dimensions of catastrophic thinking associated with pain experience and disability in patients with neuropathic pain conditions. *Pain.* 2005;113:310–315.

58. Ullrich P, Jensen MP, Loeser JD, et al. Catastrophizing mediates associations between pain severity, distress, and functional disability among persons with spinal cord injury. *Rehabil Psychol.* 2007;52:390–398.

59. Ullrich PM, Jensen MP, Loeser JD, et al. Pain among veterans with spinal cord injury. *J Rehabil Res Dev.* 2008;45:793–800.

60. Whyte A, Carroll LJ. The relationship between catastrophizing and disability in amputees experiencing phantom pain. *Disabil Rehabil.* 2004;26:649–654.

61. Asano M, Rushton P, Miller WC, et al. Predictors of quality of life among individuals who have a lower limb amputation. *Prosthet Orthot Int.* 2008;32:231–243.

62. Stroud MW, Turner JA, Jensen MP, et al. Partner responses to pain behaviors are associated with depression and activity interference among persons with chronic pain and spinal cord injury. *J Pain.* 2006;7:91–99.

63. Williams RM, Ehde DM, Smith DG, et al. A two-year longitudinal study of social support following amputation. *Disabil Rehabil.* 2004;26:862–874.

64. Ehde DM, Jensen MP. Feasibility of a cognitive restructuring intervention for treatment of chronic pain in persons with disabilities. *Rehabil Psychol.* 2004;49:254–258.

65. Budh CH, Kowalski J, Lundeberg T. A comprehensive pain management programme comprising educational, cognitive and behavioural interventions for neuropathic pain following spinal cord injury. *J Rehabil Med.* 2006;38:172–180.

66. Jensen MP, Barber J, Romano JM, et al. Effects of self-hypnosis training and EMG biofeedback relaxation training on chronic pain in persons with spinal cord injury. *Int J Clin Exper Hypnos.* 2009;57:239–268.

67. Jensen MP, Barber J, Romano JM, et al. A comparison of self-hypnosis versus progressive muscle relaxation in patients with multiple sclerosis and chronic pain. *Int J Clin Exper Hypnos.* 2009;57:198–221.

68. Turk DC. A cognitive-behavioral perspective on treatment of chronic pain patients. In: Turk DC, Gatchel RJ, eds. *Psychosocial Approaches to Pain Management: A Practitioner's Handbook.* New York: Guilford Press; 2002:138–158.

69. Elkins G, Jensen MP, Patterson DR. Hypnosis for the treatment of chronic pain. *Int J Clin Exper Hypnos.* 2007;55:275–287.

70. Patterson DR, Jensen MP. Hypnosis and clinical pain. *Psychol Bull.* 2003;29:495–521.

71. Tinazzi, M, Fiaschi A, Rosso T, et al. Neuroplastic changes related to pain occur at multiple levels of the human somatosensory system: a somatosensory-evoked potentials study in patients with cervical radicular pain. *J Neurosci.* 2000;20:9277–9283.

72. Melzack R, Coderre TJ, Katz J, et al. Central neuroplasticity and pathological pain. *Ann NY Acad Sci.* 2001;933:157–174.

73. Jensen MP, Hanley MA, Engel JM, et al. Hypnotic analgesia for chronic pain in persons with disabilities: a case series. *Int J Clin Exper Hypnos.* 2005:53:198–228.

74. Flor H, Elbert T, Knecht S, et al. Phantom-limb pain as a perceptual correlate of cortical reorganization following arm amputation. *Nature.* 1995;375:482–484.

75. Elbert T, Rockstroh B. Reorganization of human cerebral cortex: the range of changes following use and injury. *Neuroscientist.* 2004;10:129–141.

8

Pharmacotherapy of Neuropathic Pain

ROY FREEMAN

INTRODUCTION

A VARIETY OF agents from diverse pharmacological classes are used to treat neuropathic pain. Several of these have regulatory approval, while the use of others is based on data from randomized clinical trials and/or inferences about the mechanism of action. This chapter will cover the most widely used of these agents. Several approaches to the classification of the pharmacological agents used to treat neuropathic pain exist. These include (1) operational classifications, such as the World Health Organization (WHO) ladder approach based on pain severity; (2) disease-based approaches, such as drugs to treat painful diabetic peripheral neuropathy, postherpetic neuralgia, human immunodeficiency virus (HIV)-associated painful neuropathy, and so on; (3) a classification based on the primary or most widespread use of the drug, such as antidepressants, anticonvulsants, anti-inflammatories, antiarrhythmics, and so on; (4) neuroanatomical approaches, such as drugs for central neuropathic pain, spinal pain, or peripheral neuropathic pain; (5) physiological classifications, such as drugs modulating transduction, conduction, transmission, excitation, inhibition, and so on; (6) pain mechanism-based approaches, such as drugs affecting peripheral sensitization, ectopic firing, enhanced transmission, central sensitization, increased excitation, reduced inhibition, and so on; and (7) molecular target-based approaches.

In this chapter, I will adopt a molecular target-based approach while recognizing that (1) most drugs have more than one molecular target; (2) the analgesic mechanism may not be due to the primary or most widely recognized drug target; and (3) the analgesic mechanism may be related to the engagement of multiple molecular targets. Only oral and topical agents will be covered and only those that are in clinical use, although these agents are not necessarily approved by regulatory authorities for specific use in neuropathic pain. Intravenous and intrathecal agents will not be covered in this chapter.

Numerous recent expert reviews and consensus statements are available that cover treatment algorithms, suggested sequential approaches to therapy, drug stratification by weight of evidence, and neuropathic pain drug characteristics classified by the number needed to treat and the number needed to harm in clinical trials.[1–6] The interested reader is referred to those reports.

MOLECULAR TARGETS

TRPV1 Channel

BACKGROUND

The transient receptor potential (TRP) channels are a family of receptor proteins that play a role in the transduction of physical stress. These channels have a similar structure: a functional channel composed of four subunits, each consisting of six transmembrane domains with the pore-forming region between the fifth and sixth transmembrane domains (and large amino and carboxyl termini on the cytosolic side). Several of these channels (TRP vanilloid types 1–4 [V1–4], TRP melastin type 8 [M8], and TRP ankyrin type 1 [A1]) play a role in nociception. TRPV1 is the most widely studied TRP channel. This nonselective cation channel was cloned by Caterina et al. in 1997. It functions as an integrator of noxious chemical and physical stimuli. TRPV1 is expressed in small- and medium-diameter nociceptor sensory neurons, although recent reports have suggested a more widespread distribution.[7,8] There is evidence of TRPV1 expression in visceral sensory neurons including bladder, bronchopulmonary colonic, and cardiac afferents, where they play a role in visceral sensation and tissue homeostasis, most likely through the release of tachykinins and calcitonin gene related peptide (CGRP).[7,8]

TRPV1 is activated by exogenous ligands such as capsaicin and resiniferatoxin, noxious heat (>42°C), protons, and endogenous ligands including the lipid anandamide[9] (it is also activated by acid and several neuropeptides).

Activation of the TRPV1 receptor leads to the opening of the nonselective cation channel, allowing the influx of sodium and calcium ions and the consequent depolarization of nociceptor afferent neurons. The role of the TRPV1 receptor in neuropathic pain is not fully elucidated. TRPV1 null mice show impaired thermal hyperalgesia in models of inflammation but not in models of neuropathic pain.[10] Further, there is conflicting evidence as to whether TRPV1 is upregulated in neuropathic pain models and in humans with neuropathic pain.[11,12]

TRPV1 AGONISTS—CAPSAICIN

The vanilloid capsaicin, the pungent component in hot chili peppers, is widely used as a topical agent to treat neuropathic pain and also musculoskeletal pain and itch.[13] The mechanism whereby topical capsaicin leads to pain relief is unknown. This neurotoxin initially activates and then depletes substance P from the terminals of unmyelinated C fibers. Repeated application of low-concentration capsaicin[14] and a single application of high-concentration capsaicin[15] lead to impaired perception of heat and other sensory stimuli and loss of intraepidermal nerve fiber immunoreactivity. Topical application of capsaicin results in burning pain and itch mediated by discharges in C polymodal and Aδ mechano-heat nociceptors due to TRPV1 receptor activation. Physiological desensitization of the nociceptor neurons follows the initial activation; however, with repeated application, degeneration of nociceptor[14,16,17] and autonomic[18] nerves occurs. The mechanism of capsaicin-induced neurodegeneration is not fully elucidated. TRPV1-mediated calcium influx[19] with subsequent glutamate release is most likely implicated.[20,21] The desensitization and subsequent degeneration may underlie the analgesic effects of capsaicin, although this has not been definitively proven.

Topical application of capsaicin as a repeatedly applied low-concentration cream (0.075%) and application of a high-concentration patch (8%) are used therapeutically to provide pain relief in several neuropathic pain conditions.[13,22,23] There is evidence derived from randomized clinical trials that application of low-concentration capsaicin (0.025–0.075%), four to five times daily for up to 8 weeks, is effective in treating patients with neuropathic pain due to diabetic neuropathy[24-26] (although not in all studies),[27] postherpetic neuralgia,[28] postsurgical pain,[29] and postmastectomy pain.[30] Several weeks of therapy may be required to attain a therapeutic benefit (see Table 8.1).

There are more recent reports of a single application of 8% capsaicin applied as a patch to the painful site for 30 to 90 minutes. There is evidence of efficacy in postherpetic neuralgia[22,31,32] and in pain due to HIV neuropathy (following a 30 minute and 90 minute but not 60 minute application).[33] The intense pain associated with this delivery mode requires pretreatment with topical and/or oral analgesics (see Table 8.1). The potential for unblinding in all studies of capsaicin is high due to the prominent local symptoms and signs. In order to mitigate this concern, recent studies with the high-concentration (8%) capsaicin patch have used a low-concentration capsaicin (0.04%) as a control.

Systemic exposure is minimal (a mean area under the curve [AUC] value of 7.42 ng x h/mL and a maximum concentration [C_{max}] value of 1.86 ng/mL) after 60 minutes of high-concentration capsaicin patch exposure.[34] Adverse effects are primarily local and include local erythema, edema, and swelling. Sensory symptoms include pain, frequently of a stinging or burning nature, pruritus, and hyperalgesia. Aerosolization of capsaicin may lead to mucous membrane irritation, tearing, and respiratory symptoms such as coughing, sneezing, and shortness of breath due to inhalation of aerosolized capsaicin. The long-term consequences of sensory and autonomic denervation of neuropathic regions, particularly those exposed to pressure, is unknown.[17,18]

Calcium Channel—α2-δ Subunit (Ca$_v$α$_2$-δ)

BACKGROUND

Five voltage-gated calcium channels exist, each having differing biophysical and structural characteristics and nervous system distributions. Each channel consists of pore-forming α$_1$ subunits with associated auxiliary subunits.[35,36] These are subdivided into low voltage-activated T-type (Ca$_v$3.1, Ca$_v$3.2, Ca$_v$3.3) and high voltage-activated L-type (Ca$_v$1.1 through Ca$_v$1.4), N-type (Ca$_v$2.2), P/Q-type (Ca$_v$2.1), and R-type (Ca$_v$2.3) calcium channels, depending on the channel forming Ca$_v$α$_1$ subunits. The subunits regulate the

Table 8-1. The Initial and Maximal Doses of the Topical Agents

AGENT	INITIAL DOSE	MAXIMUM DOSE	COMMENTS
Lidocaine ointment (5%)	Topical application of 5 g/day (250 mg of lidocaine base). Equivalent to a 6 in. length of ointment.	17 to 20 g of ointment (850 to 1000 mg of lidocaine base) per day.	Apply to intact skin only.
Lidocaine patch (5%)	Apply up to three patches topically at one time, for up to 12 hours within a 24 hour period.		Apply to intact skin only. Patches may be cut into smaller sizes.
Capsaicin (0.025–0.075%)	Apply as a thin film to the affected area three to four times per day. Gently rub in until fully absorbed.		Apply to intact skin only. Application for up to 8 weeks may be necessary. Wash hands thoroughly immediately after use.
Capsaicin patch (8%)	Apply up to four patches every 3 months for 60 min as needed.		Apply to intact skin no more frequently than every 3 months.

biophysical properties of the channel and play a role in the expression and trafficking of the channel complex.[37] L-, N-, and P/Q-type calcium channels are expressed in sensory neurons.[35]

Gabapentin and pregabalin are structural analogs of the neurotransmitter gamma-aminobutyric acid (GABA); however, neither molecule interacts with $GABA_A$ or $GABA_B$ receptors, increases GABA availability, or influences the uptake or degradation of GABA.[38,39] The mechanism of action of these molecules in neuropathic pain is not fully elucidated, although understanding has grown substantially in the past decade. Both molecules bind with potency and selectivity to the type 1 and type 2 α_2-δ subunits of the voltage-gated calcium channel ($Ca_v\alpha_2$-δ_1 and $Ca_v\alpha_2$-δ_2).[38,40] Activity is associated with decreased calcium channel function,[41] inhibition of presynaptic vesicular release,[42] and decreased release of neurotransmitters that include glutamate, noradrenaline, and substance P.[43-45] The decreased neurotransmitter release is associated with reduced hyperexcitability in animal models of nociceptive and neuropathic pain and occurs preferentially when there is neuronal activation.[44]

There is increased expression of α_2-δ type 1 protein in rodent neuropathic pain models.[46,47] Pregabalin and gabapentin reduce pain-related behaviors in these models and others, including the formalin footpad model, the carrageenan thermal hyperalgesia model, and rodent models of postsurgical pain.[38,48] Furthermore, pregabalin activity is selectively lost in mutant mice containing a single-point mutation within the gene encoding for the auxiliary subunit to α_2-δ type 1 and type 2 proteins of voltage-dependent calcium channels. While the mice demonstrate normal pain phenotypes and typical responses to other analgesic drugs, the mutation leads to a significant reduction in the binding affinity of pregabalin in the brain and spinal cord and the loss of its analgesic efficacy, supporting the notion that the analgesic effects of these agents are mediated through the α_2-δ subunit of the calcium channel.[49-51] More recent studies show that chronic but not acute application of gabapentin inhibits calcium currents and reduces trafficking of calcium channels.[50,51] There is also evidence that gabapentin antagonizes binding of the extracellular matrix protein, thrombospondin, to α_2-δ type 1 protein, thereby inhibiting in vitro synapse formation.[52] These data suggest an additional mechanism of action for these drugs, namely, blocking the formation of new excitatory synapses.

CALCIUM CHANNEL α_2-δ SUBUNIT LIGANDS—GABAPENTIN AND PREGABALIN

The α_2-δ ligands, gabapentin and pregabalin, have shown efficacy in a number of clinical trials for the treatment of neuropathic pain including postherpetic neuralgia (gabapentin[53,54] and pregabalin[55-58]), painful diabetic peripheral neuropathy (gabapentin[59] and pregabalin[58,60-62]), and spinal cord injury pain (pregabalin[63]). However, not all neuropathic pain studies in these disorders have been positive, such as the use of gabapentin in diabetic peripheral neuropathy[64] and pregabalin in diabetic peripheral neuropathy.[65] Furthermore, efficacy has not been demonstrated in several neuropathic pain disorders, including pregabalin in HIV neuropathic pain,[66] pregabalin in radicular pain,[67] and gabapentin in chemotherapy neuropathy pain.[68]

Gabapentin is absorbed from the gastrointestinal tract by a saturable mechanism. The time to the peak concentration of immediate-release formulations is around 2 hours. This may be delayed in extended-release formulations up to 8 hours. Oral bioavailability of immediate-release formulations decreases with increasing doses; bioavailability of a 900 mg oral dose is around 60%, while bioavailability of a 3600 mg oral is around 33%. A 14% increase in the AUC and C_{max} has been reported when gabapentin is taken with food. There is minimal protein binding. Gabapentin is not metabolized and is excreted unchanged in the urine. The elimination half-life is around 6 h. The clearance of gabapentin is reduced in patients with impaired creatinine clearance, and dose adjustment is required. The plasma clearance is proportional to the creatine clearance.[69]

Pregabalin is rapidly absorbed, with a time to peak concentration of 1.5 hours. The bioavailability is greater than 90%. Food has no clinically relevant effect on total absorption but delays the time to peak concentration by

3 hours. There is no protein binding. There is no hepatic metabolism; 90% of pregabalin is excreted unchanged in the urine. The plasma clearance of pregabalin is also proportional to the creatinine clearance. The elimination half-life is 6.3 hours.[70,71]

The two α_2-δ ligands have pharmacological similarities. Neither agent binds to plasma proteins. There is no hepatic metabolism, and these agents do not compete for or inhibit the cytochrome P450 system. There are few clinically important drug-drug interactions. Both agents are excreted unchanged by the kidneys.[72] There may be some clinically important pharmacological differences between these agents. Pregabalin, in contrast to gabapentin, has linear and dose-proportional absorption in the therapeutic dose range (150–600 mg/day) due to a nonsaturable transport mechanism.[73] In addition, pregabalin has a more rapid onset of action and a more limited dosage range that requires minimal titration (gabapentin requires gradual titration to the clinically effective dose of 1800–3600 mg). Pregabalin may also be effective in a twice daily dose, although not all studies support this dosage schedule[74,75] (see Table 8.2).

Adverse effects of both agents include dose-dependent dizziness, somnolence, peripheral edema, asthenia, headache, and dry mouth. These effects may be attenuated by a lower starting dose and more gradual titration. Pregabalin is considered a Schedule V drug in the United States.

Sodium Channel

BACKGROUND

Voltage-gated sodium channels are membrane proteins that mediate the generation and transmission of electric currents in excitable cells. In response to depolarization, sodium channels activate, allow passage of sodium ions through the pore, and then inactivate rapidly.[76] Each channel is formed by four α subunits that form the ion-selective pore and one or two β subunits that modulate the channel kinetics and voltage gating. Each α subunit has six transmembrane segments connected by three intracellular loops. Nine sodium channel isoforms exist ($Na_v1.1$–$Na_v1.9$), each having unique biophysical properties and nervous system distribution.[77] $Na_v1.7$, $Na_v1.8$, and $Na_v1.9$ are expressed in peripheral sensory neurons, and $Na_v1.3$ is upregulated along pain-signaling pathways after nerve injury.[76,78–81] Several lines of evidence support a role for sodium channel channels in neuropathic pain. These include the following: (1) changes in sodium channel expression occur after nerve injury (e.g., $Na_v1.3$ expression is increased in rodent nerve injury models, and $Na_v1.3$ and $Na_v1.6$ are upregulated in a rodent model of diabetes)[76,78–81]; (2) increased sodium channel expression and lidocaine-sensitive spontaneous discharges occur at the site of nerve injury[82,83]; (3) gain-of-function missense mutations in *SCN9A*, the gene that encodes for $Na_v1.7$, have been shown to cause the inherited pain disorders primary erythermalgia and paroxysmal extreme pain disorder[84,85]; and (4) loss-of-function nonsense mutations in *SCN9A* lead to channelopathy-associated insensitivity to pain, a disorder in which affected individuals are unable to perceive physical pain.[86–88] These data not only support a potential role for sodium channel antagonists in the treatment of neuropathic pain but also provide a rationale for the use of sodium channel isoform-specific antagonists. The more specific approach to sodium channel antagonism may improve the narrow therapeutic window; dose-related adverse effects are

Table 8-2. The Initial Dose, Dose Increment, and Typical Effective Dose of the α_2–δ Subunit Ligands

AGENT	INITIAL DOSE	DOSE INCREMENT	TYPICAL EFFECTIVE DOSE
Gabapentin	100–300 mg one to three times daily	100–300 mg for 1–5 days	300–1800 mg three times daily
Pregabalin	25–75 mg one to three times daily	25–50 mg for 3 days	50–200 mg three times daily or 75–300 mg twice daily

Note: Dose increments based on efficacy and tolerability.

frequently the limiting factors when using the nonspecific sodium channel antagonists currently available. Enthusiasm for this approach to sodium channel antagonism should be tempered by the observation that neuropathic pain persists in mutant mice null for $Na_v1.3$, $Na_v1.7$, and $Na_v1.8$.[89,90]

SODIUM CHANNEL ANTAGONISTS

Topical Lidocaine. The effectiveness of topical lidocaine, applied as a 5% patch, in the treatment of postherpetic neuralgia has been demonstrated in randomized, inert, vehicle-controlled trials.[91-93] The results of these trials have led to U.S. Food and Drug Administration (FDA) approval of the 5% lidocaine patch for the treatment of postherpetic neuralgia. This agent may be more effective in postherpetic neuralgia patients with allodynia. Open-label studies have shown improvement in the treatment of neuropathic pain[94] and the quality of life in patients with painful neuropathy due to diabetes.[95] Efficacy is not demonstrated in all studies[96]

Up to three lidocaine patches may be applied, only once for up to 12 hours within a 24 hour period. Gel or ointment may be used if patches are unavailable or if the skin surface is not suitable for patch application (see Table 8.1). Adverse effects include mild skin reactions such as erythema and edema. Systemic absorption is minimal, provided that the patches are not placed over broken or inflamed skin.

Lamotrigine. Lamotrigine has been studied in a variety of neuropathic pain conditions including diabetic peripheral neuropathy, chemotherapy-induced peripheral neuropathic pain, HIV-associated neuropathic pain, mixed neuropathic pain, spinal cord injury-related pain, and poststroke pain. In smaller and/or investigator-initiated studies, this agent has shown some effectiveness in the treatment of neuropathic pain associated with HIV neuropathy[97,98] (perhaps greater effectiveness in patients on antiretroviral therapy),[98] diabetic peripheral neuropathy,[99] central poststroke pain,[100] and pain following incomplete spinal cord injury,[101] but these results were not confirmed in larger multicenter studies.[102,103]

Lamotrigine, a voltage-dependent sodium channel antagonist, attenuates repetitive firing of sodium-dependent action potentials and may inhibit the release of the excitatory neurotransmitters, glutamate and aspartate.[104] The time to peak concentration of lamotrigine is 1.4 to 4.8 hours after oral ingestion. The bioavailability is 98%. Food has no clinically relevant effect on total absorption. Protein binding is approximately 55%. There is extensive hepatic metabolism. The elimination half-life is 25–70 hours. This is increased with concurrent administration of valproic acid. Concurrent use of this agent with valproic acid should be avoided.[105,106]

The agent should be slowly titrated to doses between 200 and 400 mg daily (see Table 8.3).

Table 8-3. The Initial Dose, Dose Increment, and Typical Effective Doses of the Oral Sodium Channel Antagonists

AGENT	INITIAL DOSE	DOSE INCREMENT	TYPICAL EFFECTIVE DOSE
Lamotrigine	25 mg daily or every other day for 2 weeks	25 mg daily for 2 weeks, then increase by 25–50 mg daily every week	200–400 mg (total) once or twice a day
Topiramate	25–50 mg daily	50 mg daily, increased every week	50–200 mg twice a day
Oxcarbazepine	300 mg twice daily	300 mg every 3 days	1200–1800 mg daily
Lacosamide	50 mg once or twice daily	50 mg twice a day every week	100–200 mg twice a day
Carbamazepine	100–200 mg twice daily	100–200 mg every 2 days	200–400 mg three times a day

Note: Dose increments based on efficacy and tolerability.

Adverse effects include rash, gastrointestinal symptoms, headache, somnolence, and dizziness. Severe rash, including that of Stevens-Johnson syndrome, is a serious potential side effect of this agent.

Topiramate. The anticonvulsant and antimigraine agent, topiramate, has been extensively studied in patients with painful diabetic peripheral neuropathy. In four studies of patients with neuropathic pain due to diabetes, this agent was no more effective than placebo[107,108]; however, in one study, topiramate significantly reduced pain, measured on a visual analog scale, compared to placebo.[109] Specification of the time and location of the pain, as well as the inability to use rescue medications, may account for the differences between the positive and negative studies.

Topiramate has multiple potential mechanisms of action. It blocks voltage- activated sodium channels; blocks kainate and α-amino-3-hydroxy-5-methyisoxazole-4-propionic acid (AMPA) glutamate receptors; enhances GABA-mediated inhibition; inhibits the carbonic anhydrase enzyme, particularly isozymes II and IV; and inhibits calcium currents.[110]

Topiramate is rapidly absorbed, with a time to peak concentration of 1.5 to 4 hours after oral ingestion. Bioavailability is 80%. Protein binding is 9% to 41%. There is some hepatic metabolism, although 70% is excreted unchanged in the urine. The elimination half-life is 21 hours.[111]

The agent should be slowly titrated to doses between 50 and 200 mg twice daily (see Table 8.3). Weight loss is a common adverse effect and was observed in all studies. Nausea, somnolence, dizziness, paresthesias, and cognitive dysfunction were also frequent adverse effects. Hypohidrosis occurs rarely.[112] The paresthesias are most likely a consequence of the inhibition of carbonic acid anhydrase enzymes.[113]

Oxcarbazepine. There is limited support for the use of oxcarbazepine in the treatment of neuropathic pain. In one randomized, placebo-controlled trial, oxcarbazepine titrated to a maximum dose of 1800 mg/day was efficacious in the treatment of painful diabetic neuropathy.[114] However, in two subsequent studies, oxcarbazepine administered as 1200 and 1800 mg/day[115] and 1200 mg/day[116] failed to show a statistically significant therapeutic effect.

Oxcarbazepine is structurally related to carbamazepine and has a similar spectrum of activity in animal models of epilepsy.[117,118] The mechanism of action of oxcarbazepine is most like mediated by its 10-monohydroxy metabolite (MHD) blocking voltage-gated sodium channels, thereby stabilizing hyperexcited neuronal membranes, inhibiting repetitive neuronal discharges, and diminishing synaptic impulse propagation.

Oxcarbazepine has excellent oral bioavailability. It is completely absorbed, and there is no food effect. There is extensive hepatic metabolism to form the active MHD. Excretion is predominantly renal. The elimination half-life of oxcarbazepine is 2 hours and that of the MHD is 9 hours.[118,119]

The agent should be slowly titrated to doses between 1200 and 2400 mg daily (see Table 8.3). Common adverse effects include dizziness, somnolence, ataxia, nausea, and vomiting. Hyponatremia occurs in up to 23% of cases. Agranulocytosis, aplastic anemia, and pancytopenia may occur rarely. In two long-term safety studies in patients with painful diabetic peripheral neuropathy, approximately 20% of patients withdrew due to gastrointestinal and nervous system adverse events.[120]

Lacosamide. In three large multicenter randomized parallel trials of patients with neuropathic pain due to diabetes, 400 mg lacosamide produced equivocal results. In one study, lacosamide significantly improved neuropathic pain scores compared to placebo; in a second study, the effect in the lacosamide-treated group approached significance compared to placebo; and in a third, the effect of lacosamide failed to differentiate from that of placebo.[121–123]

Preclinical experiments suggest that lacosamide selectively enhances slow inactivation of voltage-gated sodium channels, resulting in stabilization of hyperexcitable neuronal membranes and inhibition of repetitive neuronal firing while indicating no effects on physiological neuronal excitability. Lacosamide also binds to collapsin response mediator protein 2 (CRMP-2), a phosphoprotein that is mainly expressed in the nervous system. CRMP-2 expression may be dysregulated in the central nervous system in animal models of neuropathic pain. Lacosamide has demonstrated efficacy in animal models of neuropathic pain.[124]

Lacosamide is rapidly and completely absorbed after oral administration, with a negligible first-pass effect. There is high oral bioavailability (~100%), with no food effect. Peak plasma concentrations occur between 0.5 and 4 hours after administration. Plasma concentrations are dose-proportional, with low intrasubject and intersubject variability. The plasma half-life of the unchanged drug is approximately 13 hours and is not altered by different doses or by multiple dosing. Lacosamide is largely unbound to plasma protein (<15%). About 90% of the dose is renally excreted as an unchanged compound. The major metabolic pathway is demethylation. The O-desmethyl metabolite is excreted in the urine and has no known pharmacological activity.[124]

The agent should be slowly titrated to doses between 100 and 200 mg twice a day (see Table 8.3). The most common treatment emergent adverse effects occurring with greater prevalence in the lacosamide-treated diabetic peripheral neuropathy group in these clinical trials (at the 400 mg/day dose) were dose-related dizziness (~13.6%), fatigue (~7.7%), nausea (~6.8%), ataxia, and dose-related tremor (~5.9%). Cardiac adverse effects, which occurred at low frequency, include PR interval prolongation, atrial fibrillation, and atrial flutter (0.5%).[121–123]

Mexiletine. The class 1b antiarrhythmic agent, mexiletine, an oral congener of the lidocaine blocker, has been studied in the treatment of diabetic peripheral neuropathy.[125–131]

The results obtained with this anesthetic antiarrhythmic, which is structurally similar to lidocaine, have been inconsistent. The starting dose of this agent is 150 mg daily. It can be gradually increased by 150 mg daily to a dose of 150–300 mg three or four times a day. Some have suggested that the responsiveness to this agent may be predicted based on the response to intravenous lidocaine.[126]

Side effects of this agent include gastrointestinal disturbance, headache, dizziness, and tremor. It may worsen cardiac arrhythmias. Use of this agent is contraindicated in patients with second- and third-degree heart block. The narrow therapeutic window limits extensive use of this agent.

Carbamazepine. Carbamazepine is approved by the FDA for the treatment of trigeminal neuralgia but has shown only modest success in small clinical trials in the treatment of diabetic peripheral neuropathy.[132] Carbamazepine slows the recovery rate of voltage-gated sodium channels. Side effects include dizziness, drowsiness, balance difficulties, skin rash, and, rarely, leukopenia, thrombocytopenia, and hepatic damage.[133]

Phenytoin. Phenytoin, which also slows the voltage-gated sodium channel recovery rate, has not been extensively studied in neuropathic pain. There are conflicting data on the efficacy of this agent in the treatment of painful diabetic neuropathy.[134,135] Adverse effects include rash, gingival hypertrophy, dizziness, ataxia, and teratogenicity. Frequent drug monitoring is necessary (not sure what you mean; this may be more relevant to epilepsy than PN).

The Monoamines—Norepinephrine, Serotonin, and Dopamine

BACKGROUND

A descending pain-modulating circuit, with origins in cortical and subcortical regions, projects to the spinal cord via the midbrain and plays an important role in modulating the pain experience. Projections from multiple regions including the prefrontal cortex, insula, rostral anterior cingular cortex, hypothalamus, and amygdala synapse in the midbrain periaqueductal gray. The periaqueductal gray has projections to the noradrenergic nuclei (the A5, A6 [also known as the *locus coeruleus*] and A7 nuclei) in the pons and to serotonergic nuclei, including the nucleus raphe magnus and the nucleus reticularis gigantocellularis in the rostral ventrolateral medulla. These nuclei have descending monoaminergic outputs to the spinal cord.

The monoamines—norepinephrine acting on spinal α-adrenoreceptors, serotonin acting on serotonin (5-HT) receptors, and dopamine acting on dopaminergic (D) receptors in the spinal cord—are the major neurotransmitters of these pathways. Activation of these receptors may be facilitatory or inhibitory, depending on the receptor subtype and the site of activation. For example, several lines of evidence have shown that activation of α-2 adrenoreceptors in the spinal cord leads to antinociceptive effects, as does α-1 adrenoreceptor activation of GABAergic interneurons.[136] Whereas activation of the 5-HT2 and 5-HT3 receptor subtypes is pronociceptive, activation of the 5-HT7 receptor subtype is anti-nociceptive. Further, D2 receptor activation is anti-nociceptive, while D1 receptor activation is pro-nociceptive. The balance between these inhibitory and facilitatory circuits plays a central role in the perception of pain.

The monamine reuptake inhibitors—the tricyclic antidepressants, selective serotonin reuptake inhibitors, norepinephrine and serotonin reuptake inhibitors, and triple reuptake inhibitors (which inhibit reuptake of serotonin, norepinephrine, and dopamine)—increase synaptic monoamine levels and directly influence the activity of these descending neurons. The opioids, α-2 delta ligands, and the atypical opioids (tramadol, tapentadol) interact with these pathways.[137,138]

TRICYCLIC AGENTS

The tertiary amine, amitriptyline, is the best studied of the tricyclic agents and has been shown in numerous randomized, blinded, placebo-controlled clinical trials to significantly reduce neuropathic pain.[139–141] Meta-analyses and reviews of randomized, placebo-controlled diabetic neuropathy pain and postherpetic neuralgia trials revealed that tricyclic agents are efficacious, providing at least a 50% reduction in pain intensity in 30% of individuals.[142,143] Their effectiveness in these disorders appears to be unrelated to their antidepressant effect.[139] However, tricyclic agents have not proven to be effective in HIV neuropathy,[131,144] chemotherapy neuropathy,[145] lumbar root pain,[146] spinal cord

injury pain,[147] and postamputation pain.[148] Side effects include drowsiness, confusion, constipation, dry mouth, urinary retention, weight gain, and orthostatic hypotension. The secondary amines, nortriptyline and desipramine, have a less troublesome side effect profile than the tertiary amines, amitriptyline and imipramine. The use of these secondary agents is preferable, particularly in the elderly and in side effect-prone patients.[140,149] Several studies have suggested that there is an increased risk of myocardial ischemia and arrhythmogenesis associated with tricyclic agents.[150–152] In a large retrospective cohort study, a dose-related increased risk of sudden death in patients treated with tricyclic agents was reported; this risk was produced by amitriptyline-equivalent doses of greater that 100 mg.[153] However, this finding was not confirmed in a similar study.[154] Nevertheless, because of concerns about possible cardiotoxicity, tricyclic antidepressants should be used with caution in patients with known or suspected cardiac disease A screening electrocardiogram is recommended in patients older than 40 years.[3] For dosing, see Table 8.4.

SELECTIVE SEROTONIN AND NOREPINEPHRINE REUPTAKE INHIBITORS

The selective norepinephrine and serotonin reuptake inhibitors, venlafaxine and duloxetine, have proven efficacy in neuropathic pain. These agents inhibit the reuptake of serotonin and norepinephrine without producing the muscarinic, histaminic, and adrenergic side effects that accompany the use of the tricyclic agents.

Duloxetine. Duloxetine, a secondary amine, is a balanced norepinephrine and serotonin reuptake inhibitor. This agent is FDA approved for the treatment of neuropathic pain in diabetes. In doses of 60 and 120 mg/day, duloxetine showed efficacy in the treatment of neuropathic pain due to diabetes.[155–158] The durability of the analgesic effect has been shown in a 52 week open-label study.[159] In long-term studies of duloxetine, a small increase in hemoglobin A1C was seen in duloxetine-treated diabetic

Table 8-4. The Initial Dose, Dose Increment, and Typical Effective Doses of the Monoamine Reuptake Inhibitors

AGENT	INITIAL DOSE	DOSE INCREMENT	TYPICAL EFFECTIVE DOSE
Tricyclic agents	10–25 mg daily	10–25 mg/week	25–150 mg daily
Duloxetine	20–60 mg daily	20–30 mg every 1–3 days	120 mg daily (or 60 mg twice daily)
Venlafaxine	37.5 mg daily	37.5–75 mg every 4 days	150–225 mg (total dose) taken daily (extended release) or three times a day (immediate release)
Bupropion	100 mg immediate-release or 150 mg extended-release form daily for 3 days	100–150 mg daily for several weeks	150–450 mg (total dose) taken daily (extended release) or three or four times a day (immediate release)

Note: Dose increments based on efficacy and tolerability.

subjects compared with placebo (0.52 vs. 0.19%).[160] The effectiveness of duloxetine in postherpetic neuralgia and other neuropathic pains has not been investigated.

Duloxetine potentiates serotonergic and noradrenergic activity by selectively inhibiting the reuptake of serotonin and norepinephrine. This feature differentiates this class of compounds from selective serotonin reuptake inhibitors, but there is no demonstrated evidence of efficacy in neuropathic pain. There is no significant adrenergic, dopaminergic, cholinergic, opioid, glutamate, or histaminergic receptor affinity. The oral bioavailability is around 50%. Time to peak concentration following oral administration is approximately 6 hours. There is a food effect; time to peak concentration is delayed to 10 hours, and the AUC is decreased by 10%. There is no food effect on the peak concentration. Protein binding is greater than 90%. There is extensive hepatic metabolism. Duloxetine is oxidized and conjugated in the liver. The cytochrome P450 isozymes, CYP1A2 and CYP2D6, are involved in the hepatic metabolism. Excretion is predominantly renal. Twenty percent of duloxetine is excreted unchanged in the feces. The elimination half-life is approximately 12 hours.[161,162]

Adverse events with duloxetine use include nausea, constipation, decreased appetite, dizziness, xerostomia, and hyperhidrosis. Both somnolence and insomnia may occur. Serious rare adverse events include hepatotoxicity

and abnormal bleeding. There is no significant cardiotoxicity.[159,163,164] For dosing, see Table 8.4.

Venlafaxine. Venlafaxine in doses of 150–225 mg/day has shown effectiveness in the treatment of patients with neuropathic pain of various causes[165] and painful diabetic peripheral neuropathy.[166] It may take several weeks to attain significant symptom relief. Venlafaxine was not efficacious in postmastectomy and postherpetic neuralgia clinical trials.[143,167]

Venlafaxine also selectively inhibits reuptake of the neurotransmitters norepinephrine and serotonin, although higher doses may be required for norepinephrine reuptake inhibition.[168] The bioavailability of regular-release venlafaxine following oral administration is 13%, while extended-release venlafaxine has a bioavailability of 45%. There is no significant food effect. Protein binding is around 30%. Venlafaxine undergoes extensive first-pass hepatic metabolism in the liver to the active metabolite O-desmethylvenlafaxine. This is catalyzed by the cytochrome P450 isoenzyme CYP2D6.[169,170]

Excretion is predominantly renal (82% as metabolites and 5% unchanged). The elimination half-life of venlafaxine is 5 hours and that of O-desmethylvenlafaxine is 11 hours.[161,168,171]

Adverse effects include nausea, constipation, weight loss, dizziness, tremor, erectile dysfunction, ejaculatory difficulties, xerostomia, hyperhidrosis, elevated blood pressure and heart rate, somnolence, and insomnia. In one clinical trial of extended-release venlafaxine, clinically significant electrocardiographic abnormalities were observed in about 5% of subjects.[166] Venlafaxine may lower the seizure threshold. Gradual tapering is recommended to avoid the emergence of adverse effects upon discontinuation.[172] For dosing, see Table 8.4.

OTHER MONOAMINE REUPTAKE INHIBITORS

Bupropion is an inhibitor of neuronal norepinephrine reuptake and a weak inhibitor of dopamine reuptake with no significant affinity for muscarinic, histaminergic, or α-adrenergic receptors. In a small single-center, placebo-controlled crossover trial, sustained-released bupropion at a dose of 150–300 mg/day appeared to be efficacious in the treatment of neuropathic pain of diverse etiologies.[173] For dosing, see Table 8.4. There is limited evidence for the effectiveness of selective serotonin reuptake inhibitors in the treatment of neuropathic pain[141,174,175] (with most expert consensus panels not including these agents in treatment algorithms for neuropathic pain).

Opioid Receptors

BACKGROUND

Four opioid receptors exist—the μ opioid receptor, the δ opioid receptor, the κ opioid receptor, and the opioid-like receptor 1 (ORL1). These receptors are activated by exogenous and endogenous opioid ligands. Activation of the μ receptor most consistently produces analgesia. The opioid receptors consist of seven transmembrane domains connected by short loops with an extracellular N-terminal domain and an intracellular C-terminal tail. Opioid receptors are coupled to Go/Gi inhibitory proteins. Activation of the receptor characteristically causes decreased calcium conductance and increased potassium conductance leading to decreased neural excitability. Opioid receptor activation also inhibits the cyclic adenosine monophosphate (cyclic AMP) pathway by inhibiting adenylyl cyclase.[137,138]

Opioid receptors are found throughout the central and peripheral nervous systems, on

endocrine cells, and on immune cells. They are synthesized in the small-diameter neurons of the dorsal root ganglia, from which they are transported centrally and peripherally. Within the dorsal horn, they are most prevalent in the superficial laminae (laminae I and II). In the spinal cord, opioid receptor agonists inhibit release of glutamate, substance P, and calcitonin generelated peptide. At the supraspinal level, sites of high prevalence for opioid receptors include the rostral ventrolateral medulla, the locus coeruleus, the periaqueductal gray, and the thalamus, hypothalamus, and sensory cortex.[137,138]

Fields et al. and others have proposed that μ-opioid agonists produce anti-nociception in the rostral ventrolateral medulla by activation, most likely through disinhibition, of neurons classed as OFF-cells, whereas activation of ON-cells is associated with enhanced nociception. It has been shown that local application of morphine in the rostral ventrolateral medulla leads to direct inhibition of ON-cells and indirect activation of OFF-cells, resulting in a net anti-nociceptive effect.[176]

OPIOID AND ATYPICAL OPIOID ANALGESICS

Several randomized, controlled trials have shown that opioids can effectively treat neuropathic pain due to diabetic peripheral neuropathy, postherpetic neuralgia, phantom limb, and other causes (see Table 8.5). Treatment with controlled-release oxycodone improved pain scores in patients with painful diabetic neuropathy[177] and postherpetic neuralgia[178,179] in doses ranging from 10 to 60 mg every 12 hours. In a small crossover trial of patients with postherpetic neuralgia, the efficacy of the opioids (controlled-release morphine sulfate or methadone) was similar to that of the tricyclic agents (nortriptyline or desipramine).[180] In a blinded trial, high doses (average dose, 8.9 mg/day) of the potent μ-opioid agonist, levorphanol, reduced pain in patients with refractory neuropathic pain more than low doses (average dose, 2.7 mg/day).[181] In a blinded, placebo-controlled crossover trial, low-dose (10 mg twice a day but not 5 mg twice a day) methadone was efficacious in the treatment of mixed neuropathic pain.[182] Opioids may also have a dose-sparing effect;

Table 8-5. Effective doses of opioids for neuropathic pain

AGENT	TYPICAL FIRST DOSE
Tramadol oral	25–50 mg every 6 hours
Codeine oral	30 mg every 3–4 hours
Fentanyl patch	25 μg/hour patch every 72 hours
Levorphanol oral	4 mg every 6–8 hours
Methadone oral	2.5–5 mg every 8–12 hours
Morphine IR oral	10 mg every 3–4 hours
Morphine SR oral	15 mg every 12 hours
Oxycodone IR oral	5 mg every 4–6 hours
Oxycodone CR oral	10 mg every 8–12 hours

Note: Dose increments based on efficacy and tolerability.

gabapentin and sustained-release morphine combined achieved better analgesia at lower doses of each drug than either as a single agent, but with increased adverse effects that included constipation, sedation, and dry mouth.[183]

There is also evidence that the atypical opiate analgesic, tramadol, is effective in the treatment of painful peripheral neuropathy.[184–189] This mixed opioid agonist exhibits low-affinity binding to the μ-opiate receptor.[184,185,189,190] It is biochemically distinct from other opioids in that analgesia is only partially antagonized by naloxone. Tramadol also inhibits the reuptake of norepinephrine and serotonin.[191] The side effects of tramadol are similar to those of other opioids, but tramadol may also lower the seizure threshold and lead to the serotonin syndrome when combined with serotonin receptor agonists or serotonin reuptake inhibitors. While tramadol has a low potential for abuse, it should be avoided in opioid-dependent patients and patients with a tendency to abuse drugs.

Both short- and long-acting opioids are efficacious treatments of neuropathic pain. In comparison to short-acting opioids, long-acting opioids have fewer peak-trough fluctuations. The more stable plasma level may lead to fewer periods of inadequate pain control and may attenuate end-of-dose failure. Long-acting opioids are therefore preferred for long-term therapy, although therapy may be initiated with a short-acting opioid such as morphine

(10–15 mg) every 4 hours or with an equianalgesic dose of another short-acting opioid. The synthetic opioid, methadone, which is also an N-methyl-D-aspartate antagonist, may have unique therapeutic attributes.[192] Methadone has good oral bioavailability. The duration of action is around 8 hours with repeated dosing. The elimination half-life, however, is 24–36 hours, which creates titration challenges.[193,194] The most common adverse effects associated with opioid use include gastrointestinal symptoms such as constipation, nausea, dyspepsia, and abdominal pain; headache, mental status changes including sedation, fatigue, lethargy, somnolence, and hallucinations; dry mouth; and urinary hesitancy or retention. Prolonged opioid use may lead to hypogonadism and alterations in immune function.[195] Some patients may develop hyperalgesia with long-term opioid use. The relationship between hyperalgesia and opioid tolerance is not fully elucidated.[196–198] Serious adverse effects of opioids include hypoventilation, bradypnea, and respiratory arrest.[195] There is considerable genetic variability with respect to opioid pharmacokinetics and pharmacodynamics that results in variability in the analgesic response and adverse events with specific opioids.[199]

Despite the demonstrated effectiveness of opioids in the treatment of neuropathic pain, there are ongoing concerns with respect to abuse, addiction, diversion, and other psychosocial issues.[200–202] For these reasons, opioids are generally used after the failure of agents that do not have these associated concerns; however, opioids may be used as first-line agents while titrating a tricyclic agent, a selective norepinephrine uptake inhibitor, or an α_2-δ ligand when more rapid pain relief is required. Pretreatment risk-benefit assessment and ongoing risk management strategies should be implemented prior to and during opioid therapy.[200–202]

CONCLUSION

The following general principles are applicable to the pharmacotherapy of neuropathic pain:

1. The pharmacological regimen for each patient should be individualized.

2. Pharmacotherapy should be initiated with a low dose of medication, particularly in the elderly and in patients susceptible to adverse effects of medications.

3. Topical agents should be considered in patients on multiple medications and in those susceptible to medication side effects.

4. Titrate slowly to minimize side effects.

5. Since peripheral neuropathic pain is characteristically worse at night, weight the dosing of short-acting medications to the evening hours, particularly those with somnolence as an adverse effect.

6. The onset of the therapeutic effect may be gradual. Allow sufficient time to elapse before drawing a conclusion concerning the success or failure of a drug.

7. Consider the use of drugs in combination. There is preliminary evidence that the combination of one or more drugs from different classes may result in an additive or even synergistic effect. In addition, combinations of lower doses of one or more drugs from different classes may result in analgesic efficacy, although it is not clear that this approach leads to a more favorable adverse effect profile.[183,203]

8. Comorbid conditions such as depression, anxiety, and insomnia should be considered in the choice of pharmacological agent.

9. Once patients are pain free for several months, a gradual medication taper should be considered.

Despite the availability of numerous drugs from different classes, current pharmacological approaches do not provide satisfactory pain relief for many patients. Furthermore, many patients experience intolerable adverse effects with these therapies. Recent advances in the understanding of the molecular mechanisms whereby pain is provoked after nerve injury, and knowledge of pain phenotypes and genotypes, may pave the way toward more effective treatment modalities.

REFERENCES

1. Gilron I, Watson CP, Cahill CM, et al. Neuropathic pain: a practical guide for the clinician. *CMAJ*. 2006;175:265–275.
2. Moulin DE, Clark AJ, Gilron I, et al. Pharmacological management of chronic neuropathic pain—consensus statement and guidelines from the Canadian Pain Society. *Pain Res Manag*. 2007;12:13–21.
3. Dworkin RH, O'Connor AB, Backonja M, et al. Pharmacologic management of neuropathic pain: evidence-based recommendations. *Pain*. 2007;132:237–251.
4. Dworkin RH, O'Connor AB, Audette J, et al. Recommendations for the pharmacological management of neuropathic pain: an overview and literature update. *Mayo Clin Proc*. 2010;85: S3–S14.
5. Attal N, Cruccu G, Baron R, et al. EFNS guidelines on the pharmacological treatment of neuropathic pain: 2010 revision. *Eur J Neurol*. 2010;17:1113–1123.
6. Finnerup NB, Sindrup SH, Jensen TS. The evidence for pharmacological treatment of neuropathic pain. *Pain*. 2010;150:573–581.
7. Caterina MJ. Vanilloid receptors take a TRP beyond the sensory afferent. *Pain*. 2003;105: 5–9.
8. Pingle SC, Matta JA, Ahern GP. Capsaicin receptor: TRPV1, a promiscuous TRP channel. *Handb Exp Pharmacol*. 2007;179:155–171.
9. Caterina MJ, Julius D. The vanilloid receptor: a molecular gateway to the pain pathway. *Annu Rev Neurosci*. 2001;24:487–517.
10. Caterina MJ, Leffler A, Malmberg AB, et al. Impaired nociception and pain sensation in mice lacking the capsaicin receptor. *Science*. 2000;288:306–313.
11. Facer P, Casula MA, Smith GD, et al. Differential expression of the capsaicin receptor TRPV1 and related novel receptors TRPV3, TRPV4 and TRPM8 in normal human tissues and changes in traumatic and diabetic neuropathy. *BMC Neurol*. 2007;7:11.
12. Lauria G, Morbin M, Lombardi R, et al. Expression of capsaicin receptor immunoreactivity in human peripheral nervous system and in painful neuropathies. *J Peripher Nerv Syst*. 2006;11:262–271.
13. Derry S, Lloyd R, Moore RA, et al. Topical capsaicin for chronic neuropathic pain in adults. *Cochrane Database Syst Rev*. 2009;CD007393.
14. Nolano M, Simone DA, Wendelschafer-Crabb G, et al. Topical capsaicin in humans: parallel loss of epidermal nerve fibers and pain sensation. *Pain*. 1999;81:135–145.
15. Malmberg AB, Mizisin AP, Calcutt NA, et al. Reduced heat sensitivity and epidermal nerve fiber immunostaining following single applications of a high-concentration capsaicin patch. *Pain*. 2004;111:360–367.

16. Simone DA, Nolano M, Johnson T, et al. Intradermal injection of capsaicin in humans produces degeneration and subsequent reinnervation of epidermal nerve fibers: correlation with sensory function. *J Neurosci.* 1998;18:8947–8959.

17. Polydefkis M, Hauer P, Sheth S, et al. The time course of epidermal nerve fibre regeneration: studies in normal controls and in people with diabetes, with and without neuropathy. *Brain.* 2004;127:1606–1615.

18. Gibbons CH, Wang N, Freeman R. Capsaicin induces degeneration of cutaneous autonomic nerve fibers. *Ann Neurol.* 2010;68(6):888–898.

19. Wood JN, Winter J, James IF, et al. Capsaicin-induced ion fluxes in dorsal root ganglion cells in culture. *J Neurosci.* 1988;8:3208–3220.

20. Sikand P, Premkumar LS. Potentiation of glutamatergic synaptic transmission by protein kinase C-mediated sensitization of TRPV1 at the first sensory synapse. *J Physiol.* 2007;581: 631–647.

21. Amantini C, Mosca M, Nabissi M, et al. Capsaicin-induced apoptosis of glioma cells is mediated by TRPV1 vanilloid receptor and requires p38 MAPK activation. *J Neurochem.* 2007;102: 977–990.

22. Backonja M, Wallace MS, Blonsky ER, et al. NGX-4010, a high-concentration capsaicin patch, for the treatment of postherpetic neuralgia: a randomised, double-blind study. *Lancet Neurol.* 2008;7:1106–1112.

23. Mason L, Moore RA, Derry S, et al. Systematic review of topical capsaicin for the treatment of chronic pain. *BMJ.* 2004;328:991–999.

24. Bernstein JE, Korman NJ, Bickers DR, et al. Topical capsaicin treatment of chronic postherpetic neuralgia. *J Am Acad Dermatol.* 1989;21: 265–270.

25. Capsaicin Study Group. Effect of treatment with capsaicin on daily activities of patients with painful diabetic neuropathy. *Diabetes Care.* 1992;15:159–165.

26. Tandan R, Lewis GA, Badger GB, et al. Topical capsaicin in painful diabetic neuropathy. Effect on sensory function. *Diabetes Care.* 1992;15:15–18.

27. Low PA, Opfer-Gehrking TL, Dyck PJ, et al. Double-blind, placebo-controlled study of the application of capsaicin cream in chronic distal painful polyneuropathy. *Pain.* 1995;62: 163–168.

28. Watson CP, Tyler KL, Bickers DR, et al. A randomized vehicle-controlled trial of topical capsaicin in the treatment of postherpetic neuralgia. *Clin Ther.* 1993;15:510–526.

29. Ellison N, Loprinzi CL, Kugler J, et al. Phase III placebo-controlled trial of capsaicin cream in the management of surgical neuropathic pain in cancer patients. *J Clin Oncol.* 1997;15: 2974–2980.

30. Watson CP, Evans RJ. The postmastectomy pain syndrome and topical capsaicin: a randomized trial. *Pain.* 1992;51:375–379.

31. Backonja MM, Malan TP, Vanhove GF, et al. NGX-4010, a high-concentration capsaicin patch, for the treatment of postherpetic neuralgia: a randomized, double-blind, controlled study with an open-label extension. *Pain Med.* 2010;11:600–608.

32. Irving GA, Backonja MM, Dunteman E, et al. A multicenter, randomized, double-blind, controlled study of NGX-4010, a high-concentration capsaicin patch, for the treatment of postherpetic neuralgia. *Pain Med.* 2011;12:99–109.

33. Simpson DM, Brown S, Tobias J. Controlled trial of high-concentration capsaicin patch for treatment of painful HIV neuropathy. *Neurology.* 2008;70:2305–2313.

34. Babbar S, Marier JF, Mouksassi MS, et al. Pharmacokinetic analysis of capsaicin after topical administration of a high-concentration capsaicin patch to patients with peripheral neuropathic pain. *Ther Drug Monit.* 2009;31:502–510.

35. Yaksh TL. Calcium channels as therapeutic targets in neuropathic pain. *J Pain.* 2006;7: S13–S30.

36. Perret D, Luo ZD. Targeting voltage-gated calcium channels for neuropathic pain management. *Neurotherapeutics.* 2009;6:679–692.

37. Davies A, Hendrich J, Van Minh AT, et al. Functional biology of the alpha(2)delta subunits of voltage-gated calcium channels. *Trends Pharmacol Sci.* 2007;28:220–228.

38. Taylor CP. Mechanisms of analgesia by gabapentin and pregabalin—calcium channel alpha2-delta [Cavalpha2-delta] ligands. *Pain.* 2009;142: 13–16.

39. Tuchman M, Barrett JA, Donevan S, et al. Central sensitization and Ca(V)alphadelta ligands in chronic pain syndromes: pathologic processes and pharmacologic effect. *J Pain.* 2010;11: 1241–1249.

40. Dooley DJ, Taylor CP, Donevan S, et al. Ca^{2+} channel alpha2delta ligands: novel modulators of neurotransmission. *Trends Pharmacol Sci.* 2007;28:75–82.

41. Fink K, Dooley DJ, Meder WP, et al. Inhibition of neuronal Ca(2+) influx by gabapentin and pregabalin in the human neocortex. *Neuropharmacology.* 2002;42:229–236.

42. Micheva KD, Taylor CP, Smith SJ. Pregabalin reduces the release of synaptic vesicles from cultured hippocampal neurons. *Mol Pharmacol.* 2006;70:467–476.

43. Dooley DJ, Mieske CA, Borosky SA. Inhibition of K(+)-evoked glutamate release from rat neocortical and hippocampal slices by gabapentin. *Neurosci Lett.* 2000;280:107–110.

44. Fehrenbacher JC, Taylor CP, Vasko MR. Pregabalin and gabapentin reduce release of substance P and CGRP from rat spinal tissues only after inflammation or activation of protein kinase C. *Pain.* 2003;105:133–141.

45. Dooley DJ, Donovan CM, Pugsley TA. Stimulus-dependent modulation of [(3)H]norepinephrine release from rat neocortical slices by gabapentin and pregabalin. *J Pharmacol Exp Ther.* 2000;295:1086–1093.

46. Luo ZD, Calcutt NA, Higuera ES, et al. Injury type-specific calcium channel alpha 2 delta-1 subunit up-regulation in rat neuropathic pain models correlates with antiallodynic effects of gabapentin. *J Pharmacol Exp Ther.* 2002;303:1199–1205.

47. Luo ZD, Chaplan SR, Higuera ES, et al. Upregulation of dorsal root ganglion (alpha)2(delta) calcium channel subunit and its correlation with allodynia in spinal nerve-injured rats. *J Neurosci.* 2001;21:1868–1875.

48. Field MJ, McCleary S, Hughes J, et al. Gabapentin and pregabalin, but not morphine and amitriptyline, block both static and dynamic components of mechanical allodynia induced by streptozocin in the rat. *Pain.* 1999;80:391–398.

49. Field MJ, Cox PJ, Stott E, et al. Identification of the alpha2-delta-1 subunit of voltage-dependent calcium channels as a molecular target for pain mediating the analgesic actions of pregabalin. *Proc Natl Acad Sci USA.* 2006;103: 17537–17542.

50. Hendrich J, Van Minh AT, Heblich F, et al. Pharmacological disruption of calcium channel trafficking by the alpha2delta ligand gabapentin. *Proc Natl Acad Sci USA.* 2008;105:3628–3633.

51. Heblich F, Tran Van MA, Hendrich J, et al. Time course and specificity of the pharmacological disruption of the trafficking of voltage-gated calcium channels by gabapentin. *Channels* (Austin). 2008;2:4–9.

52. Eroglu C, Allen NJ, Susman MW, et al. Gabapentin receptor alpha2delta-1 is a neuronal thrombospondin receptor responsible for excitatory CNS synaptogenesis. *Cell.* 2009;139:380–392.

53. Rice AS, Maton S. Gabapentin in postherpetic neuralgia: a randomised, double blind, placebo controlled study. *Pain.* 2001;94:215–224.

54. Rowbotham M, Harden N, Stacey B, et al. Gabapentin for the treatment of postherpetic neuralgia: a randomized controlled trial. *JAMA.* 1998;280:1837–1842.

55. Sabatowski R, Galvez R, Cherry DA, et al. Pregabalin reduces pain and improves sleep and mood disturbances in patients with post-herpetic neuralgia: results of a randomised, placebo-controlled clinical trial. *Pain.* 2004;109:26–35.

56. Dworkin RH, Corbin AE, Young JP Jr, et al. Pregabalin for the treatment of postherpetic neuralgia: a randomized, placebo-controlled trial. *Neurology.* 2003;60:1274–1283.

57. van Seventer R, Feister HA, Young JP Jr, et al. Efficacy and tolerability of twice-daily pregabalin for treating pain and related sleep interference in postherpetic neuralgia: a 13-week, randomized trial. *Curr Med Res Opin.* 2006;22: 375–384.

58. Freynhagen R, Strojek K, Griesing T, et al. Efficacy of pregabalin in neuropathic pain evaluated in a 12-week, randomised, double-blind, multicentre, placebo-controlled trial of flexible- and fixed-dose regimens. *Pain.* 2005;115: 254–263.

59. Backonja M, Beydoun A, Edwards KR, et al. Gabapentin for the symptomatic treatment of painful neuropathy in patients with diabetes mellitus: a randomized controlled trial [see comments]. *JAMA.* 1998;280:1831–1836.

60. Rosenstock J, Tuchman M, LaMoreaux L, et al. Pregabalin for the treatment of painful diabetic peripheral neuropathy: a double-blind, placebo-controlled trial. *Pain.* 2004;110:628–638.

61. Lesser H, Sharma U, LaMoreaux L, et al. Pregabalin relieves symptoms of painful diabetic neuropathy: a randomized controlled trial. *Neurology.* 2004;63:2104–2110.

62. Richter RW, Portenoy R, Sharma U, et al. Relief of painful diabetic peripheral neuropathy with pregabalin: a randomized, placebo-controlled trial. *J Pain.* 2005;6:253–260.

63. Siddall PJ, Cousins MJ, Otte A, et al. Pregabalin in central neuropathic pain associated with spinal cord injury: a placebo-controlled trial. *Neurology.* 2006;67:1792–1800.

64. Backonja M, Glanzman RL. Gabapentin dosing for neuropathic pain: evidence from randomized, placebo-controlled clinical trials. *Clin Ther.* 2003;25:81–104.

65. Pfizer Protocol No. 1008–040: a placebo-controlled trial of pregabalin and amitriptyline for treatment of painful diabetic peripheral neuropathy. http://www.clinicalstudyresults.org/drugdetails/?drug_name_id=203&sort=c.

company_name&page=2&drug_id=1952].
Accessed 3/9/2012

66. Simpson DM, Schifitto G, Clifford DB, et al. Pregabalin for painful HIV neuropathy: a randomized, double-blind, placebo-controlled trial. *Neurology*. 2010;74:413–420.

67. Baron R, Freynhagen R, Tolle TR, et al. The efficacy and safety of pregabalin in the treatment of neuropathic pain associated with chronic lumbosacral radiculopathy. *Pain*. 2010;150:420–427.

68. Rao RD, Michalak JC, Sloan JA, et al. Efficacy of gabapentin in the management of chemotherapy-induced peripheral neuropathy: a phase 3 randomized, double-blind, placebo-controlled, crossover trial (N00C3). *Cancer*. 2007;110: 2110–2118.

69. McLean MJ. Clinical pharmacokinetics of gabapentin. *Neurology*. 1994;44:S17–S22.

70. Shoji S, Suzuki M, Tomono Y, et al. Population pharmacokinetics of pregabalin in healthy subjects and patients with postherpetic neuralgia or diabetic peripheral neuropathy. *Br J Clin Pharmacol*. 2011;72(1):63–76.

71. Bockbrader HN, Wesche D, Miller R, et al. A comparison of the pharmacokinetics and pharmacodynamics of pregabalin and gabapentin. *Clin Pharmacokinet*. 2010;49:661–669.

72. McLean MJ. Gabapentin. *Epilepsia*. 1995;36 (suppl 2):S73–S86.

73. Stewart BH, Kugler AR, Thompson PR, et al. A saturable transport mechanism in the intestinal absorption of gabapentin is the underlying cause of the lack of proportionality between increasing dose and drug levels in plasma. *Pharm Res*. 1993;10:276–281.

74. Tolle T, Freynhagen R, Versavel M, et al. Pregabalin for relief of neuropathic pain associated with diabetic neuropathy: a randomized, double-blind study. *Eur J Pain*. 2008;12:203–213.

75. Freeman R, Durso-Decruz E, Emir B. Efficacy, safety and tolerability of pregabalin treatment of painful diabetic peripheral neuropathy: findings from 7 randomized, controlled trials across a range of doses. *Diabetes Care*. 2008;31(7):1448–1454.

76. Waxman SG, Cummins TR, Dib-Hajj S, et al. Sodium channels, excitability of primary sensory neurons, and the molecular basis of pain. *Muscle Nerve*. 1999;22:1177–1187.

77. Catterall WA, Goldin AL, Waxman SG. International Union of Pharmacology. XLVII. Nomenclature and structure-function relationships of voltage-gated sodium channels. *Pharmacol Rev*. 2005;57:397–409.

78. Hains BC, Saab CY, Klein JP, et al. Altered sodium channel expression in second-order spinal sensory neurons contributes to pain after peripheral nerve injury. *J Neurosci*. 2004;24: 4832–4839.

79. Craner MJ, Klein JP, Renganathan M, et al. Changes of sodium channel expression in experimental painful diabetic neuropathy. *Ann Neurol*. 2002;52:786–792.

80. Dib-Hajj SD, Fjell J, Cummins TR, et al. Plasticity of sodium channel expression in DRG neurons in the chronic constriction injury model of neuropathic pain. *Pain*. 1999;83:591–600.

81. Black JA, Cummins TR, Plumpton C, et al. Upregulation of a silent sodium channel after peripheral, but not central, nerve injury in DRG neurons. *J Neurophysiol*. 1999;82:2776–2785.

82. Devor M, Govrin-Lippmann R, Angelides K. Na⁺ channel immunolocalization in peripheral mammalian axons and changes following nerve injury and neuroma formation. *J Neurosci*. 1993;13:1976–1992.

83. Devor M, Wall PD, Catalan N. Systemic lidocaine silences ectopic neuroma and DRG discharge without blocking nerve conduction. *Pain*. 1992;48:261–268.

84. Fischer TZ, Waxman SG. Familial pain syndromes from mutations of the NaV1.7 sodium channel. *Ann NY Acad Sci*. 2010;1184:196–207.

85. Dib-Hajj SD, Rush AM, Cummins TR, et al. Gain-of-function mutation in Nav1.7 in familial erythromelalgia induces bursting of sensory neurons. *Brain*. 2005;128:1847–1854.

86. Nilsen KB, Nicholas AK, Woods CG, et al. Two novel SCN9A mutations causing insensitivity to pain. *Pain*. 2009;143:155–158.

87. Cox JJ, Reimann F, Nicholas AK, et al. An SCN9A channelopathy causes congenital inability to experience pain. *Nature*. 2006;444:894–898.

88. Cregg R, Momin A, Rugiero F, et al. Pain channelopathies. *J Physiol*. 2010;588:1897–1904.

89. Nassar MA, Baker MD, Levato A, et al. Nerve injury induces robust allodynia and ectopic discharges in Nav1.3 null mutant mice. *Mol Pain*. 2006;2:33.

90. Nassar MA, Levato A, Stirling LC, et al. Neuropathic pain develops normally in mice lacking both Na(v)1.7 and Na(v)1.8. *Mol Pain*. 2005;1:24.

91. Galer BS, Rowbotham MC, Perander J, et al. Topical lidocaine patch relieves postherpetic neuralgia more effectively than a vehicle topical patch: results of an enriched enrollment study. *Pain*. 1999;80:533–538.

92. Rowbotham MC, Davies PS, Fields HL. Topical lidocaine gel relieves postherpetic neuralgia. *Ann Neurol*. 1995;37:246–253.

93. Rowbotham MC, Davies PS, Verkempinck C, et al. Lidocaine patch: double-blind controlled study of a new treatment method for postherpetic neuralgia. *Pain.* 1996;65:39–44.

94. Baron R, Mayoral V, Leijon G, et al. 5% lidocaine medicated plaster versus pregabalin in post-herpetic neuralgia and diabetic polyneuropathy: an open-label, non-inferiority two-stage RCT study. *Curr Med Res Opin.* 2009;25:1663–1676.

95. Barbano RL, Herrmann DN, Hart-Gouleau S, et al. Effectiveness, tolerability, and impact on quality of life of the 5% lidocaine patch in diabetic polyneuropathy. *Arch Neurol.* 2004;61:914–918.

96. Ho KY, Huh BK, White WD, et al. Topical amitriptyline versus lidocaine in the treatment of neuropathic pain. *Clin J Pain.* 2008;24:51–55.

97. Simpson DM, Olney R, McArthur JC, et al. A placebo-controlled trial of lamotrigine for painful HIV-associated neuropathy. *Neurology.* 2000;54:2115–2119.

98. Simpson DM, McArthur JC, Olney R, et al. Lamotrigine for HIV-associated painful sensory neuropathies: a placebo-controlled trial. *Neurology.* 2003;60:1508–1514.

99. Eisenberg E, Lurie Y, Braker C, et al. Lamotrigine reduces painful diabetic neuropathy: a randomized, controlled study. *Neurology.* 2001;57:505–509.

100. Vestergaard K, Andersen G, Gottrup H, et al. Lamotrigine for central poststroke pain: a randomized controlled trial. *Neurology.* 2001;56:184–190.

101. Finnerup NB, Sindrup SH, Bach FW, et al. Lamotrigine in spinal cord injury pain: a randomized controlled trial. *Pain.* 2002;96:375–383.

102. Vinik AI, Tuchman M, Safirstein B, et al. Lamotrigine for treatment of pain associated with diabetic neuropathy: results of two randomized, double-blind, placebo-controlled studies. *Pain.* 2007;128:169–179.

103. Wiffen PJ, Rees J. Lamotrigine for acute and chronic pain. *Cochrane Database Syst Rev.* 2007;CD006044.

104. Cheung H, Kamp D, Harris E. An in vitro investigation of the action of lamotrigine on neuronal voltage-activated sodium channels. *Epilepsy Res.* 1992;13:107–112.

105. Rambeck B, Specht U, Wolf, P. Pharmacokinetic interactions of the new antiepileptic drugs. *Clin Pharmacokinet.* 1996;31:309–324.

106. Rambeck B, Wolf P. Lamotrigine clinical pharmacokinetics. *Clin Pharmacokinet.* 1993;25:433–443.

107. Thienel U, Neto W, Schwabe SK, et al. Topiramate in painful diabetic polyneuropathy: findings from three double-blind placebo-controlled trials. *Acta Neurol Scand.* 2004;110:221–231.

108. Freeman R, McIntosh KA, Vijapurkar U, et al. Topiramate and physiologic measures of nerve function in polyneuropathy. *Acta Neurol Scand.* 2007;115:222–231.

109. Raskin P, Donofrio PD, Rosenthal NR, et al. Topiramate vs placebo in painful diabetic neuropathy: analgesic and metabolic effects. *Neurology.* 2004;63:865–873.

110. Shank RP, Gardocki JF, Streeter AJ, et al. An overview of the preclinical aspects of topiramate: pharmacology, pharmacokinetics, and mechanism of action. *Epilepsia.* 2000;41(suppl)1:S3–S9.

111. Perucca E, Bialer M. The clinical pharmacokinetics of the newer antiepileptic drugs. Focus on topiramate, zonisamide and tiagabine. *Clin Pharmacokinet.* 1996;31:29–46.

112. de Carolis P, Magnifico F, Pierangeli G, et al. Transient hypohidrosis induced by topiramate. *Epilepsia.* 2003;44:974–976.

113. Dodgson SJ, Shank RP, Maryanoff BE. Topiramate as an inhibitor of carbonic anhydrase isoenzymes. *Epilepsia.* 2000;41(suppl 1):S35–S39.

114. Dogra S, Beydoun S, Mazzola J, et al. Oxcarbazepine in painful diabetic neuropathy: a randomized, placebo-controlled study. *Eur J Pain.* 2005;9:543–554.

115. Beydoun A, Shaibani A, Hopwood M, et al. Oxcarbazepine in painful diabetic neuropathy: results of a dose-ranging study. *Acta Neurol Scand.* 2006;113:395–404.

116. Grosskopf J, Mazzola J, Wan Y, et al. A randomized, placebo-controlled study of oxcarbazepine in painful diabetic neuropathy. *Acta Neurol Scand.* 2006;114:177–180.

117. Wamil AW, Schmutz M, Portet C, et al. Effects of oxcarbazepine and 10-hydroxycarbamazepine on action potential firing and generalized seizures. *Eur J Pharmacol.* 1994;271:301–308.

118. McLean MJ, Schmutz M, Wamil AW, et al. Oxcarbazepine: mechanisms of action. *Epilepsia.* 1994;35(suppl 3):S5–S9.

119. May TW, Korn-Merker E, Rambeck B. Clinical pharmacokinetics of oxcarbazepine. *Clin Pharmacokinet.* 2003;42:1023–1042.

120. Beydoun S, Alarcon F, Mangat S, et al. Long-term safety and tolerability of oxcarbazepine in painful diabetic neuropathy. *Acta Neurol Scand.* 2007;115:284–288.

121. Wymer JP, Simpson J, Sen D, et al. Efficacy and safety of lacosamide in diabetic neuropathic

pain: an 18-week double-blind placebo-controlled trial of fixed-dose regimens. *Clin J Pain*. 2009;25:376–385.

122. Shaibani A, Fares S, Selam JL, et al. Lacosamide in painful diabetic neuropathy: an 18-week double-blind placebo-controlled trial. *J Pain*. 2009;10(8)818–828.

123. Rauck RL, Shaibani A, Biton V, et al. Lacosamide in painful diabetic peripheral neuropathy: a phase 2 double-blind placebo-controlled study. *Clin J Pain*. 2007;23:150–158.

124. Doty P, Rudd GD, Stoehr T, et al. Lacosamide. *Neurotherapeutics*. 2007;4:145–148.

125. Stracke H, Meyer UE, Schumacher HE, et al. Mexiletine in the treatment of diabetic neuropathy. *Diabetes Care*. 1992;15:1550–1555.

126. Galer BS, Harle J, Rowbotham MC. Response to intravenous lidocaine infusion predicts subsequent response to oral mexiletine: a prospective study. *J Pain Symptom Manage*. 1996;12:161–167.

127. Oskarsson P, Ljunggren JG, Lins PE. Efficacy and safety of mexiletine in the treatment of painful diabetic neuropathy. The Mexiletine Study Group. *Diabetes Care*. 1997;20:1594–1597.

128. Dejgard A, Petersen P, Kastrup J. Mexiletine for treatment of chronic painful diabetic neuropathy. *Lancet*. 1988;1:9–11.

129. Wright JM, Oki JC, Graves L. Mexiletine in the symptomatic treatment of diabetic peripheral neuropathy. *Ann Pharmacother*. 1997;31:29–34.

130. Jarvis B, Coukell AJ. Mexiletine. A review of its therapeutic use in painful diabetic neuropathy. *Drugs*. 1998;56:691–707.

131. Kieburtz K, Simpson D, Yiannoutsos C, et al. A randomized trial of amitriptyline and mexiletine for painful neuropathy in HIV infection. AIDS Clinical Trial Group 242 Protocol Team. *Neurology*. 1998;51:1682–1688.

132. Rull JA, Quibrera R, Gonzalez-Millan H, et al. Symptomatic treatment of peripheral diabetic neuropathy with carbamazepine (Tegretol): double blind crossover trial. *Diabetologia*. 1969;5:215–218.

133. Wiffen PJ, McQuay HJ, Moore RA. Carbamazepine for acute and chronic pain. *Cochrane Database Syst Rev*. 2005;CD005451.

134. Saudek CD, Werns S, Reidenberg MM. Phenytoin in the treatment of diabetic symmetrical polyneuropathy. *Clin Pharmacol Ther*. 1977;22:196–199.

135. Chadda VS, Mathur MS. Double blind study of the effects of diphenylhydantoin sodium on diabetic neuropathy. *J Assoc Physicians India*. 1978;26:403–406.

136. Gassner M, Ruscheweyh R, Sandkuhler J. Direct excitation of spinal GABAergic interneurons by noradrenaline. *Pain*. 2009;145:204–210.

137. Pasternak GW. Molecular insights into mu opioid pharmacology: from the clinic to the bench. *Clin J Pain*. 2010;26(suppl 10):S3–S9.

138. Ossipov MH, Lai J, King T, et al. Antinociceptive and nociceptive actions of opioids. *J Neurobiol*. 2004;61:126–148.

139. Max MB, Culnane M, Schafer SC, et al. Amitriptyline relieves diabetic neuropathy pain in patients with normal or depressed mood. *Neurology*. 1987;37:589–596.

140. Max MB, Kishore-Kumar R, Schafer SC, et al. Efficacy of desipramine in painful diabetic neuropathy: a placebo-controlled trial. *Pain*. 1991;45:3–9.

141. Max MB, Lynch SA, Muir J, et al. Effects of desipramine, amitriptyline, and fluoxetine on pain in diabetic neuropathy. *N Engl J Med*. 1992;326:1250–1256.

142. Sindrup SH, Jensen TS. Pharmacologic treatment of pain in polyneuropathy. *Neurology*. 2000;55:915–920.

143. Saarto T, Wiffen PJ. Antidepressants for neuropathic pain. *Cochrane Database Syst Rev*. 2007;CD005454.

144. Shlay JC, Chaloner K, Max MB, et al. Acupuncture and amitriptyline for pain due to HIV-related peripheral neuropathy: a randomized controlled trial. Terry Beirn Community Programs for Clinical Research on AIDS. *JAMA*. 1998;280:1590–1595.

145. Hammack JE, Michalak JC, Loprinzi CL, et al. Phase III evaluation of nortriptyline for alleviation of symptoms of cis-platinum-induced peripheral neuropathy. *Pain*. 2002;98:195–203.

146. Khoromi S, Cui L, Nackers L, et al. Morphine, nortriptyline and their combination vs. placebo in patients with chronic lumbar root pain. *Pain*. 2007;130:66–75.

147. Cardenas DD, Warms CA, Turner JA, et al. Efficacy of amitriptyline for relief of pain in spinal cord injury: results of a randomized controlled trial. *Pain*. 2002;96:365–373.

148. Robinson LR, Czerniecki JM, Ehde DM, et al. Trial of amitriptyline for relief of pain in amputees: results of a randomized controlled study. *Arch Phys Med Rehabil*. 2004;85:1–6.

149. Sindrup SH, Gram LF, Skjold T, et al. Clomipramine vs desipramine vs placebo in the treatment of diabetic neuropathy symptoms.

A double-blind cross-over study. *Br J Clin Pharmacol*. 1990;30:683–691.

150. Jackson WK, Roose SP, Glassman AH. Cardiovascular toxicity of antidepressant medications. *Psychopathology*. 1987;20(suppl 1):64–74.

151. Glassman AH, Roose SP, Bigger JT Jr. The safety of tricyclic antidepressants in cardiac patients. Risk-benefit reconsidered. *JAMA*. 1993;269:2673–2675.

152. Roose SP, Glassman AH, Dalack GW. Depression, heart disease, and tricyclic antidepressants. *J Clin Psychiatry*. 1989;50(suppl): 1–18.

153. Ray WA, Meredith S, Thapa PB, et al. Cyclic antidepressants and the risk of sudden cardiac death. *Clin Pharmacol Ther*. 2004;75:234–241.

154. Tata LJ, West J, Smith C, et al. General population based study of the impact of tricyclic and selective serotonin reuptake inhibitor antidepressants on the risk of acute myocardial infarction. *Heart*. 2005;91:465–471.

155. Goldstein DJ, Lu Y, Detke MJ, et al. Duloxetine vs. placebo in patients with painful diabetic neuropathy. *Pain*. 2005;116:109–118.

156. Wernicke JF, Pritchett YL, D'Souza DN, et al. A randomized controlled trial of duloxetine in diabetic peripheral neuropathic pain. *Neurology*. 2006;67:1411–1420.

157. Raskin J, Pritchett YL, Wang F, et al. A double-blind, randomized multicenter trial comparing duloxetine with placebo in the management of diabetic peripheral neuropathic pain. *Pain Med*. 2005;6:346–356.

158. Kajdasz DK, Iyengar S, Desaiah D, et al. Duloxetine for the management of diabetic peripheral neuropathic pain: evidence-based findings from post hoc analysis of three multicenter, randomized, double-blind, placebo-controlled, parallel-group studies. *Clin Ther*. 2007;29(suppl):2536–2546.

159. Raskin J, Smith TR, Wong K, et al. Duloxetine versus routine care in the long-term management of diabetic peripheral neuropathic pain. *J Palliat Med*. 2006;9:29–40.

160. Hardy T, Sachson R, Shen S, et al. Does treatment with duloxetine for neuropathic pain impact glycemic control? *Diabetes Care*. 2007;30: 21–26.

161. Bymaster FP, Dreshfield-Ahmad LJ, Threlkeld PG, et al. Comparative affinity of duloxetine and venlafaxine for serotonin and norepinephrine transporters in vitro and in vivo, human serotonin receptor subtypes, and other neuronal receptors. *Neuropsychopharmacology*. 2001;25:871–880.

162. Bymaster FP, Lee TC, Knadler MP, et al. The dual transporter inhibitor duloxetine: a review of its preclinical pharmacology, pharmacokinetic profile, and clinical results in depression. *Curr Pharm Des*. 2005;11:1475–1493.

163. Lunn MP, Hughes RA, Wiffen PJ. Duloxetine for treating painful neuropathy or chronic pain. *Cochrane Database Syst Rev*. 2009;CD007115.

164. Gahimer J, Wernicke J, Yalcin I, et al. A retrospective pooled analysis of duloxetine safety in 23,983 subjects. *Curr Med Res Opin*. 2007;23:175–184.

165. Sindrup SH, Bach FW, Madsen C, et al. Venlafaxine versus imipramine in painful polyneuropathy: a randomized, controlled trial. *Neurology*. 2003;60:1284–1289.

166. Rowbotham MC, Goli V, Kunz NR, et al. Venlafaxine extended release in the treatment of painful diabetic neuropathy: a double-blind, placebo-controlled study. *Pain*. 2004;110:697–706.

167. Hamner JW, Morin RJ, Rudolph JL, et al. Inconsistent link between low-frequency oscillations: R-R interval responses to augmented Mayer waves. *J Appl Physiol*. 2001;90:1559–1564.

168. Harvey AT, Rudolph RL, Preskorn SH. Evidence of the dual mechanisms of action of venlafaxine. *Arch Gen Psychiatry*. 2000;57:503–509.

169. Troy SM, Parker VP, Hicks DR, et al. Pharmacokinetics and effect of food on the bioavailability of orally administered venlafaxine. *J Clin Pharmacol*. 1997;37:954–961.

170. Klamerus KJ, Maloney K, Rudolph RL, et al. Introduction of a composite parameter to the pharmacokinetics of venlafaxine and its active O-desmethyl metabolite. *J Clin Pharmacol*. 1992;32:716–724.

171. Beique JC, Lavoie N, de Montigny C, et al. Affinities of venlafaxine and various reuptake inhibitors for the serotonin and norepinephrine transporters. *Eur J Pharmacol*. 1998;349: 129–132.

172. Fava M, Mulroy R, Alpert J, et al. Emergence of adverse events following discontinuation of treatment with extended-release venlafaxine. *Am J Psychiatry*. 1997;154:1760–1762.

173. Semenchuk MR, Sherman S, Davis B. Double-blind, randomized trial of bupropion SR for the treatment of neuropathic pain. *Neurology*. 2001;57:1583–1588.

174. Sindrup SH, Bjerre U, Dejgaard A, et al. The selective serotonin reuptake inhibitor citalopram relieves the symptoms of diabetic neuropathy. *Clin Pharmacol Ther*. 1992;52:547–552.

175. Sindrup SH, Gram LF, Br:sen K, et al. The selective serotonin reuptake inhibitor paroxetine is

effective in the treatment of diabetic neuropathy symptoms. *Pain*. 1990;42:135–144.

176. Fields HL, Barbaro NM, Heinricher MM. Brain stem neuronal circuitry underlying the antinociceptive action of opiates. *Prog Brain Res*. 1988;77:245–257.

177. Gimbel JS, Richards P, Portenoy RK. Controlled-release oxycodone for pain in diabetic neuropathy: a randomized controlled trial. *Neurology*. 2003;60:927–934.

178. Watson CP, Babul N. Efficacy of oxycodone in neuropathic pain: a randomized trial in postherpetic neuralgia. *Neurology*. 1998;50:1837–1841.

179. Watson CP, Moulin D, Watt-Watson J, et al. Controlled-release oxycodone relieves neuropathic pain: a randomized controlled trial in painful diabetic neuropathy. *Pain*. 2003;105:71–78.

180. Raja SN, Haythornthwaite JA, Pappagallo M, et al. Opioids versus antidepressants in postherpetic neuralgia: a randomized, placebo-controlled trial. *Neurology*. 2002;59:1015–1021.

181. Rowbotham MC, Twilling L, Davies PS, et al. Oral opioid therapy for chronic peripheral and central neuropathic pain. *N Engl J Med*. 2003;348:1223–1232.

182. Morley JS, Bridson J, Nash TP, et al. Low-dose methadone has an analgesic effect in neuropathic pain: a double-blind randomized controlled crossover trial. *Palliat Med*. 2003;17:576–587.

183. Gilron I, Bailey JM, Tu D, et al. Morphine, gabapentin, or their combination for neuropathic pain. *N Engl J Med*. 2005;352:1324–1334.

184. Harati Y, Gooch C, Swenson M, et al. Double-blind randomized trial of tramadol for the treatment of the pain of diabetic neuropathy. *Neurology*. 1998;50:1842–1846.

185. Sindrup SH, Andersen G, Madsen C, et al. Tramadol relieves pain and allodynia in polyneuropathy: a randomised, double-blind, controlled trial. *Pain*. 1999;83:85–90.

186. Freeman R, Raskin P, Hewitt DJ, et al. Randomized study of tramadol/acetaminophen versus placebo in painful diabetic peripheral neuropathy. *Curr Med Res Opin*. 2007;23:147–161.

187. Boureau F, Legallicier P, Kabir-Ahmadi M. Tramadol in post-herpetic neuralgia: a randomized, double-blind, placebo-controlled trial. *Pain*. 2003;104:323–331.

188. Harati Y, Gooch C, Swenson M, et al. Maintenance of the long-term effectiveness of tramadol in treatment of the pain of diabetic neuropathy. *J Diabetes Complications*. 2000;14:65–70.

189. Sindrup SH, Madsen C, Brosen K, et al. The effect of tramadol in painful polyneuropathy in relation to serum drug and metabolite levels. *Clin Pharmacol Ther*. 1999;66:636–641.

190. Cohen KL, Lucibello FE, Chomiak M. Lack of effect of clonidine and pentoxifylline in short-term therapy of diabetic peripheral neuropathy [see comments]. *Diabetes Care*. 1990;13:1074–1077.

191. Raffa RB, Friderichs E, Reimann W, et al. Opioid and nonopioid components independently contribute to the mechanism of action of tramadol, an "atypical" opioid analgesic. *J Pharmacol Exp Ther*. 1992;260:275–285.

192. Gorman AL, Elliott KJ, Inturrisi CE. The D- and L-isomers of methadone bind to the non-competitive site on the N-methyl-D-aspartate (NMDA) receptor in rat forebrain and spinal cord. *Neurosci Lett*. 1997;223:5–8.

193. Russell AL, Lynch ME. A review of the use of methadone for the treatment of chronic non-cancer pain. *Pain Res Manage*. 2005;10(3):133–144. *Pain Res Manage*. 2006;11:58.

194. Moulin DE, Palma D, Watling C, et al. Methadone in the management of intractable neuropathic noncancer pain. *Can J Neurol Sci*. 2005;32:340–343.

195. Ballantyne JC, Mao J. Opioid therapy for chronic pain. *N Engl J Med*. 2003;349:1943–1953.

196. Chang G, Chen L, Mao J. Opioid tolerance and hyperalgesia. *Med Clin North Am*. 2007;91:199–211.

197. Angst MS, Clark JD. Opioid-induced hyperalgesia: a qualitative systematic review. *Anesthesiology*. 2006;104:570–587.

198. Chu LF, Clark DJ, Angst MS. Opioid tolerance and hyperalgesia in chronic pain patients after one month of oral morphine therapy: a preliminary prospective study. *J Pain*. 2006;7:43–48.

199. Tremblay J, Hamet P. Genetics of pain, opioids, and opioid responsiveness. *Metabolism*. 2010;59(suppl 1):S5–S8.

200. Hojsted J, Sjogren P. Addiction to opioids in chronic pain patients: a literature review. *Eur J Pain*. 2007;11:490–518.

201. Katz NP, Adams EH, Benneyan JC, et al. Foundations of opioid risk management. *Clin J Pain*. 2007;23:103–118.

202. Martell BA, O'Connor PG, Kerns RD, et al. Systematic review: opioid treatment for chronic back pain: prevalence, efficacy, and association with addiction. *Ann Intern Med*. 2007;146:116–127.

203. Gilron I, Bailey JM, Tu D, et al. Nortriptyline and gabapentin, alone and in combination for neuropathic pain: a double-blind, randomised controlled crossover trial. *Lancet*. 2009;374:1252–1261.

9

Understanding and Interpreting Neuropathic Pain Clinical Trials

ALEC B. O'CONNOR AND ROBERT H. DWORKIN

CLINICAL TRIALS HAVE been defined as "any research study that prospectively assigns human participants or groups of humans to one or more health-related interventions to evaluate the effects on health outcomes."[1] The double-blind randomized clinical trial (RCT) is the best study design for assessing treatment efficacy, but prospective nonrandomized or uncontrolled intervention studies are also considered clinical trials. This chapter will focus on RCTs because they are the most informative types of trials; nonrandomized or uncontrolled trials produce treatment effect estimates that can be very unreliable. However, RCTs can vary tremendously in their study quality, so attention must be paid to the methods used in an RCT in order to be able to interpret its results.

We will focus on pharmacological interventions for neuropathic pain (NP), although many of the issues we discuss also pertain to studies of other types of interventions, such as nerve blocks, spinal cord stimulation, physical therapy,

and psychological therapies. We will first provide an overview of clinical trial design issues, with emphasis on the design aspects most important for RCTs of treatments for patients with NP. We will then discuss the interpretation of trial results, including the clinical importance of the treatment response and how to approach the interpretation of negative trials.

UNDERSTANDING NP CLINICAL TRIALS: OVERVIEW OF TRIAL DESIGN ISSUES

When interpreting clinical trial results, the first issue that must be considered is the objective of the trial: what question is the trial attempting to answer? Max[2,3] emphasized the importance of distinguishing between pragmatic and explanatory clinical trials.[4] Explanatory trials seek to answer specific scientific questions (such as whether a drug might have efficacy for a disease); a trial with this purpose will seek to limit sample variability (e.g., with a large number of inclusion and exclusion criteria) and will often use methods of assessment that are not clinically practical. This type of trial typically has excellent internal validity (i.e., the research methods have been designed to limit bias and other threats to inferring drug efficacy) but often has poor external validity (i.e., the results of the trial may have limited generalizability to clinical practice). In contrast, pragmatic trials seek to answer practical clinical management questions; they are typically designed with heterogeneous patient populations and use clinically relevant endpoints and outcomes. Pragmatic trials often have less internal validity than explanatory trials (e.g., a more varied patient population does not control confounding factors as well as a more homogeneous population), but they can have greater external validity (generalizability) and produce answers that have immediate clinical relevance.

Beyond this important distinction, there are several different design features that must be considered when interpreting NP clinical trials.

Prospective Cohort Trials

In general, cohort studies can demonstrate association, but not causation; regardless of the results of a cohort study, it cannot be concluded that an intervention *caused* the observed outcomes. Since cohort trials lack randomization, the comparison groups must be assumed to be different from each other in important ways, which limits the interpretability of the results. Cohort trials are unable to distinguish between the effects of the intervention and other factors that may affect outcomes, such as the natural history of the disease (e.g., spontaneous remissions or worsening over time), placebo effects, and regression to the mean. Comparing outcomes before versus after treatment or with historical controls can produce very misleading estimates of treatment benefits or risks.

Though cohort trials have limited usefulness for establishing treatment efficacy, they can be useful for demonstrating treatment safety and tolerability. Large cohort studies may be the only method for detecting rare, serious adverse events,[5] such as those that often become apparent only after a drug is available on the market.

They can also be useful for confirming safety in samples much larger and more diverse than those studied in RCTs.

Randomized Clinical Trials

GENERAL CONSIDERATIONS

Randomized clinical trials are the best study design for determining if an intervention is efficacious. Randomization of a large group of patients tends to balance baseline factors (both measured and unmeasured differences), which results in groups that are essentially equivalent except for the study intervention. Randomized clinical trials are the only type of clinical trial for which inferences of causality are appropriate; in other words, outcome differences between the treatment and control groups in a large, well-designed RCT can be inferred to have been *caused* by the treatment.

Investigations of treatments for NP have typically compared the efficacy, tolerability, and safety of a single treatment with placebo. Few RCTs have compared different treatments to each other[6,7] or assessed the efficacy and tolerability of combinations of treatments,[8,9] which are frequently used in clinical practice.

RANDOMIZATION

Several interventions found to be effective in nonrandomized trials have been shown to be ineffective in randomized trials,[10] which highlights the importance of randomization. Randomizing subjects has two main purposes. The first is to eliminate bias (whether intentional or not) in the allocation of treatments, which has been shown to have a significant impact on the results of past clinical trials. Allocation bias is eliminated by prespecifying a protocol that randomizes patients to different groups, removing investigators from the process of allocating interventions between subjects.

In addition, randomization creates subject groups that are comparable except for the intervention. On average, randomization disperses measured and unmeasured subject variability evenly between the treatment groups; this includes characteristics such as age and sex, as well as, for example, pain-relevant genetic polymorphisms that have not yet been identified. In general, the success of randomization in creating balanced groups depends on the sample size: smaller groups may differ in potentially important ways, whereas in large randomized samples, subject variability is very likely to be dispersed evenly between groups.

BLINDING

A double-blind RCT is one in which the identity of the intervention—whether placebo or active treatment—is concealed from subjects and from investigators; placebos in pharmacotherapy studies are usually inert (unless a so-called *active placebo* is used) and formulated to be identical to the active medication in shape, size, color, taste, and even odor. The importance of blinding cannot be underestimated since interventions that have appeared highly efficacious in unblinded or *open-label* studies have been found to be ineffective in blinded studies.[10]

Rigorous attempts at blinding can be unsuccessful, however. Subjects and/or investigators can sometimes accurately guess which intervention they are receiving—for example, because of the development of side effects or because of symptom improvement. Although not routinely done, at the end of a blinded trial, subjects and investigators should be asked to identify the intervention the subject received (or, for crossover trials, to identify the treatment sequence) and to provide the basis for their guesses.[11] When subjects are able to accurately identify their treatment because of beneficial effects, such as pain relief, it is not considered a compromise of blinding; however, when subjects are able to accurately identify their treatment group based on factors unrelated to efficacy, such as side effects or taste, the integrity of the blinding is potentially compromised and the potential for bias in the results should be considered.

PARALLEL GROUP TRIALS

In parallel group trials, each subject is randomized to one of two or more treatment groups (or *treatment arms*). At the end of the trial, outcome differences between the groups are compared. Many investigators consider parallel group designs the most informative clinical trial design because, when the sample size is large enough, fewer assumptions must be made in the analysis of the data.

CROSSOVER TRIALS

In a crossover trial, the subjects receive different interventions in sequence. Each subject is randomized to a sequence order (e.g., placebo, then active treatment vs. active treatment, then placebo). Typically, a *washout period* occurs between different treatments to allow the effects of the earlier intervention to wear off prior to starting the subsequent treatment. At the conclusion of the trial, the outcomes at the end of the active treatment phase can be compared to the outcomes at the end of the placebo phase.

Crossover trials have a few major advantages. First, they are extremely efficient in terms of sample size because each subject receives one or more active and control treatments and treatment comparisons are made within patients, effectively removing between-patient variability; compared to a parallel group trial with two arms, a two-period crossover design may require only one-fourth as many subjects to show the same size treatment effect. The placebo group's response rate may be lower in crossover compared with parallel design trials, which may be associated with a greater likelihood of finding a statistically significant treatment benefit.[12] In addition, crossover trials comparing two or more active treatments make it possible to determine whether the response to one treatment predicts the response to another treatment (e.g., if a patient fails to respond to treatment A, is he or she unlikely to respond to treatment B?).[6]

Unfortunately, crossover trials also have a number of potential limitations. A central assumption of crossover trials is that outcomes in the different treatment periods are unaffected by the order of treatment. This assumption can be violated in several different ways. Outcomes in later treatment periods would be expected to differ from those in earlier periods if the underlying condition being studied is likely to evolve during the time frame of the trial (e.g., pain severity worsens over time).

If a treatment alters the natural course of the disease (e.g., treatment results in lasting benefit even after the treatment is stopped), then outcomes in later treatment periods can differ from outcomes in earlier periods. *Carryover effects*, which refer to the continuation of treatment effects after the treatment is stopped, are another important consideration. Washout periods are intended to allow all of the effects of the treatment to wear off prior to starting a subsequent treatment, but the true duration of treatment effects is usually not precisely known. If a washout period is inadequate (or if the treatment alters the underlying condition), then subjects in later periods will have different treatment responses than those in the first periods. This can result in a few different types of error that can lessen the ability of the trial to show differences in pain reduction or tolerability between the groups. There are statistical methods that can be used to assess for the presence of carryover and period effects, but these tests are typically underpowered to exclude the presence of such effects.

Despite these potential limitations, crossover trials have proven to be very informative in showing the efficacy of various NP treatments. Knowledge of the natural history of chronic NP conditions supports the assumption that little change in pain severity is likely to occur during the course of trials that typically last for several months. In addition, crossover trials examining different medications with different mechanisms of action have found little evidence of carryover or period effects.[6–8,13] It is important to recognize, however, that the results of crossover trials are difficult to compare with the results of parallel group trials; crossover trials have typically used a *completer* analysis (i.e., analyzing the responses of subjects who completed the entire trial), whereas parallel group trials typically use an intention-to-treat analysis (discussed in the "Statistical Analysis" section below).

Treatment Features

Features of the treatment administered in a clinical trial are likely to have a major effect on the results of the trial. Some trials have a *run-in period* in which subjects must comply with a treatment protocol prior to randomization; during this period, subjects may be required to fill out pain diaries daily or sometimes must take a treatment or placebo to demonstrate treatment adherence prior to randomization. Run-in periods can be used to exclude patients who fail to comply with protocol requirements (e.g., failure to record daily pain ratings), who do not have a beneficial response to the active medication, who have an especially large placebo response, who show wide variations in daily pain scales, or who have significant side effects in response to the active medication.[14] While these features may increase the likelihood of finding a significant difference between drug and placebo, they can also decrease the generalizability of the results.

Recent RCTs of NP treatments have typically included a baseline period that includes pain ratings made on several occasions, typically once daily in a diary. It is critically important to accurately establish the baseline pain level because this is the basis for comparison with the pain scores obtained while taking the treatment. Following the baseline period, patients are randomized to one of two or more treatments. In RCTs of medications for NP, the beginning of treatment often includes a period in which the dosage is titrated. The drug dosage can either be titrated to a prespecified *target* dosage or tailored flexibly as a function of the patient's pain relief and tolerability. In a flexible dosing trial, the dosing strategy or algorithm is prespecified, but the final dosage on which patients are maintained can vary; titration can, for example, increase up to a maximum as long as a patient continues to experience significant pain, but it can stop once pain relief is achieved or side effects become significant, or the dosage can be reduced if side effects are especially troubling. In theory, flexible-dosage trials account for patient variability and mimic clinical practice better than fixed-dosage trials,[15,16] although patients might not achieve adequate dosages and regulatory agencies have typically favored fixed trials so that conclusions can be clearly drawn about which specific dosages show efficacy.

The durations of the maintenance periods in RCTs for NP have typically ranged from 2 to 12 weeks. Longer durations of treatment are typically required for regulatory approval; although the results of such trials provide information regarding the durability of the treatment benefits, subject recruitment and retention are more challenging and the costs of the trial are greater.

Patient Selection

Trials may assess patients with either relatively homogeneous conditions (such as postherpetic neuralgia) or relatively heterogeneous conditions (such as peripheral neuropathic pain). In addition, many studies include a minimum level of baseline pain intensity as one of the inclusion criteria[14]; while requiring a higher pain intensity level may increase the likelihood of demonstrating the benefit of an active treatment over placebo, requiring too high a level of baseline pain may augment responses in the placebo group by increasing regression to the mean or by contributing to an escalation of baseline scores to fulfill enrollment criteria. Most recent chronic pain RCTs have required an average pain intensity of at least 4 (on a 0–10 numerical rating scale) during the baseline period. The duration of pain is also important to consider; many NP trials have required pain to be present for at least 3 to 6 months prior to enrollment. In addition, many trials have excluded patients who may have an increased risk associated with study participation due to the presence of medical or psychiatric comorbidities, allergies, or pregnancy. Some studies have also excluded patients who have previously failed to respond to prior NP treatments (e.g., those sharing a mechanism of action of the investigational drug). Although such inclusion and exclusion criteria probably increase the likelihood that a trial will demonstrate efficacy and safety, they also decrease the generalizability of the results because the study sample is not representative of the population of patients who will be treated in practice.

Treatment Outcomes

Neuropathic pain treatments can have a number of different effects besides pain relief, including a variety of side effects, additional benefits such as reduced depression or anxiety or improved sleep, and inconvenience. A primary outcome measure that would quantify the net impact of all of these potential effects on, for example, health-related quality of life would be very informative. Unfortunately, there is no outcome measure that has been shown to simultaneously capture all of these types of outcomes with demonstrated reliability and validity.

Clinical trials should clearly identify the primary outcome measure and distinguish it from the secondary endpoints. The primary outcome measure is the one that the investigators believe is the most informative with respect to testing the study's primary hypothesis, and it is used in calculating the trial's sample size. Clinical trials that report the results of several different endpoints without indicating which outcome measure was the prespecified primary endpoint are very difficult to interpret because the greater the number of statistical tests performed, the greater the probability that one or more of them will yield a statistically significant result by chance alone.

Recently, the Initiative on Methods, Measurement, and Pain Assessment in Clinical Trials (IMMPACT) recommended six core outcome domains[17] and specific outcome measures for each of these domains[18] for clinical trials of chronic pain treatments. The six recommended core outcome domains are pain, physical functioning, emotional functioning, participant ratings of improvement and satisfaction with treatment, symptoms and adverse events, and participant disposition (e.g., adherence to the treatment regimen and reasons for premature withdrawal from the trial). Specific outcome measures were recommended for four of these domains based on their appropriateness of content, reliability, validity, responsiveness, and participant burden as follows: (1) pain intensity, assessed by a 0–10 numerical rating scale; (2) physical functioning, assessed by the Multidimensional Pain Inventory or the Brief Pain Inventory interference scales; (3) emotional functioning, assessed by the Beck Depression Inventory or the Profile of Mood States; and (4) participant ratings of overall improvement, assessed by the Patient Global Impression of Change scale.[18] These recommendations are recent, and so most completed NP trials have unfortunately used different outcome measures and are therefore difficult to compare with each other. A measure of improvement in pain intensity is the most common primary endpoint in NP clinical trials, with the other outcome domains being considered secondary endpoints.

One of the most important areas to be assessed in clinical trials is the nature and severity of adverse events.[18] Trials should report how side effects were ascertained, including the wording used, which is particularly important when active ascertainment (e.g., asking about the presence of specific side effects, such as dizziness) rather than passive ascertainment (e.g., "did you develop any side effects?") is used. When comparing results from different clinical trials, it is important to realize that side effect frequency can be greatly affected by the approach used. An accurate and detailed description of the withdrawals and dropouts in a clinical trial is a critical marker of trial quality.[19,20]

Statistical Analysis

The results and interpretation of an RCT depend on the statistical analyses performed. Several specific decisions must be described in a clinical trial report. First, the primary outcome must be clearly identified; trials reporting multiple outcomes without identifying which one was prespecified as the primary outcome should be viewed critically. The sample size (or power) calculation should also be clearly described; this gives the reader information about the size of the treatment effect the investigators anticipated and believed to be a clinically meaningful response. In addition, the power calculation is especially important if a trial does not show statistical differences between groups. The specific statistical tests being used must be also described in detail.

Deviations from the trial protocol must be described and their potential impact on the results discussed. A critical factor is how patients who deviated from the trial protocol, such as those who dropped out before completion of the trial, are handled in the analysis. The best method for analyzing parallel group superiority RCTs is generally an *intention-to-treat* (ITT) analysis, in which all subjects are included in the final analysis in the group to which they were randomized. In many trials, a modified ITT analysis is used that, for example, analyzes data only from patients who took at least one dose of the study medication and completed one postbaseline pain diary; the criteria used for defining such modified ITT samples must, of course, be prospectively specified. An alternative analytic strategy, which is sometimes useful in conjunction with a primary ITT analysis, is a *per protocol* analysis, in which, for example, only subjects who completed the treatment protocol and took a certain amount of medication are included in the analysis. An ITT analysis can reflect the efficacy of a treatment in a population of patients who may or may not receive the treatment as intended, whereas a per protocol analysis of the same trial reflects efficacy among those considered most likely to respond (but in treatment groups that may be unbalanced with respect to important factors).

With an ITT analysis, subjects who do not provide a complete set of data are analyzed (e.g., those who drop out will not provide pain scores for an end of maintenance phase endpoint). The manner in which missing data are addressed is a critical factor in statistical analyses of RCTs, one that can change the results.[21] The most commonly used method in recent RCTs of NP has been the *last observation carried forward* (LOCF) approach, in which all missing data are assumed to be equal to the last results the subject provided before dropping out. However, patients with pain score improvement who drop out because they cannot tolerate a drug will be assumed to have pain score improvement at the endpoint of the trial even though they could not tolerate the drug for the duration of the trial and would therefore be expected to revert to their pretreatment pain level[22] (see Figure 9.1). As such, LOCF can misclassify patients who are truly nonresponders (because they cannot tolerate the drug) as responders, overestimating treatment benefit.

In recent medical reviews for chronic pain indications, the U.S. Food and Drug Administration (FDA) has suggested that analysis and

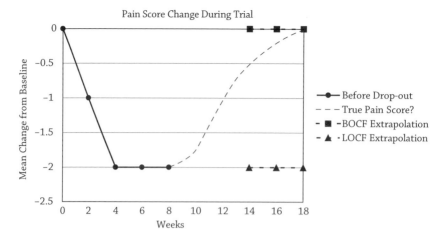

FIGURE 9.1 The graph shows the pain score change from baseline for a hypothetical patient who drops out because of side effects 8 weeks into an 18-week clinical trial. The dashed line estimates how the pain score might change if it were measured for the remainder of the clinical trial period (i.e., after the patient stops taking treatment). The triangles show how the extrapolated pain scores using a last-observation-carried-forward (LOCF) approach overestimate the patient's pain score at the endpoint (weeks 14–18). The squares show how the extrapolated pain scores using a baseline-observation-carried-forward (BOCF) approach more accurately reflects the patient's pain relief from the medication both in the trial and, more importantly, beyond the duration of the trial.

Source: Reprinted from O'Connor AB. LOCF approach to handling missing data overestimates the chronic pain scores of drop-outs. *J Pain*. 2010;11(5):500–501, with permission from Elsevier.

presentation of pivotal RCTs for chronic pain conditions should consider patients who have dropped out as nonresponders and that a *baseline observation carried forward* (BOCF) approach for handling missing data could be used for this purpose.[21] The results of LOCF analyses can overestimate the degree of pain relief when compared to the results of BOCF analyses. For patients who drop out of a trial for reasons unrelated to the treatment (e.g., change in residence), a BOCF analysis can underestimate the true treatment effect, but dropouts in NP trials are often related to poor tolerability of the medication being studied or lack of analgesic benefit. A strategy that applies BOCF to subjects who drop out due to adverse effects and LOCF to other dropouts is an appealing compromise, although the reasons for dropout can sometimes be unknown (e.g., lost to follow-up) or potentially due to more than one factor (e.g., consent revoked in part due to lack of analgesic benefit). It is important to note that a recent report recommended that

imputation methods such as LOCF and BOCF should not be used as the primary approach to missing data unless their assumptions are scientifically justified, and that analyses of existing clinical trial data should be used to determine how different models perform in different settings.[23]

Regardless of the approach used to address missing data in an RCT, the details of the analysis must be described and the limitations of the approach discussed. Ideally, alternative analyses would be presented as sensitivity analyses after clearly identifying the prespecified primary analysis.

NP CLINICAL TRIAL INTERPRETATION

There are many things to consider when interpreting the results of a clinical trial. In this section, we will discuss potential sources of bias within a clinical trial and its conclusions, interpretation of the clinical importance of between-group differences in NP trials, and the interpretation of recent negative RCTs.

Potential Sources of Bias in Clinical Trials

There are many potential sources of bias in a clinical trial, with bias often resulting in over-estimation of treatment effects. In this section, we will discuss factors that can reduce the internal and external validity of an RCT.

THREATS TO INTERNAL VALIDITY

Randomization The importance of effective randomization has been demonstrated by the fact that some interventions found to be effective in nonrandomized trials have been subsequently shown to be ineffective in randomized trials.[10] Moreover, study reports that do not clearly describe the method of randomization have been shown to, on average, overestimate treatment effects when compared to studies that clearly describe randomization methods.[10] Treatment allocation methods that are not based on random number generation (e.g., those using date of birth, date of encounter, or other methods that might allow prediction of treatment allocation) are not considered adequate methods of randomization.[19]

Dropouts Studies in which a substantial percentage of subjects drop out from one or more arms of the trial must be examined carefully to understand the reason(s) for the dropouts and their impact on the results. Dropouts that are not included in the final analysis (e.g., if a modified ITT analysis is used) alter the composition of the original randomized treatment groups, preventing the study sample from accurately representing the intended population. Nonrandom dropouts, such as those caused by treatment side effects, further imbalance the comparison groups to make them potentially dissimilar in ways other than the treatment. In addition, dropouts create missing data, which, as described above, is problematic. A trial with a large number of dropouts may not have been carefully designed or conducted. Any recent study that does not clearly account for the disposition of all study subjects using a CONSORT (Consolidated Standards of Reporting Trials) diagram[20] should be viewed critically and should be scrutinized for other evidence of poor study quality.

Blinding The adequacy of blinding is also very important to the interpretation of clinical trials. Unblinded studies tend to overestimate treatment benefit, sometimes by a large amount.[10] Blinding is especially important in pain trials since the outcomes used are subjective (e.g., pain ratings) and large placebo effects are common. Subjects' guesses about their treatment assignment should be reported, and when subjects accurately guess which treatment they received much more often than by chance, the trial results may reflect, at least in part, the effects of this unblinding; if subjects are unblinded for reasons other than efficacy, then the results may be biased, as described in the "Blinding" section above.

Statistical Analyses and Interpretation Inappropriate statistical analyses and outcome reporting of RCTs can lead to erroneous conclusions. Unfortunately, the peer review process does not consistently catch these types of errors, so readers of the medical literature must be aware of the types of errors and biases that can appear in published studies. Trial reports that do not describe the prespecified primary endpoint and statistical analysis methods may have selected statistically significant effects for emphasis on the basis of the results of the analyses (i.e., post hoc), which is not appropriate; such outcome reporting bias has been shown to result in misleading estimates of treatment benefit.[24,25] Occasionally, the primary endpoint is specified in the methods section but the results and conclusions emphasize other endpoints, presumably because analyses of the primary endpoint were not favorable; readers must be very attentive to such data presentations when interpreting the results of RCTs. As described above, the sample used in the data analyses should be clearly specified, and for a superiority trial, the primary analysis should typically be based on an ITT sample. The method of handling missing data should also be specified in advance of the data analyses, and ideally, the results using alternative methods (e.g., both BOCF and LOCF) would be reported.

Occasionally, trial reports erroneously conclude that two interventions are equivalent when an RCT fails to show superiority of either treatment group. This is not an appropriate conclusion for a trial designed to test the hypothesis that one treatment is superior to another; as noted above, trials should include a detailed description of the sample size assumptions and statistical power calculations, which will make it possible for readers to determine if assumptions about the treatment effect size (or variability) may have accounted for the lack of significant group differences. Equivalence or noninferiority of one treatment to another can only be concluded from trials specifically designed to test hypotheses of equivalence or noninferiority. These types of trials require investigators to define a prespecified equivalence or noninferiority margin (i.e., a difference between groups that is considered clinically insignificant) for the primary endpoint, power analyses based on this margin, and statistical analyses tailored to test hypotheses of equivalence or noninferiority (e.g., emphasizing the results of analyses of per protocol rather than ITT samples).

THREATS TO EXTERNAL VALIDITY

An RCT can have high internal validity yet produce estimates of treatment response that have limited applicability to clinical practice because it has poor external validity (i.e., the results of the trial may not apply to the patients treated in the community). The appropriate extrapolation of clinical trial results to patient care is challenging for many reasons, including the fact that many patients differ from the types of patients enrolled in NP trials. There are few studies demonstrating harm resulting from the extrapolation of trial results to inappropriate patient populations,[26] though it is easy to imagine that this occurs. Two aspects of RCTs commonly reduce external validity—the representativeness of the study sample and the dosing strategies used in the trial.

Study Sample Representativeness Several factors may reduce the generalizability of a

trial's results to treating patients in clinical practice. For example, the country in which an RCT is performed may impact the trial's results, presumably due to differences in subject characteristics and possibly in the treatment environment.[10,27] Furthermore, patients willing to participate in a clinical trial are probably inherently different than the broader pool of patients for whom the treatment may be prescribed. In addition, the recruitment methods investigators use (e.g., identifying patients from clinics vs. advertising in newspapers or on the Internet) can affect the types of patients enrolled in an RCT and potentially the results of the trial.[14,28,29]

The inclusion and exclusion criteria used to define an RCT's study sample frequently result in samples that differ substantially from the broader population for which the treatment is intended.[30] The study sample is such a critical factor that, strictly speaking, conclusions from a placebo-controlled trial should describe how the intervention compares with placebo or another comparator *in the specific sample studied*. The study sample is assumed to represent the population of all patients who meet the inclusion and exclusion criteria, although, as described above, factors beyond the inclusion and exclusion criteria (such as country of origin, methods of recruitment, and willingness to participate) make this an unreliable assumption. Nevertheless, the reports of RCTs often conclude that the results pertain to the entire population of patients with the disorder that has been studied, not just those who would have been eligible to participate in the trial. Trials with a run-in period that excludes patients (such as those without a beneficial response to treatment, those with a large placebo response, or those with adverse effects during the run-in period, as described in the "Treatment Features" section above) may further limit the generalizability of trial results to patient populations.

Dosing Strategy The dosing strategy employed in an RCT is another important factor to consider, since it can substantially affect both efficacy and tolerability. Two broad dosing strategies have been used in NP trials: fixed dosing, in which all subjects are ultimately treated with the same dosage unless they are unable to tolerate it, and flexible dosing, in which the patient's response is used in adjusting the dosage (e.g., if pain is relieved adequately or if poorly tolerated side effects develop, the dosage is maintained rather than increased further). These two strategies can produce different estimates of efficacy and tolerability. In addition, the rate of dosage titration and the maximum dosage administered can have major effects on the results[31] and therefore on the generalizability of the trial results to clinical practice. For example, in a trial comparing two active medications, if one medication is titrated more slowly and to a lower dosage than a second medication with comparable efficacy and tolerability, the first medication will likely be better tolerated; conversely, if one medication is titrated to relatively higher dosages than another, it can be expected to show greater efficacy, even though the medications would show comparable efficacy if tolerated to equivalent dosages.

ADDITIONAL SOURCES OF BIAS

Unwarranted Conclusions A surprising number of clinical trial reports draw conclusions that are not justified by the trial results. For example, publications describing prospective cohort studies sometimes attribute benefits to the treatment, although it is more accurate to conclude that there is an association between the treatment and the outcomes, which can be considered consistent with treatment "effectiveness" but does not provide evidence of treatment "efficacy." Reports of NP trials not infrequently summarize the results with broad statements, such as that the treatment "demonstrated efficacy for NP," despite, for example, numerous inclusion and exclusion criteria that narrow the study population to a specific disease (e.g., postherpetic neuralgia), patients who have not previously taken certain medications, and those with, for example, moderate pain severity ($\geq 4/10$) for more than 6 months. Readers should be skeptical of conclusions that are globally positive, since significant compromises are required to perform an RCT and therefore all clinical trials have important limitations.

Conflicts of Interest Clinical trial reports should always identify the source of the trial's funding and the potential conflicts of interest of the investigators. Industry-sponsored trials are predictably designed to maximize the potential for the sponsor's product to demonstrate superiority, whether via greater efficacy or tolerability, over the comparator.[31-33] A recent study, for example, found that trials sponsored by for-profit sponsors were more likely to recommend an intervention as the "treatment of choice" compared with trials sponsored by nonprofit organizations; importantly, the association between sponsorship and positive recommendations was not explained by the magnitude of the treatment effect or the occurrence of adverse events.[34] Academic investigators are also very invested in the outcomes of their research, of course, but evaluating the effects of these nonfinancial conflicts of interest on clinical trial reports is more difficult and has received far less attention than industry conflicts of interest.[35,36] Finally, it is important to remember that industry-sponsored trials undergo considerable scrutiny when they are submitted to regulatory agencies for product approval, so their quality is generally high; moreover, if the medication or device has received regulatory approval, it will often be possible to compare the results and conclusions of journal publications with analyses and interpretations of the data made by the treatment's regulatory reviewers once they become available on agency Web sites.[21]

Publication Bias Several different types of publication bias have been characterized. The fact that negative RCTs (i.e., those that fail to demonstrate adequately that an intervention is beneficial) may never be published is now widely recognized; the published literature is therefore skewed by positive trials, resulting in overestimation of the true benefits of an intervention. There are several additional forms of publication bias that are less widely recognized. Examples include pooling negative trials with positive RCTs to produce a favorable publication[24]; publishing the same positive trial multiple times[24]; and describing the results of a negative trial so that they appear positive by emphasizing secondary or post hoc outcomes.[24,25] In one example, a total of 15 RCTs were conducted to assess the efficacy of an antidepressant for major depression; 3 of these were never published, yet a total of 20 publications describing the RCTs appeared in the literature, including duplicate publications of the same trial with different authors and other seemingly intentional masking of the duplications.[24] Regulatory agencies, such as the FDA, require sponsors to submit the raw data from the trials they have conducted, and independent statisticians then analyze the data; documents summarizing these regulatory analyses have proven extremely useful in characterizing publication bias, including the potential biases introduced in statistical analyses.[21] Manipulation of statistical analyses and outcomes reporting may account for as much or even more total bias than nonpublication and multiple publication of trials.[24,25]

Clinical trial registration prior to enrolling subjects, including publicly reporting the primary outcome measure and the methods of analyses, should raise awareness of trials that are never published.[37] The registration of trial results is another positive step, but currently the reporting of results is nearly unregulated, so it is unclear how accurate and useful this will be.[21]

Interpreting the Clinical Importance of Changes in RCTs of NP Treatments

Testing of statistical significance is used to evaluate the probability that the differences between treatment groups are caused by chance (*Type I error*). Statistical significance depends on three independent factors: the magnitude of the treatment effect, the variability of the treatment effect, and the sample size. The fact that the magnitude of the treatment effect is sufficient to yield a statistically significant difference between groups does not mean that the magnitude of the treatment effect is clinically meaningful (e.g., if a trial is sufficiently large, very small between-group differences may achieve statistical significance even though they are clinically irrelevant). How then do we judge whether a statistically significant finding also has clinical importance?

Determinations of clinical significance depend upon whether one is seeking to define differences of importance to individual patients or differences between two groups of patients. Each of these issues is the topic of a recent IMMPACT consensus recommendation, the results of which will be summarized below.

CLINICAL IMPORTANCE OF CHANGES ON AN INDIVIDUAL LEVEL

Many studies have been conducted in an attempt to determine the degree of pain relief that is meaningful to patients. The available research seems to indicate that an absolute pain score improvement of approximately 2 points on a 10-point scale is clinically meaningful to patients with various chronic pain conditions; moreover, reductions in pain of ≥30% correspond to what patients would consider "moderately important" improvements in pain, whereas reductions of ≥50% can be considered "substantial" improvements.[38] Any of these cut points could reasonably be prespecified to define a patient as a *responder*.

It is important to note that pain score changes, however, should not be assumed to indicate overall patient improvement. For example, a clinically important pain score improvement could be accompanied by significant side effects, such that overall functioning and quality of life are unimproved or even worsened by the treatment; conversely, a treatment might produce a modest pain score change but might also be associated with improvements in mood, sleep, and overall function, such that a substantial net improvement results even thought the pain score reduction was modest.

For these reasons, the IMMPACT recommendations emphasized the importance of simultaneous assessment of multiple outcome domains, including measures of emotional functioning, physical functioning, sleep, other health-related quality-of-life domains, and overall improvement to augment the interpretation of pain score changes.[17] Provisional cut points for clinically meaningful changes have been proposed for the scales most commonly used to measure outcomes in NP trials, including emotional functioning, physical functioning, and overall impression of change[38] (Table 9.1).

Table 9-1. Provisional Benchmarks for Interpreting Changes in Chronic Pain Clinical Trial Outcome Measures

OUTCOME DOMAIN AND MEASURE	TYPE OF IMPROVEMENT[a]	METHOD[b]	CHANGE
	PAIN INTENSITY		
0–10 numerical rating scale	minimally important	anchor	10–20% decrease
	moderately important	anchor	≥30% decrease
	substantial	anchor	≥50% decrease
	PHYSICAL FUNCTIONING		
Multidimensional Pain Inventory Interference Scale	clinically important	distribution	≥ 0.6 point decrease
Brief Pain Inventory Interference Scale	minimally important	distribution	1 point decrease
	EMOTIONAL FUNCTIONING		
Beck Depression Inventory	clinically important	distribution	≥5 point decrease
Profile of Mood States			
Total Mood Disturbance	clinically important	distribution	≥10–15 point decrease
Specific subscales	clinically important	distribution	≥2–12 point change[c]
	GLOBAL RATING OF IMPROVEMENT		
Patient Global Impression of Change	minimally important	anchor	minimally improved
	moderately important	anchor	much improved
	substantial	anchor	very much improved

[a]Because few studies have examined the importance of worsening on these measures, benchmarks are only provided for improvement in scores.

[b]Specific method used in determining the benchmark provided in the final column; distribution-based methods were based on the use of a 0.5 standard deviation or a 1.0 standard error of measurement or both.

[c]The magnitude of a clinically important change depends on the specific subscale, as does the direction of change that reflects an improvement.

Source: Reprinted from Dworkin RH, Turk DC, Wyrwich KW, et al. Interpreting the clinical importance of treatment outcomes in chronic pain clinical trials: IMMPACT recommendations. *J Pain*. 2008;9:105–121, with permission from Elsevier.

CLINICAL IMPORTANCE OF CHANGES ON A GROUP LEVEL

IMMPACT recommendations have emphasized that the importance of group differences "can only be established in the broader context of the disease being treated, the currently available treatments, and the overall risk-benefit ratio of treatment."[38] The interpretation of primary versus secondary outcomes must be considered separately.

Primary Outcomes As noted above, a 2-point change in pain score could be used to define a clinically meaningful improvement for an individual patient, but it is *not* true that the difference between improvements in pain between a treatment and a placebo or another comparator must be at least 2 points in order for the effect of the treatment to be considered clinically meaningful. Within any treated population, there will be differences among patients in the magnitude of their response to treatment.

Critical considerations are the proportion of responders to treatment and how that proportion compares with the proportion of responders in the control group.[39] For example, in a hypothetical trial in which treatment produces a 2-point improvement and placebo produces no change in pain score (with a standard deviation of 2.5), the treatment population's average 2-point improvement should not be interpreted as meaning that each patient experienced a clinically important improvement in pain. In this example, 50% of the patients in the treatment group and 21% of the patients in the placebo group could be considered responders (i.e., ≥2-point improvement).[39] Alternatively, if the average pain score improvements in the treatment and placebo groups are 1.5 and 0.5 points, respectively, then the group difference is only 1 point. Although this magnitude of group difference is of marginal clinical importance for individual patients,[38] 42% of the patients in the treatment group could be considered responders compared to 27% of those in the placebo group.[39]

Does a group difference in the proportion of responders of 42% versus 27% have clinical importance for a population of patients in the community? How do we determine this? IMMPACT recommendations describe a number of factors that must be considered to determine whether the difference between treatments has clinical importance (Table 9.2) and conclude that "the evaluation of group differences should be carried out on a case-by-case consideration of the various characteristics of a specific treatment, the population of patients to be treated, and the risk-benefit ratio."[39]

First, the differences must be statistically significant, which is a necessary but not sufficient criterion. In addition, and possibly most significantly, the magnitude of the improvement in the primary outcome should be compared with the magnitude of improvement produced by other treatments established to produce clinically important improvements. If a new treatment produces a benefit that is comparable to or greater than that seen with established therapies, then the improvement is likely to be clinically important; if, on the other hand, the magnitude of improvement of a new treatment is substantially smaller than the improvement typically produced by established therapies, then the improvement produced by the new treatment may not be clinically important.

Table 9-2. Factors to Consider in Determining the Clinical Meaningfulness of Group Differences

- Statistical significance of the primary efficacy analysis (typically necessary but not sufficient to determine that the group difference is clinically meaningful)
- Magnitude of improvement in the primary efficacy outcome with treatment
- Results of responder analyses
- Treatment effect size compared to available treatments
- Rapidity of onset of treatment benefit
- Durability of treatment benefit
- Results for secondary efficacy endpoints (e.g., improvements in physical and/or emotional functioning)
- Safety and tolerability
- Convenience
- Patient adherence
- Cost
- Different mechanism of action vs. existing treatments
- Limitations of available treatments
- Other benefits (e.g., few or no drug interactions, availability of a test that predicts a good therapeutic response)

Source: Adapted from Dworkin RH, Turk DC, McDermott MP, et al. Interpreting the clinical importance of group differences in chronic pain clinical trials: IMMPACT recommendations. *Pain.* 2009;146:238–244.

Responder analyses, such as comparing the percentage of responders, the number needed to treat (NNT), and the cumulative proportion of responders curve,[40] can help define the benefits of a treatment to a population of patients. The NNT, which is the reciprocal of the absolute risk reduction, has been used frequently to compare the magnitude of improvement produced by different NP treatments.[41] It can be thought of as the "number of patients who must be treated to generate one more success or one less failure than would have resulted had all persons been given the comparison treatment."[42] In the example described above, the NNT for the treatment producing a 2-point difference compared to placebo is 3.45, whereas the NNT for the treatment producing a 1-point difference compared to placebo is 6.67. The NNT, however, has limitations as a means to compare the efficacy of different NP treatments.[43]

Secondary Outcomes Group level differences for secondary outcomes should generally be approached in the same way as for primary outcomes, except that secondary outcomes that fail to reach statistical significance are less easily interpreted because the sample size of a clinical trial is typically based on estimates for the primary outcome. Treatment group differences for secondary outcomes can fail to be statistically significant either because there was an inadequate clinical response or because the trial was underpowered to detect differences for the secondary outcome (e.g., there was a large amount of variability in the outcome responses). Not uncommonly, one or more secondary outcomes are found to have statistically significant improvements at the same time that the primary outcome measure fails to show a statistically significant improvement; strictly speaking, these are negative trials, although the secondary outcome improvements can be used to generate new hypotheses and may be considered supportive in considering positive results from additional trials.

Interpreting Negative RCTs of Pharmacological Treatments for NP

Randomized clinical trials for NP treatments sometimes fail to demonstrate statistically significant benefits of treatment over placebo in the primary outcome,[44] even for the most established NP treatments like tricyclic antidepressants,[9] pregabalin,[21] gabapentin,[45] and opioids.[9] There are several potential explanations for negative RCTs that must be considered.[46]

NP ETIOLOGY

First, the etiology of NP must be considered. The majority of NP trials has assessed patients with either postherpetic neuralgia (PHN) or painful diabetic peripheral neuropathy (DPN); although these patients share clinical features with patients who have NP caused by other disorders, the extent to which RCT results for these two conditions apply to other types of NP is uncertain. Lacking evidence to the contrary, the extrapolation of efficacy from one or more types of NP to other types of NP has seemed reasonable to many investigators and clinicians. It has also been suggested that medications with efficacy in multiple different NP conditions may have the greatest probability of being efficacious in additional, as yet unstudied, conditions.[44,47]

However, with the growing number of RCTs in different types of NP, there is increasing evidence suggesting that certain types of NP may be less likely to respond to the existing first-line treatments that have typically established their efficacy in RCTs of PHN and painful DPN.[48] Since 1998 there have been several placebo-controlled RCTs in human immunodeficiency virus (HIV) neuropathy, all of which have been negative, including trials assessing amitriptyline,[49,50] topical lidocaine,[51] and pregabalin.[52] Chemotherapy-induced peripheral neuropathy seems to be another NP condition that is relatively refractory to existing first-line treatments; RCTs of nortriptyline,[53] amitriptyline,[54] and gabapentin[55] have all failed to demonstrate efficacy. Finally, RCTs conducted in patients with lumbosacral radiculopathy have also failed to clearly demonstrate efficacy for pregabalin,[56] topiramate (which has had mixed results in other NP conditions),[57] and nortriptyline, morphine, and their combination.[9] Although there are multiple potential explanations for these negative RCTs, the fact that there have been few if any positive

RCTs in these conditions suggests that medications with efficacy in painful DPN—the most prevalent painful polyneuropathy—may not have efficacy in certain other painful polyneuropathies and that the extrapolation of efficacy across different NP conditions may not always be appropriate.

OTHER EXPLANATIONS FOR NEGATIVE RCTS

Although differences in NP etiology and underlying pathophysiological mechanisms of pain may explain some of the negative RCTs for potentially efficacious medications, some RCTs have been negative even with treatments established to have efficacy for a specific NP condition (based on demonstrated efficacy for the condition in multiple other RCTs). How can we explain these so-called *failed trials*? Several factors may contribute to the failure of an RCT to find benefit even with a treatment established to be efficacious for the condition being studied.

A recent study assessed 106 placebo-controlled NP trials and found that the factors that were independently associated with a positive trial (i.e., a drug response significantly greater than that of placebo for the primary outcome measure) were a larger medication response, a smaller placebo response, and a larger sample size.[12] In this study, the factors associated with larger placebo response rates were larger medication response rates and parallel group design.[12] Unfortunately, this study was, by necessity, focused on group level trial differences and was not able to assess the possible contributions of differences in many important patient characteristics that may also affect the trial outcome, so additional research in this area is needed.[12,14,29]

A number of other factors may differ among trials, potentially contributing to the likelihood that a trial will be "falsely negative."[46] The study sample is one such critical factor. The sample that is examined in an RCT is determined by the inclusion and exclusion criteria; the sample can be substantially altered by, for example, criteria defining the degree or duration of pain required for enrollment, prior experience with NP treatments, comorbidities, and other critical demographic and clinical characteristics.[14,46] In addition, the sample is further defined by the geographic location of the trial and the recruitment methods used. Sampling variability can also account for some differences.

The conduct of the trial itself can also affect its results.[46] Characteristics of the treatment intervention, such as the titration strategy and the maximum dosage, can have a major effect on the tolerability of treatment and the resulting dropout rate. The duration of a trial and how the run-in period is defined may also be important factors. Additional factors that can vary from trial to trial include subject compliance with treatment (which can be affected by the interactions of study personnel with subjects), degree of blinding, methods of pain assessment, the other outcomes used, the methods of statistical analysis, and essentially any of the factors described above in the section "Understanding NP Clinical Trials: Overview of Trial Design Issues." The amount of contact between study subjects and investigators may also affect the placebo response. Recent negative RCT results for NP and other chronic pain conditions have increased interest in the research methods used in chronic pain trials.[14,46,58–60] This increased attention to clinical trial designs will hopefully advance NP clinical trial methodology and thereby decrease the number of false-negative trials of truly efficacious medications (without increasing the rate of false-positive trials).

CONCLUSIONS

Clinical trials have become both more complex and more important as biomedical knowledge evolves. At the same time that scientific understanding of the strengths, limitations, and biases of clinical trials has reached new heights, trials have become less and less accessible to clinicians and the public. Improving awareness of what we currently know about clinical trial design and interpretation is critical to expanding the value of clinical trials and the application of the knowledge gained from them.

Advances in clinical trial designs used to study NP treatments must keep pace with the rapid evolution in understanding of pain mechanisms that is taking place.[61] A major focus of ongoing research is to identify the mechanisms underlying different NP conditions, devise methods for reliably identifying these mechanisms in individual patients, and then identify and develop treatments that will target these mechanisms. The ultimate goal of these efforts is to provide the foundation for a mechanism-based treatment approach in which therapeutic interventions target the specific mechanisms of a patient's pain. Increased knowledge of the genetic, pathophysiological, and psychosocial mechanisms of NP and its response to different treatments will require major modifications in the clinical trial designs that we have discussed in this chapter. To the extent that individualized treatments are developed, study designs in which treatments are matched to particular patient characteristics will be needed.[62,63] Patients in such clinical trials will not only be more homogeneous but may also respond more favorably to such mechanism-based treatments. Randomized clinical trials of mechanism-based treatments will be complicated by the need for sophisticated subject assessments to identify pain mechanisms and the potentially large numbers of patients who fail to meet eligibility criteria of trials targeting specific mechanisms. Fortunately, not only are efforts being made to identify factors that influence whether trials succeed in demonstrating efficacy,[12,58,64] but alternatives to the standard parallel-group RCT are also receiving increasing attention, including, for example, various enrichment and adaptive allocation designs.[65–67] We are therefore optimistic that the future management of NP will be greatly enhanced by the development of novel research methods that will accelerate the identification of treatments with greater efficacy and safety.

REFERENCES

1. World Health Organization. International Clinical Trials Registry Platform (ICTRP). http://www.who.int/ictrp/en. Accessed December 27, 2009.

2. Max MB. Neuropathic pain syndromes. In: Max M, Portenoy R, Laska E, eds. *The Design and Analysis of Analgesic Trials: Advances in Pain Research and Therapy*. Vol. 18. New York: Raven Press;1991:193–219.

3. Max MB. Divergent traditions in analgesic clinical trials. *Clin Pharmacol Ther*. 1994;56:237–241.

4. Schwartz D, Lellouch J. Explanatory and pragmatic attitudes in therapeutical trials. *J Chron Dis*. 1967;20:637–648.

5. Layton D, Pearce GL, Shakir SA. Safety profile of tolterodine as used in general practice in England: results of prescription-event monitoring. *Drug Safety*. 2001;24:703–713.

6. Raja SN, Haythornthwaite JA, Pappagallo M, et al. Opioids versus antidepressants in postherpetic neuralgia: a randomized, placebo-controlled trial. *Neurology*. 2002;59:1015–1021.

7. Sindrup SH, Bach FW, Madsen C, Gram LF, Jensen TS. Venlafaxine versus imipramine in painful polyneuropathy: a randomized, controlled trial. *Neurology*. 2003;60:1284–1289.

8. Gilron I, Bailey JM, Tu D, Holden RR, Weaver DF, Houlden RL. Morphine, gabapentin, or their combination for neuropathic pain. *N Engl J Med*. 2005;352:1324–1334.

9. Khoromi S, Cui L, Nackers L, Max MB. Morphine, nortriptyline and their combination vs. placebo in patients with chronic lumbar root pain. *Pain*. 2007;130:65–75.

10. Bandolier. Bandolier Bias Guide, 2001. http://www.medicine.ox.ac.uk/bandolier/band80/b80-2.html. Accessed December 27, 2009.

11. Moscucci M, Byrne L, Weintraub M, Cox C. Blinding, unblinding, and the placebo effect: an analysis of patients' guesses of treatment assignment in a double-blind clinical trial. *Clin Pharmacol Ther*. 1987;41:259–265.

12. Katz J, Finnerup NB, Dworkin RH. Clinical trial outcome in neuropathic pain: relationship to study characteristics. *Neurology*. 2008;70;263–272.

13. Max MB, Lynch SA, Muir J, Shoaf SF, Smoller B, Dubner R. Effects of desipramine, amitriptyline, and fluoxetine on pain in diabetic neuropathy. *N Engl J Med*. 1992;326:1250–1256.

14. Dworkin RH, Turk DC, Peirce-Sandner S, Baron R, Bellamy N, Burke LB, Chappell A, Chartier K, Cleeland CS, Costello A, Cowan P, Dimitrova R, Ellenberg S, Farrar JT, French JA, Gilron I, Hertz S, Jadad AR, Jay GW, Kalliomäki J, Katz NP, Kerns RD, Manning DC, McDermott MP, McGrath P, Narayana A, Porter L, Quessy S, Rappaport BA, Rauschkolb C, Reeve B, Rhodes T, Sampaio C, Simpson DM, Stauffer JW, Stucki G, Tobias J, White RE, Witter J. Research design considerations for confirmatory chronic pain clinical trials: IMMPACT recommendations. *Pain*. 2010;149:177–193.

15. Morello CM, Leckband SG, Stoner CP, Moorhouse DF, Sahagian GA. Randomized double-blind

study comparing the efficacy of gabapentin with amitriptyline on diabetic peripheral neuropathy pain. *Arch Intern Med.* 1999;159:1931–1937.

16. Freynhagen R, Strojek K, Griesing T, Whalen E, Balkenohl. Efficacy of pregabalin in neuropathic pain evaluated in a 12-week, randomized, double-blind, multicentre, placebo-controlled trial of flexible- and fixed-dose regimens. *Pain.* 2005;115:254–263.

17. Turk DC, Dworkin RH, Allen RR, Bellamy N, Brandenburg N, Carr DB, Cleeland C, Dionne R, Farrar JT, Galer BS, Hewitt DJ, Jadad AR, Katz NP, Kramer LD, Manning DC, McCormick CG, McDermott MP, McGrath P, Quessy S, Rappaport BA, Robinson JP, Royal MA, Simon L, Stauffer JW, Stein W, Tollett J, Witter J. Core outcome domains for chronic pain clinical trials: IMMPACT recommendations. *Pain.* 2003;106:337–345.

18. Dworkin RH, Turk DC, Farrar JT, Haythornthwaite JA, Jensen MP, Katz NP, Kerns RD, Stucki G, Allen RR, Bellamy N, Carr DB, Chandler J, Cowan P, Dionne R, Galer BS, Hertz S, Jadad AR, Kramer LD, Manning DC, Martin S, McCormick CG, McDermott MP, McGrath P, Quessy S, Rappaport BA, Robbins W, Robinson JP, Rothman M, Royal MA, Simon L, Stauffer JW, Stein W, Tollett J, Wernicke J, Witter J, IMMPACT. Core outcome measures for chronic pain clinical trials: IMMPACT recommendations. *Pain.* 2005;113:9–19.

19. Jadad AR, Moore RA, Carroll D, Jenkinson C, Reynolds DJ, Gavaghan DJ, McQuay HJ. Assessing the quality of randomized clinical trials: is blinding necessary? *Control Clin Trial.* 1996;17:1–12.

20. Moher D, Schulz KF, Altman DG. The CONSORT Statement: revised recommendations for improving the quality of reports of parallel-group randomised trials. *Lancet.* 2001;357:1191–1194.

21. O'Connor AB. The need for improved access to FDA reviews. *JAMA.* 2009;302:191–193.

22. O'Connor AB. LOCF approach to handling missing data overestimates the chronic pain scores of drop-outs. *J Pain.* 2010;15:45–46.

23. Panel on Handling Missing Data in Clinical Trials; National Research Council. The prevention and treatment of missing data in clinical trials. http://www.nap.edu/catalog/12955.html. Accessed November 1, 2010.

24. Melander H, Ahlqvist-Rastad J, Meijer G, Beerman B. Evidence b(i)ased medicine—selective reporting from studies sponsored by pharmaceutical industry: review of studies in new drug applications. *BMJ.* 2003;326:1171–1175.

25. Turner EH, Matthews AM, Linardatos E, Tell RA, Rosenthal R. Selective publication of antidepressant trials and its influence on apparent efficacy. *N Engl J Med.* 2008;358:252–260.

26. Juurlink DN, Mamdani MM, Lee DS, Kopp A, Austin PC, Laupacis A, Redelmeier DA. Rates of hyperkalemia after publication of the Randomized Aldactone Evaluation Study. *N Engl J Med.* 2004;351:543–551.

27. Vickers A, Goyal N, Harland R, Rees R. Do certain countries produce only positive results? A systematic review of controlled trials. *Controlled Clin Trials.* 1998;19:159–166.

28. Gross CP, Mallory R, Heiat A, Krumholz HM. Reporting the recruitment process in clinical trials: who are these patients and how did they get there? *Ann Intern Med.* 2002;137:10–16.

29. Polydefkis M, Raja SN. What can we learn from failed neuropathic pain trials? *Neurology.* 2008;70:250–251.

30. van Spall HGC, Toren A, Kiss A, Fowler RA. Eligibility criteria of randomized controlled trials published in high-impact general medical journals: a systematic sampling review. *JAMA.* 2007;297:1233–1240.

31. Safer DJ. Design and reporting modifications in industry-sponsored comparative psychopharmacology trials. *J Nerv Ment Dis.* 2002;190:583–592.

32. Lexchin J, Bero LA, Djulbegovic B, Clark O. Pharmaceutical industry sponsorship and research outcome and quality: systematic review. *BMJ.* 2003;326:1167–1170.

33. Chan A-W, Hrobjartsson A, Haahr MT, Gøtzsche PC, Altman DG. Empirical evidence for selective reporting of outcomes in randomized trials: comparison of protocols to published articles. *JAMA.* 2004;291:2457–2465.

34. Als-Nielsen B, Chen W, Gluud C, Kjaergard LL. Association of funding and conclusions in randomized drug trials: a reflection of treatment effect or adverse events? *JAMA.* 2003;290:921–928.

35. Lewinsky NG. Nonfinancial conflicts of interest in research. *N Engl J Med.* 2002;347:759–761.

36. Schwid SR, Gross RA. Bias, not conflict of interest, is the enemy. *Neurology.* 2005;64:1830–1831.

37. Laine C, Horton R, DeAngelis CD, Drazen JM, Frizelle FA, Godlee F, Haug C, Hébert PC, Kotzin S, Marusic A, Sahni P, Schroeder TV, Sox HC, Van Der Weyden MB, Verheugt FWA. Clinical trial registration. *BMJ.* 2007;334:1177–1178.

38. Dworkin RH, Turk DC, Wyrwich KW, Beaton D, Cleeland CS, Farrar JT, Haythornthwaite JA, Jensen MP, Kerns RD, Ader DN, Brandenburg

N, Burke LB, Cella D, Chandler J, Cowan P, Dimitrova R, Dionne R, Hertz S, Jadad AR, Katz NP, Kehlet H, Kramer LD, Manning DC, McCormick C, McDermott MP, McQuay HJ, Patel S, Porter L, Quessy S, Rappaport BA, Rauschkolb C, Revicki DA, Rothman M, Schmader KE, Stacey BR, Stauffer JW, con Stein T, White RE, Witter J, Zavisic S. Interpreting the clinical importance of treatment outcomes in chronic pain clinical trials: IMMPACT recommendations. *J Pain.* 2008;9:105–121.

39. Dworkin RH, Turk DC, McDermott MP, Peirce-Sandner S, Burke LB, Cowan P, Farrar JT, Hertz S, Raja SN, Rappaport BA, Rauschkolb C, Sampaio C. Interpreting the clinical importance of group differences in chronic pain clinical trials: IMMPACT recommendations. *Pain.* 2009;146:238–244.

40. Farrar JT, Dworkin RH, Max MB. Use of the cumulative proportion of responders analysis graph to present pain data over a range of cut-off points: making clinical trial data more understandable. *J Pain Symptom Manage.* 2006;31:369–377.

41. Finnerup NB, Sindrup SH, Jensen TS. The evidence for pharmacological treatment of neuropathic pain. *Pain.* 2010;150:573–581.

42. Kraemer HC, Morgan GA, Leech NL, Gliner JA, Vaske JJ, Harmon RJ. Measures of clinical significance. *J Am Acad Child Adolesc Psychiatry.* 2003;42:1524–1529.

43. Edelsberg J, Oster G. Summary measures of number needed to treat: how much clinical guidance do they provide in neuropathic pain? *Eur J Pain.* 2009;13:11–16.

44. Dworkin RH, O'Connor AB, Backonja M, Farrar JT, Finnerup NB, Jensen TS, Kalso EA, Loeser JD, Miaskowski C, Nurmikko TJ, Portenoy RK, Rice AS, Stacey BR, Treede RD, Turk DC, Wallace MS. Pharmacologic management of neuropathic pain: evidence-based recommendations. *Pain.* 2007;132:237–251.

45. Backonja M, Glanzman RL. Gabapentin dosing for neuropathic pain: evidence from randomized, placebo-controlled clinical trials. *Clin Ther.* 2003;25(1):81–104.

46. Dworkin RH, Turk DC, Katz NP, Rowbotham MC, Peirce-Sandner S, Cerny I, Clingman CS, Eloff BC, Farrar JT, Kamp C, McDermott MP, Rappaport BA, Sanhai WR. Evidence-based clinical trial design for chronic pain pharmacotherapy: a blueprint for ACTION. *Pain.* 2011;152 (3 Suppl):S107–115.

47. Hansson PT, Dickenson AH. Pharmacological treatment of peripheral neuropathic conditions based on shared commonalities despite multiple etiologies. *Pain.* 2005;113:251–254.

48. O'Connor AB, Dworkin RH. Treatment of neuropathic pain: an overview of recent guidelines. *Am J Med.* 2009;122:S22–S32.

49. Kieburtz K, Simpson D, Yiannoutsos C, Max MB, Hall CD, Ellis RJ, Marra CM, McKendall R, Singer E, Dal Pan GJ, Clifford DB, Tucker T, Cohen B. A randomized trial of amitriptyline and mexiletine for painful neuropathy in HIV infection. *Neurology.* 1998;51:1682–1688.

50. Shlay JC, Chaloner K, Max MB, Flaws B, Reichelderfer P, Wentworth D, Hillman S, Brizz B, Cohn DL. Acupuncture and amitriptyline for pain due to HIV-related peripheral neuropathy: a randomized controlled trial. *JAMA.* 1998;280:1590–1595.

51. Estanislao L, Carter K, McArthur J, Olney R, Simpson D. A randomized controlled trial of 5% lidocaine gel for HIV-associated distal symmetric polyneuropathy. *J Acquir Immune Defic Syndr.* 2004;37:1584–1586.

52. Simpson DM, Schifitto G, Clifford DB, Murphy TK, Durso-De Cruz E, Glue P, Whalen E, Emir B, Scott GN, Freeman R. Pregabalin for painful HIV neuropathy: a randomized, double-blind, placebo-controlled trial. *Neurology.* 2010;74:413–420.

53. Hammack JE, Michalak JC, Loprinzi CL, Sloan JA, Novotny PJ, Soori GS, Tirona MT, Rowland KM Jr, Stella PJ, Johnson JA. Phase III evaluation of nortriptyline for alleviation of symptoms of cis-platinum-induced peripheral neuropathy. *Pain.* 2002;98:195–203.

54. Kautio AL, Haanpää M, Saarto T, Kalso E. Amitriptyline in the treatment of chemotherapy-induced neuropathic symptoms. *J Pain Symptom Manage.* 2008;35:31–39.

55. Rao RD, Michalak JC, Sloan JA, Loprinzi CL, Soori GS, Nikcevich DA, Warner DO, Novotny P, Kutteh LA, Wong GY, North Central Cancer Treatment Group. Efficacy of gabapentin in the management of chemotherapy-induced peripheral neuropathy: a Phase 3 randomized, double-blind, placebo-controlled, crossover trial (N00C3). *Cancer.* 2007;110:2110–2118.

56. Baron R, Freynhagen R, Tölle TR, Cloutier C, Leon T, Murphy TK, Phillips K. The efficacy and safety of pregabalin in the treatment of neuropathic pain associated with chronic lumbosacral radiculopathy. *Pain.* 2010;150:420–427.

57. Khoromi S, Patsalides A, Parada S, Salehi V, Meegan JM, Max MB. Topiramate in chronic lumbar radicular pain. *J Pain.* 2005;6:829–836.

58. Katz N. Methodological issues in clinical trials of opioids for chronic pain. *Neurology.* 2005;65:S32–S49.

59. Quessy SN, Rowbotham MC. Placebo response in neuropathic pain trials. *Pain.* 2008;138:479–483.

60. Katz N. Enriched enrollment randomized withdrawal trial designs for analgesics: focus on methodology. *Clin J Pain.* 2009;25:979–807.

61. Campbell JN, Basbaum AI, Dray A, Dubner R, Dworkin RH, Sang CN, eds. *Emerging Strategies for the Treatment of Neuropathic Pain.* Seattle: IASP Press; 2006.

62. Turk DC. Customizing treatment for chronic pain patients: who, what, and why. *Clin J Pain.* 1990;6:255–270.

63. Woolf CJ. Pain: moving from symptom control toward mechanism-specific pharmacologic management. *Ann Intern Med.* 2004;140:441–451.

64. Dworkin RH, Turk DC, Peirce-Sandner S, McDermott MP, Farrar JT, Hertz S, Katz NP, Raja SN, Rappaport BA. Placebo and treatment group responses in postherpetic neuralgia vs. painful diabetic peripheral neuropathy clinical trials in the REPORT database. *Pain.* 2010;150:12–16.

65. Temple RJ. Special study designs: early escape, enrichment, studies in non-responders. *Commun Stat Theory Methods.* 1994;23:499–531.

66. Krishnan KRR. Efficient trial designs to reduce placebo requirements. *Biol Psychiatry.* 2000;47:724–726.

67. Berry DA. Bayesian clinical trials. *Nature Rev Drug Discovery* 2006; 5: 27–36.

10

Ethical, Legal, and Social Issues in the Management of Neuropathic Pain

KATHRYN J. ELLIOTT

INTRODUCTION

CHRONIC NONMALIGNANT NEUROPA-THIC pain burdens individuals and society, increases disability, and leads to lost productivity and increased health care utilization and health care costs.[1] Chronic noncancer neuropathic pain is present if the pain lasts longer than the normal healing time, which is commonly considered to be of 3 months' duration.[2] Neuropathic pain is complex and frustrating to treat for both patients and clinicians. This is due in part to the many gaps in our understanding of the pathophysiology of these conditions and to the fact that anti-inflammatory agents and adjuvant analgesics such as antidepressants and anticonvulsants, developed for other conditions, incompletely treat these severe pain syndromes.[3–5]

Examples of common chronic noncancer neuropathic pain syndromes include human immunodeficiency virus (HIV) neuropathy, diabetic neuropathy, and postherpetic neuralgia.[6] Identifying a safe and effective treatment for chronic neuropathic pain is a medical priority. Millions of patients in the United States suffer from chronic neuropathic pain.[7] For example, 3 million Americans have diabetic neuropathy (with an estimated prevalence of 15% of diabetics developing painful neuropathy) and more than 1 million Americans have postherpetic neuralgia.[8,9] In addition, more than half of the patients suffering from HIV develop neuropathy.[5]

Recommendations for cancer pain indicate that the severity of pain should be used as a guide to determine if opioids will be considered as part of the treatment regimen.[10,11] Many publications extol the virtues and benefits of opioids for the treatment of neuropathic pain of diverse etiologies. This chapter will review the risks of opioids, acetaminophen, aspirin (ASA), nonsteroidal anti-inflammatory agents (NSAIDs), and anticonvulsants for the treatment

Table 10-1. ELSI Issues in the Treatment of Neuropathic Pain

Risks of acetaminophen toxicity

GI hemorrhage with ASA and NSAIDs

Suicidality and anticonvulsants

Risks of opioid use

- Addiction
- Misuse
- Diversion
- Criminal charges under §841 of the Controlled Substances Act
- Cardiac risks with propxyphene and methadone

Socioeconomic stress and the "social gradient" as risk factor for addiction

of neuropathic pain. This ethical, legal, and social issues (ELSI) discussion on the management of chronic noncancer neuropathic pain will focus on changes in prescriber behavior that have contributed to societal increases in opioid prescription use that appear to be associated with increased prescription opioid abuse and inadvertent patient death.[12,13] See Table 10.1 for an overview of these ELSI issues.

ACETAMINOPHEN

More then 50 million persons in the United States use acetaminophen weekly, mostly for the treatment of diverse types of mild to moderate pain.[14] While there are no compelling data to indicate that acetaminophen has efficacy in the treatment of pain associated with peripheral neuropathy, it remains a widely used analgesic for these disorders.[15,16] There are sporadic reports of liver failure that can lead to death with therapeutic use of acetaminophen. While a systematic review of acetaminophen use has found a paucity of evidence of fulminant hepatoxicity in alcoholics, the culprit may be a toxic metabolite, N-acetyl-p-benzoquinoneimine, produced by CYP2E1-mediated acetaminophen oxidation.[17] This metabolite is detoxified in normal conditions by hepatic glutathione, an enzyme that may be reduced in alcoholics. Other conditions that stress glutathione stores, such

as malnutrition, may also be risk factors for acetaminophen liver toxicity.[18]

Randomized controlled studies of acetaminophen have been performed in alcoholics to determine the extent of risk. Hepatic failure can occur with therapeutic use of acetaminophen in alcoholics soon after alcohol intake has stopped, as this is thought to be the time of lowest glutathione levels and CYP2E1 induction. A recent study of subjects recruited at alcohol detoxification centers evaluated placebo or therapeutic dosages of acetaminophen of 4 g/day for three 3 days. There were no differences in transaminase induction between acetaminophen and placebo.[19] This study contradicted another study, which found that therapeutic dosage of 4 g/day of acetaminophen led to a threefold increase in transaminase levels in more then one-third of healthy adults.[20]

Larson and colleagues studied patients entered into the Acute Liver Failure registry.[21] Of the patients considered to have acetaminophen-related acute liver failure, one-half used acetaminophen therapeutically. Two-thirds of these individuals described using acetaminophen in combination with an opioid. Most of the patients who used acetaminophen therapeutically ingested an overdose (mean dose of 7.5 g/day). There was a wide dosage range, with patients taking from 1 to 78 g/day (4 g is recommended as the maximum daily dosage). Therefore, despite the therapeutic intent, most patients in this study with acute liver failure overdosed on acetaminophen, even if unintentionally.

The Food and Drug Adminstration (FDA) has responded to the above information identifying acetaminophen as a major cause of acute liver failure. Since 2002, the FDA has been engaged in repeated educational attempts to decrease the number of such cases. It has recently established a working group to study the issue further.[22] A new final rule requires new labeling on over-the-counter (OTC) products containing acetaminophen identifying the potential risk of liver injury.[23] This action was based on the results of acute liver failure studies published by the U.S. Acute Liver Failure Study Group and on case series. It was determined that unintentional acetaminophen overdosage leads to large numbers of emergency room and hospital admissions and approximately 100 deaths per year in the United States. One recent study shows that while the risk of acetaminophen remains low and has not changed in recent years, toxicity is persistently occurring despite educational efforts. In metropolitan Atlanta, a 5-year prospective surveillance study of acute liver failure identified 94 patients hospitalized in this period with acute liver failure. Of these patients, 65 agreed to participate in the study. Forty-nine of the 65 were adults. Of these 49 adults, 29 (41%) had acetaminophen-related acute liver failure. This is evidence that acetaminophen may be the most common cause of acute liver failure in adults. Further study of these 29 subjects revealed that 45% were intentional overdosers. Extrapolating these data to the United States as a whole,, it is estimated that 640 adult cases of acute liver failure will occur each year in the United States from acetaminophen overdosage.[24]

ASPIRIN AND NSAIDS

Aspirin (ASA) and NSAIDs are very commonly used and available in many OTC preparations for the treatment of both acute and chronic mild to moderate pain syndromes. In spite of minimal data demonstrating efficacy, they are often used as a first-line agent in the management of neuropathic pain.[4] There are persistent and high levels of risk, especially of gastrointestinal (GI) bleeding, that leads to substantial medical care and even death with the use of these agents. It is estimated that more than 100,000 persons in the United States each year are hospitalized with bleeding from ASA or NSAIDs, and that of these, at least 16,000 die. The deaths are due to GI hemorrhage, bleeding ulcers, and perforation of the stomach and bowel.[25] These complications, unlike the liver injury risk seen with acetaminophen, occur at therapeutic dosages. The use of NSAIDs increases GI bleeds, especially within 1 week of starting treatment.[26] The FDA requires these risks to be stated explicitly in the product package insert.

ANTICONVULSANTS

Certain anticonvulsants, particularly gabapentin and pregabalin, have efficacy and are widely used in the treatment of neuropathic pain.[27,28] In 2008 the FDA caused a stir in the medical community, particularly in the fields of epilepsy, pain and psychiatry, when it warned of the suicide risk associated with anticonvulsants. At that time, the FDA published a systematic review indicating that persons taking anticonvulsants were at a twofold increased risk of suicidality.[29] In 2010, Patorno and colleagues corroborated the FDA findings by identifying the same agents (especially gabapentin, lamotrigine, oxcarbazepine, and tiagabine) with a twofold increase in attempted or completed suicide, using topiramate as a reference anticonvulsant. This was a cohort study with subjects aged 15 or older taking anticonvulsants from 2001 to 2006. The medical and prescription data were from the Health Core Integrated Research Database, which represents all filled prescriptions and clinical encounters from health plans in the southeastern, Mid-Atlantic, central, and western United States. Suicide attempts were identified from emergency room visits and hospitalizations. This study identified 300,000 new treatment periods with anticonvulsants. The most frequently prescribed anticonvulsants were gabapentin (48%), topiramate (19.4%), lamotrigine (7.5%), and valproate (6.2%). New users of anticonvulsants other then topiramate were likely to have diagnoses other than epilepsy, which included psychiatric disorders such as bipolar disorder, anxiety, depression, and neuropathic pain syndromes. When the disorder was not epilepsy, patients were also likely to be taking antidepressants, antipsychotics, and analgesics. A total of 868 patients attempted or completed suicide within 180 days of starting anticonvulsant therapy. This study found that the increased risk for suicidal acts began within 14 days of starting treatment.[30] The anticonvulsants gabapentin, lamotrigine, oxcarbazepine, and tiagabine were associated with an increased risk of suicidality compared to topiramate.

The methods used in this study and in the FDA 2008 systematic review have been questioned.[31] Many of the anticonvulsants identified as associated with increased suicidality are used primarily for other indications, such as a mood stabilizer for conditions that have an underlying suicidal risk, while topiramate is used primarily for migraine therapy.[32] It might not be the drugs themselves but the underlying condition for which they are being prescribed that may be associated with the increased risk of suicidality.

A recent study from health researchers in Spain found that anticonvulsants' link to suicide is not found in patients receiving these drugs as treatment for epilepsy.[33] Arana and colleagues had a longer follow-up period than the FDA meta-analysis. Data on antiepileptic drug use was collected as part of clinical practice from the United Kingdom, and the researchers focused on the drugs identified by the FDA in 2008. Patients with a prior or family history of suicidality were excluded, and data from over 5 million patients were examined. Of 8212 attempted suicides, 464 were completed. The rate varied from 38.2 per 100,000 person-years in patients with epilepsy not on anticonvulsants to 441.3 per 100,000 person-years in patients with bipolar disorder taking anticonvulsants for psychiatric indications. The authors found that the underlying illness was more strongly associated with suicidality than the use or nonuse of anticonvulsants. They concluded that the use of anticonvulsants slightly increased the risk of suicidality in patients with depression and who were using these agents for indications other than epilepsy.

Andersohn and colleagues examined whether suicidality varied by anticonvulsant type or class.[34] In this study, 44,300 patients with epilepsy from the United Kingdom treated with anticonvulsants were followed for 5 years. Data on suicidal behavior and self-harm were collected. A total of 453 persons with suicidality or self-harm were compared to 8962 age-matched controls. The use of the newer anticonvulsants with a high risk of depression (levetiracetam, tiagabine, topiramate, and vigabitrin) showed a threefold increased risk of suicidality compared to other classes of anticonvulsants. This translated into 6/453 persons (1.3%) who harmed themselves or attempted suicide when taking these newer anticonvulsants compared to 45/8962 (0.5%) of those who were not taking the newer anticonvulsants with a high risk of depression.

In 2010 the FDA warned of the risk of lamotrigine causing aseptic meningitis, reporting 40 cases in children and adults. The condition typically began 1 to 42 days after starting lamotrigine with headache, fever, nausea, vomiting, nuchal rigidity, rash, photophobia, and myalgias. Thirty-five patients had to be hospitalized, and most resolved with drug discontinuation. Fifteen patients were rechallenged, and the clinical syndrome of aseptic meningitis returned within 1 day. The cerebrospinal fluid (CSF) showed a neutrophil-predominant mild to moderate pleocytosis with elevation of protein. This syndrome is considered most likely to be a hypersensitivity reaction.[35]

OPIOIDS

Chronic neuropathic pain may respond to opioids. Opioid use requires a balance of efficacy against the risks of opioid side effects and misuse. Kalso et al. identified 15 studies of opioids for the treatment of chronic noncancer pain with a placebo arm.[36] Studies ranged in duration from 4 days to 8 weeks. Opioids demonstrated short-term efficacy for the treatment of chronic noncancer pain. Of the 388 subjects who continued with an open-label extension, only a minority (44%) were on opioids 7 to 24 months later. These studies do not answer the question of whether opioids have long-term efficacy, nor do they establish the risk of side effects, misuse, and opioid addiction.

Eisenberg and colleagues conducted a similar review of opioid trials but focused on chronic neuropathic pain.[37] Of the 22 articles they reviewed describing research trials on opioids in neuropathic pain, 14 were short-term (brief infusions of treatment periods if 24 h or less), and the results concerning analgesic efficacy were mixed.[37] The other eight studies were of intermediate duration, with opioids given for 8 to 56 days. Two of these studies found a dose-dependent reduction in pain severity with opioids (methadone and levorphanol).[38,39] Four of the studies found a significant reduction in pain severity when opioids (oxycodone in three studies, morphine in one study) were compared to placebo.[40-43] Two of these eight intermediate-duration studies showed either no benefit of opioids (morphine) compared to placebo or no difference between opioids and tricyclic antidepressants.[44,45] Overall, opioids reduced pain severity from 20% to 30% compared to placebo, a result comparable to that produced by nonopioid adjuvants used to treat neuropathic pain.[46,47] Misuse was not assessed.[41-45] Long-term evidence showing that opioids remain an effective treatment for neuropathic pain is lacking, and no long-term data shows superiority of opioids over other adjuvants for neuropathic pain.[48] In other chronic pain syndromes, long-term use of opioids has been questioned.

The long-term efficacy of opioids, when defined as use for more than 16 weeks, in treating low back pain is now in doubt.[49] Patients with low back pain are more likely to be prescribed opioids if there is a neuropathic pain component.[50] The Martell et al. meta-analysis found only two studies in which a standardized instrument was used to identify substance abuse.[49] The lifetime estimate for substance abuse was 54%, with an estimate of current substance abuse of 23% in chronic back pain patients.[51] Such data are not available for neuropathic pain syndromes. Opioid trial subjects are usually selected based on a lack of risk factors (e.g., substance abuse histories are often exclusionary). Thus, there is a need for long-term studies of analgesic efficacy balanced with a study of risk.

The use of opioids is controversial for the treatment of chronic neuropathic pain because patient misuse, side effects, and diversion may be opioid-specific.[52] Many new opioid analgesics are available.[53] Increased access to prescription opioids has led to an increase in the problem of prescription opioid abuse.

National surveys illustrate the problem.[54-56] One national survey of 55,023 individuals found a 5% nonmedical use of prescription opioids in the past year by self-report.[57] This occurs with a patient's own prescriptions for pain, and it is a growing problem with women.[58]

Accompanying opioid prescription misuse/addiction are unintentional deaths from prescription opioids. This comprises 90% of unintentional poisonings in some locations.[59] Prescription opioid overdose deaths accounted for 153 of 256 overdose deaths in 2008 in Washington State, more than twice the number of any other drug of abuse.[60] Methadone was the most commonly identified agent.[60] Treatment admissions for prescription opioid addiction in Washington State also rose from 87 in 1999 to 614 in 2008, an increase of more than 700%.[60] More than half of these admissions were young persons aged 18–29.[60] There are few data available on teenage prescription opioid addicts, but teenagers seeking treatment are highly likely to abuse multiple substances, have a major mood disorder, be in trouble with the law, and experience school failure.[61] The number of teenage prescription opioid addicts is increasing; they tend to be suburban, white, and male, with early marijuana and alcohol experience.[61] These data have captured the attention of both public health authorities and law enforcement agencies.[62]

There is no consensus on how to select patients for an opioid trial, and whether a behavioral contract is necessary, or even if opioids can be used for chronic noncancer neuropathic pain without additional treatment of function and mood.[63-67] See Table 10.2 for recent trends in prescription opioid use/misuse.

Ethical Issues

The most important ethical issues surrounding opioid use include the potential of harm to patients by creating an addiction disorder. The potential harm that may be caused by opioid side effects is similar to that of acetaminophen, ASA, and NSAIDs and anticonvulsant use and requires an informed discussion between the clinician and patient about the acceptable risk.

Table 10-2. Trends in Prescription Opioid Use/Misuse

5% of patients admit to misuse

Opioids make up an increasing number of unintentional poisonings

700% increase in admissions for opioid addiction in the past 10 years

Addicted physicians have high death rates and do not return to practice

CAUSING HARM: DEVELOPMENT OF AN IATROGENIC OPIOID ADDICTION DISORDER

The use of opioids for chronic nonmalignant neuropathic pain has become widespread, without data on the long-term risks of creating iatrogenic opioid addiction, misuse, or diversion. Opioid trials of short-term or intermediate-term duration in neuropathic pain make some estimates of addiction risks. Fishbain et al. identified patients treated with chronic opioids and reviewed 67 studies.[68] This review defined chronic use as at least 1 month's duration, while the data on low back pain use defined long-term use as 16 weeks or more, so it is questionable whether 4 weeks of opioid therapy is chronic.[68] Most of the studies were retrospective. Three percent of patients were determined by the clinician to have developed abuse or addiction, although this was inconsistently defined.[68] Of the patients with no history of prior opioid exposure, 4.4% developed addiction as defined by the clinician.[68] Eleven percent of patients showed aberrant drug-taking behaviors as determined by their clinicians, and there was a twofold increase in the identification of such behaviors with the use of urine toxicology.[68] These data support at least a 20% risk of new problems with opioid use/abuse developing de novo in this mix of chronic pain patients, as identified by clinicians. Passik and Kirsh reported that the use of a standardized tool (Pain Assessment and Documentation Tool) identified five times as many aberrant opioid-taking behaviors as the patients' treating physicians, suggesting that aberrant misuse of opioids is much more common than the literature suggests.[69] The signs and symptoms of addictive illness can be very subtle.[70] Whether certain pain syndromes and opioids pose higher risks of misuse/addiction was not examined. Katz et al. found that nearly one-half of the patients in their study of a chronic pain clinic population showed aberrant behaviors.[71]

RISKS OF DEVELOPING ADDICTION AND NOT RESPONDING TO ADDICTION TREATMENT

Physicians are the group most extensively studied for opioid addiction risk factors and for outcomes of opioid addiction. One in 10 clinicians will develop a substance use disorder.[72] Physicians have better access to treatment and long-term support than other patients with substance abuse disorders.[72] Anesthesiologists have the highest risk of opioid addiction.[73]

Physician opioid addiction informs the understanding of opioid addiction in general. Menk and colleagues found that two-thirds of the physicians addicted to opioids relapsed upon return to practice, despite intensive treatment.[74] Fourteen of 79 died (16% of relapses), with their death being the initial presentation of relapse.[74] These data have led to a "one strike and you're out" approach to opioid-addicted anesthesiologists and nurse anesthetists.

Access is the driving factor for untreatable opioid addiction.[75] Of the physicians who do not die from their opioid addiction, only a minority return to clinical practice.[73,74] Berge and colleagues described a 100% relapse rate and lack of response to treatment in 12 nurse anesthetists with opioid addiction.[76] Similar data are not available for patients prescribed opioids for chronic neuropathic pain who develop aberrant behaviors that may indicate opioid addiction; thus, the risks in nonphysician populations are not known.

Domino et al.[77] found that in physicians, a personal or family history of substance abuse, especially of alcohol, a major psychiatric disorder, and strong opioid abuse, such as with oxycodone, increases the risk of substance abuse relapse 13-fold. Applying these data to nonmedical populations suffering from chronic neuropathic pain suggests that clinicians in general are not skilled at identifying opioid addiction and abuse. The Berge and Domino data on physician opioid addicts also highlight the fact that treatment options for potent opioid addictions are poor and the relapse rate is high.

It is unclear what a physician should do when faced with a patient who wishes to try opioids for chronic neuropathic pain management. The ethical requirement is to make sure that the patient can give *informed consent*, which includes discussion of possible future harm with opioid use in the presence of uncertainty about the potential to treat opioid addiction. This caution must be balanced against the ethical requirement to treat pain.

Legal Issues

GUIDELINES

Guidelines are pieces of evidence presented to the trier of fact (jury or judge) to determine the standard of medical care in an action in tort for civil malpractice.[78–80] There are several professional guidelines for the use of opioids in chronic noncancer pain. A systematic review of the evidence for using opioids in chronic pain syndromes was recently completed by the American Pain Society and the American Academy of Pain Medicine.[65] While there is consensus among the authors of this document concerning the risk-benefit assessment of each patient prior to prescribing opioids, there is only low-quality evidence to stratify patients on risk.[65] This is because the burden of a risk-benefit assessment rests on a truthful patient. Clinicians are not skilled at identifying patients who are faking their medical conditions (they have a "truth bias"), Munchausen's syndrome patients who are falsifying their medical conditions, or undercover Drug Enforcement Administration (DEA) agents, who are also faking pain.[81]

The Chou et al. guideline also suggests an informed consent process that includes a management plan with goals of therapy, expectations for patient follow-up, and instructions on how opioids should be taken.[65] Written management plans can help manage expectations and provide structure for the patient whom the provider considers to be at some risk of opioid misuse.[65] The contract also provides written notification to the patient that certain behaviors are grounds for opioid discontinuation. Such *exit rules* may include behaviors such as doctor shopping, using multiple pharmacies, using opioids outside of the prescribed dose range, and other aberrant drug-related behaviors. Guidelines generated by experts for the use of opioids for chronic pain provide limited protection against legal risks. Opioid contracts do not protect physicians criminally prosecuted under §841 of the Controlled Substances Act (CSA; see below).[82]

LEGAL ACTIONS AGAINST PHYSICIANS FOR PAIN MANAGEMENT

The underlying legal risks in using acetaminophen, ASA, NSAIDs, and anticonvulsants for pain management are related to a failure to follow the accepted standard of care, which is based on a civil medical malpractice tort claim. For example a clinician who did not pay attention to the ceiling dosage of acetaminophen in a combination product such as Percocet could potentially face such a risk, as the liver failure seen with acetaminophen is known to be dosage-related. The legal risks with prescribing opioids are different. This is because in the field of opioid use for chronic noncancer pain, there are no civil malpractice actions against physicians for underprescribing opioids. There is a small body of case law involving the undertreatment of cancer pain that is legally distinguishable from the claim of undertreatment of nonmalignant neuropathic pain.[83] The case law for undertreatment of cancer pain does not comprise the typical tort action of medical malpractice but involves an unusual cause of action under the California elder abuse statute. In *Bergman v. Eden Medical Center*, the family of Mr. Bergman was awarded monetary damages for pain and suffering for undertreatment of his cancer pain. Another civil case litigated under the elder abuse statute was settled prior to trial and also involved an elderly man with cancer, Mr. Lester Tomlinson. Both of these unfortunate patients were dying from terminal lung cancer, and their clinicians either withheld opioids altogether or permitted only small amounts of intermittent opioids for documented metastatic cancer pain.[83,84]

To prevail in a civil action requires a lower standard of proof than in a criminal trial, and most clinicians prevail in a civil medical malpractice action. Thus, the civil malpractice action that a physician prescribing opioids is most likely to face will be a charge of overprescribing these drugs. This follows evidence presented at a criminal trial under §841 of the CSA. Following a professional guideline is not a protective shield in such a civil action, as the clinician will have already been found guilty under a criminal standard. Clinicians need to know the elements of a CSA claim. Under the CSA, clinicians face felony charges and jail time.

THE CSA

The CSA is a federal criminal statute regulating drug abuse and trafficking of controlled substances, which includes prescription opioids.[85] The federal DEA enforces the federal CSA. Opioid providers must comply with the federal CSA, the Code of Federal Regulations (CFR), which operationalizes the CSA, and state regulations. The CSA defines an addict as "any individual who habitually uses any narcotic drug so as to endanger the public morals, health, safety, or welfare, or who is so far addicted to the use of narcotic drugs as to have lost the power of self-control with reference to his addiction."[85] Most individuals describing nonmedical use of prescription opioids obtained their opioids from a medical provider. Such nonmedical use of prescription opioids often is the trigger for a DEA investigation of the prescribing physician. The DEA estimates that in any given year, 0.01% of all DEA-registered providers (a total of 750,000) lose their DEA registration and are criminal charged following a DEA investigation for improper prescribing. Only a small number of DEA-registered physicians undergo DEA investigations. This is confirmed by a recent systemic review of physicians criminally or administratively charged with alleged offenses involving opioid prescribing encompassing the time period 1998–2006. During this period, 335 criminal cases were identified.[86] Goldenbaum and colleagues found a 31.6% increase in DEA criminal investigations of physicians from 2003 to 2006. Of the physicians ultimately prosecuted, 91% either pled guilty or were ultimately found guilty on at least one criminal charge. The most common criminal charges included drug trafficking, illegal distribution, and racketeering. The classical criminal prosecution of these providers includes charges of multiple felonies from violations of the CSA and legal accusations that the clinicians act as "pill mills."

CRIMINAL PROSECUTIONS OF PHYSICIANS UNDER §841 OF THE CSA

Section (§) 841 of the CSA states that "...it shall be unlawful for any person knowingly or intentionally...to...distribute, or dispense, or possess with intent to...distribute, or dispense, a controlled substance" unless "authorized" to do so.[87] To be authorized, a physician must be registered by the U.S. Attorney General

(i.e., registered with the DEA). The conditions under which physicians can prescribe controlled substances are defined in the implementing regulations of the CSA, which require a "legitimate medical purpose."[88] To stay within the law, a physician prescribing opioids for pain must prescribe for a legitimate medical purpose in the usual course of his or her professional practice.[89]

United States v. Moore defines the legal parameters of a §841 physician prosecution.[90] Under *Moore*, the U.S. Supreme Court determined that the federal statute, the CSA, permitted federal prosecution of physicians who prescribed control substance opioids "unlawfully." *Moore* extended the control of medical practice from the states to the federal government and established the federal CSA as the mechanism to do this. Moore was a physician prescribing methadone and billing patients based on the quantity of methadone prescribed rather than for medical services provided, a behavior the Supreme Court described as acting like a pill mill. The Court first established in *Moore* that physicians faced prosecution if their prescribing practices "fell outside the usual course of professional practice." The Court also found that the intent behind the CSA was to limit a physician's prescribing authority. The Court determined that Moore was acting as a "pusher" (i.e., a drug trafficker subject to felony charges) and referenced an earlier pre-CSA case in which the physician, Behrman, prescribed opioids to a known opioid addict as an example of unlawful or "unauthorized" acts.[91] Table 10.3 summarizes the elements of a §841 claim.

The newer §841 cases describe physicians whose behavior is not so obviously unlawful.

Table 10-3. Elements of a CSA §841 Claim

Unauthorized prescribing

No legitimate medical purpose

Outside the usual course of professional practice

Acting like a pill mill (e.g., in the *Behrman* case, providing opioids to a known opioid addict was considered "unauthorized," and in the *Moore* case, providing methadone pills for money was characterized as "drug dealing")

The appellate court in *McIver* referred to the large numbers of opioid pills prescribed and described instances of aberrant drug-taking behavior that the defendant tolerated, such as continuing to prescribe opioids to an addict and to patients' claims to loss of opioids, and to patients with early requests for refills.[82] However, although McIver treated chronic pain with higher than normal dosages of opioids, he examined his patients and established pain

Table 10-4. Compassionate Physician or Pill Mill?

United States v Moore 423 US 122 (1975)

United States v Carroll 518 F.2d 187 (6th Cir. 1975)

United States v Seelig 622 F.2d 207 (6th Cir. 1980)

United States v Voorhies 663 F.2d 30 (6th Cir. 1981)

United States v Hayes 794 F.2d 1348 (9th Cir. 1986)

United States v Norris 780 F.2d 1207 (5th Cir.1986)

United States v Vamos 797 F.2d 1146 (2nd Cir.1986)

United States v Hughes 895 F.2d 1135 (6th Cir.1990)

United States v Polan 970 F 2d 1280 (3rd Cir. 1992)

United States v Daniel 3 F.3d 775 (4th Cir. 1993)

United States v Tran Trong Cuong 18 F.3d 1132 (4th Cir. 1994)

United States v Singh 54 F.3d 1182 (4th Cir. 1995)

United States v Steele 147 F.3d 1316 (11th Cir. 1998 en banc)

United States v Alerre 430 F.3d 681 (4th Cir. 2005)

United States v Hurwitz 459 F.3d 463 (4th Cir. 2006)

United States v McIver 470 F.3d 550 (4th Cir. 2006)

United States v Williams 445 F 3d 1302 (11th Cir. 2006)

United States v Feingold 454 F.3d 1001 (2006)

contracts, unlike the "pill mill" physicians in *Moore* and *Behrman*. See Table 10.4 for a recent listing (in chronological order) of higher court decisions, published and publicly available, that discuss the reasoning in finding physician opioid prescribing criminally actionable.

CARDIAC RISKS WITH PROPOXYPHENE AND METHADONE

Propoxyphene (Darvon® or Darvocet®) was recently removed from the U.S. market by the request of the FDA based on a study in healthy volunteers showing significant cardiac changes of prolonged PR, widened QRS, and prolonged QT intervals.[92] These cardiac changes predispose to polymorphic ventricular tachycardia, or Torsade des pointes (TDP). Propoxyphene shares cardiac risks with methadone.

Methadone is an off-patent synthetic opioid that costs pennies per tablet. It is a racemic mixture of two isomeric forms, D-isomer and L-isomer.[93,94] Both isomers have noncompetitive antagonist activity at the *N*-methyl-D-aspartate (NMDA) receptor.[94] Mu opioid analgesia is attributed to the L-isomer. For multiple reasons, most likely reflecting its dual mechanism of action (as an NMDA receptor and a mu opioid receptor) and its off-patent low cost, methadone use for noncancer chronic pain has markedly increased in the past decade.

The DEA considers the increasing use of methadone to treat pain a public health crisis,[52] describing a 700% increase in methadone prescriptions in the last decade alone. Data from 2006 from the DEA National Forensic Laboratory Information System finds that on a per prescription basis, methadone is more likely to be diverted and abused than either hydrocodone or oxycodone. The DEA has evidence that most of the methadone that is diverted and the increase in methadone deaths are associated with providers' prescriptions for pain management rather than diversion from methadone maintenance clinics.

Some of the increased death rate from methadone results from the complicated pharmacokinetics and pharmacodynamics of methadone. Methadone has a short serum half-life for analgesia complicated with a serum half-life for respiratory depression that can be up to

1 week in duration, requiring sophistication and extreme care when methadone therapy is first started.[95] An additional concern about methadone is its nonopioid receptor-mediated cardiac toxicity. Recent data suggest that some of the sudden deaths associated with methadone use may be a methadone-specific induction of a fatal arrhythmia.

Methadone causes cardiac arrhythmia via suppression of a specific cardiac gene. Methadone affects the human ether a go-go-related gene (hERG) in a nonopioid manner.[96] There are increasing data on clinical Torsades des Pointes (TDP) and methadone. Krantz et al. described this risk in a retrospective case series of patients presenting with TDP while on methadone. Of these 17 patients, 9 were on methadone for treatment of opioid dependence and 8 for the treatment of chronic pain. The mean methadone dose in the opioid dependence group was 269 mg (±316 mg/day), and in the chronic pain group it was 541 mg (±156 mg/day). All of the patients had very abnormal prolongation of their QTc on electrocardiography (ECG).[97]

The FDA MedWatch system identified 59 additional cases of abnormal QTc prolongation and TDP associated with methadone use, of which 8% were fatal. Most patients reported in MedWatch were taking more than 100 mg of methadone per day, but not all (range, 29–1680 mg methadone per day).[98]

Methadone is an old and inexpensive off-patent analgesic, which explains both the benefits and problems with its use. The lack of patent protection results in methadone's low cost, and it can be prescribed to many more patients in settings where cost is a barrier. The potential for cardiac toxicity can be masked by lack of preexistent ECGs and by the likelihood that medical examiners cannot differentiate a sudden death from a primary respiratory cause from one due to a ventricular arrhythmia. Table 10.5 summarizes the risks with methadone use.

Social Issues

U.K. VIEW OF SOCIOECONOMIC STRESS

Two pivotal long-term studies first identified some of the social determinants of health.[99,100]

Table 10-5. Risks with Methadone

700% increase in methadone prescriptions in the past 10 years

Complicated pharmacokinetics and pharmacodynamics: half-life for analgesia different than half-life for respiratory depression, making initiation of use potentially dangerous

Commonly diverted

Nonopioid induction of ventricular tachycardia may be a cause of sudden death

Progressive prolongation of the QTc interval suggests that ECGs are required for use

Whitehall examined the prevalence of cardiovascular disease and mortality in British civil servants. This study described a strong association of both overall health and lower mortality with a higher grade of civil servant employment. Civil servants at the lower grades, including doormen and messengers, had four times as much cardiac mortality as the highest-grade civil servants once comorbidities were controlled for.

The second Whitehall study attempted to determine what elements in the social context of work explained these findings.[100] This study evaluated the psychosocial work environment by looking at factors such as amount of control, variety and use of skills, pace of work, and amount of support at work. The results showed a social gradient, defined as a variation in health outcomes across a social hierarchy, with persons in the lower positions in the hierarchy having greater health risk.

One possible mechanism for this social gradient is the concept of *social stressors*. Social stressors are factors in the psychosocial work environment that trigger the two pathways that modulate the fight-or-flight response to stress: the sympathetico-adrenaline pathway and the hypothalamic-pituitary-adrenal axiss. These two stress hormone pathways lead to increased corticosteroid production; when repeatedly activated, these pathways may lead to increased susceptibility to disease[101]

Patients who develop opioid addiction acknowledge using opioids because of the way opioids "make them feel" and not to relieve pain. Especially in this time of economic recession when many people are very stressed, as well as located on the low rungs of the social gradient or off it entirely, it is likely that future addicts will begin using opioids to manage social, economic, or personal stress.

CONCLUSION

The benefits of pain relief must be balanced against the risks to patients and clinicians. While this risk-benefit calculus is particularly difficult with opioids there are identified risks with anti-inflammatory agents and anticonvulsants. The risk of addiction appears to be opioid specific. Long-term outcomes research on addiction and risks of addiction, and data on the long-term efficacy of opioids in specific neuropathic pain syndromes, would help clarify treatment choices and clinician risks.

ACKNOWLEDGMENTS

Supported in part by the Manhattan Brain Bank (MHBB) (PI Susan Morgello).

REFERENCES

1. McDermott AM, Toelle TR, Rowbotham DJ, et al. The burden of neuropathic pain: results from a cross-sectional survey. *Eur J Pain.* 2006;10:127–135.
2. International Association for the Study of Pain. Classification of chronic pain: descriptions of chronic pain syndromes and definitions of pain terms. Prepared by the International Association for the Study of Pain, Subcommittee on Taxonomy. *Pain Suppl.* 1986;S1–S226.
3. Elliott KJ. Taxonomy and mechanisms of neuropathic pain. *Semin Neurol.* 1994;14;195–205.
4. Elliott KJ. Management of postherpetic pain. In: Arvin AM, Gershon AA, eds. *Varicella-Zoster Virus: Virology and Clinical Management.* Cambridge: Cambridge University Press; 2000:412–427.
5. Elliott KJ, Simpson DM. Neurotoxic dideoxynucleoside antiretroviral therapy is not associated with progression of painful distal neuropathy. Priority paper evaluation. *HIV Ther.* 2009;3:35–38.
6. Sadosky A, McDermott AM, Brandenburg NA, et al. A review of the epidemiology of painful diabetic peripheral neuropathy, postherpetic neuralgia, and less commonly studied neuropathic pain conditions. *Pain Practice.* 2008;8:45–56.
7. Foley KM. Opioids and chronic neuropathic pain [editorial]. *N Engl J Med.* 2003;348:1279–1281.
8. Bowsher D. The lifetime occurrence of herpes zoster and prevalence of postherpetic neuralgia: a retrospective survey in an elderly population. *Eur J Pain.* 1999;3:335–342.
9. Schmader KE. Epidemiology and impact on quality of life of postherpetic neuralgia and painful diabetic neuropathy. *Clin J Pain.* 2002;18:350–354.
10. Elliott KJ, Portenoy RK. Cancer pain: pathophysiology and syndromes. In: Yaksh TL, ed. *Anesthesia: Biologic Foundations.* New York: Raven Press; 1997:803–817.
11. Elliott KJ, Pasternak G. Section 1: symptomatic care pending diagnosis. In: Rakel RR, ed. *Conn's Current Therapy.* New York: W.B.Saunders Co; 1996:1–4.
12. Compton WM, Volkow ND. Major increases in opioid analgesic abuse in the United States: concerns and strategies. *Drug Alcohol Depend.* 2006;81:103–107.
13. Centers for Disease Control and Prevention, National Drug Intelligence Center. National prescription drug threat assessment 2009: executive summary. http://www.usdoj.gov/ndic/pubs33/33775/execsum.htm. Accessed July 20, 2009.
14. Kaufman DW, Kelly JP, Rosenberg L, et al. Recent patterns of medication use in the ambulatory adult population of the U.S.: the Slone survey. *JAMA.* 2002;287:337–344.
15. Argoff CE, Sivershein DI. A comparison of long and short acting opioids for the treatment of chronic noncancer pain: tailoring therapy to meet patient needs. *Mayo Clinic Proc.* 2009;84:602–612.
16. Gloth FM 3rd. Pharmacological management of persistent pain in older persons: focus on opioids and nonopioids. *J Pain.* 2011;12:S14–S20.
17. Dart RC, Kuffner EK, Rumakc BH. Treatment of pain or fever with paracetamol (acetaminophen) in the alcoholic patient: a systematic review *Am J Ther.* 2000;7:123–134.
18. Nelson SD. Molecular mechanisms of the hepatoxicity caused by acetaminophen. *Semin Liver Dis.* 1990;10:267–278.
19. Kuffner EK, Green JL, Bogdan GM, et al. The effect of acetaminophen (four grams a day for three consecutive days) on hepatic tests in alcoholic patients—a multicenter randomized study. *BMC Med.* 2007;5:13.

20. Watkins PB, Kaplowitz N, Slattery JT, et al. Aminotransferase elevations in healthy adults receiving 4 grams of acetaminophen daily. *JAMA*. 2006;296:87–96.
21. Larson AM, Poison J, Fontana RJ, et al. Acetaminophen-induced acute liver failure: result of the U.S. Multicenter Prospective Study. *Hepatology*. 2005;42:1364–1372.
22. Food and Drug Administration 2009 meetings materials Web page. http://www.fda.gov. Accessed December 20, 2010.
23. 21 CFR Part 201, *Federal Register*, vol. 74 (81), April 29, 2010.
24. Bower WA, Johns M, Margolis HS, et al. Population based surveillance for acute liver failure. *Am J Gastroenterol*. 2007;102:2459–2463. [E-pub June 29, 2007.]
25. Blot WJ, McLaughlin JK. Over the counter nonsteroidal anti-inflammatory drugs and risk of gastrointestinal bleeding. *J Epidemiol Biostat*. 2000;5:137–147.
26. Lewis SC, Langman MJ, Laporte JR, Jr, et al. Dose-response relationships between individual nonaspirin nonsteroidal anti-inflammatory drugs (NANSAIDS) and serious upper gastrointestinal bleeding: a meta-analysis based on individual patient data. *Br J Pharmacol*. 2002;54:320–326.
27. Sabatowski R, Galvez R, Cherry DA, et al. Pregabalin reduces pain and improves sleep and mood disturbances in patients with post-herpetic neuralgia: results of a randomized, placebo-controlled clinical trial. *Pain*. 2005;109:26–35.
28. Finnerup NB, Otto M, McQuay HJ, et al. Alogorithm for neuropathic pain treatment: an evidence based proposal. *Pain*. 2005;118:289–305.
29. *Statistical Review and Evaluation: Antiepilpetic Drugs and Suicidality*. Washington, DC: U.S. Department of Health and Human Services, Food and Drug Administration, Center for Drug Evaluation and Research, Office of Translational Sciences, Office of Biostatistics. http://www.fda.gov. Accessed May 23, 2010.
30. Patorno E, Bohn RL, Wahl PM, et al. Anticonvulsant medications and the risk of suicide, attempted suicide or violent death. *JAMA*. 2010;303:1401–1409.
31. Hesdorffer DC, Kanner AM. The FDA alert on suicidality and antiepileptic drugs: fire or false alarm? *Epilepsia*. 2009;50:978–986; Mula M, Sander JW. Antiepileptic drugs and suicidality. Much ado about very little? *Neurology*. 2010;75:300–301; Mula M, Bell GS, Sander JW. Suicidality in epilepsy and possible effects of antiepileptic drugs. *Curr Neurol Neurosci Rep*. 2010;4:327–332.
32. Craven R. Antiepilpetic drugs and suicidality: finding ways forward. *Lancet Neurol*. 2010;9:568–569.
33. Arana A, Wentworth CE, Ayuso-Mateos JL, et al. Suicide related events in patients treated with antiepileptic drugs. *N Engl J Med*. 2010;363:542–551.
34. Andersohn F, Schade R, Garbe E, et al. Use of antiepileptic drugs in epilepsy and the risk of self harm or suicidal behavior. *Neurology*. 2010;75:335–340.
35. In the FDA Web site, see *lamotrigine* under *drugs*. http://www.fda.gov. Accessed October 31, 2010.
36. Kalso E, Edwards JE, Moore RA, et al. Opioids in chronic noncancer pain: systematic review of efficacy and safety. *Pain*. 2004;112:372–380.
37. Eisenberg E, McNicol ED, Carr DB. Efficacy and safety of opioid agonists in the treatment of neuropathic pain of nonmalignant origin. *JAMA*. 2005;293:3043–3052.
38. Morley JS, Bridson J, Nash TP, et al. Low-dose methadone has an analgesic effect in neuropathic pain: a double-blind randomized controlled crossover trial. *Palliat Med*. 2003;17;576–587.
39. Rowbotham MC, Twilling L, Davies PS, et al. Oral opioid therapy for chronic peripheral and central neuropathic pain. *N Engl J Med*. 2003;348:1223–1232.
40. Watson CP, Babul N. Efficacy of oxycodone in neuropathic pain: a randomized trial in postherpetic neuralgia. *Neurology*. 1998;50:1837–1841.
41. Huse E, Larbig W, Flor H, et al. The effect of opioids on phantom limb pain and cortical reorganization. *Pain*. 2001;90:47–55.
42. Gimbel JS, Richards P, Portenoy RK. Controlled release oxycodone for pain in diabetic neuropathy: a randomized controlled trial. *Neurology*. 2003;60:927–934.
43. Watson CP, Moulin D, Watt-Watson J, et al. Controlled-release oxycodone relieves neuropathic pain: a randomized controlled trial in painful diabetic neuropathy. *Pain*. 2003;105:71–78.
44. Raja SN, Haythornthwaite JA, Pappagallo M, et al. Opioids versus antidepressants in postherpetic neuralgia: a randomized, placebo-controlled trial. *Neurology*. 2002;59:1015–1021.
45. Harke O. The response of neuropathic pain and pain in complex regional pain syndrome 1 to carbamezepine and sustained-release morphine I patients pretreated with spinal cord stimulation: a double-blinded randomized study. *Anesth Analg*. 2001;92:488–495.
46. Saarto T, Wiffen PJ. Antidepressants for neuropathic pain [review]. http://www.thecochranelibrary.com. Accessed May 10, 2010.
47. Backonja M, Beydoun A, Edwards KR, et al. Gabapentin for the symptomatic treatment of

painful neuropathy in patients with diabetes mellitus: a randomized controlled trial. *JAMA*. 1998;280:1831–1836.

48. Dworkin RH, O'Connor AB, Backonja M, et al. Pharmacologic management of neuropathic pain: evidence-based recommendations. *Pain*. 2007;132:237–251.

49. Martell BA, O'Connor PG, Kerns RD, et al. Systemic review: opioid treatment for chronic back pain: prevalence, efficacy, and association with addiction. *Ann Intern Med*. 2007;146:116–127.

50. Fanciullo GJ, Ball PA, Girault G, et al. An observational study on the prevalence and pattern of opioid use in 25,479 patients with spine and radicular pain. *Spine*. 2002;27:201–205.

51. Brown RL, Patterson JJ, Rounds LA, et al. Substance abuse among patients with chronic low back pain. *J Family Pract*. 1996;43:152–160.

52. Methadone: Methadone Mortality Working Group, Drug Enforcement Agency, Office of Diversion Control, April 2007. http://www.deadiversion.usdoj.gov/drugs_concern/methadone/methadone_presentation0407_revised.pdf. Accessed June 15, 2009.

53. Markman JD. Not so fast: the reformulation of fentanyl and breakthrough chronic non-cancer pain. *Pain*. 2008;136:227–229.

54. Substance Abuse and Mental Health Services Administration (SAMHSA). National Survey on Drug Use and Health. Washington, DC: Office of Applied Studies (OAS), Department of Health and Human Services (DHHS); 2006.

55. Cicero TJ, Inciardi JA, Munoz A. Trends in abuse of oxycontin and other opioid analgesics in the United States: 2002–2004. *J Pain*. 2005;6:662–672.

56. Dasgupta N, Brason WSA II, Albert S, et al. Project Lazarus: Overdose Prevention and Responsible Pain Management. *NCMB Forum*. 2008;1:8–12.

57. Tetrault M, Desai RA, Becker WC, et al. Gender and non-medical use of prescription opioids: results from a national U.S. survey. *Addiction*. 2008;108:258–268.

58. Green TC, Serrano JM, Licari A, et al. Women who abuse prescription opioids: findings from the Addiction Severity Index-Multimedia Version Connect prescription opioid database. *Drug Alcohol Depend*. 2009;103;65–73.

59. Hall AJ, Logan RL, Toblin JA, et al. Patterns of abuse among unintentional pharmaceutical overdose fatalities. *JAMA*. 2008;200: 2613–2620.

60. Banta-Green C, Jackson R, Albert D, et al. Drug trends in the Seattle–King County area, 2008. http://depts.washington.edu/adai/pubs/tr/cewg/CEWG_Seattle_July2009.pdf. Accessed July 23, 2009.

61. Subramaniam GA, Stitzer MA. Clinical characteristics of treatment-seeking prescription opioid vs. heroin-using adolescents with opioid use disorder. *Drug Alcohol Depend*. 2009;101:13–19.

62. Van Zee A. The promotion and marketing of oxycontin: commercial triumph, public health tragedy. *Am J Public Health*. 2009;99;221–227.

63. Dworkin RH, Backonja M, Rowbotham MC, et al. Advances in neuropathic pain. diagnosis, mechanisms and treatment recommendations. *Arch Neurol*. 2003;60:1524–1534.

64. Gourlay DH, Heit HA, Almahrezi A. Universal precautions in pain medicine: a rational approach to the treatment of chronic pain. *Pain Med*. 2005;6:107–112.

65. Chou R, Fanciullo GJ, Fine PG, et al. Opioid treatment guidelines. Clinical guidelines for the use of chronic opioid therapy in chronic noncancer pain. *J Pain*. 2009;10: 113–130.

66. Passik SD. Issues in long-term opioid therapy: unmet needs, risks and solutions. *Mayo Clin Proc*. 2009;84:593–601.

67. Lanier WL, Kharasch ED. Contemporary clinical opioid use: opportunities and challenges [editorial]. *Mayo Clin Proc*. 2009;84:572–575.

68. Fishbain DA, Cole B, Lewis J, et al. What percentage of chronic nonmalignant pain patients exposed to chronic opioid analgesic therapy develop abuse/addiction and/or aberrant drug-related behaviors? A structured evidence-based review. *Pain Med*. 2008;9:444–459.

69. Passik SD, Kirsh KL. The need to identify predictors of aberrant drug-related behavior and addiction in patients being treated with opioids for pain. *Pain Med*. 2003;4:186–189.

70. Berge KJ, Seppala MD, Schipper AM. Chemical dependency and the physician. *Mayo Clin Proc*. 2009;84:625–631.

71. Katz NP, Sherburne S, Beach M, et al. Behavioral monitoring and urine toxicology testing in patients receiving long-term opioid therapy. *Anesth Analg*. 2003;97:1097–1102.

72. Baldisseri MR. Impaired healthcare professional. *Crit Care Med*. 2007;35(suppl 2): 706–716.

73. Oreskovich MR, Caldeiro RM. Anesthesiologists recovering from chemical dependency: can they safely return to the operating room? *Mayo Clin Proc*. 2009;84:576–580.

74. Menk EJ, Baumgarten RK, Kinsley CP, et al. Success of reentry into anesthesiology training programs by residents with a history of substance abuse. *JAMA*. 1990;263:3060–3062.

75. Bryson EO, Silverstein JH. Addiction and substance abuse in anesthesiology. *Anesthesiology*. 2008;109:905–917.

76. Berge KH, Seppala MD, Lanier WL. The anesthesiology community's approach to opioid and anesthetic abusing personnel: time to change course. *Anesthesiology*. 2008;109:762–764.

77. Domino KB, Hornbein TF, Polissar NL, et al. Risk factors for relapse I health care professionals with substance use disorders. *JAMA*. 2005;293;1453–1460.

78. Vidmar N. *Medical Malpractice and the American Jury: Confronting the Myths about Jury Incompetence, Deep Pockets, and Outrageous Jury Awards*. Ann Arbor: University of Michigan Press; 1995.

79. Vidmar N. Expert evidence, the adversary system, and the jury. *Am J Public Health*. 2005;95:S137–S143.

80. Pegalis SE. *American Law of Medical Malpractice*. 3rd ed. Eagen, MN: West Thomson Reuters; 2009.

81. Jung B, Reidenberg MM. Physicians being deceived. *Pain Med*. 2007;8:433–437.

82. *United States v McIver*, 470 F.3d 550 (4th Cir. 2006).

83. Tucker KL. Medico-legal case report and commentary: inadequate pain management in the context of terminal cancer. The case of Lester Tomlinson. *Pain Med*. 2004;5:214–218.

84. *Bergman v Eden Medical Center*, No H205732–1, Superior Court, Alameda County, CA.

85. 21 U.S.C. §801 et seq.

86. Goldenbaum DM, Christopher M, Gallagher RM, et al., Physicians charged with opioid-analgesic prescribing offenses. *Pain Med*. 2008;9(6):737–747.

87. 21 U.S.C.A. §841 (a) (1).

88. 21 C.F.R. §1306.04 (a) (2006).

89. Rannazzisi JT. The DEA's balancing act to ensure public health and safety. *Clin Pharmacol Ther*. 2007;81;805–806.

90. *United States v Moore*, 423 US 122 (1975).

91. *United States v Behrman*, 258 US 280 (1922).

92. In the FDA Web site, see *propoxyphene*. http://www.fda.gov/Drugs/DrugSafety/ucm234338.htm. Accessed November 20, 2010.

93. Ebert B, Andersen S, Krogsgaard-Larsen P. Ketobemidone, methadone and pethidine are non-competitive *N*-methyl-D-aspartate (NMDA) antagonists in the rat cortex and spinal cord. *Neurosci Lett*. 1995;187:165–168.

94. Gorman AL, Elliott KJ, Inturrisi CE. The D- and L-isomers of methadone bind to the non-competitive site on the *N*-methyl-D-aspartate (NMDA) receptor in rat forebrain and spinal cord. *Neurosci Lett*. 1997;223:5–8.

95. Hunt G, Bruera E. Respiratory depression in a patient receiving oral methadone for cancer pain. *J Pain Symptom Manage*. 1995;10:401–404.

96. Krantz MJ, Martin J, Stimmel B, et al. QTc interval screening in methadone treatment. Clinical guidelines. *Ann Intern Med*. 2009;150:387–395.

97. Krantz MJ, Lewkowiez L, Hays H, et al. Torsades de pointes associated with very high dose methadone. *Ann Intern Med*. 2002;137:501–504.

98. Pearson EC, Woolsey RL. QT prolongation and torsade de pointes among methadone users: reports to the FDA spontaneous reporting system. *Pharmacoepidemiol Drug Safety*. 2005;14:747–753.

99. Marmot MG, Rose G, Shipley M, et al. Employment grade and coronary heart disease in British civil servants. *J Epidemiol Commun Health*. 1978;32:244–249.

100. Marmot MG, Smith GD, Stansfeld S, et al. Health inequalities among British civil servants: the Whitehall II study. *Lancet*. 1991;337:1387–1393.

101. Wilkinson R, Marmot M, eds. *Social Determinants of Health: The Solid Facts*. 2nd ed. Copenhagen: World Health Organization Regional Office for Europe; 2003.

11

Painful Diabetic Neuropathy

HSINLIN T. CHENG, BRIAN CALLAGHAN, AND EVA L. FELDMAN

EPIDEMIOLOGY

DIABETES MELLITUS IS one of the most common chronic medical conditions in the general population worldwide. The two types of diabetes mellitus are caused by very different mechanisms. Type 1 diabetes is a genetically linked autoimmune disease that results in the destruction of β cells in the pancreas and diminished ability to produce insulin. In contrast, type 2 diabetes is a condition associated with obesity, hyperinsulinemia, and insulin resistance and accounts for 90%–95% of the diabetic population. In general, these two distinct diseases affect separate patient populations: type 1 diabetes strikes a younger age group, while the incidence of type 2 diabetes is higher in older generations (http://diabetes.niddk.nih.gov). The combined global prevalence was estimated to be 2.8% in 2000. However, with the rapidly increasing incidence of type 2 diabetes, the prevalence is expect

to rise to 4.4% in the year 2030.[1] This trend has been dramatically observed in the United States, where it has been reported that 65% of the American population is overweight and at least 30% is clinically obese.[2] Currently, body mass index (BMI) defines people as overweight (preobese) when their BMI is between 25 and 30 kg/m^2 and as obese when it is greater than 30 kg/m^2.[3] There were 23.6 million Americans (7.8% of the population) with diabetes in 2007, making the United States among the countries with the highest prevalence of diabetes (http://www.cdc.org).

Although type 1 and type 2 diabetes are very different in their pathophysiology, they share similar symptoms and complications resulting from chronic hyperglycemia. Both commonly result in vasculopathy, retinopathy, nephropathy, neuropathy, and various symptoms generated from these secondary complications. A frequent complication of diabetes is neuropathy, affecting about 60% of patients.

In the United States, diabetic neuropathy is the leading cause of diabetes-related hospital admissions and nontraumatic amputations.[3-5] Although many types of neuropathy are associated with diabetes, the most common neuropathy is a distal symmetric neuropathy, or polyneuropathy.[6] This neuropathy is an axonal length-dependent process with loss of distal sensation, yielding a "stocking-glove" sensory loss. Other presentations of diabetic neuropathy include focal and multifocal neuropathies, as well as a higher incidence of pressure palsies and superimposed acquired inflammatory demyelinating neuropathies.[7] Currently, no approved treatment exists in the United States for diabetic neuropathy outside of strict glycemic control.[8]

Pain is the most common symptom associated with diabetic neuropathy. According to the literature, diabetic neuropathic pain (DNP) develops in 10% to 20% of the diabetic population and can be found in 40% to 50% of diabetics with documented neuropathies.[9] Diabetic neuropathic pain is an early manifestation of diabetic neuropathy and frequently presents in patients with the prediabetic states of impaired fasting glucose (IFG) or impaired glucose tolerance (IGT).[8,10,11] Ziegler et al. reported that the prevalence of DNP is 13.3% (8.9%–18.9%) in diabetic subjects, 8.7% (2.4%–20.0%) in those with IGT, 4.2% (0.9%–11.9%) in those with IFG, and 1.2% (0.03%–6.7%) in those with normal glucose tolerance.[11] In addition, several recent studies suggest that nearly one-third of patients with IGT seek medical attention for a pain syndrome identical to DNP.[12,13] While DNP is a prevalent symptom in epidemiological studies of patients with type 2 diabetes (about 26%), it is less common in type 1 diabetes (about 16%).[14-17] In addition, the intensity of DNP varies between type 1 and type 2 diabetes. The Diabetic Cardiovascular Autonomic Neuropathy Multicenter Study Group reported significantly less pain in both the lower and upper extremities in patients with type 1 compared with type 2 diabetes.[18] Judging from the rising prevalence of type 2 diabetes, it is anticipated that DNP will become a significant social burden worldwide in the near future.

NATURAL HISTORY

Diabetic neuropathic pain (DNP) frequently is diagnosed before the diagnosis of diabetes.[19] Often DNP is described by patients as a continuously burning, tingling, electricity-like, crampy, or achy pain beginning in the feet and extending proximally over time. Patients with DNP also experience allodynia and hyperalgesia. *Allodynia* occurs when normally nonpainful stimuli become painful, whereas *hyperalgesia* is an increased sensitivity to normally painful stimuli. These symptoms are frequently exacerbated at night and can disturb sleep. Adding all these symptoms together, DNP becomes a major factor in decreasing the quality of life for patients with diabetes.[20-22]

Diabetic neuropathic pain can be caused by either an acute sensory neuropathy or a chronic sensorimotor neuropathy.[23] Acute sensory neuropathy usually occurs in patients with poorly controlled type 1 diabetes. The acute onset of pain has features of severe burning, aching, and sometimes electricity-like shooting pains. It is suggested that the acute pain is associated with sudden blood glucose fluxes and related ischemic changes in the nerves.[24] In contrast, chronic sensorimotor neuropathy is gradual in onset and is believed to result from diabetes-related metabolic damage to the peripheral nervous system.[23] The most common cause of DNP is a chronic sensorimotor neuropathy.[14] However, DNP can result from numerous diabetic neuropathies including plexopathy,[25] mononeuropathy from diabetes-induced entrapment syndromes,[26,27] and mononeuropathy multiplex.[25] Over a period of time that can last for several years, DNP subsides and the disabling pain is replaced by a loss of sensation, leading to the numb, insensate diabetic foot.[10,28]

SOCIETAL IMPACT

Previously accepted medical approaches to diabetes lack clearly defined mechanisms of action and, as a result, are only partially successful and are often ineffective.[20,21] Recently, due to many evidence-based studies, effective treatments have become available. Over the last two decades, multiple pain-modifying medications have been tested to treat DNP, including anticonvulsants, antidepressants, topical analgesics, and opioids.[29] Many multi-ticenter, double-blinded, placebo-controlled trials have proven the efficacy of these medications for DNP.[30] However, only 30%–50% of treated patients reported a 50% improvement in symptoms,,[31] and a combination of multiple regimens is usually required to control the pain adequately.[32] In addition, the annual cost for treating this chronic disabling condition is extremely high.[14] As a result, patients with DNP commonly develop insomnia, depression, anxiety, decreased mobility, and psychomotor impairment from uncontrolled symptoms, medication side effects, and associated psychosocial stress.[20–22] These comorbidities negatively impact their quality of life and significantly increase the annual cost of their medical care.[33] Recently, significant effort has been devoted to improving the management of DNP. Evidence based-guidelines have been established for treating neuropathic pain, including DNP.[30,34] Although DNP is a common and disabling problem, its pathogenesis remains unclear.[10,28] This lack of knowledge prevents the development of mechanism-specific therapies that can target the genes, proteins, and/or signaling cascades underlying DNP. Clearly, more basic science research involving animal models and clinical studies is urgently needed to reveal the molecular mechanisms of DNP. Such studies would allow these specific mechanisms to be targeted in the development of effective treatments for this common and highly morbid health problem.

PATHOGENESIS

Animal Models of Type 1 Diabetes

Animal models have been used extensively to try to understand the mechanisms behind DNP. Streptozotocin (STZ)-treated rodents are the most commonly used animal models for type 1 diabetes. Administration of STZ damages pancreatic islet cells and decreases insulin secretion in response to glucose loading. Several behavioral assays are routinely used to assess different aspects of neuropathic pain in this animal model of diabetes, including mechanical allodynia and heat hyperalgesia. *Mechanical allodynia* is defined as the ability to elicit pain at lower mechanical thresholds and can be demonstrated by increased responsiveness to stimulation with von Frey filaments. *Thermal hyperalgesia*, defined as an excessive sensation of pain in response to heat stimulation, is detected by the quicker responsiveness of the diabetic animals to a radiant heat source than control animals.[35] Typically, STZ-treated animal develop diabetes 3 days after treatment, and features of neuropathic pain start 4 weeks after the STZ treatment.[35]

In addition to STZ treatment, there are also other animal models for type 1 diabetes using genetically modified animals like the BB/Wor rat.[36] Similar to human patients, the BB/Wor rat has impaired insulin secretion via autoimmune mechanisms and gradually develops features of type 1 diabetes.[37] There is also evidence to suggest that this rat develops peripheral neuropathy[38] and neuropathic pain.[39]

Animal Models of Type 2 Diabetes

ZUCKER DIABETIC FATTY RAT

The Zucker Diabetic Fatty (ZDF) rat carries a homozygous mutation (fa/fa) of the leptin receptor.[40,41] These rats develop features of type 2 diabetes when they are fed with a high-energy rodent diet for 8–10 weeks.[42] The ZDF rats initially develop hyperinsulinemia and insulin resistance but later develop hypoinsulinemia from beta cell failure, similar to patients with type 2 diabetes. The ZDF rats have been shown to develop neuropathy and pain behaviors.[43,44] Thermal hyperalgesia develops at 8 weeks of age, at about the same time as the initiation of diabetes, and diminishes by 12 weeks of age. In contrast, mechanical allodynia develops at 18 weeks of age and lasts for up to 36 weeks.[45] Mechanical allodynia begins prior to the development of type 2 diabetes and lasts from the prediabetic stage until full development of diabetes, suggesting that it could be used as an animal model of prediabetic pain.[44]

SAND RAT

The desert gerbil *Psammomys obesus* (fat sand rat) has emerged as a useful model of type 2 diabetes. Innately insulin resistant, these animals develop moderate obesity and hyperglycemia when fed a high-energy diet, a condition associated first with compensatory hyperinsulinemia, followed by hypoinsulinemia related to β-cell failure.[46] Sand rats develop pain behavior at an early age that correlates inversely with their respective HbA1c levels.[47] In addition, sand rats develop evidence of peripheral neuropathy.

BBZDR/WOR RAT

The BBZDR/Wor rat is another genetically modified strain with a leptin receptor mutation. Only the obese male rats are used as models of type 2 diabetes. They develop hyperinsulinemia, hyperglycemia, and obesity. BBZDR/Wor rats also develop evidence of peripheral neuropathy.[39] In addition, thermal hyperalgesia has been reported in the BBZDR/Wor rat.[48]

OB/OB MICE

Ob/ob mice carry a homozygous mutation of leptin that induces leptin deficiency and a phenotype mimicking type 2 diabetes. Like ZDF and BBZDR/Wor rats that have the mutation of the leptin receptor (fa/fa), ob/ob mice develop an uncontrolled appetite and metabolic syndromes mimicking those of patients with type 2 diabetes. Ob/ob mice developed evident diabetic neuropathy.[49,50] Interestingly, these animals develop tactile allodynia, but not thermal hyperalgesia, at 11 weeks of age.[50]

DB/DB MICE

Another model of type 2 diabetes is the BKS. Cg-m+/+lepr^db^/J (commonly known as the db/db) mouse. Db/db mice are well characterized; they develop insulin resistance and hyperglycemia at approximately 4 weeks of age, with persistent blood glucose levels above 400 mg/dL.[51-54] The db/db mice display all the key features of type 2 diabetes, including hyperphagia, dyslipidemia, and obesity.[55-58] They develop hyperglycemia and increased body weight, as well as decreased fasting glycosylated hemoglobin and insulin levels at 5 weeks of age.[59] In addition, mechanical allodynia is detected from 6 to 12 weeks of age.[59] The pain behaviors subside after 16 weeks of age and are replaced by sensory loss, a sequence that is typical of diabetic neuropathy.[59,60]

Etiology of DNP

The cause of DNP is still under debate. Previously, it was believed that DNP is caused by hyperglycemia, since transient hyperglycemia from excess glucose injection reduced pain thresholds in animals.[61] In addition, normalization of hyperglycemia improves acute diabetic pain.[62,63] Recently, this concept has been challenged in light of new studies. Romanovsky and colleagues compared the mechanical thresholds of STZ-treated rats with euglycemia to those with hyperglycemia, even though both groups developed insulin deficiency. There was no difference in the pain behaviors of these two groups of animals. Therefore, they concluded that hypoinsulinemia, rather than hyperglycemia, is the main factor contributing to DNP caused by type 1 diabetes.[64] In support of their findings, Hoybergs and colleagues treated STZ rats with low-dose insulin after the induction of diabetes and neuropathy. The low-dose insulin treatment normalized pain behaviors even though severe hyperglycemia persisted. This study supports the hypothesis that the deficit of insulin and its associated neurotrophic support, rather than hyperglycemia, plays an essential role in the pathophysiology of DNP.[65]

The relative roles of hyperglycemia and hyperinsulinemia in the development of DNP in type 2 diabetes have been a topic of debate over the last few years. Rosiglitazone, an antidiabetic drug in the thiazolidinedione class, given prior to the development of diabetes, prevents the progression of impaired glucose tolerance to nonfasting hyperglycemia in ZDF rats.[66] However, even though rosiglitazone normalizes fasting glucose levels, it has no effect on the development of thermal hyperalgesia, suggesting that hyperglycemia is not a main cause of DNP in type 2 diabetes. Thus, abnormal insulin signaling has become the current hypothesis for the etiology of DNP in type 2 diabetes.

Molecular Mechanisms of DNP

Animal studies have revealed multiple molecular mechanisms for the development of DNP. Several nociceptive molecules, including ion channels, cell surface receptors for neurotrophic factors, and neurotransmitters have been demonstrated to play important roles in the development of DNP (Figure 11.1).

SODIUM CHANNELS

The upregulation of certain voltage-gated (Na(v)) sodium channels[67] has been studied in animal models of DNP. [68,69] These channels are normally expressed in the nociceptive dorsal root ganglion (DRG) neurons that supply either Aδ or C fibers and play critical roles in the initiation and propagation of pain signals from the periphery to the spinal cord. Increased excitability of these sodium channels contributes to allodynia and hyperalgesia in pain states.[69,70] Based on their affinity to tetrodotoxin (TTX), these sodium channels can be divided to two groups: tetrodotoxin-resistant (TTX-R) and tetrodotoxin-sensitive (TTX-S). Craner and colleagues reported that there are significant increases in the expression of Na(v)1.3 (TTX-S) and Na(v) 1.7 (TTX-S) and decreases in the expression of Na(v) 1.6 (TTX-S) and Na(v)1.8 (TTX-R) in diabetic rats.[69] In agreement with Craner et al, Hong and colleagues reported increased levels of serine/threonine phosphorylation of Na(v) 1.6 and of Na(v)1.8 and tyrosine phosphorylation of Na(v)1.6 and Na(v)1.7 in diabetic DRG.[68] These results suggest that serine/threonine and tyrosine phosphorylation of both TTX-S and TTX-R sodium channels play important roles in DNP. Blocking these sodium channels has been shown to decrease DNP in animal models and patients.[71] Targeting the Na(v) channels is a new approach for treating DNP; however, effective and selective antagonists for these channels are still under development.[70]

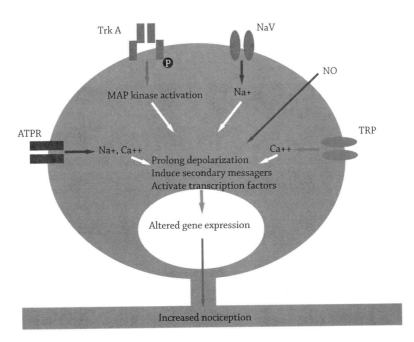

FIGURE 11.1   Molecular mechanisms of DNP in a nociceptive DRG neuron. To cause DNP, diabetes induces changes in several pathways to enhance nociception. First, NGF phosphorylates the Trk A receptor to induce downstream signaling cascades, including the MAP kinase pathway. Second, the upregulation of Navs and ATP receptors (ATPR) promotes membrane depolarization by increasing Na$^+$ inflow. Third, both ATPR and TRP receptors increase intracellular Ca^{2+}. Fourth, NO directly diffuses into the cytoplasm. Altogether, these events prolong action potentials and activate secondary messenger systems and transcription factors to alter gene expression.

ADENOSINE TRIPHOSPHATE RECEPTORS

Purines, such as adenosine and adenosine triphosphate (ATP), are endogenous ligands that modulate pain transmission and pain hypersensitivity by acting on P1 and P2 purinoceptors in both the peripheral and central nervous systems. For P1 (adenosine) receptors, both clinical studies in humans and experimental animal studies have demonstrated that activation of the A1 subtype reduces both inflammatory and neuropathic types of chronic pain.[72] There is a growing body of evidence indicating that multiple receptor subtypes of the P2 receptor are differentially involved in pain processing.[72] The most well known of the P2 receptors is the P2X$_3$ subtype, which is found in primary sensory neurons. Inhibition of the P2X$_3$ receptor is effective in reducing pain behaviors in animal models of chronic inflammatory and neuropathic pain.[72] The P2X$_3$ receptor is expressed by the nociceptive small to medium-sized DRG isolectin-B4-positive neurons, which also express the transient receptor potential vanilloid 1 (TRPV1) receptor.[72] On the cell membrane, P2X receptors form cation-selective channels with not only almost equal permeability to Na$^+$ and K$^+$, but also significant permeability to Ca^{2+}.[73,74] Site-specific injection of broadly acting P2X receptor agonists and antagonists has been shown to modulate nociceptive behavior in rodents.[75,76] The levels of P2X$_2$ and P2X$_3$ receptor mRNA were significantly increased in diabetic mice 14 days after the intravenous injection of STZ.[77] Intrathecal administration of P2X receptor antagonists (PPADS and TNP-ATP) inhibits the mechanical allodynia in STZ-treated diabetic mice, suggesting that the upregulation of P2X$_2$, P2X$_3$, and/or P2X$_{(2/3)}$ receptors in DRG neurons is associated with mechanical allodynia in STZ-induced diabetic mice.[77] Unfortunately, the availability of pharmacological tools with which to study the roles of specific P2X receptor subunits in the mechanism of pain is still limited, as most currently available ligands have low affinity and/or selectivity for their corresponding P2X receptors.[72] Understanding the mechanisms for regulating P2X receptor expression will lead to more efficient pharmacological approaches to relieve P2X receptor-mediated pain.

TRANSIENT RECEPTOR POTENTIAL RECEPTORS

The transient receptor potential (TRP) receptors respond to different chemical or physical stimuli.[78] TRPV1 is the most widely studied in regard to pain. It is a nonselective calcium channel that responds to capsaicin, the spicy component of hot pepper. TRPV1 expression correlates with the level of thermal hyperalgesia in STZ-treated animals.[79] In addition, TRPV1 is activated by other nociceptive mediators, including prostaglandins, bradykinin, glutamate, histamine, and nerve growth factor.[80–83] These data contribute to the clinical application of capsaicin for treating DNP.[30,84]

NERVE GROWTH FACTOR

Nerve growth factor (NGF) belongs to the neurotrophin family of growth factors, which regulate the development and survival of neurons in the central and peripheral nervous systems. The neurotrophin family members share homology, but individual neurotrophins mediate molecule-specific actions by binding to corresponding receptors, known as *Trks*.[85,86] Trk A is the high-affinity receptor for NGF and is expressed on small and medium-sized DRG neurons that project unmyelinated and thinly myelinated nerve fibers. These Trk A-expressing, NGF-responsive DRG neurons are the key generators of neuropathic pain[85,86] and are affected early in the course of diabetes.[85] Nerve growth factor is produced and released from target organs, binds to receptors on the unmyelinated and thinly myelinated nerve fibers, and is retrogradely transported to DRG neurons. Gene expression of NGF is increased in DRG neurons in animal models of spinal cord injury[87] and in human sural nerves as a result of various peripheral neuropathies.[88] The increased neuronal NGF expression suggests potential autocrine or paracrine mechanisms of NGF, similar to those of brain-derived neurotrophic factor, during noxious insults to the nervous system.[89]

Multiple studies confirm that NGF is vital in the development of nociception. During embryonic development, all unmyelinated and thinly myelinated sensory fibers from small and medium-sized DRGs are NGF-dependent. Postnatally, roughly half of DRG sensory neurons remain NGF-responsive; these DRG neurons express nociceptive neuropeptides.[90] In animals genetically deficient in NGF and Trk A, pain sensation is essentially absent,[85] suggesting that NGF signaling is central to the development of nociception. In parallel, NGF is expressed locally in DRG neurons following nerve injury.[85,86]

Accumulating evidence suggests that NGF is important in the pathogenesis of DNP.[91,92] In the STZ model of type 1 diabetes, NGF gene expression in sciatic nerves is upregulated by 1.65-fold[93] and higher NGF levels are detected in the superior mesenteric ganglia and celiac ganglia.[94] Elevated NGF levels could serve to mediate the early reduced mechanical and thermal thresholds reported in these animals.[95] Following nerve injury, NGF is expressed locally in the DRG neuron and is considered a source of postinjury pain.[85,86] As diabetes progresses, NGF levels are reduced in the DRG due to impaired axonal transport.[92] The long-term loss of NGF neurotrophism is considered a major cause of sensory loss in diabetic neuropathy.[92,96] Insulin treatment normalizes the NGF deficiency, reduces the expression of nociceptive molecules[96] and reverses the conduction deficits in STZ-treated animals.[97] Collectively, these studies suggest that during the early stages of diabetes-induced nervous system injury, NGF expression is elevated and mediates the signaling cascades that underlie the development of DNP. It has been recently reported that increased NGF expression in both the target organs of the DRG and the DRG neurons themselves activates Trk A receptors, mediating downstream signaling pathways to enhance nociception.[59] Over time and with continued injury, there is a loss of NGF expression and neurotrophism, leading to permanent nerve injury and the signs and symptoms of diabetic neuropathy (Figure 11.2).[10]

NITRIC OXIDE

Nitric oxide (NO) is an important regulator for vascular perfusion to tissues. In addition, it mediates a variety of inflammatory reactions. Due to its high lipophilicity, NO serves as a diffusible molecule across the cell membrane. It activates cyclic guanosine monophosphate (GMP)-mediated intracellular signaling. There are three nitric oxide synthases (NOSs): neuronal

NOS (nNOS or NOS1), inducible NOS (iNOS or NOS2), and endothelial NOS (eNOS or NOS3). Both nNOS and iNOS are localized in the DRG in either neuron or satellite cells.[98] Among the NOSs, current evidence indicates that nNOS does not mediate DNP.[99,100] In contrast, iNOS knockout mice have increased resistance to diabetic neuropathic complications, including impaired nerve conduction velocities and small-fiber sensory neuropathy. These findings indicate that iNOS could be an important mediator for DNP.[100,101] There is also evidence to imply that diabetes-induced increased NO levels are due to advanced glycation and lipoxidation end products (AGEs/ALEs).[102] The increased NO levels likely contribute to tactile hyperalgesia in the STZ model of type 1 diabetes.[103] To date, the role for eNOS in the pathogenesis of DNP is still unknown.

N-METHTL-D-ASPARTATE RECEPTOR ACTIVATION

There is strong evidence that peripheral nerve insults increase the excitability of spinal cord neurons, resulting in enhanced pain. This process involves the alteration of multiple neurotransmitters and intracellular signaling events in the spinal cord dorsal horn (SCDH) and is termed *central sensitization*.[104,105]

Once SCDH sensory neurons are activated by an initial peripheral noxious stimulus, the depolarization of postsynaptic terminals in SCDH neurons triggers the activation of the *N*-methyl-D-aspartate (NMDA) receptor, one of the receptors for glutamate.[104,106] Membrane depolarization activates the NMDA receptor, removing magnesium blockade from the ion channel and allowing the influx of calcium. The elevation of the intracellular calcium triggers a series of calcium-sensitive signal cascades, including protein kinase C (PKC) and mitogen-activated protein kinase (MAPK), and ultimately leads to altered gene expression.[106–108] The end result of central sensitization is a prolonged postsynaptic depolarization in SCDH neurons that enhances nociceptive messages.

The role of NMDA receptor activation in DNP is unknown. MK801, an NMDA receptor inhibitor, and magnesium administration were

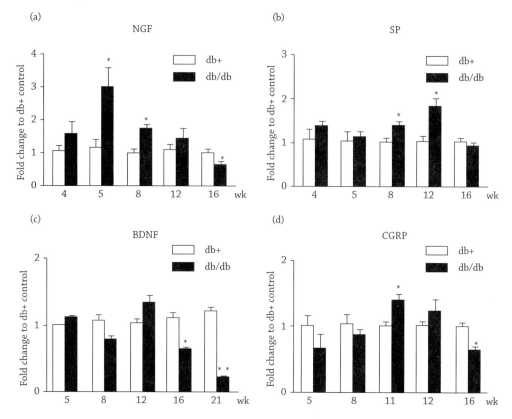

FIGURE 11.2   Increased NGF and SP gene expression in db/db mice during the period of mechanical allodynia. NGF (A) and SP (B) gene expression was measured by real time RT-PCR. A: NGF gene expression was upregulated at 5 and 8 wk of age in L 4-6 DRG of db/db mice. This upregulation of NGF expression diminished by 12 wk of age, and NGF gene expression fell below the control level at 16 wk of age. B: SP gene expression was enhanced at 8 and 12 wk of age in db/db mice. C: BDNF expression was not affected during the period of mechanical allodynia but decreased at 16 wk and 21 wk of age in db/db mice. D: Increased CGRP gene expression was detected in db/db mice at 11 wk of age. Data are normalized to that of db+ mice of the same age as mean + SEM from 4 animals of each group (*, p < 0.05; **, p < 0.001, compared with db+ of the same age).

Source: Reprinted with permission from Cheng HT, Dauch JR, Hayes JM, Hong Y, Feldman EL. Nerve growth factor mediates mechanical allodynia in a mouse model of type 2 diabetes. *J Neuropathol Exp Neurol*. 2009;68(11):1229–1243.

reported to inhibit the DNP from STZ-treated rats.[109] However, a later study demonstrated that MK801 treatment did not affect the mechanical allodynia in STZ rats.[110] These two studies varied in duration and in routes of MK801 treatment, which could have contributed to the conflicting results. Memantine is a noncompetitive NMDA antagonist that is approved by the U.S. Food and Drug Administration (FDA) for dementia. To date, memantine does not appear to be useful as therapy for chronic neuropathic pain, but it may be a useful acute adjunctive agent such as in the initial phases of phantom limb pain or soon after surgery in opioid-tolerant subjects.[111]

CLINICAL AND DIAGNOSTIC FEATURES

History

Patients with DNP may develop pain before or after the diagnosis of diabetes. Most patients are found to have impaired glucose tolerance during the workup for DNP but without clinical evidence of diabetes.[112] Most patients with DNP follow a similar course of polyneuropathic progression. The burning and tingling pain associated with DNP frequently starts in distal portions of the feet. Over time, the symptoms spread to the legs and increase in intensity. Frequently, the pain is worse at night and while walking. Contact of clothing or pressure from the shoe during walking may trigger or enhance the symptoms (allodynia). In addition, normally comfortable thermal stimuli frequently become painful (hyperalgesia). Over time, the pain becomes spontaneous, with increased intensity. Patients then begin to lose sensation in both feet and develop characteristic features of the diabetic foot. The progression of the symptoms is closely associated with the quality of blood glucose control. Sudden elevations or decreases in blood glucose levels frequently exacerbate the pain.[113,114] However, the typical course of DNP varies for patients with significant peripheral vascular disease, a common comorbidity with DNP.[115] In this group of patients, the duration of DNP is relatively short and is followed quickly by loss of sensation.[115]

Clinical Examination

Diagnosis of DNP is based primarily on clinical evaluations. Patients with DNP may have various clinical presentations. These patients can be divided into two major groups. Group 1 is associated with small-fiber neuropathy, usually characterized by distal symmetric DNP in both feet. Most of these patients have IFG, IGT, or established diabetes. They commonly have intact large nerve fibers and normal nerve conduction studies. Like most patients with DNP, these patients develops features of spontaneous pain, allodynia, and hyperalgesia. Consequently, they exhibit hypersensitivity to clinical sensory testing including light touch, pinprick, and mechanical stimulation with von Frey filaments. Vibratory sense and joint sensations are frequently intact, however. Group 2 consists of patients with large-fiber damage in addition to small-fiber neuropathy. They frequently have loss of sensation to light touch, pinprick, and vibratory and joint sensations on affected limbs. They also frequently lose deep tendon reflexes in the affected areas. This group

of patients usually has long-term diabetes with poorly controlled blood glucose and elevated glycosylated hemoglobin.

Laboratory Evaluation, Pain Questionnaires, and Other Diagnostic Tests

As mentioned, DNP frequently occurs in the prediabetic states of IFG and IGT. Impaired fasting glucose is defined as 12 hour fasting glucose levels ranging from 100 to 125 mg/dL. Impaired glucose tolerance is present with a 2-hour glucose level of 140 to 199 mg/dL on the 75 g oral glucose tolerance test.[116] Diabetes is present when the fasting glucose level exceeds 126 mg/dL. Currently, there is no direct objective assessment for DNP. Diabetic neuropathic pain is diagnosed by the presence of neuropathic pain symptoms concurrent with clinical evidence of diabetes or prediabetes. The intensity and quality of the pain component are usually assessed subjectively by questionnaires. A frequently used questionnaire for neuropathic pain is the McGill Pain Questionnaire.[117] Recently, an expanded and revised version of the Short-form McGill Pain Questionnaire (SF-MPQ) was created that includes more descriptive symptoms relevant to neuropathic pain and has a wider range of numerical possibilities (0–10). These changes allow for increased responsiveness when the questionnaire is used for longitudinal studies and clinical trials on neuropathic pain.[118] The Neuropathic Pain Questionnaire is another assessment designed for neuropathic pain.[119] The short version of this questionnaire provides a more efficient way of determining the features of neuropathic pain.[120] In addition, the Brief Pain Inventory has been modified to specifically assess DNP.[121] The Neuropathic Pain Symptom Inventory provides evaluation for features of neuropathic pain as well as the effects of pharmacological treatments or other therapies.[122]

Small-fiber neuropathy can be measured by nerve axon reflex-related vasodilation.[123] Intraepidermal nerve fiber (IENF)[124] measurement has also been used to evaluate the degree of C-fiber loss from diabetic neuropathy. However, the number of IENFs does not reflect the degree of DNP or predict its occurrence.[125,126]

Mechanical and thermal thresholds can be measured by von Frey monofilaments and a radiant heat source, respectively. Nerve conduction velocity (NCV) studies usually have limited use in diagnosing small-fiber neuropathy. However, they have great value in diagnosing patients with large-fiber involvement in polyneuropathy, plexopathy, mononeuropathy, and mononeuropathy multiplex. In addition, NCV can monitor the degree and progression of DNP in patients with large-fiber involvement.

PATHOLOGY OF DIABETIC NEUROPATHY

The characteristic pathological features of diabetic neuropathy are microangiopathic changes in the endoneurial capillaries (Figure 11.3).[127–129] These alterations include thickening of the basement membrane, swelling of the endothelial cells, and reduction in the caliber of the capillary lumen.[129] Microvascular changes observed in proximity to nerves are similar to the pathology related to other diabetic complications such as retinopathy and nephropathy. The importance of the microvascular abnormalities is underscored by the fact that they precede the nerve fiber loss seen in advanced diabetic neuropathy.[130,131] These changes also appear to parallel the changes seen in nerve fiber density, with both becoming more severe with worsening neuropathy.[128] Early changes seen in the nerve itself include paranodal changes, segmental demyelination, and remyelination followed by axonal degeneration.[130] The changes are more severe distally than proximally, which parallels the clinical presentation of a length-dependent neuropathy.

TREATMENT OF DNP

Over the last 3 decades, several effective treatments have been studied by placebo-controlled double blinded clinical trials (Table 11.1).

Calcium Channel α2-δ Ligands

Gabapentin is widely used for neuropathic pain due to its effectiveness and relatively fewer side effects than tricylic and tetracylic

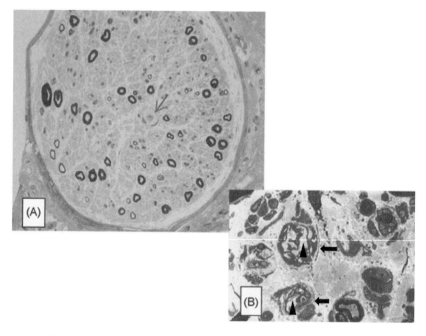

FIGURE 11.3 Pathological changes in peripheral nerves in diabetic neuropathy. (A) Microscopic image of a semithin transverse section through a sural nerve biopsy specimen from a patient with diabetic neuropathy. There is a gross loss of myelinated nerve fibers (arrowhead). In addition, the endoneurial capillaries (arrow) have considerably thickened walls. (B) Electron micrograph of a degenerating nerve; demyelination (arrows) and axonal degeneration (arrowheads) are prominent.

Table 11-1. Pharmaceutical Therapies for Diabetic Neuropathy

DRUG	NUMBER OF PATIENTS	DAILY DOSES	DURATION	OUTCOME	NNT	REFERENCE
CALCIUM CHANNEL α2-δ AGONISTS						
Gabapentin	165	<3600 mg	Parallel, 8 wks	Gabapentin > palcebo	4	187
Pregabalin	146	300 mg	Parallel, 8 wks	Pregabalin > placebo	3.9	130
Pregabalin	338	75, 300, 600 mg	Parallel, 5 wks	Pregabalin (300, 600 mg) > placebo	300 mg: 3.6 600 mg: 3.3	129
Pregabalin	246	150, 600 mg	Parallel, 6 wks	Pregabalin (600 mg) > placebo	600 mg: 4.2	188
TCAs						
Amitriptyline	29	≤150mg	Crossover, 2x6 wks	Amitriptyline > placebo	2.1	189
Desipramine	20	Average 201 mg	Crossover, 2x6 wks	Desipramine > placebo	2.2	190
Imipramine	19	25–350 mg	Crossover, 3x2 wks	Imipramine > placebo	4	191
Clomipramine	18	50–200 mg	Crossover, 3x2 wks	Clomipramine> placebo	4.5	136
SNRIs						
Venlafaxine	244	150–225 mg	Parallel, 6 wks	Venlafaxine > placebo	4.5	144
Duloxetine	457	20, 60, 120 mg	Parallel, 12 wks	Duloxetine (60, 120 mg) > placebo	60 mg: 4.3 120 mg: 3.8	192
Duloxetine	348	60, 120 mg	Parallel, 12 wks	Duloxetine (60, 120 mg) > placebo	60 mg: 11 120 mg: 5	142
Duloxetine	334	60, 120 mg	Parallel, 12 wks	Duloxetine (60, 120 mg) > placebo	60 mg: 6.3 120 mg: 3.8	193
SSRIs						
Paroxetine	26	40 mg	Crossover, 3x2 wks	Paroxetine > placebo	5	194
Citalopram	18	40 mg	Crossover, 3x2 wks	Citalopram > placebo	3	195
Fluoxetine	46	40 mg	Crossover, 2x6 wks	Fluoxetine = placebo	NA	190

(continued)

Table 11-1. (continued)

DRUG	NUMBER OF PATIENTS	DAILY DOSES	DURATION	OUTCOME	NNT	REFERENCE
Anticonvulsants						
Carbamazepine	40	400 mg	Crossover, 2 wks	Carbamazepine > placebo	2.3	196
Lamotrigine	59	<400 mg	Parallel, 8 wks	Lomotrigine > placebo	4	149
Oxcarbazepine	146	<1800 mg	Parallel, 16 wks	Oxcarbazepine > palcebo	6	153
Topiramate	323	<400 mg	Parallel, 12 wks	Topiramate > placebo	7.4	152
Lacosamide	370	400 mg	2 week run-in; 6-week titration; 12 wks maintenance	Lacosamide > placebo	NA	155
μ-RECEPTOR AGONISTS						
Tramadol	127	100–400 mg	Parallel, 6 wks	Tramadol > placebo	3.1	197
Oxycodon CR	159	10–100 mg	Parallel, 6 wks	Oxycodon > placebo	NA	159
NMDA antagonists						
Dextromethorphan	19	400 mg	Crossover, 9 wks	Dextromethorphan > placebo	3.2	161
Memantine	19	55 mg	Crossover, 9 wks	Memantine = placebo	NS	161
TOPICAL AGENTS						
Capsaicin cream	252	0.075% qid	8 wks	Capsaicin > placebo	NA	198

TCAs: tricyclic and tetracyclic antidepressants, SNRIs: serotonin-norepinephrine reuptake inhibitors, SSRIs: selective serotonin reuptake inhibitors, NNT: number needed to treat, NA: not available. NS: not significant, Qid: four times a day.

Source: Reprinted from Edwards JL, Vincent AM, Cheng HT, Feldman EL. Diabetic neuropathy: mechanisms to management. *Pharmacol Ther.* 2008;120(1):1–34, with permission from Elsevier.

antidepressants (TCAs) and other anticonvulsants. Gabapentin produces analgesia by binding to the α2-δ site of L-type voltage-gated calcium channels and decreasing calcium influx. Gabapentin ≤2400 mg/day is effective in treating DNP compared to amitryptyline (≤90 mg/day) according to a randomized control trial of 165 patients.[132,133] The efficacy of gabapentin (900–1800 mg/day) for DNP is comparable to that of amitriptyline (25–75 mg/day).[134] Gabapentin is usually well tolerated with slow titration. Common side effects of gabapentin include dizziness, ataxia, sedation, euphoria, ankle edema, and weight gain. Moreover, it usually takes weeks of titration to reach the maximal effective dose, and dosing three times per day is often necessary.

Like gabapentin, pregabalin acts by binding to the α2-δ subunit of calcium channels. As demonstrated in four randomized, placebo-controlled trials, pregabalin (300–600 mg/day) is significantly more effective in alleviating DNP than placebo.[135–137] Unlike gabapentin, pregabalin has better gastrointestinal absorption and can be administered twice per day. Its linear pharmacokinetics provide a rapid (<2 weeks) onset of maximal pain relief.[138] However, the side effects are similar to those of gabapentin, including dizziness, ataxia, sedation, euphoria, ankle edema, and weight gain. Among these side effects, weight gain is especially of concern for patients with type 2 diabetes. Like duloxetine, pregabalin is approved by the FDA for treating DNP.

Tricylic and Tetracyclic Reagents

The TCAs are considered first-line treatments for neuropathic pain. The therapeutic actions of these agents are mediated by inhibition of the reuptake of norepinephrine and serotonin. These antidepressants not only control pain, but also pain-related symptoms such as insomnia and depression. Max et al. reported that amitriptyline (150 mg/day) is superior to placebo in relieving DNP after 6 weeks of treatment.[139] Desipramine at 111 mg/day is as effective as amitriptyline in alleviating DNP.[139] Another TCA, imipramine, also significantly improves DNP at a dose of 50 and 75 mg/day.[140,141] In addition, clomipramine relieves the symptoms of DNP.[142] Pooling the data from all of these trials suggests that approximately one in three patients experience at least 50% relief of pain by using these drugs.[143] However, the use of TCAs is limited by their side effects,[144] which include dry mouth, sedation, and blurred vision. Overall, secondary amines (nortriptyline, desipramine) are better tolerated than tertiary amines (amytriptyline, imipramine).[145] The TCAs are not well tolerated by older patients and should be used with great caution (or avoided altogether) in patients with cardiac arrhythmias, congestive heart failure, orthostatic hypotension, urinary retention, or angle-closure glaucoma.[146] It is important to note that TCAs are contraindicated in patients taking monoamine oxidase (MAO) inhibitors. The usual dosage schedule for TCAs is 10 to 25 mg at bedtime initially, titrating as tolerated up to 100 or 150 mg as a single bedtime dose. In addition, their analgesic effects require several weeks to develop, which limits their utility for acute pain.

Serotonin-Norepinephrine Reuptake Inhibitors

The serotonin-norepinephrine reuptake inhibitors (SNRIs) have greater efficacy against DNP than the selective serotonin reuptake inhibitors (SSRIs). Duloxetine has been approved by the FDA for treating DNP following three large randomized, placebo-controlled trials.[147–149] In these trials, duloxetine 60 and 120 mg daily provided significant relief from DNP. The higher dose provides greater relief but is associated with increased side effects. In general, duloxetine is better tolerated, in terms of gastrointestinal and cardiac side effects, than other SNRIs. Another SNRI, venlafaxine 150–225 mg/day, alleviates DNP but produces unacceptable cardiac side effects with an increased risk of electrocardiographic changes.[150]

SELECTIVE SEROTONIN REUPTAKE INHIBITORS

The SSRIs are newer antidepressants that have largely replaced TCAs for the treatment of depression because they are better tolerated. However, in contrast to TCAs, the efficacy of SSRIs is limited in DNP. For example, fluoxetine 40 mg/day has no efficacy compared to placebo.[139] In general, SSRIs demonstrate no significant efficacy in DPN pain control, but they provide significant improvement in mood that results in better compliance with other treatments and an improved quality of life.[151] In the literature, only citalopram 40 mg/day was reported to be more effective than placebo for treating DNP.[152]

Anticonvulsants

Anticonvulsants control neuronal excitability by blocking sodium and/or calcium channels.[153] Originally developed for preventing seizures, they are in broad use for the treatment of neuropathic pain.

Sodium valproate enhances gamma-aminobutyric acid (GABA) levels in the central nervous system, inhibits T-type calcium channels, and increases potassium inward currents. However, the side effects, including hair loss, weight again, hepatotoxicity, and cognitive dysfunction, are not insignificant and increase with long-term use, although a dose of 500 mg/day decreases DNP.[154]

Lamotrigine is an anticonvulsant that blocks voltage-gated sodium channels, decreases presynaptic calcium currents to inhibit the release of glutamate, and increases GABA levels in the brain. Eisenberg et al. reported favorable results of lamotrigine ($\leq$400 mg/day) against DNP.[155] In addition, two large-scale ($n = 360$) randomized, double-blind, placebo-controlled trials also demonstrated some efficacy for lamotrigine in treating DNP.[156] However, the results are not as promising. Although there is was a reduction on the pain scale in one trial after a 19 week trial of lamotrigine (400 mg/day), there was no difference between lamotrigine and the placebo group at the end of the trial. Taken together, these findings indicate that lamotrigine is well tolerated but its efficacy against DNP is still questionable.

Another anticonvulsant that has undergone clinical trials for DNP is topiramate. Topiramate has multiple actions: (1) blocking activity-dependent, voltage-gated sodium channels; (2) inhibiting L-type voltage-gated calcium channels; and (3) blocking postsynaptic kainite/α-amino-3-hydroxy-5-methyl-4-isoxazolepropionic acid (AMPA) excitatory amino acid receptors. Raskin et al. reported a randomized, double-blind, placebo-controlled study that involved 323 patients with DNP. In that study, topiramate $\leq$400 mg/day was usually well tolerated and significantly alleviated DNP in approximately one out of six patients.[157,158]

Oxcarbazepine is a keto analog of carbamazepine that blocks sodium channels. In one study, a dose of $\leq$1800 mg/day significantly reduced DNP,[159] but in a larger study, no significant reduction of DNP was seen with 1200 and 1800 mg/day.[160] Oxcarbazepine has a good side effect profile and is well tolerated. However, more studies are necessary to clarify its potential for treating DNP.

Lacosamide is a newly developed anticonvulsant. It acts by enhancing the slow inactivation of voltage-gated sodium channels and binding to collapsin response mediator protein-2 (CRMP-2), which is part of the signal transduction cascade of neurotrophic factors. Wymer and colleagues reported a multicenter, randomized, placebo-controlled, double-blinded trial confirming the efficacy of lacosamide for treating DNP.[161] In their study, lacosamide, at a daily dose of 400 mg, was effective in treating DNP after a 6 week titration phase and 12 weeks of maintenance therapy.[161] In addition, Ziegler et al. reported similar results using lacosamide at 400 and 600 mg/day.[162] Common side effects associated with lacosamide include, nausea, vomiting, ataxia, dizziness, tremor, and headache.

Tramadol

Tramadol is a weak μ-receptor agonist that also inhibits reuptake of serotonin. A double-blind, randomized, placebo-controlled trial using an average dose of 210 mg/day for 6 weeks produced significantly reduced pain scores in patients with DNP.[163] Nausea, constipation, headache, and dyspepsia were common side effects. Tramadol is well tolerated, with only mild side effects. In addition, a combination of tramadol and acetaminophen (37.5/325 mg) when taken as one to two tablets four times a day, is effective in alleviating DNP.[164]

Opiates

Slow-release oxycodone 20 mg/day relieves DNP over a 6-week period.[165] In a crossover design treatment strategy, slow-release oxycodone was effective against DNP at a maximum dose of 80 mg/day.[166] Although opioids are effective against DNP, long-term use will result in side effects including constipation, urinary retention, impaired cognitive function, impaired immune function, and many other issues associated with tolerance and addiction.

NMDA Antagonists

Two NMDA receptor antagonists, dextromethorphan and memantine, have been tested in DNP.[167] These placebo-controlled crossover studies involved 23 patients with diabetic neuropathy. The studies were designed with a 7 week titration period followed by a 2 week maintenance period for lorazepam, an active placebo, or one of the NMDA inhibitors. Both high and low doses of the inhibitors were assessed. Treatment with dextromethorphan, but not memantine, produced a significant dose-dependent decrease in DNP. However, the NMDA inhibitors have significant side effects including, sedation, dry mouth, and gastrointestinal distress.

Topical Agents

Capsaicin is an extract of capsicum peppers. Capsaicin binds to the TRPV1 receptor and exhausts substance P in the peripheral nerves to achieve its analgesic effects. In the study published by the Capsaicin Study Group, 0.075% capsaicin cream applied three times a day for 6 weeks was more effective in alleviating DNP than placebo.[168] Burning was the most common side effect, which tended to decrease as therapy continued. The therapeutic effects of capsaicin started weeks after the cream's application. Recently, a patch containing highly concentrated capsaicin has demonstrated promising effects in treating diabetic pain.

Because impaired NO generation leading to reduced blood flow may be involved in DNP, a small trial using isosorbide dinitrate, an NO donor, was performed. In a 12 week double-blind, placebo-controlled crossover study with 22 patients, isosorbide dinitrate spray significantly relieved DNP.[169] Patients in the trial reported minor headaches. A larger study is necessary to evaluate the potential use of this treatment for DNP.

Topical lidocaine 5% patches have been reported in several studies to relieve DNP. In an open-label study, up to four 5% lidocaine patches applied for up to 18 h/day were well tolerated in patients with painful diabetic polyneuropathy. Lidocaine patches significantly improved pain and quality-of-life ratings and may allow tapering of concomitant analgesic therapy.[170] Given the open-label design of this trial, a randomized, controlled trial is necessary to confirm these results.

Combination Drug Therapies

Recently, trials using a combination of drug therapies have proven to provide additive effects of pain relief in comparison to single-drug treatment. Gilron et al. tested patients with neuropathic pain from DNP and postherpetic neuralgia using maximally tolerated doses of morphine, gabapentin, or both. The combination of drugs achieved more potent pain relief than either individual treatment.[171] However, the maximal tolerated dose of each drug was lower in the patient group with combination therapy, suggesting increased side effects with drug combination. In Gilron et al.'s recent report, the combination of nortriptyline and gabapentin also achieved more efficacy against DNP than either drug alone.[32] Combination pharmacotherapy has been used widely in clinical practice, but more studies are needed to establish its safety, efficacy, compliance, and cost effectiveness; to determine optimal drug combinations and dose ratios; to compare concurrent with sequential combination therapy; and to explore the results of combining more than two drugs.

Alternative Pharmacological Treatment

ALPHA-LIPOIC ACID

Alpha-lipoic acid (ALA) is a potent antioxidant that has been used in Europe for the treatment of diabetic neuropathy. Alpha-lipoic acid can reduce diabetic neuropathy by (1) normalizing NO production,[172] (2) decreasing lipid peroxidation and normalizing sodium/calcium adenosine triphosphatase activity,[173] (3) increasing glucose uptake, as well as myo-inositol and glutathione levels in the peripheral nerves,[174] (4) increasing blood flow, and (5) reducing oxidative stress.[175] Three Alpha-Lipoic Acid in Diabetic Neuropathy (ALADIN) trials have demonstrated the efficacy of ALA in reducing symptoms of diabetic neuropathy. The first 3 week trial used an intravenous infusion of ALA at doses of 600 or 1200 mg/day. A total of 328 patients with type 2 diabetes participated in the study. The ALA treatment significantly alleviated DNP more effectively than placebo, with 600 mg/day slightly better than 1200 mg/day.[176] It was well tolerated at both dosages.

The ALADIN II trial studied whether ALA could improve diabetic neuropathy by following nerve conduction studies and the Neuropathic Disability Score (NDS).[177] Sixty- five patients with type 1 or type 2 diabetes enrolled in this 2 year trial. Alpha-lipoic acid was administered as 600 mg twice daily, 600 mg once daily with placebo once daily, or placebo twice daily by intravenous (IV) infusion for 5 days. The IV treatments were followed by corresponding oral regimens of the same dosage for the rest of the trial. The ALA treatment significantly improved sural NCV and amplitudes as well as tibial motor NCV. There was no significant change in tibial nerve distal motor latencies or the NDS.

The ALADIN III trial involved 509 patients with type 2 diabetes. The patients were treated with ALA 600 mg or placebo IV three times a day for 3 weeks, followed by placebo three times a day for 6 months.[178] No significant difference in total symptom score (TSS) and neuropathy impairment score (NIS) were detected between the placebo and ALA groups.

In a meta-analysis of four trials with a total of 1258 patients given ALA 600 mg/day for 3 weeks,[179] the TSS and NIS of the ALA group were significantly better than those of the control group. Among the individual components of the TSS, pain, burning, and numbness decreased in favor of ALA compared with placebo, while among the NIS-LL components, pinprick and touch-pressure sensation as well as ankle reflexes were improved in favor of ALA after 3 weeks. The rates of adverse effects did not differ between the groups.

ACETYL-L-CARNITINE

Acetyl-L-carnitine (ALC) is another antioxidant that has been tested in large clinical trials of diabetic neuropathy. Sima et al. reported two double-blind, placebo-controlled trials. A total of 1346 patients enrolled in these trials and were treated with placebo or ALC at dosages of 500 or 1000 mg/day three times a day for 1 year. One study involved centers in the United States, Canada, and Europe (UCES). The other trial included centers in the United States and Canada (UCS). In the UCS group, 1000 mg ALC taken three times a day significantly improved pain but did not have this effect in the UCES group. After analyzing the subgroups, the authors concluded that ALC is more effective in patients with type 2 diabetes and those with a shorter duration of neuropathy.[180]

OTHER TREATMENT MODALITIES

Acupuncture is a commonly used alternative treatment for many medical conditions. It has been widely accepted and used in Asian countries for centuries. Recently, acupuncture therapy has gained more popularity in the U.S. pain management community and has been widely accepted as an effective treatment modality. The National Institutes of Health have recognized acupuncture as an effective treatment for a variety of painful conditions.[a1] Acupuncture analgesia is likely mediated through increased descending inhibitory control from the brain, including endogenous opioids, serotonin, and norepinephrine systems.[181,182] However, studies of DNP treatment with acupuncture are limited. In a long-term study, Abuaisha and colleagues reported on patients who initially received up to six courses of classical acupuncture analgesia over a period of 10 weeks. All but one patient completed the study, and 77% of patients showed significant improvement in their primary and/or secondary symptoms. These patients were followed up for a period of 18–52 weeks, during which 67% of them were able to stop or reduce their medications significantly. In the responding group, only 21% noted that their symptoms cleared completely.

1 [a]http://nccam.nih.gov/health/acupuncture/acupuncture-for-pain.htm

Table 11-2. Management of Neuropathic Pain. Stepwise instructions for treatment of the symptoms for painful diabetic neuropathy based on multiple levels of medications, pain scores and evaluations

STEPWISE PHARMACOLOGICAL MANAGEMENT OF NEUROPATHIC PAIN (NP)

Step 1
- Assess pain and establish the diagnosis of NP; if uncertain about diagnosis, refer to pain specialist or neurologist
- Establish & treat cause of NP; if uncertain about availability of treatments addressing NP etiology, refer to appropriate specialist
- Identify relevant co-morbidities (e.g. cardiac, renal, or hepatic disease, depression, gait instability that might be relieved or exacerbated by NP treatment, or that might require dosage adjustment or additional monitoring of therapy
- Explain diagnosis and treatment plan to patient and establish realistic expectations

Step 2
- Initiate therapy of disease causing NP, if applicable
- Initiate symptom treatment with one or more of the following:
    - Secondary amine TCA (nortriptyline, desipramine or an SSNRI (duloxetine, venlafaxine)
    - Calcium channel α2-δ ligand, either pregabalin or gabapentin
    - For localized peripheral NP; topical lidocaine used alone or in combination with one of the other 1st line therapies
    - For patients with acute NP, neuropathic cancer pain or episodic exacerbations of sever pain, and when prompt pain relief during titration of a 1st line medication to an efficacious dosage is required, opioid analgesics or tramadol may be used alone or in combination with one of the 1st line therapies
- Evaluate patient for non-pharmacologic treatments and initiate if appropriate

Step 3
- Reassess pain and health-related quality of life frequently
- If substantial pain relief (e.g. average pain reduced to <3/10) and tolerable side effects, continue treatment
- If partial pain relief (e.g. average pain remains >4/10) after an adequate trial, add one of the other 1st line medications
- If no or inadequate pain relief (e.g. <30% reduction) at target doseage after an adequate trial, switch to alternateive 1st line medication

Step 4
- If trials of 1st line medications alone and in combination fail, consider 2nd and 3rd line medications or referral to a pain specialist or multidisciplinary pain center

Source: Reprinted from Edwards JL, Vincent AM, Cheng HT, Feldman EL. Diabetic neuropathy: mechanisms to management. *Pharmacol Ther*. 2008;120(1):1–34, with permission from Elsevier.

These data suggest that acupuncture is a safe and effective therapy for the long-term management of DPN.[183]

Spinal cord stimulators (SCS) apply pulsed electrical signals to the spinal cord to achieve analgesia. An SCS typically consists of stimulating electrodes implanted in the epidural space at a higher level than the affected limbs. The electrodes are powered by an electrical pulse generator that is usually implanted in the lower abdominal or gluteal region. The mechanisms for using SCS to treat pain are based on evidence that SCS alters the local neurochemistry in the dorsal horn, suppressing the hyperexcitability of the nociceptive neurons. Specifically, there is some evidence for increased levels GABA and serotonin, and perhaps for suppression of levels of excitatory amino acids, including glutamate and aspartate.[184] Kumar and colleagues reported that long-term treatment with SCS significantly improves pain control in patients with failed back syndrome.[185] Trials using SCS in treating DPN are very limited. Only trials with limited numbers of patients are available in the current literature.[186,187]

External high-frequency muscle stimulation (EHFMS) is also reported to have efficacy in treating DNP.[188] In this pilot study, EHFMS was demonstrated to be more effective than transcutaneous electrical nerve stimulation (TENS) in controlling symptoms associated with both nonpainful and painful neuropathies caused by diabetes after 3 days of treatment.[188]

Monochromatic infrared photo energy (MIRE) treatment has been tested for treating DNP. Harkless et al. reported that MIRE treatment significantly improved foot sensation and reduced pain levels by up to 67% on an 11-point visual analog pain scale in patients with DNP.[189] However, the mechanism for this treatment is still unclear.

Current Practice

The typical treatment approach to the patient with DNP is to start with a TCA, an SNRI, or a calcium channel ligand such as gabapentin or pregabalin (Table 11-2). Only duloxetine (an SNRI) and pregabalin are FDA approved for the treatment of DNP, but all of these medications are believed to have similar efficacy and relatively low side effect profiles (the number needed to treat to obtain a 50% reduction in pain ranges from three to six[153,190–192]). The initial choice among these agents is largely based on the individual patient's comorbidities. Patients with depression are often started on TCAs or SNRIs, whereas patients with a history of seizures are started on an anticonvulsant. Patients with renal disease or peripheral edema typically are not prescribed calcium channel ligands. Conversely, patients with cardiac conduction disease usually are not treated with TCAs and SNRIs. Given the lack of consensus on the treatment of DNP, many physicians use these other patient factors to aid in making the decision concerning the first-line medication. Clearly, more clinical trials comparing these agents are needed to help guide these common clinical decisions.

FUTURE DIRECTIONS

Recently discovered molecular mechanisms of neuropathic pain from animals studies have led to the development of multiple novel pharmacological treatments for DNP. Even with this tremendous effort, satisfactory treatments for DNP are still under development. Although animal studies provide scientifically based approaches for the development of treatments, clinical trials for these new treatments have not been as promising as the animal studies due to the multifactorial variation in human patients and the complicated nature of human disease. Current evidence-based practice has improved the pain control of DNP. However, evidence in the literature indicates that a single agent usually is not sufficient to improve the variety of symptoms occurring in DNP. A combination of different drugs and various treatment modalities is the current trend in the treatment of DNP. Future studies for understanding the complex molecular mechanisms of DNP are urgently needed to improve the medical management of this devastating condition.

ACKNOWLEDGEMENTS

The authors would like to thank the support from National Institutes of Health [UO1-DK60994 (ELF); 1K08NS061039 (HTC)] and the Juvenile Diabetes Research Foundation Center for the Study of Complications in Diabetes.

REFERENCES

1. Wild S et al. Global prevalence of diabetes: estimates for the year 2000 and projections for 2030. *Diabetes Care*. 2004;27(5):1047–1053.
2. Hedley AA et al. Prevalence of overweight and obesity among US children, adolescents,

and adults, 1999–2002. *JAMA*. 2004;291(23): 2847–2850.

3. Feldman EL et al. Diabetic neuropathy. In: Simeon I, Taylor MD, eds. *Current Review of Diabetes*. Current Medicine. 1999:71–83.

4. Feldman EL et al. Diabetic neuropathy. In: Mario UD, Leonetti F, Pugliese C, Sbraccia P, Signore A eds. *Diabetes in the New Millennium*. Sydney: The Endocrinology and Diabetes Research Foundation of the University of Sydney; 1999:387–402.

5. Feldman EL et al. Diabetic neuropathy. In Becker KL, ed. *Principles and Practice of Endocrinology and Metabolism*. 2001, Philadelphia: Lippincott Williams & Wilkins; 2001:1391–1399.

6. Boulton AJ, Malik RA. Diabetic neuropathy. *Med Clin North Am*. 1998;82(4):909–929.

7. Thomas PK. Classification of the diabetic neuropathies. In Gries FA, Low PA, Ziegler D, eds. *Textbook of Diabetic Neuropathy*. Stuttgart: Thieme; 2003:175–177.

8. Boulton AJ et al. Diabetic neuropathies: a statement by the American Diabetes Association. *Diabetes Care*. 2005;28:956–962.

9. Galer BS et al. Painful diabetic polyneuropathy: epidemiology, pain description, and quality of life. *Diabetes Res Clin Pract*. 2000;47(2):123–128.

10. Feldman EL et al. Somatosensory neuropathy. In: Inzucchi S ed. *The Diabetes Mellitus Manual*. New York: McGraw-Hill; 2005:366–384.

11. Ziegler D et al. Neuropathic pain in diabetes, prediabetes and normal glucose tolerance: the MONICA/KORA Augsburg Surveys S2 and S3. *Pain Med*. 2009;10(2):393–400.

12. Singleton JR et al. Microvascular complications of impaired glucose tolerance. *Diabetes*. 2003;52:2867–2873.

13. Singleton JR et al. Polyneuropathy with impaired glucose tolerance: implications for diagnosis and therapy. *Curr Treat Options Neurol*. 2005;7: 33–42.

14. Barrett AM et al. Epidemiology, public health burden, and treatment of diabetic peripheral neuropathic pain: a review. *Pain Med*. 2007;8 (suppl 2):S50–S62.

15. Clarke P, Gray A, Holman R. Estimating utility values for health states of type 2 diabetic patients using the EQ-5D (UKPDS 62). *Med Decis Making*. 2002;22(4):340–349.

16. Currie CJ et al. *The financial costs of healthcare treatment for people with Type 1 or Type 2 diabetes in the UK with particular reference to differing severity of peripheral neuropathy*. Diabetes Med. 2007;24(2):187–194.

17. Martin CL et al. Neuropathy among the diabetes control and complications trial cohort 8 years after trial completion. *Diabetes Care*. 2006;29(2):340–344.

18. Ziegler D et al. The epidemiology of diabetic neuropathy. Diabetic Cardiovascular Autonomic Neuropathy Multicenter Study Group. *J Diabetes Complications*. 1992;6(1):49–57.

19. Singleton JR, Smith AG, Bromberg MB. Painful sensory polyneuropathy associated with impaired glucose tolerance. *Muscle Nerve*. 2001;24(9):1225–1228.

20. Dworkin RH et al. Symptom profiles differ in patients with neuropathic versus non-neuropathic pain. *J Pain*. 2007;8:118–126.

21. Dworkin RH et al. Core outcome measures for chronic pain clinical trials: IMMPACT recommendations. *Pain*. 2005;113:9–19.

22. Jensen MP et al. Do pain qualities and spatial characteristics make independent contributions to interference with physical and emotional functioning? *J Pain*. 2006;7:644–653.

23. Boulton AJ. Painful diabetic neuropathies. In: Cervero F, Jensen TS, eds. *Handbook of Clinical Neurology*. Oxford: Elsevier; 2006:609–619.

24. Tesfaye S et al. Prevalence of diabetic peripheral neuropathy and its relation to glycaemic control and potential risk factors: the EURODIAB IDDM Complications Study. *Diabetologia*. 1996;39(11):1377–1384.

25. Thomas PK, Tomlinson DR. Diabetic and hypoglycemic neuropathy. In: Dyck DJ, Thomas PK, eds. *Peripheral Neuropathy*. Philadelphia: WB Saunders;1993:1219–1241.

26. Wilbourn AJ, Dyck PJ, Thomas PK. Diabetic entrapment and compression neuropathies. In: Dyck DJ, Thomas PK, eds. *Diabetic Neuropathy*. Philadelphia: WB Saunders; 1999:481–508.

27. Thomas PK, Ochoa J. Clinical features and differential diagnosis. In: *Peripheral Neuropathy*, In: Dyck PJ, Thomas PK, Griffin JW, Low PA, Poduslo JF, eds. *Peripheral Neuropathy*. Philadelphia: WB Saunders; 1993:749–774.

28. Feldman, EL et al. Diabetic peripheral and autonomic neuropathy. In: *Contemporary Endocrinology*. New York: Humana Press; 2002.

29. Ziegler D. Treatment of diabetic polyneuropathy: update 2006. *Ann NY Acad Sci*. 2006;1084: 250–266.

30. Edwards JL et al. Diabetic neuropathy: mechanisms to management. *Pharmacol Ther*. 2008; 120(1):1–34.

31. Jensen TS et al. New perspectives on the management of diabetic peripheral neuropathic pain. *Diabetes Vasc Dis Res*. 2006;3:108–119.

32. Gilron I et al. Nortriptyline and gabapentin, alone and in combination for neuropathic pain:

a double-blind, randomised controlled crossover trial. *Lancet*. 2009;374(9697):1252–261.

33. Boulanger L et al. Impact of comorbid depression or anxiety on patterns of treatment and economic outcomes among patients with diabetic peripheral neuropathic pain. *Curr Med Res Opin*. 2009;25(7):1763–1773.

34. Dworkin RH et al. Pharmacologic management of neuropathic pain: evidence-based recommendations. *Pain*. 2007;132(3):237–251.

35. Morrow TJ. Animal models of painful diabetic neuropathy: the STZ rat model. *Curr Protoc Neurosci*. 2004;chap 9:unit 9. 18.

36. Nakhooda AF et al. The spontaneously diabetic Wistar rat. Metabolic and morphologic studies. *Diabetes*. 1977;26(2):100–112.

37. Marliss EB et al. The diabetic syndrome of the "BB" Wistar rat: possible relevance to type 1 (insulin-dependent) diabetes in man. *Diabetologia*. 1982;22(4):225–232.

38. Sima AA et al. A comparison of diabetic polyneuropathy in type II diabetic BBZDR/Wor rats and in type I diabetic BB/Wor rats. *Diabetologia*. 2000;43(6):786–793.

39. Kamiya H et al. Unmyelinated fiber sensory neuropathy differs in type 1 and type 2 diabetes. *Diabetes Metab Res Rev*. 2005;21(5):448–458.

40. Friedman JE et al. Altered expression of muscle glucose transporter GLUT-4 in diabetic fatty Zucker rats (ZDF/Drt-fa). *Am J Physiol*. 1991;261(6 pt 1):E782–E788.

41. Clark JB, Palmer CJ, Shaw WN. The diabetic Zucker fatty rat. *Proc Soc Exp Biol Med*. 1983;173(1):68–75.

42. Chen D, Wang MW. Development and application of rodent models for type 2 diabetes. *Diabetes Obes Metab*. 2005;7(4):307–317.

43. Brussee V et al. Distal degenerative sensory neuropathy in a long-term type 2 diabetes rat model. *Diabetes*. 2008;57(6):1664–1673.

44. Romanovsky D, Walker JC, Dobretsov M. Pressure pain precedes development of type 2 disease in Zucker rat model of diabetes. Neurosci Lett. 2008;445(3):220–223.

45. Sugimoto K et al. Time course of pain sensation in rat models of insulin resistance, type 2 diabetes, and exogenous hyperinsulinaemia. *Diabetes Metab Res Rev*. 2008;24(8):642–650.

46. Shafrir E, Ziv E, Kalman R. Nutritionally induced diabetes in desert rodents as models of type 2 diabetes: *Acomys cahirinus* (spiny mice) and *Psammomys obesus* (desert gerbil). *Ilar J*. 2006;47(3):212–224.

47. Wuarin-Bierman L et al. Hyperalgesia in spontaneous and experimental animal models of diabetic neuropathy. *Diabetologia*. 1987;30(8): 653–658.

48. Obrosova IG. Diabetic painful and insensate neuropathy: pathogenesis and potential treatments. *Neurotherapeutics*. 2009;6(4):638–647.

49. Drel VR et al. The leptin-deficient (ob/ob) mouse: a new animal model of peripheral neuropathy of type 2 diabetes and obesity. *Diabetes*. 2006;55(12):3335–3343.

50. Vareniuk I et al. Nitrosative stress and peripheral diabetic neuropathy in leptin-deficient (ob/ob) mice. *Exp Neurol*. 2007;205(2):425–436.

51. Sima AAF, Shafrir E. *Animal Models in Diabetes: A Primer*. Amsterdam: Taylor and Francis; 2000.

52. Chua SC Jr et al. Phenotypes of mouse diabetes and rat fatty due to mutations in the OB (leptin) receptor. *Science*. 1996;271:994–996.

53. Hummel KP, Dickie MM, Coleman DL. Diabetes, a new mutation in the mouse. *Science*. 1966;153:1127–1128.

54. Chen H et al. Evidence that the diabetes gene encodes the leptin receptor: identification of a mutation in the leptin receptor gene in db/db mice. *Cell*. 1996;84:491–495.

55. Walwyn WM et al. HSV-1-mediated NGF delivery delays nociceptive deficits in a genetic model of diabetic neuropathy. *Exp Neurol*. 2006;198: 260–270.

56. Miwa I, Kanbara M, Okuda J. Improvement of nerve conduction velocity in mutant diabetic mice by aldose reductase inhibitor without affecting nerve myo-inositol content. *Chem Pharm Bull (Tokyo)*. 1989;37:1581–1582.

57. Sima AA, Robertson DM. Peripheral neuropathy in mutant diabetic mouse [C57BL/Ks (db/db)]. *Acta Neuropathol (Berl)*. 1978;41:85–89.

58. Moore SA et al. Reduced sensory and motor conduction velocity in 25-week-old diabetic [C57BL/Ks (db/db)] mice. *Exp Neurol*. 1980;70:548–555.

59. Cheng HT et al. Nerve growth factor mediates mechanical allodynia in a mouse model of type 2 diabetes. *J Neuropathol Exp Neurol*. 2009;68(11):1229–243.

60. Sullivan KA et al. Mouse models of diabetic neuropathy. *Neurobiol Dis*. 2007;28(3):276–285.

61. Raz I et al. Effect of hyperglycemia on pain perception and on efficacy of morphine analgesia in rats. *Diabetes*. 1988;37(9):1253–1259.

62. Tesfaye S et al. Arterio-venous shunting and proliferating new vessels in acute painful neuropathy of rapid glycaemic control (insulin neuritis). *Diabetologia*. 1996;39:329–335.

63. Lee JH, McCarty R. Glycemic control of pain threshold in diabetic and control rats. *Physiol Behav*. 1990;47(2):225–230.

64. Romanovsky D et al. Mechanical hyperalgesia correlates with insulin deficiency in normoglycemic streptozotocin-treated rats. *Neurobiol Dis*. 2006;24(2):384–394.

65. Hoybergs YM, Meert TF. The effect of low-dose insulin on mechanical sensitivity and allodynia in type I diabetes neuropathy. *Neurosci Lett*. 2007;417(2):149–154.

66. Piercy V et al. Thermal, but not mechanical, nociceptive behavior is altered in the Zucker Diabetic Fatty rat and is independent of glycemic status. *J Diabetes Complications*. 1999;13(3):163–169.

67. Alusik S, Trnavsky K. [Pharmacotherapy of pain in rheumatic disease]. *Vnitr Lek*. 2003;49(6): 490–495.

68. Hong S et al. Early painful diabetic neuropathy is associated with differential changes in tetrodotoxin-sensitive and -resistant sodium channels in dorsal root ganglion neurons in the rat. *J Biol Chem*. 2004;279(28):29341–29350.

69. Craner MJ et al. Changes of sodium channel expression in experimental painful diabetic neuropathy. *Ann Neurol*. 2002;52(6):786–792.

70. Birch PJ et al. Strategies to identify ion channel modulators: current and novel approaches to target neuropathic pain. *Drug Discov Today*. 2004;9(9):410–418.

71. Dick IE et al. Sodium channel blockade may contribute to the analgesic efficacy of antidepressants. *J Pain*. 2007;8(4):315–324.

72. Liu XJ, Salter MW. Purines and pain mechanisms: recent developments. *Curr Opin Investig Drugs*. 2005;6(1):65–75.

73. North RA. Molecular physiology of P2X receptors. *Physiol Rev*. 2002;82(4):1013–1067.

74. Jacobson KA, Jarvis MF, Williams M. Purine and pyrimidine (P2) receptors as drug targets. *J Med Chem*. 2002;45(19):4057–4093.

75. Tsuda M et al. Mechanical allodynia caused by intraplantar injection of P2X receptor agonist in rats: involvement of heteromeric P2X2/3 receptor signaling in capsaicin-insensitive primary afferent neurons. *J Neurosci*. 2000; 20(15):RC90.

76. Jarvis MF et al. Modulation of BzATP and formalin induced nociception: attenuation by the P2X receptor antagonist, TNP-ATP and enhancement by the P2X(3) allosteric modulator, cibacron blue. *Br J Pharmacol*. 2001;132(1):259–269.

77. Migita K et al. Modulation of P2X receptors in dorsal root ganglion neurons of streptozotocin-induced diabetic neuropathy. *Neurosci Lett*. 2009;452(2):200–203.

78. Clapham DE. TRP channels as cellular sensors. *Nature*. 2003;426(6966):517–524.

79. Pabbidi RM et al. Influence of TRPV1 on diabetes-induced alterations in thermal pain sensitivity. *Mol Pain*. 2008;4:9.

80. Lopshire JC, Nicol GD. The cAMP transduction cascade mediates the prostaglandin E2 enhancement of the capsaicin-elicited current in rat sensory neurons: whole-cell and single-channel studies. *J Neurosci*. 1998;18(16):6081–6092.

81. Cesare P, McNaughton P. A novel heat-activated current in nociceptive neurons and its sensitization by bradykinin. *Proc Natl Acad Sci USA*. 1996;93(26):15435–15439.

82. Sugiuar T, Bielefeldt K, Gebhart GF. TRPV1 function in mouse colon sensory neurons is enhanced by metabotropic 5-hydroxytryptamine receptor activation. *J Neurosci*. 2004;24(43):9521–9530.

83. Shu X, Mendell LM. Acute sensitization by NGF of the response of small-diameter sensory neurons to capsaicin. *J Neurophysiol*. 2001;86(6):2931–2938.

84. The Capsaicin Study Group. Treatment of painful diabetic neuropathy with topical capsaicin. A multicenter, double-blind, vehicle-controlled study. The Capsaicin Study Group. *Arch Intern Med*. 1991;151:2225–2229.

85. Pezet S, McMahon SB. Neurotrophins: mediators and modulators of pain. *Annu Rev Neurosci*. 2006;29:507–538.

86. Leinninger GM, Vincent AM, Feldman EL. The role of growth factors in diabetic peripheral neuropathy. *J Periph Nerv Syst*. 2004;9:26–53.

87. Brown A, Ricci MJ, Weaver LC. NGF mRNA is expressed in the dorsal root ganglia after spinal cord injury in the rat. *Exp Neurol*. 2007;205(1): 283–286.

88. Yamamoto M et al. Expression of mRNAs for neurotrophic factors (NGF, BDNF, NT-3, and GDNF) and their receptors (p75NGFR, trkA, trkB, and trkC) in the adult human peripheral nervous system and nonneural tissues. *Neurochem Res*. 1996;21(8):929–938.

89. Lindsay RM. Role of neurotrophins and trk receptors in the development and maintenance of sensory neurons: an overview. *Philos Trans R Soc Lond B Biol Sci*. 1996;351(1338):365–373.

90. McMahon SB NGF as a mediator of inflammatory pain. *Philos Trans R Soc Lond B Biol Sci*. 1996;351:431–440.

91. Unger JW et al. Nerve growth factor (NGF) and diabetic neuropathy in the rat: morphological investigations of the sural nerve, dorsal root ganglion, and spinal cord. *Exp Neurol*. 1998;153:23–34.

92. Tomlinson DR, Fernyhough P, Diemel LT. Neurotrophins and peripheral neuropathy. *Philos Trans R Soc Lond B Biol Sci*. 1996;351:455–462.

93. Fernyhough P et al. Altered neurotrophin mRNA levels in peripheral nerve and skeletal muscle of experimentally diabetic rats. *J Neurochem.* 1995;64:1231–1237.

94. Schmidt RE et al. Effect of streptozotocin-induced diabetes on NGF, P75(NTR) and TrkA content of prevertebral and paravertebral rat sympathetic ganglia. *Brain Res.* 2000;867:149–156.

95. Christianson JA, Riekhof JT, Wright DE. Restorative effects of neurotrophin treatment on diabetes-induced cutaneous axon loss in mice. *Exp Neurol.* 2003; 179:188–199.

96. Tomlinson DR, Fernyhough P, Diemel LT. Role of neurotrophins in diabetic neuropathy and treatment with nerve growth factors. *Diabetes.* 1997;46:S43–S49.

97. Biessels GJ et al. Insulin partially reverses deficits in peripheral nerve blood flow and conduction in experimental diabetes. *J Neurol Sci.* 1996;140:12–20.

98. Abe S et al. Nitric oxide synthase expressions in rat dorsal root ganglion after a hind limb tourniquet. *Neuroreport.* 2003;14(17): 2267–2270.

99. Vareniuk I et al. Peripheral neuropathy in mice with neuronal nitric oxide synthase gene deficiency. *Int J Mol Med.* 2009;23(5):571–580.

100. Bujalska M et al. Effect of cyclooxygenase and nitric oxide synthase inhibitors on streptozotocin-induced hyperalgesia in rats. *Pharmacology.* 2008;81(2):151–157.

101. Vareniuk I, Pavlov IA, Obrosova IG. Inducible nitric oxide synthase gene deficiency counteracts multiple manifestations of peripheral neuropathy in a streptozotocin-induced mouse model of diabetes. *Diabetologia.* 2008;51(11): 2126–2133.

102. Cameron NE et al. *Inhibitors of advanced glycation end product formation and neurovascular dysfunction in experimental diabetes. Ann NY Acad Sci.* 2005;1043:784–792.

103. Khan N et al. Ameliorative potential of spironolactone in diabetes induced hyperalgesia in mice. *Yakugaku Zasshi.* 2009;129(5):593–599.

104. Woolf CJ, Salter MW. Neuronal plasticity: increasing the gain in pain. *Science.* 2000; 288(5472):1765–1769.

105. Woolf CJ. Central sensitization: uncovering the relation between pain and plasticity. *Anesthesiology.* 2007;106(4):864–867.

106. Costigan M, Woolf CJ. Pain: molecular mechanisms. *J Pain.* 2000;1(3 suppl):35–44.

107. Haddad JJ. *N*-methyl-D-aspartate (NMDA) and the regulation of mitogen-activated protein kinase (MAPK) signaling pathways: a revolving neurochemical axis for therapeutic intervention? *Prog Neurobiol.* 2005;77(4):252–282.

108. Cheng HT et al. Inflammatory pain-induced signaling events following a conditional deletion of the *N*-methyl-D-aspartate receptor in spinal cord dorsal horn. *Neuroscience.* 2008;155(3): 948–958.

109. Begon S et al. Magnesium and MK-801 have a similar effect in two experimental models of neuropathic pain. *Brain Res.* 2000;887(2):436–439.

110. Aley KO, Levine JD. Different peripheral mechanisms mediate enhanced nociception in metabolic/toxic and traumatic painful peripheral neuropathies in the rat. *Neuroscience.* 2002;111(2):389–397.

111. Buvanendran A, Kroin JS. Early use of memantine for neuropathic pain. *Anesth Analg.* 2008;107(4):1093–1094.

112. Singleton, JR, Smith AG. Neuropathy associated with prediabetes: what is new in 2007? *Curr Diabetes Rep.* 2007;7(6):420–424.

113. Llewelyn JG, et al. Acute painful diabetic neuropathy precipitated by strict glycaemic control. *Acta Neuropathol.* 1986;72(2):157–163.

114. Steel JM et al. Clinically apparent eating disorders in young diabetic women: associations with painful neuropathy and other complications. *Br Med J (Clin Res Ed).* 1987;294(6576):859–862.

115. Benbow SJ et al. A prospective study of painful symptoms, small-fibre function and peripheral vascular disease in chronic painful diabetic neuropathy. *Diabetes Med.* 1994;11(1):17–21.

116. Rao SS, Disraeli P, McGregor T. Impaired glucose tolerance and impaired fasting glucose. *Am Fam Physician.* 2004;69(8):1961–1968.

117. Melzack R The McGill Pain Questionnaire: major properties and scoring methods. *Pain.* 1975;1(3):277–299.

118. Dworkin RH et al. Development and initial validation of an expanded and revised version of the Short-form McGill Pain Questionnaire (SF-MPQ-2). Pain. 2009;144(1–2):35–42.

119. Krause SJ, Backonja MM. Development of a neuropathic pain questionnaire. *Clin J Pain.* 2003;19(5):306–314.

120. Backonja MM, Krause SJ. *Neuropathic pain questionnaire—short* form. Clin J Pain. 2003; 19(5):315–316.

121. Zelman DC et al. Validation of a modified version of the Brief Pain Inventory for painful diabetic peripheral neuropathy. *J Vasc Nurs.* 2005;23(3):97–104.

122. Bouhassira D et al. Development and validation of the Neuropathic Pain Symptom Inventory. *Pain.* 2004; 108(3):248–257.

123. Caselli A et al. Role of C-nociceptive fibers in the nerve axon reflex-related vasodilation in diabetes. *Neurology*. 2003;60(2):297–300.

124. Catalan V et al. *Proinflammatory cytokines in obesity: impact of type 2 diabetes mellitus and gastric bypass. Obes Surg.* 2007;17(11): 1464–1474.

125. Sorensen L, Molyneaux L, Yue DK. The relationship among pain, sensory loss, and small nerve fibers in diabetes. *Diabetes Care*. 2006;29(4): 883–887.

126. Sorensen L, Molyneaux L, Yue DK. The level of small nerve fiber dysfunction does not predict pain in diabetic neuropathy: a study using quantitative sensory testing. *Clin J Pain*. 2006;22(3):261–265.

127. Said G. Diabetic neuropathy—a review. *Nat Clin Pract Neurol*. 2007;3(6):331–340.

128. Yagihashi S. Pathology and pathogenetic mechanisms of diabetic neuropathy. *Diabetes Metab Rev*. 1995;11(3):193–225.

129. Yagihashi S, Yamagishi S, Wada R. Pathology and pathogenetic mechanisms of diabetic neuropathy: correlation with clinical signs and symptoms. *Diabetes Res Clin Pract*. 2007;77(suppl 1): S184–S189.

130. Malik RA, et al. Sural nerve pathology in diabetic patients with minimal but progressive neuropathy. *Diabetologia*. 2005;48(3):578–585.

131. Thrainsdottir S et al. Endoneurial capillary abnormalities presage deterioration of glucose tolerance and accompany peripheral neuropathy in man. *Diabetes*. 2003;52(10): 2615–2622.

132. Backonja M et al. Gabapentin for the symptomatic treatment of painful neuropathy in patients with diabetes mellitus: a randomized controlled trial. *JAMA*. 1998;280(21):1831–1836.

133. Dallocchio C et al. Gabapentin vs. amitriptyline in painful diabetic neuropathy: an open-label pilot study. *J Pain Symptom Manage*. 2000;20(4):280–285.

134. Morello CM et al. Randomized double-blind study comparing the efficacy of gabapentin with amitriptyline on diabetic peripheral neuropathy pain. *Arch Intern Med*. 1999;159(16): 1931–1937.

135. Lesser H et al. Pregabalin relieves symptoms of painful diabetic neuropathy: a randomized controlled trial. *Neurology*. 2004;63(11): 2104–2110.

136. Rosenstock J et al. Pregabalin for the treatment of painful diabetic peripheral neuropathy: a double-blind, placebo-controlled trial. *Pain*. 2004;110(3):628–638.

137. Freynhagen R et al. Efficacy of pregabalin in neuropathic pain evaluated in a 12-week, randomised, double-blind, multicentre, placebo-controlled trial of flexible- and fixed-dose regimens. *Pain*. 2005;115(3):254–263.

138. Stacey BR et al. Pregabalin in the treatment of refractory neuropathic pain: results of a 15-month open-label trial. *Pain Med*. 2008;9(8):1202–1208.

139. Max MB et al. Effects of desipramine, amitriptyline, and fluoxetine on pain in diabetic neuropathy. *N Engl J Med*. 1992;326(19):1250–1256.

140. Sindrup SH et al. Imipramine treatment in diabetic neuropathy: relief of subjective symptoms without changes in peripheral and autonomic nerve function. *Eur J Clin Pharmacol*. 1989;37(2):151–153.

141. Sindrup SH, Jensen TS. Efficacy of pharmacological treatments of neuropathic pain: an update and effect related to mechanism of drug action. *Pain*. 1999;83(3):389–400.

142. Sindrup SH et al. Clomipramine vs. desipramine vs. placebo in the treatment of diabetic neuropathy symptoms. A double-blind cross-over study. *Br J Clin Pharmacol*. 1990; 30(5):683–691.

143. Collins SL et al. Antidepressants and anticonvulsants for diabetic neuropathy and postherpetic neuralgia: a quantitative systematic review. *J Pain Symptom Manage*. 2000;20(6):449–458.

144. Jann MW, Slade JH. Antidepressant agents for the treatment of chronic pain and depression. *Pharmacotherapy*. 2007;27(11):1571–1587.

145. Jensen MP, Chodroff MJ, Dworkin RH. The impact of neuropathic pain on health-related quality of life: review and implications. *Neurology*. 2007;68(15):1178–1182.

146. Simmons Z, Feldman EL. Update on diabetic neuropathy. *Curr Opin Neurol*. 2002;15(5):595–603.

147. Goldstein DJ et al. Duloxetine vs. placebo in patients with painful diabetic neuropathy. *Pain*. 2005;116(1–2):109–118.

148. Raskin J et al. A double-blind, randomized multicenter trial comparing duloxetine with placebo in the management of diabetic peripheral neuropathic pain. *Pain Med*. 2005;6(5):346–356.

149. Wernicke JF et al. A randomized controlled trial of duloxetine in diabetic peripheral neuropathic pain. *Neurology*. 2006;67(8):1411–1420.

150. Rowbotham MC et al. Venlafaxine extended release in the treatment of painful diabetic neuropathy: a double-blind, placebo-controlled study. *Pain*. 2004;110(3):697–706.

151. Giannopoulos S et al. Patient compliance with SSRIs and gabapentin in painful diabetic neuropathy. *Clin J Pain*. 2007;23(3):267–269.

152. Brosen K et al. Pharmacogenetics of tricyclic and novel antidepressants: recent developments. *Clin Neuropharmacol.* 1992;15(suppl 1 pt A): 80A–81A.

153. Wiffen P et al. Anticonvulsant drugs for acute and chronic pain. *Cochrane Database Syst Rev.* 2005(3):CD001133.

154. Kochar DK et al. Sodium valproate for painful diabetic neuropathy: a randomized double-blind placebo-controlled study. *QJM.* 2004; 97(1):33–38.

155. Eisenberg E et al. Lamotrigine reduces painful diabetic neuropathy: a randomized, controlled study. *Neurology.* 2001;57(3):505–509.

156. Vinik AI et al. Lamotrigine for treatment of pain associated with diabetic neuropathy: results of two randomized, double-blind, placebo-controlled studies. *Pain.* 2007;128(1–2):169–179.

157. Donofrio PD et al. Safety and effectiveness of topiramate for the management of painful diabetic peripheral neuropathy in an open-label extension study. *Clin Ther.* 2005;27(9): 1420–1431.

158. Raskin P et al. Topiramate vs. placebo in painful diabetic neuropathy: analgesic and metabolic effects. *Neurology.* 2004;63(5): 865–873.

159. Dogra S et al. Oxcarbazepine in painful diabetic neuropathy: a randomized, placebo-controlled study. *Eur J Pain.* 2005;9(5):543–554.

160. Beydoun A et al. Oxcarbazepine in painful diabetic neuropathy: results of a dose-ranging study. *Acta Neurol Scand.* 2006;113(6):395–404.

161. Wymer JP et al. Efficacy and safety of lacosamide in diabetic neuropathic pain: an 18-week double-blind placebo-controlled trial of fixed-dose regimens. *Clin J Pain.* 2009;25(5): 376–385.

162. Ziegler D et al. *Efficacy and safety of lacosamide in painful diabetic neuropathy. Diabetes Care.* 2010;33(4):839–841.

163. Harati Y et al. Double-blind randomized trial of tramadol for the treatment of the pain of diabetic neuropathy. *Neurology.* 1998;50(6): 1842–1846.

164. Freeman R et al. Randomized study of tramadol/acetaminophen versus placebo in painful diabetic peripheral neuropathy. *Curr Med Res Opin.* 2007;23(1):147–161.

165. Gimbel JS, Richards P, Portenoy RK. Controlled-release oxycodone for pain in diabetic neuropathy: a randomized controlled trial. *Neurology.* 2003;60(6):927–934.

166. Watson CP et al. Controlled-release oxycodone relieves neuropathic pain: a randomized controlled trial in painful diabetic neuropathy. *Pain.* 2003;105(1–2):71–78.

167. Sang CN et al. Dextromethorphan and memantine in painful diabetic neuropathy and posttherpetic neuralgia: efficacy and dose-response trials. *Anesthesiology.* 2002;96(5):1053–1061.

168. Effect of treatment with capsaicin on daily activities of patients with painful diabetic neuropathy. Capsaicin Study Group. *Diabetes Care.* 1992;15(2):159–165.

169. Yuen KC, Baker NR, Rayman G. Treatment of chronic painful diabetic neuropathy with isosorbide dinitrate spray: a double-blind placebo-controlled cross-over study. *Diabetes Care.* 2002;25(10):1699–1703.

170. Barbano RL et al. Effectiveness, tolerability, and impact on quality of life of the 5% lidocaine patch in diabetic polyneuropathy. *Arch Neurol.* 2004;61(6):914–918.

171. Gilron I et al. Morphine, gabapentin, or their combination for neuropathic pain. *N Engl J Med.* 2005;352(13):1324–1334.

172. Strokov IA et al. The function of endogenous protective systems in patients with insulin-dependent diabetes mellitus and polyneuropathy: effect of antioxidant therapy. *Bull Exp Biol Med.* 2000;130(10):986–990.

173. Jain SK, Lim G. Lipoic acid decreases lipid peroxidation and protein glycosylation and increases (Na(+) + K(+))- and Ca(++)-ATPase activities in high glucose-treated human erythrocytes. *Free Radic Biol Med.* 2000;29(11):1122–1128.

174. Kishi Y et al. Alpha-lipoic acid: effect on glucose uptake, sorbitol pathway, and energy metabolism in experimental diabetic neuropathy. *Diabetes.* 1999;48(10):2045–2051.

175. Stevens MJ et al. Effects of DL-alpha-lipoic acid on peripheral nerve conduction, blood flow, energy metabolism, and oxidative stress in experimental diabetic neuropathy. *Diabetes.* 2000;49(6):1006–1015.

176. Ziegler D et al. Treatment of symptomatic diabetic peripheral neuropathy with the antioxidant α-lipoic acid—a 3-week multicentre randomized controlled trial (ALADIN study). *Diabetologia.* 1995;38:1425–1433.

177. Reljanovic M et al. Treatment of diabetic polyneuropathy with the antioxidant thioctic acid (alpha-lipoic acid): a two year multicenter randomized double-blind placebo-controlled trial (ALADIN II). Alpha Lipoic Acid in Diabetic Neuropathy. *Free Radic Res.* 1999;31(3): 171–179.

178. Ziegler D et al. Treatment of symptomatic diabetic polyneuropathy with the antioxidant

alpha-lipoic acid: a 7-month multicenter randomized controlled trial (ALADIN III Study). ALADIN III Study Group. Alpha-Lipoic Acid in Diabetic Neuropathy. *Diabetes Care*. 1999;22:1296–1301.

179. Ziegler D et al. Treatment of symptomatic diabetic polyneuropathy with the antioxidant alpha-lipoic acid: a meta-analysis. *Diabetes Med*. 2004;21(2):114–121.

180. Sima AA et al. Acetyl-L-carnitine improves pain, nerve regeneration, and vibratory perception in patients with chronic diabetic neuropathy: an analysis of two randomized placebo-controlled trials. *Diabetes Care*. 2005;28(1):89–94.

181. Harris RE et al. Traditional Chinese acupuncture and placebo (sham) acupuncture are differentiated by their effects on mu-opioid receptors (MORs). *Neuroimage*. 2009;47(3):1077–1085.

182. Okada K, Kawakita K. Analgesic action of acupuncture and moxibustion: a review of unique approaches in Japan. *Evid Based Complement Alternat Med*. 2009;6(1):11–17.

183. Abuaisha BB, Costanzi JB, Boulton AJ. Acupuncture for the treatment of chronic painful peripheral diabetic neuropathy: a long-term study. *Diabetes Res Clin Pract*. 1998;39(2):115–121.

184. Kunnumpurath S, Srinivasagopalan R, Vadivelu N. Spinal cord stimulation: principles of past, present and future practice: a review. *J Clin Monit Comput*. 2009;23(5):333–339.

185. Kumar K et al. The effects of spinal cord stimulation in neuropathic pain are sustained: a 24-month follow-up of the prospective randomized controlled multicenter trial of the effectiveness of spinal cord stimulation. *Neurosurgery*. 2008;63(4):762–770; discussion 770.

186. de Vos CC et al. Effect and safety of spinal cord stimulation for treatment of chronic pain caused by diabetic neuropathy. *J Diabetes Complications*. 2009;23(1):40–45.

187. Daousi C.-, Benbow SJ, MacFarlane IA. Electrical spinal cord stimulation in the long-term treatment of chronic painful diabetic neuropathy. *Diabetes Med*. 2005;22(4):393–398.

188. Reichstein L et al. Effective treatment of symptomatic diabetic polyneuropathy by high-frequency external muscle stimulation. *Diabetologia*. 2005;48(5):824–828.

189. Harkless LB et al. Improved foot sensitivity and pain reduction in patients with peripheral neuropathy after treatment with monochromatic infrared photo energy—MIRE. *J Diabetes Complications*. 2006;20(2):81–87.

190. Moore RA et al. Pregabalin for acute and chronic pain in adults. *Cochrane Database Syst Rev*. 2009(3):CD007076.

191. Lunn MP, Hughes RA, Wiffen PJ. Duloxetine for treating painful neuropathy or chronic pain. *Cochrane Database Syst Rev*. 2009(4):CD007115.

192. Saarto T, Wiffen PJ. Antidepressants for neuropathic pain. *Cochrane Database Syst Rev*. 2007(4):CD005454.

12

HIV-Associated Distal Symmetric Polyneuropathy

JESSICA ROBINSON-PAPP, JUSTIN C. MCARTHUR, AND DAVID M. SIMPSON

INTRODUCTION

NEARLY 30 YEARS have passed since the beginning of the acquired immune deficiency syndrome (AIDS) epidemic in the United States. In that time, remarkable progress has been made in treating patients infected with the human immunodeficiency virus (HIV). Highly active antiretroviral therapy (HAART) has made HIV a manageable chronic illness for many patients. This progress has led to a change in the neurological manifestations of HIV. Dramatic neurological disorders associated with profound immunosuppression, such as primary central nervous system lymphoma, cryptococcal meningitis, and cytomegalovirus-induced progressive polyradiculopathy, have become less common. The neurological disorders that have persisted, even among patients who have responded well to HAART, are more insidious and chronic. Of these, HIV-associated distal symmetric polyneuropathy (HIV-DSP) is the most common.

While HIV-DSP is not a life-threatening condition, it can be a source of significant morbidity and reduction in the quality of life, primarily due to neuropathic pain. The management of neuropathic pain is difficult, and certain factors common in the HIV-positive population create even greater challenges. HIV disproportionately affects minority persons of low socioeconomic status who have historically had poorer access to medical care and greater mistrust of the health care system. This can impede the establishment of the strong therapeutic relationship between patient and provider needed to best treat chronic pain. Patients frequently report social instability and isolation, a history of physical or sexual abuse, substance use disorders, and other psychiatric illnesses, all of which may reduce their ability to cope with chronic pain and limit the provider's therapeutic options. Comorbid conditions are very common in HIV, some of which, like diabetes, renal failure, hepatitis C, and poor nutritional status, can worsen neuropathy and chronic pain.

This chapter will address HIV-DSP including the epidemiology, clinical presentation, diagnostic evaluation, and pathophysiology. The treatments for neuropathic pain due to HIV-DSP are similar to those used for other forms of neuropathic pain. These will be addressed briefly, with emphasis on data specific to HIV and the assessment and treatment of pain in high-risk populations.

EPIDEMIOLOGY

HIV is one of the greatest global public health challenges. It is estimated that in the United States, approximately 339 per 100,000 people are infected with HIV. In certain populations, rates are much higher—for example, those in cities such as New York City, Washington, D.C., and Miami. Minorities are also disproportionately affected. African-Americans and Hispanics represent 48% and 17% of people living with HIV/AIDS, respectively, but only 13% and 12% of the total population.[1] HIV-DSP is very common among patients with HIV. Between one-half and two-thirds of patients have signs of HIV-DSP on neurological examination. The prevalence of symptomatic HIV-DSP is 25%–50%.[2-5] A toxic neuropathy due to antiretrovirals such as stavudine (d4T), didanosine (ddI), and zalcitabine (ddC), referred to as *d-drugs*, is also well described but has become relatively rare as these agents have fallen into disuse in resource-rich environments.[6] However, d4T is still widely used in the developing world and is included in fixed-dose generic antiretroviral combinations. Data emerging from those areas suggest a persistently high prevalence of toxic neuropathy, thought to be due to mitochondrial toxicity.[7] Recent data also suggest that ethnicity and certain genetic profiles may represent risk factors for the development of toxic neuropathy.[8,9]

Prior to the advent of HAART, HIV-DSP was associated with markers of advanced HIV infection, such as a low CD4 count and a high plasma HIV viral load.[10] Today the importance of these risk factors is less clear. In general, HAART-era studies have demonstrated either no association between CD4 count and HIV-DSP or a negative correlation in which a higher CD4 count was associated with HIV-DSP.[3,4] Other studies have found demographic variables such as older age, height, male gender, and white race to be associated with HIV-DSP.[3,5,11] Recent data from the CNS HIV Antiviral Therapy Effects Research (CHARTER) study indicate that increasing age is a very important risk factor,[12] corroborating data from numerous prior studies.[3,5]

NATURAL HISTORY AND SOCIETAL IMPACT

HIV-DSP may develop at any time during the course of infection. In one study, the mean time to development of neuropathy was 9.5 years after HIV diagnosis.[9] Onset is typically insidious except in the case of toxic neuropathy, which can be more rapid in onset. HIV-DSP is not necessarily progressive. In a cohort study that followed patients with and without HIV-DSP over 48 weeks,[5] 10 of 28 (36%) participants without HIV-DSP at baseline developed it during the study. Participants who had HIV-DSP at baseline experienced no worsening during the study, as measured by a change in the mean total neuropathy score (TNS). Notably, 10 of 53 (19%) participants with symptomatic HIV-DSP at baseline improved.

There is scant research addressing the effect of HIV-DSP on quality of life. One study showed a reduced quality of life in patients with HIV-DSP in multiple domains including general overall perception of health, physical functioning, level of pain, energy level, and role functioning.[13] While there is no research addressing the impact of HIV-DSP on patients' communities or on society as a whole, the impact of HIV itself has been studied extensively. In European studies, HIV infection has been associated with high rates of unemployment, especially among those with lower positions in the labor market.[14] In the United States, the impact of HIV is especially marked in the African-American community. African-Americans have the highest rates of new infection and high rates of comorbid diseases such as liver, kidney, and metabolic disease and depression. Sociocultural factors including poverty, lack of health insurance, mistrust of the medical establishment, and stigmatization of HIV are also likely to contribute to the poorer health outcomes experienced by African-Americans with HIV.[15] Many of these factors may interact with one another to increase risks. For example, poverty and associated hopelessness are linked to increased risk-taking behaviors.[16] One manifestation of mistrust of the medical establishment is genocidal conspiracy theories about the origins of HIV, which have also been associated with risky behaviors such as decreased condom use.[17] These issues have a clear detrimental impact on the African-American community, but the ethical and public health implications have a negative impact on American society as a whole.[18]

CLINICAL FEATURES AND DIAGNOSTIC EVALUATION

HIV-DSP typically presents with predominantly sensory symptoms in a distal, symmetric distribution. Patients may experience "negative" symptoms such as numbness, tightness, or clumsiness or "positive" symptoms such as pain, burning, or sensitivity. These symptoms may be spontaneous or evoked by mechanical stimulation. As HIV-DSP progresses, the more proximal lower extremities and ultimately the hands may be involved, producing the classic "stocking and glove" distribution. Neurological examination may reveal one or more of the following signs: decreased distal vibratory, temperature, or pinprick sensation; distal hyperalgesia; or ankle deep tendon reflexes that are absent or reduced compared to those of the knees. Proprioception and strength are often normal. Relatively hyperactive patellar reflexes may be elicited and likely reflect the high prevalence of coexisting central nervous system disease in HIV.

HIV-DSP presenting with typical signs and symptoms is often not extensively evaluated, partly due to its high prevalence. It is advisable to conduct a limited search for common comorbidities that might contribute to HIV-DSP and be amenable to treatment. Demographic shifts, longer life, and overall improved well-being have changed the health challenges faced by the HIV-positive community. In addition to increasing the disease burden, many of the comorbid conditions affecting HIV-positive

patients can cause or worsen neuropathy and neuropathic pain.

Diabetes mellitus and vitamin deficiencies, especially of vitamin B_{12}, are well-known risk factors for neuropathy and are prevalent in HIV. Diabetes is associated with HAART, although HIV itself and other factors, such as the obesity epidemic and the shift of HIV to ethnic groups with a propensity for diabetes, may also be contributory.[19] Dietary factors are also likely to be important. Dietary habits simultaneously conducive to obesity and poor in vitamin content, such as low consumption of fruits and vegetables and high consumption of processed foods, are associated with low socioeconomic status.[20] A large study of HIV-positive patients in the HAART era revealed that nutritional deficiencies were common and were correlated with lower socioeconomic status rather than with stage of disease.[21] Other systemic conditions associated with HIV that may contribute to neuropathy include renal failure, hepatitis C coinfection, and rheumatological disorders.

Numerous drugs used in the treatment of HIV and associated conditions are potentially neurotoxic. The toxic neuropathy associated with the d-drug antiretrovirals is discussed above. Other potentially neurotoxic medications used for HIV-related conditions include chloramphenicol, dapsone, ethambutol, etoposide, isoniazid, metronidazole, pyridoxine, thalidomide, and vincristine.[22]

Diagnostic evaluation for HIV-DSP should include blood tests to exclude glucose intolerance or diabetes and vitamin B_{12} deficiency, and inquiry concerning the use of any neurotoxic drugs or alcohol consumption. Nerve conduction studies and electromyography (EMG) are helpful to confirm the diagnosis and document the severity of the condition, but these may be normal in mild cases or if small fibers are preferentially involved. Nerve biopsy is reserved for highly atypical cases.

Other tests, including quantitative sensory testing (QST), intraepidermal nerve fiber density (INFD) measurement, and quantitative sudomotor axon reflex testing (QSART), may be helpful in documenting small-fiber neuropathy. These diagnostic techniques are particularly useful in cases where objective evidence of neuropathy is important, such as in clinical research trials, or when contemplating opioid treatment in high-risk patients without other objective evidence of HIV-DSP.

Quantitative sensory testing has been used extensively in studies of HIV-DSP and other neuropathies.[5,11] In this procedure, sensory stimuli are applied to standardized sites, such as the great toe. Available stimuli include cold sensation, warm sensation, heat/pain, and vibration. For each modality, a computer-driven algorithm is used to determine a sensory threshold defined as the minimal intensity stimulus that the patient is reliably able to detect. This threshold can be compared to age-adjusted normal values and followed over time.

Intraepidermal nrve fiber density is measured in skin biopsy specimens. The technique requires that small punch biopsy specimens be taken from the skin on the thigh and leg. The specimens are then examined microscopically and compared between the two sites and to standardized values. In general, INFD in the distal lower extremity correlates well with the clinical and electrophysiological severity of HIV-DSP.[23] However, some patients with clinical signs consistent with HIV-DSP have normal INFD.[24] This potentially reflects the length-dependent nature of the neuropathy; thus, if biopsy is performed proximal to the location of nerve fiber injury, the biopsy will perforce be normal. Quantitative sudomotor axon reflex testing is an alternative approach to the assessment of small-fiber neuropathy. This test measures the integrity of the postganglionic sympathetic sudomotor axon. Acetylcholine is iontophoresed into the skin at four standardized sites (forearm, proximal lateral leg, medial distal leg, and proximal foot). The sweat response is measured and compared to normal values. Loss of sudomotor axons leads to decreased sweating, which is correlated with distal small-fiber neuropathy.[25] Although QSART is a widely used technique in the investigation of neuropathy, there are limited data about its use specifically in HIV-DSP.

Several measures have been used to screen for and quantify HIV-DSP, particularly in the research setting. The TNS incorporates neuropathic symptoms (sensory, motor, and autonomic), elements of the neurological examination (pinprick and vibration sensation, strength, and deep tendon reflexes), and neurophysiological testing (QST and nerve conduction studies) to produce a quantitative measure of neuropathy severity.[26] The brief peripheral neuropathy screen (BPNS) was designed for use by nonneurologists for the detection of HIV-DSP. The BPNS consists of questions about pain, paresthesias, and numbness in the distal lower extremities and examination of vibratory sense and ankle reflexes.[5]

PATHOGENESIS

The peripheral nerve pathology of HIV-DSP has not been comprehensively studied in the HAART era. Studies from the late 1980s and early 1990s reported variable and inconsistent pathological features including axonal loss, demyelination, and macrophagic or lymphocytic inflammation.[27–31] Examination of the peripheral nerves included biopsy and autopsy specimens from patients with different types of neuropathy including HIV-DSP, inflammatory demyelinating polyneuropathy, and mononeuropathy. Correlation with clinical signs and symptoms was inconsistent, with some studies noting sural nerve abnormalities in patient with no neuropathy, or without clinical data.[28,31] Other studies focused on dorsal root ganglia (DRG) and demonstrated variable amounts of inflammation with lymphocytes and HIV-infected activated macrophages.[32,33]

The observation of inflammatory cells in peripheral nerve and DRG, and the lack of demonstrable HIV virus in many of these tissues, has led to a proposed immunological basis for the pathogenesis of HIV-DSP. In this theory, HIV leads to activation of immune cells such as macrophages and microglia, which then produce cytokines and excitatory amino acids that lead to axonal injury.[34] Some support for this mechanism has come from animal and in vitro models. Many of these models make use of the HIV envelope protein, gp120, which binds to epitopes present on peripheral nerve and DRG neurons and is thought to be pathogenic in HIV-DSP.[35,36]

In the rodent model, the sciatic nerve is exposed to gp120. This produces persistent mechanical hypersensitivity, as reflected by hind paw withdrawal in response to application of a filament. Pathological findings in this model resemble those documented in humans: decreased INFD in the distal limb, macrophage infiltration in the nerve and the DRG, and activated microglia in the dorsal horn of the spinal cord.[37] In vitro models have used DRG cell cultures that may be compartmentalized to expose the cell bodies and axons to different experimental conditions. These models have suggested that gp120-mediated neurotoxicity is caused by an interaction between the Schwann cell and the sensory neuron. Specifically, gp120 induces the Schwann cell to release chemokines, which in turn activate an apoptotic pathway in the sensory neuron.[38] There may also be an additional independent mechanism by which gp120 causes toxicity directly to the axon.[39]

The microglial cell is of particular interest in HIV-DSP and its associated neuropathic pain because of its role both in other neurological complications of HIV, such as HIV encephalitis, and in non-HIV models of neuropathic pain. Microglia are resident central nervous system macrophages that are productively infected by HIV.[40] Infection of microglia and other mononuclear phagocytes by HIV leads to a predisposition toward immune activation. In the brain, the subsequent production of neurotoxins, such as pro-inflammatory cytokines, is associated with astrogliosis and synaptic loss and clinically with HIV-associated dementia.[41]

Activation of microglia in the dorsal horn of the spinal cord is characteristic of animal models of non-HIV neuropathy, including the induced diabetes and spared nerve injury models in rats.[42,43] Microglia respond to a wide variety of central nervous system insults; however, in the case of experimental peripheral nerve injury, microglia are activated in the dorsal horn of the spinal cord in the absence of a local precipitating event.[43] Microglial activation is a subacute process, occurring one to several weeks after nerve injury, and is characterized by an increase in the number of microglial cells via both proliferation and infiltration, as well as changes in gene expression and morphology.[44] This results in the release of pro-inflammatory cytokines and other mediators, such as brain-derived neurotrophic factor (BDNF), which may serve as signaling molecules from microglia

to neurons and lead to the establishment of central sensitization.[45]

Several mechanisms by which damaged neurons could recruit microglia to the dorsal horn have been proposed. The neuronal transmembrane protein fractalkine may do so via its interaction with the CXCR1 receptor present on the microglia. A role for fractalkine and its interaction with CXCR1 in the development of neuropathic pain has been supported by experimental data. Intrathecal injection of fractalkine causes allodynia, whereas administration of an anti-CX3CR1 antibody delays the development of allodynia.[46] The chemokine CCL2 has also been implicated. The central terminals of sensory neurons release CCL2 in response to peripheral nerve injury, leading to microglial activation.[47] Mice lacking the CCL2 receptor, CCCR2, show diminished monocyte recruitment and reduced neuropathic pain behavior.[48] Finally, it has been suggested that damaged sensory neurons activate spinal cord glial cells via toll-like receptors (TLR) 2 and 4. Experiments in mice have shown that the development of microglial activation and neuropathic pain is inhibited in TLR2 and TLR4 knockout mice.[49,50]

Many of the same microglial chemokine receptors that have been implicated in the establishment of central sensitization in neuropathic pain models are also HIV coreceptors that play a role in HIV infection of the cell. The association of genetic polymorphisms in these receptors with differences in susceptibility to HIV-1 infection has been studied.[51] Considering the known role of HIV-infected microglia in the pathogenesis of HIV encephalitis, it is interesting to postulate a unique role for microglia in central sensitization at the level of the spinal cord in HIV-DSP, above and beyond that observed in other forms of neuropathic pain.

Similar to the microglial cell, opioids and their receptors are an area of overlap between research in spinal sensitization in neuropathic pain and research relevant to another disorder common in HIV, substance abuse. The μ-opioid receptor (MOR) is a transmembrane G-protein-coupled receptor that reduces neuronal excitability by inhibiting calcium channel currents and activating inward rectifier potassium channel currents.[52] Opioid receptors are present in multiple locations throughout the dorsal horn and play a complex role in pain transmission. Presynaptic opioid receptors inhibit transmission of pain from the primary to the secondary sensory afferent.[53] However, there is also a mechanism by which opioids may facilitate pain transmission. Inhibitory interneurons in the dorsal horn act tonically to inhibit spinothalamic tract neurons. Opioids may inhibit the interneuron, effectively releasing these neurons.[54] Animal models of neuropathic pain have demonstrated a discrete loss of MORs in the dorsal horn at the spinal level corresponding to experimental nerve injury and have proposed this loss as a mechanism for neuropathic pain.[55,56]

The substance abuse literature has described a phenomenon of opioid-induced hyperalgesia in humans and animal models. In human studies, methadone-maintained opiate addicts had decreased cold pressor tolerance compared to controls.[57] In animal models, exposure to opioids either locally, spinally, or systemically results in hyperalgesia. Mechanisms involving multiple sites throughout the nervous system have been proposed, including sensitization of the primary afferents in peripheral nerves, an increase in excitatory neurotransmitters in the dorsal horn, sensitization of secondary afferents to excitatory neurotransmitters, and supraspinal changes.[58] It is interesting to hypothesize that opiate addicts with HIV-DSP may have unique mechanisms contributing to neuropathic pain. There are little human data to support this hypothesis, although one study showed that DSP associated with antiretroviral use was more common in HIV-positive patients with a history of intravenous drug use.[9]

Other mechanisms of neuropathic pain that have been described in experimental models may also play a role, albeit nonspecific, in the neuropathic pain associated with HIV-DSP. These mechanisms involve both the peripheral and central nervous systems. In the periphery after axonal injury, changes occur in the surviving axons. Intact nociceptive afferents (C fibers) may begin to discharge spontaneously. A fibers typically conduct nonnoxious stimuli but may begin to express neuromodulators normally expressed only by C fibers, such as substance P, in effect phenotypically switching to pain-conducting neurons.[59]

In the central nervous system, in addition to the mechanisms described above, increased release of excitatory neurotransmitters (e.g., glutamate, substance P), and enhanced synaptic efficacy have been important in animal models of neuropathic pain. Presynaptic changes demonstrated in rats include upregulation of the α-2-δ subunit of the voltage-gated calcium channel, leading to increased release of excitatory neurotransmitters, which in turn can cause long-term potentiation.[60] Postsynaptic mechanisms include upregulation of α-amino-3-hydroxy-5-methyl-4-isoxazolepropionate (AMPA) and *N*-methyl-D-aspartate (NDMA) receptors leading to a decreased depolarization threshold.[61,62] Other proposed mechanisms include long-term depression (LTD) and selective apoptosis of inhibitory interneurons.[59]

MANAGEMENT, TREATMENT, AND PREVENTION

There is currently no U.S. Food and Drug Administration (FDA)-approved treatment for HIV-DSP or its painful symptoms. Comorbid factors, such as vitamin deficiency or alcohol abuse, should be modified if possible. If the patient is taking neurotoxic medications that can safely be stopped or changed, it may be helpful to do so. As in other forms of neuropathy, clinical trials of potentially neuroregenerative therapies in HIV-DSP have been disappointing. Recombinant human nerve growth factor and prosaptide, agents that were neurotrophic in vitro and in animal models, were not in humans.[63,64] Peptide T, an in vitro inhibitor of gp-120 binding, also failed to show efficacy.[65]

Treatment of HIV-DSP is currently focused on the symptomatic management of neuropathic pain. Since the available treatments do not alter the course of disease, some patients choose to forgo treatment, preferring not to take more medications. For others, neuropathic pain is so debilitating that aggressive management is desired. Neuropathic pain is difficult to treat. Even with aggressive management it is rarely eliminated, and many experts consider a 30%–50% reduction in pain to be a clinically significant response.[66] Recent clinical trials of agents that have shown efficacy

Table 12-1. Potential Barriers to Management of Neuropathic Pain in HIV Patients

TYPE OF BARRIER	POTENTIAL BARRIERS
Medical	Lack of highly efficacious treatments
	Complicated medical illnesses and medication regimens limiting choices of neuropathic pain agents
	Undertreatment of pain in minorities
Psychiatric/psychological	Limited choice of neuropathic pain agents because of drug interactions
	Poorer coping mechanisms
	Complicated therapeutic relationship with provider
	Substance use disorders complicating the use of certain pain medications
	Low self-efficacy
Sociocultural	Poor social support and isolation
	Underutilization of care due to mistrust of the medical establishment
	Poorer access to care due to low socioeconomic status

for neuropathic pain, such as duloxetine and pregabalin, typically report such improvement in approximately 50% of patients.[67,68] Accordingly, a 50% improvement in 50% of patients may be a reasonable, albeit less than ideal, goal for clinicians managing neuropathic pain. This response rate to treatment is important to bear in mind when counseling patients so that realistic expectations can be set (Table 12.1).

In addition to the lack of highly efficacious therapies, there are other potential barriers to effective treatment of neuropathic pain more specific to HIV patients. HIV patients typically have complicated medical conditions that may preclude the use of certain agents due to concern about side effects or drug interactions. Psychiatric disorders, which are prevalent among HIV patients, may also complicate treatment. Patients may already be taking medications used in the treatment of neuropathic pain for psychiatric indications, limiting treatment options. Psychiatric disorders may also interfere with the establishment of an effective therapeutic relationship between the patient and the health care provider that is needed for the optimum management of chronic pain. Substance abuse disorders raise similar issues, with the additional complexity of provider concern over the legal, ethical, and therapeutic implications of prescribing opiates in this population.

Even in the absence of overt psychiatric disease, psychological factors affect the course of disability and pain in chronic pain disorders. Patients with strong perceived self-efficacy, that is, a personal conviction of their ability to perform required behaviors in a given situation, are more likely to develop active, constructive mechanisms for coping with pain.[69] Such mechanisms include willfully distracting attention from pain and continuing activities in spite of pain. In contrast, in patients with low self-efficacy, fear of pain and of the underlying disorder may lead to hypervigilance, preoccupation with bodily symptoms, and avoidance of activities, which in turn lead to deconditioning, worsening pain, and increased disability.[70] HIV occurs most often in disenfranchised populations, in which risk factors for low self-efficacy, such as prior victimization, are prevalent.[71,72] Therefore, low self-efficacy may be a mechanism by which chronic pain due to HIV-DSP may be even more debilitating than other types of neuropathic pain. Self-efficacy has been studied in other HIV-related health outcomes. Higher self-efficacy has been associated with increased condom use[73,74] and adherence to antiretroviral drug regimens.[75]

Social, cultural, and economic factors are also important. Good social support is associated with better physical and emotional health in HIV patients,[76] whereas poor social support is associated with greater pain and disability in chronic pain patients.[70,77] Many patients suffering from HIV are socially isolated. A recent study of older adults with HIV in New York City found that only one in three have a life partner and 71% live by themselves.[78] Networks made up primarily of friends are the primary source of informal caregiving and social support. These friendships replace those lost through stigma and rejection related to HIV and confer the benefits of safety, support, mentorship, and inspiration. However, these networks are inherently fragile due to uncertain health, and high levels of unmet needs for support still exist.[79] Lack of adequate social support likely impairs the ability of HIV patients to cope with chronic neuropathic pain.

There are also cultural barriers to pain control that are important among HIV patients because of the disproportionate number of minority patients affected. There is a historic mistrust of the medical establishment in some minority communities, which is partially founded in long-standing disparities in the health care system.[80] This may lead to patient-dependent disparities including underutilization of care and poorer adherence to medical advice. Clinician-dependent factors also play a role. Hispanic and African-American patients receive less analgesia than white patients with similar pain conditions.[81,82]

Economic disadvantage is yet another barrier to adequate pain management. Due to their low-income status, many HIV patients are dependent on Medicaid for health insurance. Key components of Medicaid are controlled at the state level, including eligibility, service coverage, and provider payments. This leads to great variability in programs by state. Although studies have shown that patients covered by Medicaid do not typically receive poorer care than comparable low-income privately insured patients, it is unlikely that these patients have the same access to medical care as higher-income groups.[83] This may lead to poorer access to the specialty providers most experienced in the care of neuropathic pain.

Treatment recommendations for neuropathic pain due to HIV-DSP are based not only on studies done specifically in HIV but also on inference from the larger diabetic neuropathy and postherpetic neuralgia literature. Clinical trials on the treatment of neuropathic pain due to HIV-DSP are summarized in Table 12-2. In addition to the social considerations discussed above, special concerns in the HIV population include drug-drug interactions and the use of opiates in high-risk populations. Five main classes of agents are used in the treatment of neuropathic pain: anticonvulsants, antidepressants, nonspecific analgesics, topical treatments, and alternative/complementary therapies.

Nearly all of the available anticonvulsants have been used for neuropathic pain. Some are considered especially efficacious for certain types of neuropathic pain, such as carbamazepine for trigeminal neuralgia. Others, such as gabapentin, are used much more broadly. Mechanisms of action vary among the anticonvulsants, but most are related to modification of ion channels. For example, pregabalin binds to voltage-gated calcium channels inhibiting the release of excitatory neurotransmitters including glutamate, substance P, and calcitonin gene-related peptide.[68] Among the anticonvulsants, gabapentin and lamotrigine have shown some efficacy in clinical trials in painful HIV-DSP.[84,85] Pregabalin is also commonly used based on its efficacy in diabetic neuropathy,[68,86] despite the negative results of a recent clinical trial in HIV.[87] Pregabalin and gabapentin are excreted by the kidney, which is advantageous in HIV patients who are often taking hepatically metabolized antiretrovirals. Lamotrigine is metabolized in the liver but does not have known cytochrome P450 interactions. It is used less frequently in clinical practice due in part to the potential side effect of rash and a long titration schedule.

Among the antidepressants, the tricyclic compounds and the selective norepinepherine serotonin reuptake inhibitors are most often used for neuropathic pain. Both classes of drugs undergo hepatic metabolism via cytochome P450 and therefore have potential for interaction with antiretrovirals. Amitriptyline was studied in a placebo-controlled trial in HIV-DSP but failed to show efficacy.[88,89] Duloxetine is commonly used off label in HIV based on the literature in diabetic neuropathy, and studies in HIV-DSP are underway.[67,90] A topical patch containing high-dose capsaicin has shown efficacy

Table 12-2. Clinical Trials in the Treatment of HIV-DSP

TREATMENT	REFERENCE	TRIAL DESIGN AND OUTCOME
Peptide T	Simpson et al.[65]	Placebo-controlled trial of 81 subjects, with change in the Gracely pain score as the primary outcome measure. Peptide T was safe but ineffective.
Amytriptyline and mexiletine	Kieburtz et al.[89]	Compared amytriptyline and mexiletine to placebo in 145 patients using the Gracely pain score. Neither agent was superior to placebo.
Amytriptyline and acupuncture	Shlay et al.[88]	Complicated design with a total of 239 patients receiving combinations of acupucture, amitriptyline, control points, or placebo. Neither intervention was superior to placebo.
Recombinant human nerve growth factor	McArthur et al.[98] Schifitto et al.[63]	Placebo-controlled trial of 270 patients showed improvement on the Gracely pain scale. A subsequent open-label trial with 200 patients confirmed the findings of improved pain but did not show improvement in DSP severity.
Lamotrigine	Simpson et al.[84]	Compared lamotrigine to placebo in 42 patients. Patients receiving lamotrigine had greater improvement in neuropathic pain as measured by the modified Gracely pain scale.
Gabapentin	Hahn et al.[85]	Placebo-controlled trial of 26 patients showed improvement in pain and sleep as measured by the visual analog scale.
Lidocaine gel	Estanislao et al.[92]	Placebo-controlled trial of 64 subjects showed that lidocaine gel was safe but ineffective in relieving pain as measured by the Gracely pain scale.
Prosaptide	Evans et al.[64]	Used the Gracely pain scale in an electronic diary form to monitor pain in 237 patients. Prosaptide was safe but ineffective.
Smoked cannabis	Abrams et al.[95] Ellis et al.[94]	Placebo-controlled trial of 50 patients showed that smoked cannabis was well tolerated and effective. The primary outcome was improvement in the visual analog scale. A subsequent study showed superiority to placebo in 28 patients using the descriptor differential scale.
High-dose capsaicin patch	Simpson et al.[91]	Controlled trial of 307 patients using change in the numeric pain rating score as a primary outcome measure showed reduction in pain for up to 12 weeks.
Hypnosis	Dorfman et al.[93]	Uncontrolled trial of hypnosis in 38 patients showed improvement in pain as measured by the Short Form McGill questionnaire.
Pregabalin	Simpson et al.[99]	Placebo-controlled trial of 302 patients showed no superiority to placebo in pain reduction as measured by a numeric rating score.

in HIV-DSP, and has recently been approved for use in peripheral neuropathic pain in Europe and for postherpetic neuralgia in the United States.[91] Topical lidocaine failed to show superiority to placebo in HIV-DSP but is nonetheless commonly used.[92] Alternative/complementary therapies include hypnosis[93] and smoked cannabis,[94,95] which have both shown efficacy in clinical trials. However, for reasons of access for the former and regulatory concerns for the latter, these treatments are not typically employed in clinical practice. Acupuncture was not efficacious in a controlled clinical trial.[88] Nonspecific analgesics include the nonsteroidal anti-inflammatory drugs (NSAIDs), acetaminophen and opiates. The NSAIDs and acetaminophen are typically ineffective in the management of neuropathic pain, but they may be tried.

The use of opioids in chronic noncancer pain is controversial. Recent guidelines commissioned by the American Pain Society and the American Academy of Pain Medicine acknowledged that evidence for the use of opioids in these patients is limited. The panel stated that opioids may be appropriate for moderate to severe chronic noncancer pain, but it emphasized careful patient selection with an assessment of potential benefits and harms.[96] Risk factors for developing a substance use disorder after receiving opioids for pain include a personal or family history of substance abuse, a personal history of preadolescent sexual abuse, or psychiatric illness of any kind.[97] These factors are highly prevalent in the HIV population, and while they do not entirely preclude the use of opiates, they require the clinician to exercise particular caution. The guidelines described above recommend more frequent and stringent monitoring in high-risk patients and ongoing evaluation for aberrant drug-related behaviors, such as the use of cocaine, the use of unprescribed opioids, or obtaining opioids from multiple sources. A multidisciplinary approach, including involvement of addiction and mental health specialists, may be necessary.[96]

FUTURE DIRECTIONS

The current treatment of HIV-DSP and neuropathic pain has significant limitations. There are no neuroregenerative therapies, and efforts to control neuropathic pain are only partially successful. Thus, there are many potential avenues for future research. Future investigations should explore all aspects of this disease, including the pathogenesis of HIV-DSP and associated pain; targeted neuroregenerative and neuropathic pain drug development; the optimum tools to quantify the signs and symptoms of HIV-DSP in order to improve clinical trial design and communication with patients; and the best use of nonpharmacological interventions for pain including psychosocial interventions and alternative/complementary therapies. This multidisciplinary approach will hopefully provide patients with HIV-DSP with more effective tools to reduce pain and disability and improve their quality of life.

REFERENCES

1. Centers for Disease Control and Prevention. HIV/AIDS surveillance report, 2007. Vol. 19.<http://www.cdc.gov/hiv/topics/surveillance/resources/reports/>. U.S. Department of Health and Human Services, Centers for Disease Control and Prevention, Atlanta. Accessed May 14, 2009.
2. Schifitto G, McDermott MP, McArthur JC, et al. Incidence of and risk factors for HIV-associated distal sensory polyneuropathy. *Neurology*. 2002;58(12):1764–1768.
3. Morgello S, Estanislao L, Simpson D, et al. HIV-associated distal sensory polyneuropathy in the era of highly active antiretroviral therapy: the Manhattan HIV brain bank. *Arch Neurol*. 2004;61(4):546–551.
4. Schifitto G, McDermott MP, McArthur JC, et al. Markers of immune activation and viral load in HIV-associated sensory neuropathy. *Neurology*. 2005;64(5):842–848.
5. Simpson DM, Kitch D, Evans SR, et al. HIV neuropathy natural history cohort study: assessment measures and risk factors. *Neurology*. 2006; 66(11):1679–1687.
6. Simpson DM, Tagliati M. Nucleoside analogue-associated peripheral neuropathy in human immunodeficiency virus infection. *J Acquir Immune Defic Syndr Hum Retrovirol*. 1995;9(2):153–161.
7. Wright E, Brew B, Arayawichanont A, et al. Neurologic disorders are prevalent in HIV-positive outpatients in the Asia-Pacific region. *Neurology*. 2008;71(1):50–56.
8. Cherry CL, Rosenow A, Affandi JS, McArthur JC, Wesselingh SL, Price P. Cytokine genotype suggests a role for inflammation in nucleoside analog-associated sensory neuropathy (NRTI-SN) and predicts an individual's NRTI-SN risk. *AIDS Res Hum Retroviruses*. 2008;24(2):117–123.
9. Robinson-Papp J, Gonzalez-Duarte A, Simpson DM, Rivera-Mindt M, Morgello S. The roles of ethnicity and antiretrovirals in HIV-associated polyneuropathy: a pilot study. *J Acquir Immune Defic Syndr*. 2009;51(5):569–573.
10. Childs EA, Lyles RH, Selnes OA, et al. Plasma viral load and CD4 lymphocytes predict HIV-associated dementia and sensory neuropathy. *Neurology*. 1999;52(3):607–613.

11. Cherry CL, Skolasky RL, Lal L, et al. Antiretroviral use and other risks for HIV-associated neuropathies in an international cohort. *Neurology*. 2006;66(6):867–873.

12. Evans SR, Ellis RJ, Chen H, et al. Peripheral neuropathy in HIV: prevalence and risk factors. *AIDS*. 2011;25(7):919–928.

13. Pandya R, Krentz HB, Gill MJ, Power C. HIV-related neurological syndromes reduce health-related quality of life. *Can J Neurol Sci*. 2005;32(2):201–204.

14. Dray-Spira R, Gueguen A, Lert F, VESPA Study Group. Disease severity, self-reported experience of workplace discrimination and employment loss during the course of chronic HIV disease: differences according to gender and education. *Occup Environ Med*. 2008;65(2):112–119.

15. Rawlings MK, Masters HL 3rd. Comorbidities and challenges affecting African Americans with HIV infection. *J Natl Med Assoc*. 2008;100(12):1477–1481.

16. Bolland JM. Hopelessness and risk behaviour among adolescents living in high-poverty inner-city neighbourhoods. *J Adolesc*. 2003;26(2):145–158.

17. Ross MW, Essien EJ, Torres I. Conspiracy beliefs about the origin of HIV/AIDS in four racial/ethnic groups. *J Acquir Immune Defic Syndr*. 2006;41(3):342–344.

18. Plowden K, Miller JL, James T. HIV health crisis and African Americans: a cultural perspective. *ABNF J*. 2000;11(4):88–93.

19. Samaras K. Prevalence and pathogenesis of diabetes mellitus in HIV-1 infection treated with combined antiretroviral therapy. *J Acquir Immune Defic Syndr*. 2009;50(5):499–505.

20. Cade J. The low income diet and nutrition survey: implications for relationships between diet and disease. *Proc Nutr Soc*. 2008;67(OCE):E89.

21. Kim JH, Spiegelman D, Rimm E, Gorbach SL. The correlates of dietary intake among HIV-positive adults. *Am J Clin Nutr*. 2001;74(6):852–861.

22. Estanislao L, Geraci A, Di Rocco A, Simpson DS. HIV myelopathy, peripheral neuropathy and myopathy. In: Nath A, Berger J, eds. *Clinical Neurovirology*. New York: Marcel Dekker; 2003:315–335.

23. Zhou L, Kitch DW, Evans SR, et al. Correlates of epidermal nerve fiber densities in HIV-associated distal sensory polyneuropathy. *Neurology*. 2007;68(24):2113–2119.

24. Polydefkis M, Yiannoutsos CT, Cohen BA, et al. Reduced intraepidermal nerve fiber density in HIV-associated sensory neuropathy. *Neurology*. 2002;58(1):115–119.

25. Low VA, Sandroni P, Fealey RD, Low PA. Detection of small-fiber neuropathy by sudomotor testing. *Muscle Nerve*. 2006;34(1):57–61.

26. Cornblath DR, Chaudhry V, Carter K, et al. Total neuropathy score: validation and reliability study. *Neurology*. 1999;53(8):1660–1664.

27. Chaunu MP, Ratinahirana H, Raphael M, et al. The spectrum of changes on 20 nerve biopsies in patients with HIV infection. *Muscle Nerve*. 1989;12(6):452–459.

28. de la Monte SM, Gabuzda DH, Ho DD, et al. Peripheral neuropathy in the acquired immunodeficiency syndrome. *Ann Neurol*. 1988;23(5):485–492.

29. Leger JM, Bouche P, Bolgert F, et al. The spectrum of polyneuropathies in patients infected with HIV. *J Neurol Neurosurg Psychiatry*. 1989;52(12):1369–1374.

30. Mah V, Vartavarian LM, Akers MA, Vinters HV. Abnormalities of peripheral nerve in patients with human immunodeficiency virus infection. *Ann Neurol*. 1988;24(6):713–717.

31. Winer JB, Bang B, Clarke JR, et al. A study of neuropathy in HIV infection. *Q J Med*. 1992;83(302):473–488.

32. Pardo CA, McArthur JC, Griffin JW. HIV neuropathy: insights in the pathology of HIV peripheral nerve disease. *J Peripher Nerv Syst*. 2001;6(1):21–27.

33. Rizzuto N, Cavallaro T, Monaco S, et al. Role of HIV in the pathogenesis of distal symmetrical peripheral neuropathy. *Acta Neuropathol*. 1995;90(3):244–250.

34. Herzberg U, Sagen J. Peripheral nerve exposure to HIV viral envelope protein gp120 induces neuropathic pain and spinal gliosis. *J Neuroimmunol*. 2001;116(1):29–39.

35. van den Berg LH, Sadiq SA, Lederman S, Latov N. The gp120 glycoprotein of HIV-1 binds to sulfatide and to the myelin associated glycoprotein. *J Neurosci Res*. 1992;33(4):513–518.

36. Apostolski S, McAlarney T, Quattrini A, et al. The gp120 glycoprotein of human immunodeficiency virus type 1 binds to sensory ganglion neurons. *Ann Neurol*. 1993;34(6):855–863.

37. Wallace VC, Blackbeard J, Pheby T, et al. Pharmacological, behavioural and mechanistic analysis of HIV-1 gp120 induced painful neuropathy. *Pain*. 2007;133(1–3):47–63.

38. Keswani SC, Polley M, Pardo CA, Griffin JW, McArthur JC, Hoke A. Schwann cell chemokine receptors mediate HIV-1 gp120 toxicity to sensory neurons. *Ann Neurol*. 2003;54(3):287–296.

39. Melli G, Keswani SC, Fischer A, Chen W, Hoke A. Spatially distinct and functionally independent

mechanisms of axonal degeneration in a model of HIV-associated sensory neuropathy. *Brain*. 2006;129(pt 5):1330–1338.

40. Cosenza MA, Zhao ML, Si Q, Lee SC. Human brain parenchymal microglia express CD14 and CD45 and are productively infected by HIV-1 in HIV-1 encephalitis. *Brain Pathol*. 2002;12(4):442–455.

41. Kim MO, Suh HS, Si Q, Terman BI, Lee SC. Anti-CD45RO suppresses human immunodeficiency virus type 1 replication in microglia: role of hck tyrosine kinase and implications for AIDS dementia. *J Virol*. 2006;80(1):62–72.

42. Tsuda M, Ueno H, Kataoka A, Tozaki-Saitoh H, Inoue K. Activation of dorsal horn microglia contributes to diabetes-induced tactile allodynia via extracellular signal-regulated protein kinase signaling. *Glia*. 2008;56(4):378–386.

43. Beggs S, Salter MW. Stereological and somatotopic analysis of the spinal microglial response to peripheral nerve injury. *Brain Behav Immun*. 2007;21(5):624–633.

44. Scholz J, Woolf CJ. The neuropathic pain triad: neurons, immune cells and glia. *Nat Neurosci*. 2007;10(11):1361–1368.

45. Coull JA, Beggs S, Boudreau D, et al. BDNF from microglia causes the shift in neuronal anion gradient underlying neuropathic pain. *Nature*. 2005;438(7070):1017–1021.

46. Zhuang ZY, Kawasaki Y, Tan PH, Wen YR, Huang J, Ji RR. Role of the CX3CR1/p38 MAPK pathway in spinal microglia for the development of neuropathic pain following nerve injury-induced cleavage of fractalkine. *Brain Behav Immun*. 2007;21(5):642–651.

47. Thacker MA, Clark AK, Bishop T, et al. CCL2 is a key mediator of microglia activation in neuropathic pain states. *Eur J Pain*. 2009;13(3):263–272.

48. Abbadie C, Lindia JA, Cumiskey AM, et al. Impaired neuropathic pain responses in mice lacking the chemokine receptor CCR2. *Proc Natl Acad Sci USA*. 2003;100(13):7947–7952.

49. Kim D, Kim MA, Cho IH, et al. A critical role of toll-like receptor 2 in nerve injury-induced spinal cord glial cell activation and pain hypersensitivity. *J Biol Chem*. 2007;282(20):14975–14983.

50. Tanga FY, Nutile-McMenemy N, DeLeo JA. The CNS role of toll-like receptor 4 in innate neuroimmunity and painful neuropathy. *Proc Natl Acad Sci USA*. 2005;102(16):5856–5861.

51. Parczewski M, Leszczyszyn-Pynka M, Kaczmarczyk M, et al. Sequence variants of chemokine receptor genes and susceptibility to HIV-1 infection. *J Appl Genet*. 2009;50(2):159–166.

52. Connor M, Christie MD. Opioid receptor signalling mechanisms. *Clin Exp Pharmacol Physiol*. 1999;26(7):493–499.

53. Glaum SR, Miller RJ, Hammond DL. Inhibitory actions of delta 1-, delta 2-, and mu-opioid receptor agonists on excitatory transmission in lamina II neurons of adult rat spinal cord. *J Neurosci*. 1994;14(8):4965–4971.

54. Holden JE, Jeong Y, Forrest JM. The endogenous opioid system and clinical pain management. *AACN Clin Issues*. 2005;16(3):291–301.

55. Kohno T, Ji RR, Ito N, et al. Peripheral axonal injury results in reduced mu opioid receptor pre- and post-synaptic action in the spinal cord. *Pain*. 2005;117(1–2):77–87.

56. Porreca F, Tang QB, Bian D, Riedl M, Elde R, Lai J. Spinal opioid mu receptor expression in lumbar spinal cord of rats following nerve injury. *Brain Res*. 1998;795(1–2):197–203.

57. Pud D, Cohen D, Lawental E, Eisenberg E. Opioids and abnormal pain perception: new evidence from a study of chronic opioid addicts and healthy subjects. *Drug Alcohol Depend*. 2006;82(3):218–223.

58. Chu LF, Angst MS, Clark D. Opioid-induced hyperalgesia in humans: molecular mechanisms and clinical considerations. *Clin J Pain*. 2008;24(6):479–496.

59. Campbell JN, Meyer RA. Mechanisms of neuropathic pain. *Neuron*. 2006;52(1):77–92.

60. Li CY, Song YH, Higuera ES, Luo ZD. Spinal dorsal horn calcium channel alpha2delta-1 subunit upregulation contributes to peripheral nerve injury-induced tactile allodynia. *J Neurosci*. 2004;24(39):8494–8499.

61. Gu JG, Albuquerque C, Lee CJ, MacDermott AB. Synaptic strengthening through activation of Ca^{2+}-permeable AMPA receptors. *Nature*. 1996;381(6585):793–796.

62. Yoshimura M, Yonehara N. Alteration in sensitivity of ionotropic glutamate receptors and tachykinin receptors in spinal cord contribute to development and maintenance of nerve injury-evoked neuropathic pain. *Neurosci Res*. 2006;56(1):21–28.

63. Schifitto G, Yiannoutsos C, Simpson DM, et al. Long-term treatment with recombinant nerve growth factor for HIV-associated sensory neuropathy. *Neurology*. 2001;57(7):1313–1316.

64. Evans SR, Simpson DM, Kitch DW, et al. A randomized trial evaluating prosaptide for HIV-associated sensory neuropathies: use of an electronic diary to record neuropathic pain. *PLoS One*. 2007;2(6):e551.

65. Simpson DM, Dorfman D, Olney RK, et al. Peptide T in the treatment of painful distal neuropathy associated with AIDS: results of a placebo-controlled trial. The Peptide T Neuropathy Study Group. *Neurology*. 1996;47(5):1254–1259.

66. Sindrup SH, Jensen TS. Efficacy of pharmacological treatments of neuropathic pain: an update and effect related to mechanism of drug action. *Pain*. 1999;83(3):389–400.

67. Raskin J, Pritchett YL, Wang F, et al. A double-blind, randomized multicenter trial comparing duloxetine with placebo in the management of diabetic peripheral neuropathic pain. *Pain Med*. 2005;6(5):346–356.

68. Lesser H, Sharma U, LaMoreaux L, Poole RM. Pregabalin relieves symptoms of painful diabetic neuropathy: a randomized controlled trial. *Neurology*. 2004;63(11):2104–2110.

69. Turk DC, Okifuji A. Psychological factors in chronic pain: evolution and revolution. *J Consult Clin Psychol*. 2002;70(3):678–690.

70. Evers AW, Kraaimaat FW, Geenen R, Jacobs JW, Bijlsma JW. Pain coping and social support as predictors of long-term functional disability and pain in early rheumatoid arthritis. *Behav Res Ther*. 2003;41(11):1295–1310.

71. Hovsepian SL, Blais M, Manseau H, Otis J, Girard ME. Prior victimization and sexual and contraceptive self-efficacy among adolescent females under child protective services care. *Health Educ Behav*. 2010;37(1):65–83.

72. Martinez J, Hosek SG, Carleton RA. Screening and assessing violence and mental health disorders in a cohort of inner city HIV-positive youth between 1998–2006. *AIDS Patient Care STDS*. 2009;23(6):469–475.

73. Strathdee SA, Mausbach B, Lozada R, et al. Predictors of sexual risk reduction among Mexican female sex workers enrolled in a behavioral intervention study. *J Acquir Immune Defic Syndr*. 2009;51(suppl 1):S42–S46.

74. Basen-Engquist K, Parcel GS. Attitudes, norms, and self-efficacy: A model of adolescents' HIV-related sexual risk behavior. *Health Educ Q*. 1992;19(2):263–277.

75. Ammassari A, Trotta MP, Murri R, et al. Correlates and predictors of adherence to highly active antiretroviral therapy: overview of published literature. *J Acquir Immune Defic Syndr*. 2002; 31 Suppl 3:S123–7.

76. Gielen AC, McDonnell KA, Wu AW, O'Campo P, Faden R. Quality of life among women living with HIV: the importance violence, social support, and self care behaviors. *Soc Sci Med*. 2001;52(2):315–322.

77. Feldman SI, Downey G, Schaffer-Neitz R. Pain, negative mood, and perceived support in chronic pain patients: a daily diary study of people with reflex sympathetic dystrophy syndrome. *J Consult Clin Psychol*. 1999;67(5):776–785.

78. Shippy RA, Karpiak SE. The aging HIV/AIDS population: fragile social networks. *Aging Ment Health*. 2005;9(3):246–254.

79. Poindexter C, Shippy RA. Networks of older New Yorkers with HIV: fragility, resilience, and transformation. *AIDS Patient Care STDS*. 2008;22(9):723–733.

80. Suite DH, La Bril R, Primm A, Harrison-Ross P. Beyond misdiagnosis, misunderstanding and mistrust: relevance of the historical perspective in the medical and mental health treatment of people of color. *J Natl Med Assoc*. 2007;99(8):879–885.

81. Todd KH, Deaton C, D'Adamo AP, Goe L. Ethnicity and analgesic practice. *Ann Emerg Med*. 2000;35(1):11–16.

82. Todd KH, Samaroo N, Hoffman JR. Ethnicity as a risk factor for inadequate emergency department analgesia. *JAMA*. 1993;269(12):1537–1539.

83. Coughlin TA, Long SK, Shen YC. Assessing access to care under Medicaid: evidence for the nation and thirteen states. *Health Aff (Millwood)*. 2005;24(4):1073–1083.

84. Simpson DM, McArthur JC, Olney R, et al. Lamotrigine for HIV-associated painful sensory neuropathies: a placebo-controlled trial. *Neurology*. 2003;60(9):1508–1514.

85. Hahn K, Arendt G, Braun JS, et al. A placebo-controlled trial of gabapentin for painful HIV-associated sensory neuropathies. *J Neurol*. 2004;251(10):1260–1266.

86. Richter RW, Portenoy R, Sharma U, Lamoreaux L, Bockbrader H, Knapp LE. Relief of painful diabetic peripheral neuropathy with pregabalin: a randomized, placebo-controlled trial. *J Pain*. 2005;6(4):253–260.

87. Simpson DM, Murphy TK, Durso-De Cruz E, Glue P, Whalen E. A Randomized, Double-Blind, Placebo-Controlled, Multicenter Trial of Pregabalin Vs Placebo in the Treatment of Neuropathic Pain Associated with HIV Neuropathy. Program and abstracts of the XVII International AIDS Conference, August 3–8, 2008; Mexico City. Abstract THAB0301.

88. Shlay JC, Chaloner K, Max MB, et al. Acupuncture and amitriptyline for pain due to HIV-related peripheral neuropathy: a randomized controlled trial. Terry Beirn community programs for clinical research on AIDS. *JAMA*. 1998;280(18):1590–1595.

89. Kieburtz K, Simpson D, Yiannoutsos C, et al. A randomized trial of amitriptyline and mexiletine for painful neuropathy in HIV infection. AIDS Clinical Trial Group 242 Protocol Team. *Neurology*. 1998;51(6):1682–1688.

90. Goldstein DJ, Lu Y, Detke MJ, Lee TC, Iyengar S. Duloxetine vs. placebo in patients with painful diabetic neuropathy. *Pain*. 2005;116(1–2):109–118.

91. Simpson DM, Brown S, Tobias J, NGX-4010 C107 Study Group. Controlled trial of high-concentration capsaicin patch for treatment of painful HIV neuropathy. *Neurology*. 2008;70(24):2305–2313.

92. Estanislao L, Carter K, McArthur J, Olney R, Simpson D, Lidoderm-HIV Neuropathy Group. A randomized controlled trial of 5% lidocaine gel for HIV-associated distal symmetric polyneuropathy. *J Acquir Immune Defic Syndr*. 2004;37(5):1584–1586.

93. Dorfman D, Montgomery G, George M, et al. Hypnosis for the treatment of HIV neuropathic pain. *J Pain*. 2008;9(4 suppl 2):59.

94. Ellis RJ, Toperoff W, Vaida F, et al. Smoked medicinal cannabis for neuropathic pain in HIV: a randomized, crossover clinical trial. *Neuropsychopharmacology*. 2009;34(3):672–680.

95. Abrams DI, Jay CA, Shade SB, et al. Cannabis in painful HIV-associated sensory neuropathy: a randomized placebo-controlled trial. *Neurology*. 2007;68(7):515–521.

96. Chou R, Fanciullo GJ, Fine PG, et al. Clinical guidelines for the use of chronic opioid therapy in chronic noncancer pain. *J Pain*. 2009;10(2):113–130.

97. Nicholson B, Passik SD. Management of chronic noncancer pain in the primary care setting. *South Med J*. 2007;100(10):1028–1036.

98. McArthur JC, Yiannoutsos C, Simpson DM, et al. A phase II trial of nerve growth factor for sensory neuropathy associated with HIV infection. AIDS Clinical Trials Group Team 291. *Neurology*. 2000;54(5):1080–1088.

99. Simpson DM, Schifitto G, Clifford DB, et al. Pregabalin for painful HIV neuropathy: a randomized, double-blind, placebo-controlled trial. *Neurology*. 2010;74(5):413–420.

13

Heritable Neuropathies

JOHN W. GRIFFIN†

INTRODUCTION

TAKEN TOGETHER, THE many distinct heritable neuropathies form one of the most prevalent groups of inherited neurological diseases. In most inherited nerve disorders the symptom of pain is overshadowed by other sensory manifestations or by weakness, but in a small number neuropathic pain is the primary or a prominent manifestation. This chapter will review Fabry's disease, familial amyloidotic polyneuropathy (FAP), erythromelalgia, and selected types of hereditary sensory and autonomic neuropathy (HSAN). It will contrast these disorders with the most prevalent heritable neuropathy, the Charcot-Marie-Tooth (CMT) complex of diseases, in which true neuropathic pain is less prominent.

In spite of their low prevalence, the heritable painful neuropathies are disproportionately important for four reasons. First,

from the clinical standpoint, successful early diagnosis of two of these disorders—FAP and Fabry's disease—can potentially lead to life-prolonging therapies. Second, in all four diseases, accurate diagnosis can end fruitless testing and inappropriate therapies, and lead to focused symptomatic therapy and genetic counseling. Third, taken as a group, these diseases are teaching important lessons about the mechanisms of neuropathic pain in general. For example, the familial erythromelalgia/ paroxysmal extreme pain (PEP) complex of disorders have identified new ion channel-mediated mechanisms that can lead to spontaneous neuropathic pain.

Fourth, all of these disorders—Fabry's disease, erythromelalgia/PEP, FAP, and the relevant types of HSAN—involve small-caliber sensory fibers out of proportion to their effects on large sensory fibers. They thereby combine to reinforce the point that disorders of small fibers are sufficient to drive neuropathic pain. This pattern

†Deceased - April 16, 2011.

conforms to that seen in many acquired painful neuropathies, such as diabetic polyneuropathy and amyloidosis associated with monoclonal gammopathies, that have prominent small-fiber involvement and spontaneous neuropathic pain. These small-fiber disorders in patients, in turn, complement experimental data showing that injury or disease of the nociceptor, particularly disorders that lead to spontaneous electrical activity,[1] can be sufficient to produce neuropathic pain. Few of the small-fiber neuropathies are limited to small-fiber disease alone; most have some degree of large-fiber involvement, and this typically increases with time and severity. In addition, small-fiber disease is probably not the only substrate that can lead to the development of neuropathic pain. Experimental data from animal models of nerve injury indicate that allodynia can also be driven by spontaneous activity arising within the cell bodies of large neurons giving rise to Aβ fibers.[2] However, the four painful disorders reviewed here reinforce the concept that disease that is largely restricted to small fibers can be sufficient to induce neuropathic pain.

Finally, there is new evidence that the frequency and severity of pain experienced by individuals with neuropathic disorders appear to be influenced by genetic background in humans[3] as well as in mice.[4,5] In patients with low back pain, certain patterns of single nucleotide polymorphisms (SNPs) are associated with greater severity and poor therapy responses than are seen in other patterns.[3] Similarly, in mice, strain differences produce variation in the susceptibility to developing allodynia after nerve injury.[4,5] Individuals with nerve disorders are just beginning to be stratified in terms of their susceptibility to developing pain disorders, as reviewed below. Individualized targeted therapies, including prophylaxis, are a realistic future goal of this work.

The number of genes that could potentially affect nociception and contribute to spontaneous pain is suggested by the rapidly growing list of genetically engineered mice that have altered pain responses. Some of the targeted genes in these mice influence the responses of primary nociceptors. These genes include examples that encode neuronal sodium, potassium, and calcium channels, as well as several neuronal

growth factors and their receptors. Some growth factors augment pain responses, including nerve growth factor (NGF), produced by target and supportive cells, and brain-derived neurotrophic factor (BDNF), produced by the primary nociceptors themselves.[6] Some cytokines, chemokines, and other molecules, such as tumor necrosis factor-α, that are usually associated with inflammatory responses have been found to alter the perception of noxious stimuli and can probably drive spontaneous pain. Importantly, some of these inflammatory factors can be produced by the primary nociceptive neuron. Some nociceptor products, including BDNF, are known to influence neurotransmission to second-order sensory neurons in the dorsal horn.[6,7] Other influences on the second-order neurons include glutamate and the N-methyl-D-aspartate (NMDA) and α-amino-3-hydroxy-5-methyl-4-isoxazolepropionate (AMPA) receptors, neuropeptides, and proton-mediated neurotransmission. Other relevant molecules include gamma-aminobutyric acid (GABA) and a variety of G-protein-coupled receptors, specific protein kinases, and other elements of signaling systems, as well as members of the opiate/opiate receptor systems. Reasoning from this known complexity, a great many more genes producing neuropathic pain probably remain to be identified.

FABRY'S DISEASE

Fabry's disease is an X-linked lysosomal storage disease caused by missense mutations in the gene encoding for the α-galactosidase A enzyme. It can produce painful neuropathies in both men and women. Early diagnosis followed by enzyme replacement therapy may not only improve the symptoms but may retard life-threatening complications including renal failure, stroke, and myocardial injury.

GENETIC DEFECT

The incidence of disease-causing mutations in α-galactosidase A has recently been estimated to be as high as 1 in 3100 births.[8] The known mutations in α-galactosidase A that can cause Fabry's disease now number in the hundreds. All of these mutations produce a loss of function in the enzyme, and a mouse model has been made by knocking out the gene.[9]

Deficiency of the enzyme results in accumulation of the three-sugar neutral glycosphingolipid triaosylceramide (Gal(α1 → 4)Gal(β1 → 4)Glc-Cer) or Gb3.[10] Gb3 is a member of the globo- series of glycosphingolipids. Globose (Gb4) was named for its prominence in erythrocyte membranes, and Gb3 as well is a constituent of red blood cell and many other nonneural membranes, including endothelial cells. In its metabolism, the terminal α-linked galactose is removed by α-galactosidase A. Gb3 is normally organized in specific lipid microdomains within membranes. Gb3 is a receptor for the bacterial toxins produced by Shigella and the Shiga-like toxins of some *Escherichia coli* strains.[11,12] As a consequence, mice lacking the *a-GalA* gene are resistant to the lethal effects of the Shiga toxin-2.[11] Such mice have markedly elevated levels of Gb3 in the circulation, and this circulating "receptor" presumably competes for and interferes with binding of the toxin to tissues. Gb3 is also necessary for the cell fusion events in human immune deficiency virus (HIV) that are mediated by interactions of the chemokine receptor CXCR4 on CD4+ lymphocytes. α-Galactosidase A also removes the terminal α-galactose from other glycoproteins and glycolipids. Because of the large number of identified mutations in the gene, including many private mutations, determination of enzyme activity rather than mutation analysis is the key to diagnosis.

PATHOLOGY

Fabry's disease is a true small-fiber neuropathy, with much greater involvement of small-caliber sensory fibers than large-caliber myelinated fibers.[13-18] Within the small-fiber population, the unmyelinated C fibers are lost out of proportion to the small myelinated Aδ fibers.[13,14,18] As would be expected, on skin biopsy specimens the density of sensory fibers within the epidermis is reduced, more so in distal regions of the extremities than in proximal areas.[14,19] This pattern indicates that there is a component of length-dependent axonal degeneration and loss. However, the small sensory fibers to the cornea are also reduced, as assessed by

corneal confocal microscopy,[15] demonstrating that even short C fibers can be affected. The cellular pathology of Fabry's disease is dominated by the accumulation of multilamellated lysosomal inclusions within endothelial cells, pericytes, and perineurial cells[13,18] (Figure 13.1). In the peripheral nervous system (PNS), accumulations also occur in dorsal root ganglion (DRG) neurons.[13] These accumulations can produce perikaryal distention and neuronal loss, but distally predominant axonal loss is much more severe than neuronal loss. Unmyelinated autonomic fibers, including postganglionic sympathetic fibers, are involved, and hypohidrosis can

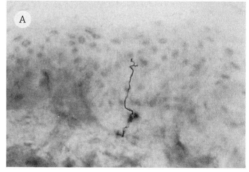
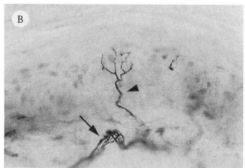

FIGURE 13.1   Photomicrograph of a punch skin biopsy specimen from a leg. Innervation of epidermis in normal control subjects. (A) A single, simple fiber can be seen to enter into and terminate within the epidermis. (B) A subepithelial nerve (arrow) sends off a small bundle of axons, which penetrate the basal lamina of the epidermis (arrowhead). Once within the epidermis, individual axons branch off the bundle to form a candelabra pattern of innervation, which we refer to as the complex form of innervation.

Source: Reprinted with permission from Scott LJ, Griffin JW, Luciano C, et al. Quantitative analysis of epidermal innervation in Fabry disease. *Neurology.* 1999;52(6):1249–1254.

be prominent.[20] Large neurons are preserved at stages when Aδ and especially C nociceptors are lost.[13,14,17,18] The mouse model produced by *a-GalA* gene knockout has a similar loss of small fibers with preservation of myelinated fibers.[9]

In nerve biopsy specimens and in mouse models, the major changes are in the endothelial cells, pericytes, and perineurial cells (Figure 13.1). Small inclusions are occasionally found within axons and in Schwann cells. In skin biopsy specimens, the eccrine sweat glands as well as the blood vessels may contain inclusions. Importantly, skin biopsies are useful for identifying involvement of small sensory and autonomic fibers, but they are not sufficient for excluding the diagnosis of Fabry's disease, because they can lack the diagnostic inclusions.[21]

CLINICAL MANIFESTATIONS

Neuropathic pain, typically beginning in the feet and hands, is the most frequent presenting symptom. In males, onset before age 10 is typical. In boys and in teenagers of either sex who present with painful acral neuropathies, Fabry's disease should be a major diagnostic concern and must be excluded. The persistent spontaneous neuropathic pain is typically accompanied by abrupt lancinating or "lightning" pains. Crises of pain can occur. The pain is often increased by exercise and by elevated body temperature, and occasional patients have heat hyperalgesia. Punctate mechanical and stroking hyperalgesia are not seen. Quantitative sensory testing demonstrates elevated warmth and cooling detection thresholds and decreased perception of heat pain.[22-24] These changes undoubtedly reflect the loss of C- and Aδ-fiber nociceptors. However, painless lesions and injuries of the type seen in FAP, diabetes, and other anesthetic neuropathies are uncommon in Fabry's disease patients.

The single most distinctive feature is the early and disproportionate loss of cold detection.[22-24] It is strikingly prominent compared to other neuropathies and should be sufficient to raise the diagnostic possibility of Fabry's disease. Loss of cold sensibility is best demonstrated using quantitative thermal sensory testing.[22,23,28] Unfortunately, cold hypesthesia is easily overlooked during a standard clinical sensory examination. Autonomic dysfunction, including hypohidrosis in the hands and feet,[20,25] also occurs in Fabry's disease. Occasional patients present with cramps and fasciculations as the primary symptoms.[21]

The systemic aspects of Fabry's disease can include flat dark blue or purple papules (angiokeratomas), typically in a bathing suit distribution. Corneal clouding can begin relatively early. Elevation of the erythrocyte sedimentation rate may erroneously suggest a rheumatic disease, especially when coupled with arthralgias.[16] Death can result from renal failure and vascular complications, especially stroke. Premature stroke in a patient with sensory neuropathy should also suggest the possibility of Fabry's disease.[20] Cardiac disease in patients with Fabry's disease can include myocardial infarction and arrhythmias.

From a diagnostic standpoint, determination of α-galactosidase A activity in leukocytes is the test of choice. Because so many of the *α-gal A* mutations are private, mutation analysis is not a realistic clinical test.

PATHOPHYSIOLOGY

The pathological hallmarks of Fabry's disease, inclusions in endothelial and perivascular cells, probably result in the vascular dysfunction that underlies many of the disease manifestations. Endothelial cells derived from patients with Fabry's disease have been cultured and fed Gb3. They produce increased reactive oxygen species and augment their expression of adhesion molecules, including intercellular adhesion molecule 1 (ICAM-1) and vascular cell adhesion molecule 1 (VCAM).[26,27] If these same changes occur in vivo, they are likely to contribute to the widespread angiopathy and vessel occlusion characteristic of Fabry's disease. There is a strong suggestion that Fabry's disease patients can have accelerated atherosclerosis that may contribute to the large-vessel occlusions that produce stroke and myocardial infarction. An autopsy of a young male with Fabry's disease on enzyme replacement therapy demonstrated that inclusions had been largely cleared from the endothelial cells throughout the body, but not from the cells that surrounded the vessels.[28] He had severe atherosclerosis[28] and died of his vascular disease.

A second candidate mechanism is likely to contribute to the small-fiber neuropathy of Fabry's disease. The sensory and sympathetic ganglia accumulate intraneuronal Gb3 in the characteristic lysosomal inclusions, and some of these neurons die.[13] Death of the neuronal cell body—a primary neuronopathy—might be expected to produce length-independent involvement, yet the clinical and pathological data indicate that long axons are lost to a much greater extent than small ones. Because small axons are differentially susceptible to ischemic injury, it is attractive to postulate that the endothelial cell dysfunction in Fabry's disease produces widespread angiopathic injury of nerves and that this is the predominant pathophysiological process. Because ischemic injury should accumulate with axonal length, longer nerves should, in principle, be at greater risk than shorter ones.

SYMPTOMATIC TREATMENT

Treatment for the neuropathic pain symptoms involves the same symptomatic approaches used in other painful small-fiber neuropathies, reviewed in Chapter 6 Medications include anticonvulsants such as gabapentin and pregabalin, as well as selective norepinephrine reuptake inhibitors (SNRIs). Because of its low prevalence, Fabry's disease has not had systematic clinical trials of any of these agents.

ENZYME REPLACEMENT THERAPY (ERT)

Fabry's disease was one of the first disorders in which enzyme replacement therapy (ERT) was utilized. Currently, two preparations are available, one produced in an immortalized human cell line and one in which the human enzyme is expressed in Chinese hamster ovary cells. Enzyme replacement therapy has been reported to reduce Gb3 levels in plasma and, in some studies, in tissue. Compared to placebo, ERT appears to reduce spontaneous pain, as reflected in pain scores.[29] In additional, just noticeable detection thresholds for warming

and cooling have small improvements.[29] These changes are not reflected in improvements in the density of epidermal fibers.[30] This measure was unchanged by 18 months of ERT, suggesting that the benefit does not depend on regeneration of nociceptors.[30] Sudomotor function also improves.[29] Sweating can improve transiently a few days after ERT, indicating that not all of this improvement is unlikely to reflect increased sympathetic innervation.[29] Rather, it has been interpreted as probably reflecting a direct effect of ERT on Gb3 accumulation in the sweat glands themselves.[29,31] Some data suggest that blood flow, including cerebrovascular flow, returns toward normal with ERT. The degree of effect on long-term renal and cardiac function and on mortality remains to be demonstrated.

FAMILIAL AMYLOIDOTIC POLYNEUROPATHY

Transthyretin Amyloidosis

Mutations in transthyretin are the most frequent cause of FAP. Of these mutations the val30met substitution is the most prevalent, but more than 90 other mutations have been described.

CLINICAL MANIFESTATIONS

Familial neuropathic amyloidosis is an autosomal dominant disease with highly variable penetrance. The disorder was first described in a classic report by Corina Andrade of families in the fishing villages of Povoa de Varzim and Vila do Conde in northwest Portugal.[32] Before the identification of the genetic mutation this type of FAP was often termed *Portuguese amyloidosis*, but there are also regions of high frequency in Sweden and Japan, as well as epidemiological clues that the disease may have reached Portugal through the Vikings. The disease is also prevalent in foci in Japan, and it occurs worldwide.

The disease typically begins in the third decade, but it can become symptomatic in childhood or the first manifestations can occur late in life. The sensorimotor neuropathy is the most frequent presenting manifestation, but cardiac and renal involvement typically follows, resulting in weight loss and death after about 10 years. The central clinical feature is dissociated sensory loss, with loss of small-fiber sensibilities and preservation of touch, positions sense, kinesthesia, and vibration. Classical studies by Dyck and Lambert[33] confirmed that small-fiber modalities and autonomic function were disproportionately lost compared to strength, reflexes, and large-fiber sensory functions. The clinical and electrophysiological pictures correlate well with the pathological changes described below. The presentation can consist of gastrointestinal symptoms including nausea, vomiting, and weight loss, and autonomic crises can occur.

A major consequence of the sensory loss is the predilection for painless injuries, a particularly disabling condition for workers in an industry as demanding as commercial fishing. Autonomic impairment includes impotence and cardio-regulatory abnormalities, often associated with orthostatic hypotension.[34,35] Length-dependent sudomotor failure is also seen.[25] The degree of spontaneous pain differs among individuals. Overall, the pattern is often one of more prominent pain early, with less pain as the sensory loss progresses. In addition to the length-dependent pain in the hands and feet, there is a predilection for nerve entrapments.[34] Carpal tunnel syndrome can be the presenting picture, with polyneuropathy becoming symptomatic only later[34] (also see Chapter 17). Thus, a history of earlier carpal tunnel surgery in a patient presenting with polyneuropathy should prompt consideration of FAP.

The initial description[32] identified the marked variability in severity of neuropathic and systemic manifestations. In some populations, maternal inheritance of the gene is associated with more penetrant disease.[36] This pattern may be explained by polymorphisms in mitochondrial DNA.[36] A particularly important distinction has been identified in Japan, where there are epidemiologically distinct endemic foci.[37] The disease associated with these foci has the expected early age of onset (the 20s and 30s) and the typical dissociated sensory loss and autonomic insufficiency. However, individuals not associated with these endemic areas may present with onset after age 50 and a particularly challenging diagnostic picture.

In these older-onset FAP patients, once the disease becomes symptomatic, it can progress rapidly. This sequence was illustrated in a personal patient who presented after age 60 with a new polyneuropathy, with spontaneous pain and prominent small-fiber loss as judged by skin biopsies, and with large-fiber involvement reflected in loss of tendon reflexes at the ankle and abnormalities on his electrodiagnostic studies. He had no autonomic symptoms and only distal sudomotor loss on examination. Over the next 8 years he developed impotence, orthostatic hypotension, and more severe pain. His nerve biopsy identified small transthyretin (TTR)-positive amyloid deposits, and the val30met mutation was found on genetic testing. He died 3 years later of heart failure due to amyloid cardiomyopathy.

This population of older men without family histories, but with val30met mutations, represents a special diagnostic challenge, because they may have only mild autonomic dysfunction and less dissociated sensory involvement. The diagnosis can be established by TTR genetic testing if common mutations are present, but the initial diagnosis of some form of amyloid deposition is often still made through nerve and muscle biopsies. These older men often have little autonomic dysfunction at the onset, a more generalized polyneuropathy, and often no family history.[35,37] Their pathology differs as well; there is less bright congophilia with shorter fibrils in the late-onset cases, compared to more florid congophilic, and TTR-bright amyloid and long amyloid fibrils in the early-onset cases. In addition, mass spectroscopy has shown that in the early-onset cases, most of the TTR in deposits was mutant, as expected. In the late-onset cases, more wild-type TTR was found in the amyloid deposits. Because some *senile amyloid* due to TTR deposition can develop with age in individuals with no identified mutations, these late-onset patients suggest that that they may become symptomatic as a result of age-related changes combined with the TTR mutation. The data on late onset indicate a substantial male predominance, similar to that in senile in senile amyloidosis.[35]

PATHOPHYSIOLOGY

The TTR protein was first recognized by Elvin Kabat and colleagues in 1942 as they assessed electrophoretic patterns in the cerebrospinal fluid (CSF) of normal individuals and of patients with a variety of neurological diseases.[38] From its characteristics on charge-based electrophoresis, the protein was initially termed *prealbumin*. Because the protein binds thyroid hormone and retinol, it was renamed *transthyretin*. The protein is made in the liver and the choroid plexus and circulates in the blood.

The mechanism of injury to nerve by mutant TTR remains controversial, but it is likely to share common features with other types of amyloid fibrillogenesis, including Aβ deposition in Alzheimer's disease. All of the diverse proteins that are deposited in the amyloidoses share the characteristic of becoming misfolded, forming β-pleated sheets, and producing fibrils. This can occur when the concentration of susceptible proteins is sufficiently high, which presumably contributes to immunoglobulin light chain deposition in multiple myeloma to produce neuropathic amyloid. Instructively, light chain and TTR deposition in peripheral nerve produce very similar amyloid pathology and clinical consequences. Both the acquired amyloidotic polyneuropathy associated with monoclonal gammopathies and the TTR mutations share the features of predominant small-fiber involvement with a predilection for painless injuries, autonomic insufficiency, and a variable degree of spontaneous neuropathic pain.

In TTR the amyloid deposition is not driven by an excessive serum concentration of TTR, but rather by protein misfolding due to the underlying mutation. In the val30met TTR, it has been noted that other proteins can bind directly to TTR and inhibit fibril formation. Among these proteins is the holo- form of the retinol binding protein (RBP). Small molecules including thyroxine can have a similar effect. The capacity to modify fibrillogenesis by molecules that bind TTR is the target of much of the therapeutic research on FAP.

TREATMENT

Transthyretin amyloidosis is an ominous diagnosis with a markedly reduced life expectancy; from the time of neuropathic diagnosis, life expectancy averages only 10.8 years.[39] The mortality reflects cardiac and other systemic complications. Because much of the protein is made in the liver, removal of the liver with orthotopic[34,40] or partial[41,42] liver transplantation directly reduces amyloidogenesis. The efficacy of these procedures for the neuropathy has been assessed in a few studies that have used baseline and posttransplantation examination, electrophysiology, and nerve biopsies. The data, for the most part, show stabilization of the nerve disease.[34,40,42] Adams and colleagues[34] studied 25 patients followed for 2 or more years after liver transplantation. The serum levels of mutant TTR fell 40-fold, as expected. The autonomic function and motor scores remained unchanged. Seven of these patients had biopsies before and after transplantation and were compared to nontransplanted patients. The rate of fiber loss was slowed in the transplanted group. One case report[41] describes higher fiber densities in a sural nerve taken after transplantation compared to the opposite side before transplantation. Although side-to-side differences alone might account for this pattern, this report suggests that occasionally there may be substantial regeneration after transplantation. These and other data[37,40,42] indicate that survival and nerve function may be better when diagnosis is made early in the disease course. Mortality and disability are higher in patients with more advanced disease, including urinary incontinence and severe gastrointestinal dysfunction.[34,42]

There are surprisingly little data on the effect of liver transplantation on neuropathic pain. Currently, the mainstay of symptomatic therapy for patients with TTR amyloidosis remains standard drug regimens for neuropathic pain coupled with education in preventing painless injuries to anesthetic limbs. There is great interest in interfering with fibrillogenesis and in the possibility that suppression of TTR mRNA production might be accomplished by antisense or other gene-silencing strategies. The possibility that immunization with mutant proteins might produce clearance of tissue deposits has been suggested by the demonstrated capacity to reduce the amount of cerebral Aβ-amyloid by immunization.

Gelsolin Amyloidosis

This dominantly inherited amyloidosis was first described in patients from Finland. It results from mutations in gelsolin, an actin-binding protein. Gelsolin mutations produce a distinctive neuropathy, with less neuropathic pain and autonomic dysfunction than in TTR amyloidosis or the amyloidosis produced by light chain deposition. Instead, affected individuals have cranial nerve involvement with facial paralyses and sensory loss, and with large-fiber nerve involvement that produces weakness and gait disorders out of proportion to small-fiber involvement or pain. Nerve biopsies confirm the prominence of large-fiber loss.[43] The amyloid is found predominantly around vessels and in the perineurium, with little endoneurial deposition.[43] The contrast between the small-fiber involvement prominent in the often painful TTR neuropathy and the large motor fiber involvement in the largely painless gelsolin neuropathy reinforces the role of small sensory fiber injury in the pathogenesis of neuropathic pain.

HERITABLE ERYTHROMELALGIA

Erythromelalgia, described over a century ago, was long regarded as a poorly defined and controversial entity. In the last few years, familial erythromelalgia has abruptly become one of the most instructive of the painful nerve diseases, as reflected in the explosion of publications on the topic. The prominence of this syndrome has been driven by the identification of its molecular basis in heritable cases.[44,45]

The genetic story of the relevant chanellopathies began with a northern Pakistani family that had an inborn inability to experience pain.[46] Strikingly, these individuals had, within limits of the available testing, preserved thermal and cooling sensibility, touch, vibration, proprioception, and kinesthetic sensibilities.[46] In addition, autonomic function appeared to be normal.[46] In contrast, affected individuals all had a selective deficit in perception of pain to noxious stimuli. This proved to be due to a mutation in the *SCN9A* gene that encodes one type of voltage-gated sodium channel, Nav1.7.[44,46] This channel is expressed in a variety of dorsal root and ganglia neurons as well as in the sympathetic ganglia. Importantly, most of these ganglion populations also express other sodium channels. The experience with this initial Pakistani family and with subsequent families with loss-of-function mutations indicated that this channel is singularly important in the function of nociceptors in normal perception of nociceptive pain. Its loss can be compensated for in autonomic and other sensory neurons[44] but not in the nociceptors.

The relevance of this story to neuropathic pain came with the identification of a series of families with dominant mutations in *SCN9A* that had familial erythromelalgia. The symptoms usually begin in childhood with episodes of intense burning pain in the feet and/or hands, typically accompanied by a feeling of warmth and by visible redness.[44] The pain in these individuals is often increased by heat and activity, and they experience relief with cooling. From a pathophysiological standpoint, these patients have evidence of a small-fiber neuropathy.[47] One family from Taiwan had a substantial loss of epidermal nerve fibers in affected individuals. This family had a confirmed mutation in *SCN9A* (I136V).[48] In a series of skin biopsies from individuals with the sporadic form of erythromelalgia syndrome but without identified genetic mutations, reduced epidermal nerve fiber density was also identified, as were reduced perivascular innervation, presumably representing loss of sympathetic fibers, and abnormalities on sudomotor testing. These fibers all support the presence of a small-caliber fiber neuropathy.[47]

PATHOPHYSIOLOGY

The mutations of heritable erythromelalgia have been tested by transfection of the human mutant genes into rodent DRG neurons in vitro.[49,50] The expressing neurons are hyperexcitable and can attain higher than normal rates of firing to suprathreshold stimuli.[49,50] This provides a satisfying correlation with the findings of microneurographic studies of human patients with erythromelalgia.[51] Some mechanically sensitive cutaneous C fibers demonstrated spontaneous activity and an increased response to mechanical stimulation,[49,50] providing a physiological underpinning to the spontaneous pain and the mechanical allodynia experienced by patients. The cellular physiology varies somewhat among the different mutations, but usually includes altered voltage-dependent activation with a shift toward hyperpolarization, slower deactivation, and larger ramp currents, although the cellular physiology varies somewhat among the different mutations. These characteristics are consistent with the clinical impression of hyperexcitability.

TREATMENT

Treatment of erythromelalgia in general and the heritable syndromes in particular remains unsatisfactory. In an encouraging approach, clinicians noted that members of a family with a mutation in *SCN9A* responded to carbamazepine, and rodent DRG neurons transfected with the mutant channel in vitro[52] had the abnormalities in activation, deactivation, steady state, and ramp currents partially normalized by carbamezipine in culture.[52] Thus, in this instance, the in vitro response was predicted by the response of the family members to this agent. Similarly, in vitro data suggested that the lidocaine analog mexilitene might be effective in some patients,[53] and clinical improvement with this agent was subsequently reported.[54] Such patterns may presage a future of mechanism-based selection of therapeutics for different neuropathic pain syndromes, and of individualized therapy, based on analysis of the specific mutations.

The story of the *SCN9A* mutations and their relationship to pain appreciation has recently been extended in a study of SNPs in a variety of pain disorders including lumbar radiculopathy, osteoarthritis, and pancreatitis.[55] One polymorphism, an A for G substitution in one SNP, was associated with greater susceptibility to these chronic pain states. Expressing this substitution in the $Na_v1.7$ protein in vitro produced increased excitability of the channel in a fashion reminiscent of that seen in the erythromelalgia mutations.[55] This approach brings together the issue of genetic heterogeneity in pain responsiveness and the disease of primary nociceptors.[3]

HEREDITARY AND SENSORY AUTONOMIC NEUROPATHIES

The brunt of the involvement in these genetically heterogeneous disorders is borne by small sensory and autonomic neurons. Dominantly inherited forms of HSAN typically present in adulthood, whereas many of the recessive forms begin in childhood. All of the HSANs are predominantly axonal/neuronal disorders rather than demyelinating diseases. Importantly, in most of them, the sensory problems are predominantly loss of protective sensibility with acral ulcers, Charcot joints, and other complications of anesthetic limbs. In about one third of HSAN patients, neuropathic pain is a feature. Lightning or lancinating pains may occur. Tingling and paresthesias are not a feature of these disorders.

The form of HSAN that is most relevant to neuropathic pain was described by Dyck and colleagues.[56] They found families who had mild sensory neuropathy, apparently dominantly inherited, presenting in midlife and characterized by burning feet and mild autonomic dysfunction with preserved large-fiber functions and normal nerve conduction studies.[56] An analysis of a large German kindred[57] confirmed the mildness of large myelinated fiber involvement and documented moderately severe loss of unmyelinated fibers in the sural nerve. To date, no genetic abnormality has been identified in this pattern of HSAN1. Undoubtedly, many more genetic alterations remain to be determined in the whole HSAN category.

The two most prevalent dominantly inherited defects in HSAN1 are mutations in serine palmitoyltransferase long chain 1 (SPTLC1) and the small guanine triphosphate-ase (GTPase, Rab 7. The latter is a component of the signaling endosome involved in transport and signaling of the activated receptor for nerve growth factor, TrkA.[58] The genotype-phenotype correlations that have been reported make it clear that the Rab7 mutation usually presents as a heritable motor-sensory neuropathy with a tendency for painless acral injuries.[59] Klein and colleagues examined 25 previously undiagnosed families for mutations in the known HSAN I genes and identified only one mutation in *SPTLC1* and one in Rab7-9.[60] In addition, in 92 patients presenting with idiopathic painful sensory neuropathies, no mutations were found. Taken together, these data indicate that many genetic causes of HSAN1 remain to be discovered.

Charcot-Marie-Tooth Disease (CMT)

This group of disorders accounts for a high proportion of inherited neuropathies. A daunting and growing list of genetic abnormalities are included within this "umbrella" diagnosis of CMT. Some genotypes affect myelination. These include the autosomal dominant forms termed CMT1 and the X-linked known as CMTX. All of them affect proteins of the Schwann cells and myelin of the PNS. From early life, individuals affected with CMT1 and CMTX usually have profoundly reduced conduction velocities in motor and sensory myelinated nerve fibers. The best-known clinical manifestations of these demyelinating forms of CMT are distally predominant muscle weakness and wasting, high arches, hammertoes, and sensory loss, particularly that mediated by large nerve fibers. Even though the genetic defects are in myelin-forming cells and there are lifelong abnormalities in the myelin sheaths, the clinical manifestations reflect length-dependent axonal degeneration and loss. Such late progressive axonal loss in the setting of long-standing abnormalities of myelination is termed *secondary axonal degeneration*.

Another class of CMT, termed CMT2, is characterized by length-dependent axonal loss in the absence of abnormalities in myelin, without the early and severe reduction in nerve conduction velocities characteristic of CMT1 and CMTX. Many of the disorders in the class of CMT2 have molecular defects in neuronal proteins, such as the neurofilament light chain (NF-L). In some disorders the tidy classification of demyelinating versus primarily axonal breaks down, because individuals within a single family can appear to have different patterns of involvement.

In all forms of CMT the motor signs and symptoms, including weakness of the intrinsic muscles of the foot, foot drop, and hand weakness, predominate. Sensory abnormalities on examination as well as electrophysiological changes in sensory nerves are found. The exception is a few uncommon purely motor forms, often termed *distal spinal muscular atrophy* (SMA). One form of almost purely motor involvement has recently been linked to mutations in the gene *TrpV4*, an ion channel.[61,62]

The prevalence of pain in CMT has been addressed in a few studies. The first was a retrospective questionnaire survey with responses from 400 individuals.[63] Pain was present in 70%, and was reported equally frequently in CMT1 and CMT2. However, the nature of this study prohibited the differentiation of musculoskeletal nociceptive pain from arthritis or tendinitis related to changes in muscle usage from neuropathic pain. Much of the reported discomfort appears to have been consistent with joint and tendon problems. For example, low back, knee, and ankle pains were the most frequently reported types of pain. The second study[61] was smaller but had the advantage of direct patient interviews. The results suggested that nociceptive pain—including low back and joint pains—were more frequent in CMT1, whereas true paresthesias and dysesthesias were more frequent in CMT2. In both studies, the adjectives such as *burning* that are often used to describe neuropathic pain were not prominent.

More recently, Pazzaglia and colleagues used a questionnaire designed to identify neuropathic pain more appropriately in CMT1A and correlated the results with laser-evoked potential (LEP) recordings.[64] There was a relatively high incidence of pain interpreted as neuropathic in the feet and hands in the CMT1A patients and a significant correlation with the degree of reduction in the LEP potentials.[64] These results were interpreted to reflect loss of Aδ fibers. A correlate may be found in mice with knockout of periaxin, a Schwann cell pdz protein that contributes to stabilization of PNS myelin. In its absence, the nerves undergo demyelination.[65] These mice also had spontaneous firing in the small fibers of the saphenous nerves, as well as hyperalgesia to mechanical stimulation of the feet, a finding that is usually interpreted as suggestive of neuropathic pain.[65] Like the LEP abnormalities in CMT1A, the hyperalgesia was interpreted as a consequence of the loss of Aδ fibers with resulting central sensitization.[64,65] It is likely that the pain in

CMT represents a combination of the weakness and gait disorders, with consequent abnormal usage of joints and tendons and a predisposition to neuropathic pain.

In both CMT1 and CMT2, the development of a second cause of nerve disease can produce much more severe pain and weakness than expected in either disorder alone. The most frequent such second injury to nerves is caused by the use of neurotoxic agents for cancer or antiviral chemotherapy. For example, the antimitotic chemotherapy agent vincristine, when used in standard doses in normal individuals, is well known to produce some paresthesias, neuropathic pain, and distally predominant weakness. In individuals with CMT1 or CMT2 all three manifestations may be markedly amplified, leading to severe neuropathic pain requiring intensive medication regimens, as well as weakness and gait ataxia that may preclude walking for months.

REFERENCES

1. Wu G, Ringkamp M, Hartke TV, et al. Early onset of spontaneous activity in uninjured c-fiber nociceptors after injury to neighboring nerve fibers. J Neurosci, 2001;21(8):RC140.
2. Devor M. Ectopic discharge in A beta afferents as a source of neuropathic pain. Exp Brain Res, 2009;196(1):115–128.
3. Max MB, Wu T, Atlas SJ, et al. A clinical genetic method to identify mechanisms by which pain causes depression and anxiety. Mol Pain. 2006;2:14.
4. Mogil JS, Wilson SG, Bon K, et al. Heritability of nociception I: responses of 11 inbred mouse strains on 12 measures of nociception. Pain. 1999;80(1–2):67–82.
5. Persson AK, Gebauer M, Jordan S, et al. Correlational analysis for identifying genes whose regulation contributes to chronic neuropathic pain. Mol Pain. 2009;5:7.
6. Fukuoka T, Kondo E, Dai Y, Hashimoto N, Noguchi K. Brain-derived neurotrophic factor increases in the uninjured dorsal root ganglion neurons in selective spinal nerve ligation model. J Neurosci. 2001;21(13):4891–900.
7. Dai Y, Iwata K, Fukuoka T, et al. Phosphorylation of extracellular signal-regulated kinase in primary afferent neurons by noxious stimuli and its involvement in peripheral sensitization. J Neurosci. 2002;22(17):7737–7745.
8. Spada M, Pagliardini S, Yasuda M, et al. High incidence of later-onset Fabry disease revealed by newborn screening. Am J Hum Genet. 2006;79(1):31–40.
9. Rodrigues LG, Ferraz MJ, Rodrigues D, et al. Neurophysiological, behavioral and morphological abnormalities in the Fabry knockout mice. Neurobiol Dis. 2009;33(1):48–56.
10. Wiegandt H. Glycolipids. In: Wiegandt H, ed. New Comprehensive Biochemistry, Vol. 10. Amsterdam: Elsevier Science; 1985:199–260.
11. Keusch GT, Jacewicz M, Acheson DW, Donohue-Rolfe A, Kane AV, McCluer RH. Globotriaosylceramide, Gb3, is an alternative functional receptor for Shiga-like toxin 2e. Infect Immun. 1995;63(3):1138–1141.
12. Ren J, Utsunomiya I, Taguchi K, et al. Localization of verotoxin receptors in nervous system. Brain Res. 1999;825(1–2):183–188.
13. Ohnishi A, Dyck PJ. Loss of small peripheral sensory neurons in Fabry's disease. Arch Neurol. 1974;31:120–127.
14. Scott LJ, Griffin JW, Luciano C, et al. Quantitative analysis of epidermal innervation in Fabry disease. Neurology. 1999;52(6):1249–1254.
15. Malik RA, Kallinikos P, Abbott CA, et al. Corneal confocal microscopy: a non-invasive surrogate of nerve fibre damage and repair in diabetic patients. Diabetologia. 2003;46(5):683–688.
16. Lacomis D, Roeske-Anderson L, Mathie L. Neuropathy and Fabry's disease. Muscle Nerve. 2005;31(1):102–107.
17. Toyooka K, Said G. Nerve biopsy findings in hemizygous and heterozygous patients with Fabry's disease. J Neurol. 1997;244(7):464–468.
18. Dutsch M, Marthol H, Stemper B, Brys M, Haendl T, Hilz MJ. Small fiber dysfunction predominates in Fabry neuropathy. J Clin Neurophysiol. 2002;19(6):575–586.
19. Liguori R, Di Stasi, V, Bugiardini E, et al. Small fiber neuropathy in female patients with fabry disease. Muscle Nerve. 2010;41(3):409–412.
20. Shimizu J, Hashimoto M, Murayama S, Tsuji S. A 52-year-old man with hypohidrosis. Neuropathology. 2006;26(6):592–594.
21. Nance CS, Klein CJ, Banikazemi M, et al. Later-onset Fabry disease: an adult variant presenting with the cramp-fasciculation syndrome. Arch Neurol. 2006;63(3):453–457.
22. Moller AT, Jensen TS. Neurological manifestations in Fabry's disease. Nat Clin Pract Neurol. 2007;3(2):95–106.
23. Naleschinski D, Arning K, Baron R. Fabry disease—pain doctors have to find the missing ones. Pain. 2009;145(1–2):10–11.

24. Torvin MA, Winther BF, Feldt-Rasmussen U, et al. Functional and structural nerve fiber findings in heterozygote patients with Fabry disease. *Pain.* 2009;145(1–2):237–245.

25. Ohnishi A, Yamamoto T, Murai Y, et al. Denervation of eccrine glands in patients with familial amyloidotic polyneuropathy type I. *Neurology.* 1998;51(3):714–721.

26. Shen JS, Meng XL, Schiffmann R, Brady RO, Kaneski CR. Establishment and characterization of Fabry disease endothelial cells with an extended lifespan. *Mol Genet Metab.* 2007;92 (1–2):137–144.

27. Shen JS, Meng XL, Moore DF, et al. Globotriaosylceramide induces oxidative stress and up-regulates cell adhesion molecule expression in Fabry disease endothelial cells. *Mol Genet Metab.* 2008;95(3):163–168.

28. Schiffmann R, Rapkiewicz A, bu-Asab M, et al. Pathological findings in a patient with Fabry disease who died after 2.5 years of enzyme replacement. *Virchows Arch.* 2006;448(3):337–343.

29. Schiffmann R, Floeter MK, Dambrosia JM, et al. Enzyme replacement therapy improves peripheral nerve and sweat function in Fabry disease. *Muscle Nerve.* 2003;28(6):703–710.

30. Schiffmann R, Hauer P, Freeman B, et al. Enzyme replacement therapy and intraepidermal innervation density in Fabry disease. *Muscle Nerve.* 2006;34(1):53–56.

31. Gupta SN, Ries M, Murray GJ, et al. Skin-impedance in Fabry disease: a prospective, controlled, non-randomized clinical study. *BMC Neurol.* 2008;8:41.

32. Andrade C. A peculiar form of peripheral neuropathy; familiar atypical generalized amyloidosis with special involvement of the peripheral nerves. *Brain.* 1952;75(3):408–427.

33. Dyck PJ, Lambert EH. Dissociated sensation in amyloidosis: compound action potentials; quantitative histologic and teased fibers; and electron microscopic studies of sural nerve biopsies. *Trans Am Neurol Assoc.* 1968;93:112–115.

34. Adams D, Samuel D, Goulon-Goeau C, et al. The course and prognostic factors of familial amyloid polyneuropathy after liver transplantation. *Brain.* 2000;123(pt 7):1495–1504.

35. Koike H, Ando Y, Ueda M, et al. Distinct characteristics of amyloid deposits in early- and late-onset transthyretin Val30Met familial amyloid polyneuropathy. *J Neurol Sci.* 2009;287(1–2): 178–184.

36. Bonaiti B, Olsson M, Hellman U, Suhr O, Bonaiti-Pellie C, Plante-Bordeneuve V. TTR familial amyloid polyneuropathy: does a mitochondrial polymorphism entirely explain the parent-of-origin difference in penetrance? *Eur J Hum Genet.* 2010;18(8):948–952. [E-pub March 17, 2010.]

37. Rudolph T, Kurz MW, Farbu E. Late-onset familial amyloid polyneuropathy (FAP) Val30-Met without family history. *Clin Med Res.* 2008;6(2):80–82.

38. Kabat EA, Moore DH, Landow H. An electrophoretic study of the protein components in cerebrospinal fluid and their relationship to the serum proteins. *J Clin Invest.* 1942;21(5):571–577.

39. Coutinho P, Martins da Silva A, Lopes Lima J, Resende Barbosa A. Forty years of experience with type I amyloid neuropathy. Review of 483 cases. In: Glenner GG, Pinho e Costa P, Falcao de Freitas A, eds. *Amyloid and Amyloidosis.* Amsterdam: Excerpta Medica; 1980:88–98.

40. Okamoto S, Wixner J, Obayashi K, et al. Liver transplantation for familial amyloidotic polyneuropathy: impact on Swedish patients' survival. *Liver Transplant.* 2009;15(10):1229–1235.

41. Ikeda S, Takei Y, Yanagisawa N, et al. Peripheral nerves regenerated in familial amyloid polyneuropathy after liver transplantation. *Ann Intern Med.* 1997;127(8 pt 1):618–620.

42. Takei Y, Ikeda S, Hashikura Y, Ikegami T, Kawasaki S. Partial-liver transplantation to treat familial amyloid polyneuropathy: follow-up of 11 patients. *Ann Intern Med.* 1999;131(8):592–595.

43. Kiuru-Enari S, Somer H, Seppalainen AM, Notkola IL, Haltia M. Neuromuscular pathology in hereditary gelsolin amyloidosis. *J Neuropathol Exp Neurol.* 2002;61(6):565–571.

44. Cummins TR, Sheets PL, Waxman SG. The roles of sodium channels in nociception: implications for mechanisms of pain. *Pain.* 2007;131(3): 243–257.

45. Dib-Hajj SD, Yang Y, Waxman SG. Genetics and molecular pathophysiology of Na(v)1.7-related pain syndromes. *Adv Genet.* 2008;63:85–110.

46. Cox JJ, Reimann F, Nicholas AK, et al. An SCN9A channelopathy causes congenital inability to experience pain. *Nature.* 2006;444(7121): 894–898.

47. Davis MD, Weenig RH, Genebriera J, Wendelschafer-Crabb G, Kennedy WR, Sandroni P. Histopathologic findings in primary erythromelalgia are nonspecific: special studies show a decrease in small nerve fiber density. *J Am Acad Dermatol.* 2006;55(3):519–522.

48. Lee MJ, Yu HS, Hsieh ST, Stephenson DA, Lu CJ, Yang CC. Characterization of a familial case with primary erythromelalgia from Taiwan. *J Neurol.* 2007;254(2):210–214.

49. Estacion M, Dib-Hajj SD, Benke PJ, et al. NaV1.7 gain-of-function mutations as a continuum: A1632E displays physiological changes associated with erythromelalgia and paroxysmal extreme pain disorder mutations and produces symptoms of both disorders. *J Neurosci.* 2008;28(43):11079–11088.

50. Han C, Dib-Hajj SD, Lin Z, et al. Early- and late-onset inherited erythromelalgia: genotype-phenotype correlation. *Brain.* 2009;132(pt 7): 1711–1722.

51. Orstavik K, Weidner C, Schmidt R, et al. Pathological C-fibres in patients with a chronic painful condition. *Brain.* 2003;126(pt 3):567–578.

52. Fischer TZ, Gilmore ES, Estacion M. et al. A novel Nav1.7 mutation producing carbamazepine-responsive erythromelalgia. *Ann Neurol.* 2009; 65(6):733–741.

53. Choi JS, Zhang L, Dib-Hajj SD, et al. Mexiletine-responsive erythromelalgia due to a new Na(v)1.7 mutation showing use-dependent current fall-off. *Exp Neurol.* 2009;216(2):383–389.

54. Iqbal J, Bhat MI, Charoo BA, Syed WA, Sheikh MA, Bhat IN. Experience with oral mexiletine in primary erythromelalgia in children. *Ann Saudi Med.* 2009;29(4):316–318.

55. Reimann F, Cox JJ, Belfer I, et al. Pain perception is altered by a nucleotide polymorphism in SCN9A. *Proc Natl Acad Sci USA.* 2010;107(11):5148–5153.

56. Dyck PJ, Low PA, Stevens JC. Burning feet as the only manifestation of dominantly inherited sensory neuropathy. *Mayo Clin Proc.* 1983;58:426–429.

57. Stogbauer F, Young P, Kuhlenbaumer G, et al. Autosomal dominant burning feet syndrome. *J Neurol Neurosurg Psychiatry.* 1999;67(1):78–81.

58. Cogli L, Piro F, Bucci C. Rab7 and the CMT2B disease. *Biochem Soc Trans.* 2009;37(pt 5):1027–1031.

59. Rotthier A, Baets J, De VE, et al. Genes for hereditary sensory and autonomic neuropathies: a genotype-phenotype correlation. *Brain.* 2009;132(pt 10):2699–2711.

60. Klein CJ, Wu Y, Kruckeberg KE, et al. SPTLC1 and RAB7 mutation analysis in dominantly inherited and idiopathic sensory neuropathies. *J Neurol Neurosurg Psychiatry.* 2005;76(7): 1022–1024.

61. Deng HX, Klein CJ, Yan J, et al. Scapuloperoneal spinal muscular atrophy and CMT2C are allelic disorders caused by alterations in TRPV4. *Nat Genet.* 2010;42(2):165–169.

62. Landoure G, Zdebik AA, Martinez TL, et al. Mutations in TRPV4 cause Charcot-Marie-Tooth disease type 2C. *Nat Genet.* 2010;42(2): 170–174.

63. Carter GT, Jensen MP, Galer BS, et al. Neuropathic pain in Charcot-Marie-Tooth disease. *Arch Phys Med Rehabil.* 1998;79(12):1560–1564.

64. Pazzaglia C, Vollono C, Ferraro D, et al. Mechanisms of neuropathic pain in patients with Charcot-Marie-Tooth 1 A: a laser-evoked potential study. *Pain.* 2010;149(2):379–385.

65. Gillespie CS, Sherman DL, Fleetwood-Walker SM, et al. Peripheral demyelination and neuropathic pain behavior in periaxin-deficient mice. *Neuron.* 2000;26(2):523–531.

14

Cancer-Associated Neuropathic Pain and Paraneoplastic Syndromes

ADITYA BARDIA, ROSS DONEHOWER, AND VINAY CHAUDHRY

PAIN IS THE most common and one of the most feared symptoms of cancer. Cancer-associated pain is estimated to occur in more than 75% of hospitalized patients. It is one of the most common reasons for inpatient oncology admission and is often referred to as the *fifth vital sign* of cancer patients. Optimal management of cancer-related pain is widely recognized as a quality benchmark in oncology. A deeper understanding of the pathophysiology and cause of cancer-related pain is crucial.

While somatic pain due to cancer infiltration of the tissues is the most common type of cancer pain, neuropathic pain is also common among patients with cancer and is often refractory to standard opioid and pain medications. We will focus on cancer-associated neuropathic pain in this chapter.

Conceptually, cancer-associated neuropathic pain can occur due to the direct infiltrative effect of the cancer itself or can be due indirectly to adverse effects of treatment or the presence of a paraneoplastic syndrome (Table 14.1). Of the treatment-induced neuropathies, those due to chemotherapy are most common and will be discussed in detail below. This would be followed by a discussion of radiation-induced plexopathies and, finally, paraneoplastic syndromes. Neuropathies asso-ciated with mono-clonal gammopathies, amyloid neuropathies, and toxic neuropathies (besides chemotherapy-induced neuropathies) are covered elsewhere in this book (Chapters 13, 16, and 24).

CHEMOTHERAPY-INDUCED PERIPHERAL NEUROPATHY

Chemotherapy-induced peripheral neuropathy (CIPN) is a common, often dose-limiting side effect of many chemotherapeutic agents, including cisplatin, taxols, and newer agents such as ixabepilone.[1] The incidence of CIPN is variable and ranges from 10% to 100%, depending on

Table 14-1. Causes of Cancer-Associated Neuropathic Pain Syndromes

1. Direct effect of cancer infiltrating nerve roots, plexus, nerves
2. Treatment-associated neuropathic pain syndromes
    a. Chemotherapy-induced peripheral neuropathy
        i. Cisplatin, carboplatin, and oxaliplatin
        ii. Taxanes (paclitaxel and docetaxel) and epothilones
        iii. Bortezomib
        iv. Vinca alkaloids
        v. Others: thalidomide, suramin
    b. Radiation-induced peripheral neuropathy
3. Paraneoplastic neuropathic pain syndromes
    a. Stiff person syndrome
    b. Sensory neuronopathy
    c. Sensorimotor neuropathy—acute and chronic
    d. Mononeuropathy multiplex-vasculitic neuropathy
    e. Autonomic neuropathy
    f. Neuromyotonic syndrome
4. Others
    a. Immune-mediated neuropathy
    b. Compressive (entrapment) neuropathy
    c. Toxicity from other drugs (e.g., pyridoxine) neuropathy
    d. Associated metabolic disorders (diabetes, e.g., induced by steroid use, vitamin B_{12} deficiency, alcohol abuse)
    e. Infections (e.g., zoster)

the criteria used for diagnosis and whether a neuromuscular evaluation including neurophysiological testing was done at baseline and then again after chemotherapy. Typical risk factors include the following: (1) the presence of preexisting symptomatic or asymptomatic neuropathy—such as diabetes, alcohol abuse, or a family history of hereditary neuropathy such as Charcot-Marie-Tooth neuropathy (hereditary motor and sensory neuropathy [HMSN])—may make CIPN appear earlier or be more severe; (2) the type of chemotherapy and combinations of drugs, if used (e.g., a combination of paclitaxel and cisplatin), may cause a more severe CIPN than either drug alone; (3) the chemotherapy regimen, including the dose (and rate of infusion) per cycle, the duration and frequency of chemotherapy cycles, and the total cumulative dose) is an important factor. In general, a lower dose over a longer period of time is less toxic than a higher dose for a short period even if the eventual cumulative dose might be similar (also see Chapter 24, Toxic Neuropathy/Peltier, Figure 24.1).

Clinically, three different presentations of neuropathy are recognized. The clinical features are determined by the pathophysiology and the type of fibers affected, as outlined in Table 14.2 and 14.3. The most common type of CIPN is a *stocking-glove sensory > motor polyneuropathy.* Sensory symptoms arise from small-caliber nerve fiber dysfunction and include severe pain, tingling, burning, and sensitivity (resulting in allodynia); sensory symptoms from large-fiber sensory dysfunction include numbness, proprioceptive dysfunction, and gait problems (Table 14.2). The symptoms are usually noted in the feet, gradually ascend up the leg, and may eventually involve the fingers and hand. Motor symptoms occur late and are predominantly distal, with foot and hand weakness. Autonomic symptoms of light-headedness, sweating problems, ileus, and bladder or sexual dysfunction are uncommon with toxic neuropathies but have been described with the use of vincristine, paclitaxel, and bortezomib. Examination reveals abnormalities that depend on the fiber types affected. Small-fiber sensory

Table 14-2. Key Clinical and Diagnostic Features of Chemotherapy-Induced Peripheral Neuropathies Based on Pathophysiology

	DEMYELINATING	AXONAL	NEURONAL
Pattern	Proximal =Distal	Distal > proximal; length dependent	Non-length-dependent; UE, LE, face
Onset	Acute/subacute	Slow evolution	Rapid
Symptoms	paresthesias and weakness	Dysesthesias and distal weakness	Paresthesias, gait ataxia
Sensory signs	Vibration and proprioception > pain and temperature	Pain and temperature affected > vibration and proprioception	Vibration and proprioception > pain and temperature
Motor	Distal and proximal weakness	Distal weakness	Proprioceptive weakness
Deep tendon reflexes	Areflexia	Distal areflexia	Areflexia
Nerve conduction studies	Velocity affected > amplitude	Amplitudes affected > velocity	Only sensory amplitudes affected
Nerve biopsy	Demyelination and remyelination	Axonal degeneration and regeneration	Axonal degeneration but no regeneration
Prognosis	Rapid recovery	Slow recovery	Poor recovery
Chemotherapy	Suramin, bortezomib	Taxol, vincristine, bortezomib	Cisplatin, oxalaplatin, paraneoplastic

LE= lower extremity; UE = upper extremity.

Table 14-3. Key Clinical and Diagnostic Features of Chemotherapy-Induced Peripheral Neuropathies Based on Type of Fibers Affected

	LARGE FIBER	SMALL FIBER	MOTOR	AUTONOMIC
Symptoms	Numbness, pins and needles, tingling, poor balance	Burning pain, shock-like, stabbing, prickling sensation, shooting, lancinating pain Allodynia (touch/clothing induce pain)	Cramps, weak grip, foot drop, twitching	Sweating decreased or increased Dry eyes, mouth, Erectile dysfunction Gastroparesis/diarrhea Faintness, light-headedness
Signs	Decreased vibration and joint position sense Reduced/absent reflexes	Decreased pinprick and temperature sensations	Reduced strength distally and reduced reflexes	Orthostasis Poor pupil light reaction
Test	NCS: reduced sensory amplitudes	NCS: normal Skin biopsy: reduced fiber density	NCS: reduced motor amplitudes; may show reduced velocities	QSART Tilt table R-R interval Valsalva test

neuropathies cause distal pinprick, temperature loss, and allodynia, while large-fiber sensory neuropathies result in loss of vibration and proprioception with a positive Romberg's test. Stretch reflexes are reduced or absent at the ankles. Weakness of toe and foot extensors and flexors may be found. The nerve conduction study shows a pattern of axonal neuropathy affecting sensory more than motor fibers in a length-dependent fashion if large fibers are involved (Table 14.2). Skin biopsy has been increasingly used to determine the density of intraepidermal fibers to assess the small fibers. Quantitative sensory testing has been used to assess the large fibers (vibration thresholds) and small fibers (thermal thresholds). The second pattern of neuropathy occurs when there is involvement of the dorsal root ganglion called *ganglionopathy or sensory neuronopathy*. Generally, this occurs with higher dosages of toxic drugs.

Cisplatin is known to be particularly associated with this pattern of nerve involvement. Clinically, numbness in the feet, clumsiness, and gait problems, especially when the eyes are closed, typify the presenting symptoms. Some patients may volunteer a Lhermitte's phenomenon of tingling going down the spine triggered by neck flexion. Examination shows large-fiber sensory loss (decreased vibration and position joint sense) and more diffuse loss of reflexes. A positive Romberg's sign and pseudoathetoid movements of the toes and fingers may be observed if there is severe proprioceptive loss. Strength is normal since the motor neurons and nerve fibers are spared. The nerve conduction study shows a non-length-dependent pattern of sensory axonal loss. Sensory neuronopathy is generally associated with a poor prognosis, and in some cases symptoms may even worsen after discontinuation of therapy (*coasting*), such as with cisplatin. The third pattern is a *demyelinating neuropathy* that is associated with more diffuse involvement, with weakness (proximal and distal), sensory loss, and generalized loss of reflexes. Bortezomib, suramin, and vincristine have rarely been reported to cause an acute or subacute Guillain-Barré-like demyelinating polyneuropathy. In general, demyelinating CIPN recovers faster than axonal CIPN.

Treatment of CIPN involves stopping the toxic agent and management of neuropathic pain, which can be significant and affect activities of daily living. Withdrawal of the offending agent results in improvement of symptoms in some but not all cases. If the damage is at the level of axons, reversibility can occur; however, if the cell body (sensory neuron) is affected, reversibility is less likely. Several neuroprotective agents including neurotrophic factors (nerve growth factor [NGF], glutamine/glutamate, acetyl-L-carnitine), antioxidants (amifostine, glutathione, *N*-acetylcystine, vitamin E, adrenocorticotrop ic hormone [ACTH] analog ORG 2766), chelating agents, calcium gluconate, and magnesium sulfate have all been tried but proved ineffective for CIPN. Close monitoring, with early recognition of CIPN and adjustment of the dose and number of cycles if necessary, remains the cornerstone of therapy to prevent CIPN, being mindful of the primary goal of chemotherapy. Perhaps more than with any other pharmacotherapy, constant vigilance and maintaining a balance between risks and benefits as they relate to antitumor efficacy, CIPN, and alternative treatment strategies is essential.

Monitoring for peripheral neuropathy should include a directed neurological evaluation, including a history, an examination, and, if available, nerve conduction studies, quantitative sensory testing, and skin biopsy. An attempt should be made to define all characteristics of the neuropathy, including (1) *fiber types affected*: sensory (small or large fibers), motor, sensorimotor, or autonomic small or large fibers; (2) *pathophysiology*: axonal, demyelinating, or neuronal;(3) *pattern of neuropathy*: length-dependent (distal axonopathy) or -independent (neuronopathy); (4) *dose relationships*: single dose, number of cycles, and cumulative dose; (5) *severity*: mild, moderate, severe; and (6) *time course of evolution*: acute, subacute, or chronic.

Clinical trials and research in CIPN have been somewhat limited by lack of consensus criteria that define these measures in a single scoring system. Several scales have been used for measuring CIPN, including the National Cancer Institute-Common Toxicity Scale (NCI-CTC), World Health Organization grading, Eastern

Cooperative Group (ECOG) grading, and Ajani criteria (Table 14.4). In general, these scales rely on limited 5-point rating systems of neuromotor (graded from none [0] to paralysis [4]) and neurosensory (graded from none [0] to debilitating paresthesias [4]) deficits. Scores of 0 to 4 are assigned from subjective (patient reports) or objective (clinical examination) reports or both. Discrimination between grade 2 (mild paresthesias, loss of deep tendon reflexes) and grade 3 (mild or moderate objective sensory loss, moderate paresthesias) may vary between providers and methods of evaluation because criteria for assigning a score are not given. Because of the use of broad categories, these scales are limited in their ability to detect incremental changes in impairment. In addition, the highest score cannot discriminate between the most severe cases of peripheral neurotoxicity, thereby introducing a ceiling effect for the measures. Symptoms may be located in different parts of the body and may be equally disabling, resulting in the same score. Pain due to thermal hypoesthesia or ataxias with joint position impairment reflecting the involvement of two different fiber types are not distinguished.

The total neuropathy score (TNS), composed of 10 component parts or measures, each of which is graded from 0 to 4, overcomes most of the above-noted drawbacks. The 10 measures are abstracted from neurological symptoms, the neurological examination, nerve conduction studies, and quantitative sensory tests (Table 14.5). Psychometric testing of the TNS revealed high reliability estimates and demonstrated criterion validity. Shorter versions of the TNS have been developed: TNSr, TNS without the quantitative determination of vibration threshold but including the neurophysiological investigation of peripheral nerves, and TNSc, exclusively clinically-based, without nerve conduction studies or quantitative vibration threshold testing. A correlation between the severity and measuring changes of CIPN, assessed using the TNS, TNSr, or TNSc and NCI-CTC, ECOG, and Ajani criteria, have been demonstrated, with acceptable reliability and validity estimates. The TNS is becoming a widely accepted, validated, comparable, sensitive, and clinically relevant method for assessing the presence of CIPN, assessing its severity,

and documenting the changes in severity during the course of chemotherapy.

The key features of individual CIPNs are outlined in Table 14.6 and discussed in detail below.

CISPLATIN

Epidemiology and Pathophysiology

Cisplatin (*cis*-diaminodichloroplatinum) was the first heavy metal used as a chemotherapeutic drug and is widely used in the treatment of head and neck, lung, esophageal, ovarian, and breast cancer. Like other heavy metals, cisplatin can be neurotoxic. The primary site of toxicity is the dorsal root ganglia neurons, which results in a large-fiber sensory neuropathy (neuronopathy). The mechanism of action of toxicity is probably similar to its chemotherapeutic action, that is, DNA binding and inhibition of DNA synthesis. The sensory neuropathy is dose related and usually occurs after a cumulative cisplatin dose of at least 300 mg/m^2.[2] However, preexisting neuropathy such as diabetic neuropathy is a risk factor, and in such cases the toxic neuropathy may occur at lower doses of cisplatin.

Clinical Features

The clinical features mimic those of a symmetric large-fiber sensory neuropathy. The onset is usually subacute, and symptoms typically start distally in the hands and feet. The classical symptoms include distal paresthesias and numbness, decreased sensation in fingers and toes, reduced vibration and joint position sensations, and ataxia. Lhermitte's sign may occur due to posterior column degeneration secondary to proximal axonal degeneration of the centrally directed portion of the bipolar sensory neuron. Small-fiber sensation (i.e., pain and temperature) and strength are generally spared. Deep tendon reflexes are absent. Most patients with cisplatin-induced sensory neuropathy experience only mild neuropathy symptoms that do not interfere with their activities of daily living, but for some patients the symptoms can be disabling, requiring cessation of chemotherapy. Even after cessation, in some patients the

Table 14-4. Various Grading Scales for Chemotherapy-Induced Peripheral Neuropathies

GRADE	0	1	2	3	4
CTC 2.0 Revised June 1999 (Neuropathy-**sensory**)	None	Loss of deep tendon reflexes (DTR) or paresthesias not interfering with activities of daily living	Objective sensory loss or paresthesias not interfering with activities of daily living (ADLs)	Sensory loss or paresthesias interfering with ADLs	Permanent sensory loss that interferes with function
CTC 2.0 Revised June 1999 (**Motor**)	Normal	Subjective weakness but no objective findings	Mild objective weakness interfering with function but not interfering with ADLs	Objective weakness interfering with ADLs	Paralysis
CTC 3.0 Revised, June 2003 (**Sensory**) *5 = death	None	Asymptomatic; loss of DTR or paresthesias (including tingling) but not interfering with function	Sensory alteration or paresthesias (including tingling) interfering with function but not with ADLs	Sensory alteration or paresthesias interfering with ADLs	Disabling
CTC 3.0 Revised June, 2003 (**Motor**) *5 = death	None	Asymptomatic; weakness on exam/testing only	Symptomatic; weakness interfering with function but not with ADLs	Weakness interfering with ADLs; bracing or assistance to walk (e.g., cane or walker) indicated	Life-threatening; disabling (e.g., paralysis)
ECOG—Neurosensory	None or no change	Mild paresthesias; loss of DTR, mild constipation	Mild or moderate objective sensory loss; moderate paresthesias	Severe objective sensory loss or paresthesias that interfere with function	
ECOG—Neuromotor	None or no change	Subjective weakness; no objective findings	Mild objective weakness without significant impairment of function	Objective weakness with impairment of function	Paralysis
Ajani sensory neuropathy	None	Paresthesias and decreased DTR	Mild objective abnormalities, absent DTR, mild to moderate functional abnormality	Severe paresthesias, moderate objective abnormality, severe functional abnormality	Complete sensory loss, loss of function
Ajani motor neuropathy	None	Mild transient muscle weakness	Persistent moderate weakness, but ambulatory	Unable to ambulate	Complete paralysis
World Health Organization grade	None	Paresthesias and/or decreased DTR	Severe paresthesias and or/or mild weakness	Intolerable paresthesias and/or marked motor loss	paralysis

Table 14-5. Total Neuropathy Score (TNS)

TNS	0	1	2	3	4
Sensory symptoms	None	Limited to fingers or toes	Extend to ankle or wrist	Extend to knee or elbow	Extend to above knee or elbow or functionally disabling
Motor symptoms	None	Slight difficulty	Moderate difficulty	Require help/assistance	Total loss of function
Autonomic symptoms[a]	None	1 yes	2 yes	3 yes	4 or 5 yes
Pinprick sensibility	Normal	Reduced in fingers/toes	Reduced up to wrist/ankle	Reduced up to elbow/knee	Reduced to above elbow/knee
Vibration sensibility	Normal	Reduced in fingers/toes	Reduced up to wrist/ankle	Reduced up to to elbow/knee	Reduced to above elbow/knee
Strength	Normal	Mild weakness (MRC 4)	Moderate weakness (MRC 3)	Severe weakness (MRC 2)	Paralysis (MRC 0 or 1)
Tendon reflexes	Normal	Ankle reflex reduced	Ankle reflex absent	All reflexes reduced	All reflexes absent
Sural amplitude	Normal/reduced <5% of the lower limit of normal (LLN)	76%–95% of LLN	51%–75% of LLN	26%–50% of LLN	0%–25% of LLN
Peroneal amplitude	Normal/reduced <5% LLN	76%–95% of LLN	51%–75% of LLN	26%–50% of LLN	0%–25% of LLN

MRC = Medical Research Council

[a]Autonomic symptoms: 1. Postural fainting, 2. Impotence in males, 3. Loss of urinary control, 4. Night diarrhea, 5. Gastroparesis.

symptoms may continue to progress, a condition known as *coasting*.

Laboratory Findings

Classical nerve conduction study-electromyographic-EMG findings include progressive reduction in sensory nerve action potential (SNAP) amplitudes, with little or no change in motor nerve conduction studies. The findings may not be length dependent. For example, the sural amplitude may be preserved, asymmetrically affected, or less affected than the radial sensory amplitude. Sural nerve biopsy usually shows Wallerian-like axonal degeneration with little evidence of regeneration, confirming that the pathology is more proximal at the level of the dorsal root ganglia.

Treatment

There is no effective treatment for cisplatin-induced neuropathy, and withdrawal of the drug is recommended in patients with bothersome or disabling symptoms. Although the neuropathy is largely irreversible, cessation of cisplatin use results in improvement of symptoms in a large number of cases.[3] Recovery usually occurs slowly over many months and in a minority of patients, particularly those with higher cumulative dosages; the symptoms may continue to worsen even when cisplatin

Table 14-6. Key Features of Individual Chemotherapy-Induced Peripheral Neuropathies

CHEMOTHERAPY	CANCERS	MECHANISM OF ACTION	NEUROPATHY	DOSE	COMMENT
Cisplatin, carboplatin, and oxaliplatin	Lung, colorectal, pancreatic, bladder, testicular	Induce crosslinks in DNA—apoptotic cell death; voltage-dependent sodium channels (only oxaliplatin)	Sensory neuronopathy Acute transient paresthesia and cold sensitivity (oxaliplatin only)	Cisplatin >300 mg/m² Carboplatin >400 mg/m² Oxalaplatin >750 mg/m² (coasting effect)	Coasting can be seen up to 6 months; sensory neuronopathy irreversible Reversible in most patients
Taxanes (paclitaxel and docetaxel) and epothilones (ixabepilone)	Breast, ovarian, lung, stomach, colon	Stabilize microtubules and interfere with their normal breakdown during cell division, leading to cell cycle arrest and death	Sensory motor neuropathy Higher single doses may cause sensory neuronopathy	Paclitaxel >750 mg/m² Docetaxel >600 mg/m² Ixabepilone >40 mg/²	
Proteasome inhibitor (Bortezomib)	Multiple myeloma, lymphomas	Inhibits proteasome—cell-cycle arrest and apoptosis	Sensory > motor axonal neuropathy Rare demyelinating neuropathy	After third cycle with dose per day of each cycle of 1.3 mg/m² worsening with each cycle. Cumulative dose of 30 mg/m² per cycle.	Reversible if recognized early and treatment stopped
Vinca alkaloids (vincristine, vinorelbine)	Leukemias, lymphomas, ovarian, testicular, breast, lung, colorectal	Inhibits microtubules	Sensory > motor axonal neuropathy; autonomic neuropathy (paralyzed ileum)	Vincristine >1.4 mg/m² Vinorelbine 25–30 mg/m²	Acute demyelinating neuropathy described with vincristine
Thalidomide Lenalidomide	Multiple myeloma		Sensory > motor neuropathy Neuronopathy described	Thalidomide >60 g	May be irreversible if neuronopathy

therapy stops (coasting). Various preventive therapies have been proposed, including vitamin E and amifostine, but the clinical trials studying these agents have reported mixed results. A comprehensive Cochrane systematic review and meta-analyses concluded that currently there are insufficient data to recommend any preventive therapy, including amifostine, diethyldithiocarbamate, glutathione, or ORG 2766, to prevent or limit the neurotoxicity of cisplatin.[4] Recently, a randomized clinical trial has reported that administration of vitamin E (400 IU daily orally) during and for 3 months after cisplatin treatment was associated with a lower incidence and reduced severity of cisplatin-induced neuropathy compared to placebo. However, the trial had a large number of dropouts (>50%) and currently, vitamin E cannot be recommended.[5]

OXALIPLATIN

Epidemiology and Pathophysiology

Oxaliplatin is a third-generation platinum that is widely used in the treatment of metastatic as well as stage II–III colon cancer. As with cisplatin, neurotoxicity is the most frequent dose-limiting toxicity of oxaliplatin. Two distinct neuropathy syndromes related to oxaliplatin use have been defined[6]: early acute neuropathy and chronic neuropathy. The pathophysiology is postulated to be related to functional channelopathy of axonal sodium channels.[7] The chronic neuropathy is an ataxic neuropathy, similar to cisplatin-induced toxic neuropathy, and usually occurs after a cumulative dose of greater than 800 mg/m^2, that is, usually after eight or nine treatments cycles.

Clinical Features and Laboratory Findings

The early acute neuropathy typically begins during infusion, within minutes to hours, or within 1–2 days of administration and is characterized by paresthesias in the hands or feet, mouth, or throat.[8] Myalgias, cramps, stiffness, and sometimes shortness of breath or difficulty swallowing may occur. The symptoms are often triggered by exposure to cold, including even simple daily activities such as holding a glass of cold water. The symptoms are usually self-limited, often resolving within days. The nerve conduction study may show repetitive discharges on compound muscle action potential (CMAP). Needle EMG shows multiple discharges or neuromyotonia, a pattern seen with Isaac's syndrome, in which voltage-gated potassium channels are implicated. Given this finding, oxaliplatin-induced acute neuropathy may be a channelopathy.

The clinical features of the chronic neuropathy are similar to those of cisplatin neuropathy, with paresthesias from distal sensory loss and gait imbalance from proprioceptive dysfunction. Studies have suggested that sensory axonal excitability techniques may provide a means to identify preclinical oxaliplatin-induced nerve dysfunction prior to the onset of chronic neuropathy.[9]

Treatment

Slowing the rate of infusion has been reported to reduce the incidence of the acute neuropathy.[10] Patients need to be reassured that the acute side effects are transient and should disappear within a week or so. While there is no effective treatment for oxaliplatin-induced chronic neuropathy, withdrawal of the drug usually results in improvement in symptoms within 2–3 months in the majority of cases.[11] Various preventive therapies have been proposed including calcium, magnesium, glutathione, carbamazepine, and amifostine. Of the various preventive agents, calcium and magnesium intravenous supplementation with oxaliplatin chemotherapy appear to the most promising[12,13]; however, they should be used with caution, as concerns exist regarding the lower response to chemotherapy with the supplementation. Avoiding cold liquids or cold exposure during acute dosing of oxaliplatin may avert some of the worrisome acute side effects.

PACLITAXEL (TAXOL®) AND DOCETAXEL (TAXOTERE®)

Epidemiology and Pathophysiology

Paclitaxel, a plant alkaloid derived from the yew tree (*Taxus brevifolia*), and its semisynthetic analog, docetaxel, are widely used chemotherapeutic agents for the treatment of breast, ovarian, head and neck, esophageal, and lung cancers. The taxols bind to microtubules and stabilize them to inhibit cell division. Peripheral neuropathy is a frequent and major dose-limiting toxicity of taxols.[14] The pathophysiology is related to disruption of axonal transport due to interference with microtubule assembly and a resultant "dying-back" axonal neuropathy.[15] The peripheral neuropathy is both dose dependent (with a higher incidence at doses >250 mg/m^2 of paclitaxel) and frequency dependent (higher with one weekly than with three weekly administrations) with a cumulative dose of >750 mg/m^2.[16] The cumulative dose of docetaxel associated with CIPN has been variable, but significant neuropathy is associated with doses >600 mg/m^2.

Clinical Features and Laboratory Findings

Taxol-induced neuropathy is characterized as a symmetric, sensory (large > small fiber) and motor, length-dependent axonal neuropathy.[17] Clinical symptoms include burning paresthesias, weakness in the arms and legs, and perioral numbness. Myalgias are not considered part of the neuropathy and are generally transient. Examination shows distal sensory loss and weakness. Nerve conduction studies have shown a reduction of sensory > motor amplitudes with preservation of latency and velocities. Autonomic features such as orthostatic hypotension have been noted in some studies. The peripheral neuropathy can be severe and functionally disabling. Awareness of dose dependence (both cumulative and single-dose) toxicity, and keeping the dose level lower than for neuropathy, has helped avoid the neuropathy.

Treatment

Dose reduction or withdrawal of the drug should be considered in appropriate cases. While various preventive therapies have been proposed, currently no therapy can be recommended for prophylaxis or treatment of taxol-induced neuropathy.[18] Nab-paclitaxel (Abraxane) is albumin nanoparticle-bound encapsulated paclitaxel that is reported to have overall lower toxicity, but the incidence of peripheral neuropathy is similar to that of paclitaxel.[19]

VINCRISTINE

Epidemiology and Pathophysiology

Vincristine, an alkaloid derived from the periwinkle plant, *Catharanthus roseus* (formerly called *vinca rosea*), is a chemotherapeutic agent used in the treatment of lymphomas, leukemias, lung cancer, and breast cancer. Vincristine is an antimicrotubule agent and inhibits the assembly of microtubule structures. Peripheral neuropathy is the main dose-limiting side effect of vincristine chemotherapy. The pathophysiology is similar to that of taxol neuropathy, that is, disruption of axonal transport due to interference with microtubule assembly and a resultant axonal neuropathy. The peripheral neuropathy occurs frequently (up to one-third of patients may experience grade 3 or 4 toxicity) and is both dose dependent and cumulative.[20,21]

Clinical Features and Laboratory Findings

Clinically, vincristine neuropathy is characterized as a sensorimotor neuropathy. Lower cumulative doses (4–10 mg) cause only reflex changes, while higher doses progressively cause paresthesias followed by sensory loss, weakness (foot drop is one of the first symptoms), and loss of deep tendon reflexes. Autonomic neuropathy can also occur, and symptoms such constipation, bladder dysfunction, postural hypotension, and even cardiac arrhythmias are not uncommon. Cranial neuropathies may also occur.[22]

Treatment

Dose reduction or withdrawal of the drug should be considered in appropriate cases. However, recovery can be slow (months), and in some cases the neuropathy may even wor-sen despite cessation of therapy.[23] Preventive therapies such as glutamine and pyridoxine have been reported to offer benefit and are under study.[24] Two other vinka alkaloids, vinblastine and vinorelbine, are associated with less peripheral neurotoxicity (5%–10%), possibly because it has less neural affinity than vincristine.[25]

THALIDOMIDE

Epidemiology and Pathophysiology

Thalidomide represents a classical example of the rebirth of an old drug with many new uses, including anticancer therapy. It was originally used as a sedative but was withdrawn over concerns of teratogenicity in the 1960s. Its immune-modulatory and antiangiogenesis properties have created renewed interest in thalidomide.[26] Currently, thalidomide, and the newer-generation analog, lenalidomide (Revlimid®), are widely used in the treatment of multiple myeloma.[27,28] Peripheral neuropathy is a major dose-limiting toxicity of thalidomide. The pathophysiology of the peripheral neuropathy is not fully understood, and multiple mechanisms including direct toxicity to nerves and reduced blood supply due to antiangiogenesis have been proposed.[29] Thalidomide-induced neuropathy is both dose dependent (cumulative doses of 100 g or more) and time-dependent; up to two-thirds of the patients receiving thalidomide over 1 year will develop neuropathy.[30,31]

Clinical Features and Laboratory Findings

Clinically, thalidomide is associated with a length-dependent distal axonal polyneuropathy that predominantly affects large fibers.[32] While the neuropathy is mostly sensory, motor neuropathy or demyelinating polyneuropathy may develop in a minority of cases. It is important to distinguish the neuropathy from direct neurotoxicity due to multiple myeloma. Serial sensory action potential measurements can allow early detection of the neuropathy.

Treatment

Use of a lower dose (≤150 mg/day) or withdrawal of the drug in severe cases is recommended. However, the improvement can be partial and may take months. Lenalidomide is associated with lower neurotoxicity than thalidomide.

BORTEZOMIB (VELCADE®)

Epidemiology and Pathophysiology

Bortezomib is a proteasome inhibitor used in the treatment of multiple myeloma, either alone or in combination with other chemotherapeutic agents.[33,34] Peripheral neuropathy is one of the most common adverse effects of bortezomib therapy, occurring in up to two-thirds of patients receiving therapy, and can be dose-limiting in up to one-third of patients.[35] The precise pathophysiology of the neuropathy is unknown but appears to be immune-mediated. The neuropathy is dependent on both the dose and the duration of therapy. Like other chemotherapy-associated neuropathies, traditional risk factors for bortezomib-associated neuropathy include baseline neuropathy, the presence of diabetes, and previous use of thalidomide.[36,37] Genetic predictors based on pharmacogenomics are being developed.[38]

Clinical Features and Laboratory Findings

Clinically, bortezomib is associated with a length-dependent mixed axonal neuropathy, although demyelinating neuropathy can also occur.[36,39] The neuropathy affects both small and large fibers, and painful paresthesias are not uncommon.

Treatment

Unlike thalidomide neuropathy, bortezomib-associated neuropathy is generally reversible, and discontinuation of the drug results in improvement of symptoms within a few weeks.[40] Currently, there is no recommended therapy for prophylaxis or treatment of bortezomib-associated neuropathy, although there have been anecdotal reports of success with a TRPM8 activator, menthol.[41]

OTHER AGENTS

Ixabepilone

Ixabepilone, an epothilone derived from *Sorangium cellulosum*, is a relatively new chemotherapeutic agent used in the treatment of refractory metastatic breast cancer.[42,43] Like the taxols, ixabepilone binds to microtubules and promotes tubulin stabilization and inhibition of cell division.[44] The microtubule binding property also contributes to ixabepilone-induced neurotoxicity similar to that of the taxols. Ixabepilone-associated peripheral neuropathy is cumulative, usually occurring after four to six cycles of treatment.[45] Clinically, ixabepilone-induced neurotoxicity manifests as a sensorimotor neuropathy (sensory > motor). Dose reduction or treatment discontinuation is effective in most cases and recovery is usually rapid (within weeks), unlike the case of vinca alkaloids.[46,47] Currently, there is no recommended therapy for prophylaxis or treatment of ixabepilone-induced neuropathy.[48]

Other chemotherapeutic agents that have been associated with CIPN include 5-fluorouracil, etoposide, gemcitabine, cytarabine, and ifosfamide (Table 14.7). Indeed, there are case reports of virtually every chemotherapeutic agent as an etiological factor for CIPN. Careful attention must be paid to differentiating CIPN from direct neoplastic effects of cancer, paraneoplastic syndromes, and toxic neuropathy due to other causes.

Table 14-7. Chemotherapy Agents Associated with Peripheral Neuropathies

Common
- Cisplatin
- Oxaplatin
- Vincristine
- Vinblastine
- Paclitaxel
- Docetaxel
- Thalidomide
- Bortezomib
- Ixabepilone

Rare
- 5-Fluorouracil
- Etoposide
- Gemcitabine
- Cytarabine
- Carmustine (BCNU)
- Fludarabine
- L-Asparaginase
- Procarbazine
- Ifosfamide
- Suramin

Radiation Plexopathy

Radiation-induced plexopathy is a relatively rare but well-described adverse effect of radiation therapy. Brachial and lumbosacral plexopathies are the most common.[49] The pathophysiology of the plexopathy is related to direct radiation injury to the nerve bundle or indirect ischemic injury due to radiation-induced toxicity to the blood vessels supplying the nerves. The injury is dose related, usually occurring after a radiation dose of >4500 cGy, with a median duration of 1 year after radiation therapy.[50]

Clinically, radiation-induced plexopathy can be difficult to distinguish from the direct effects of cancer infiltration, and careful clinical assessment is needed. Unlike neoplastic plexopathies, in radiation-induced plexopathies tingling and numbness symptoms usually occur early, pain symptoms occur late, and the involvement of the plexus is usually complete and bilateral.[51,52] Weakness also usually occurs early, and the absence of impaired hand function has high sensitivity in excluding radiation-induced brachial plexopathies.[53] (Hoeller 04). The presence of myokymic discharges on EMG suggests the presence of radiation-induced plexopathy rather than neoplastic plexopathy.[51] Imaging studies such as computed tomography (CT) and positron emission tomography (PET) scans can be helpful in identifying the presence of tumor plexopathy. Newer techniques such as magnetic resonance neurography (MRN) are being developed.[54] The treatment is largely supportive. In severe cases, neurolysis and/or omental transplant can be employed.[55] Small studies have reported successful results with anticoagulation (heparin) and vascular agents (pentoxifylline, vitamin E), highlighting the role of ischemic injury in the pathogenesis of radiation-induced plexopathies.[56,57]

Paraneoplastic Peripheral Neuropathic Syndromes

Paraneoplastic neurological syndromes (PNS) are a heterogeneous group of disorders characterized by various neurological manifestations that cannot be explained directly by the cancer, its metastases, infection, ischemic or metabolic effects, or treatment-related abnormalities.[58] These syndromes may appear before, concurrent with, or after the diagnosis of cancer. Paraneoplastic syndromes may prompt identification and treatment of the primary tumors and their recurrence, since the natural history of the PNS tends to follow that of the tumor.

The past few years have seen an increase in identification of various antibodies associated with these syndromes. The antibodies can be directed at neural antigens expressed by the cancer and are called *onconeural antibodies*. The identification of these antibodies, the presence of inflammatory response, and the observed response (in some syndromes) to immune modulation suggest that these disorders, at least in part, are immune mediated. In some respects, all PNS are autoimmune disorders thought to be initiated by the immune system response to cancer whether an onconeural antibody is identified or not.

Cancers causing symptomatic PNS are often asymptomatic and sometimes remain occult. At the time of presentation of neurological syndromes, the tumors are usually small and confined to a single organ or lymph nodes. Demonstration of these tumors may require appropriate periodic imaging including CT, MRI (magnetic resonance imaging), or, most importantly, PET imaging to uncover these malignancies.

Paraneoplastic neurological syndromes can be broadly divided into those associated with the central nervous system or the peripheral nervous system (Table 14.8). In conjunction with the theme of this book, this chapter will focus on the PNS associated with the peripheral nervous system (PPNS) concentrating on those syndromes presenting with neuropathic pain as the major manifestation.

Definition Given the lack of uniform criteria to diagnose PNS, an international panel of neurologists called the Paraneoplastic Neurological Syndrome Euronetwork (EFNS) Task Force developed guidelines for the diagnosis of suspected PNS.[59] The experts identified all the PNS and classified them as *classical* or *nonclassical* and by the presence or absence of onconeural antibodies. The classical syndromes include central nervous system disorders (encephalomyelitis, limbic encephalitis, subacute cerebellar degeneration, and opsoclonus-myoclonus) and peripheral

---

Table 14-8. Paraneoplastic Neurological Syndrome Euronetwork (EFNS) Task Force Criteria for the Diagnosis of Suspected PNS

Criteria for Definite PNS

1. Classical presentations (such as encephalomyelitis, cerebellar degeneration, limbic encephalitis, degeneration, sensory neuronopathy, opsoclonus-myoclonus, chronic gastrointestinal pseudoobstruction, Lambert-Eaton myasthenic syndrome or dermatomyositis) accompanied by cancer developing within 5 years of diagnosis of the neurological disorder.
2. A nonclassical presentation that remits following cancer treatment without concomitant immunotherapy.
3. A nonclassical presentations with onconeural antibodies and cancer developing within 5 years of neurological diagnosis.
4. A neurological disorder, classical or otherwise, in which well-characterized onconeural antibodies (Hu-Ab, Yo-Ab, CV2-Ab, Ri-Ab, Ma2-Ab or anphiphysin-Ab) are present but no cancer can be found.

Criteria for Possible PNS

1. Classical presentations without onconeural antibodies or identified cancer but with high risk of an underlying neoplasia.
2. A neurological syndrome (classical or otherwise) with partially characterized onconeural antibodies and no cancer.
3. A non-classical neurological condition without onconeural antibodies, but with cancer identified.

nervous system disorders (subacute sensory neuropathy, chronic gastrointestinal pseudo-obstruction, Lambert-Eaton myasthenic syndromes, and dermatomyositis).

The nonclassical syndromes include the following in the central nervous system: brainstem encephalitis, optic neuritis, myeloma-associated retinopathy, stiff person syndrome, and necrotizing myelopathy; and the following in the peripheral nervous system: motor neuron disease, Guillain-Barré syndrome, brachial neuritis, subacute/chronic sensorimotor neuropathy, paraproteinimic neuropathy, vasculitic neuropathy, autonomic neuropathies, acquired neuromyotonia, and acute necrotizing myopathy.

Onconeural Antibodies Several well-characterized onconeural antibodies have been identified with both classical and nonclassical syndromes. Some of these are specific markers of cancer and include anti-Hu-Ab (antineuronal antibody type 1, ANNA-1) for small cell lung cancer (SCLC); anti-Yo-Ab (PCA1-AB) for gynecological and breast cancers; anti-CV2 Ab (CRMP5 antibody-Ab) for SCLC and thymoma; Ri antibody-Ab (ANNA2 antibody) for breast cancer, gynecological cancer, and SCLC; Ma2-Ab (Ta-Ab) for testicular germ cell cancer; Amiphysin-Ab for breast cancer and SCLC; Tr-Ab for Hodgkin's lymphoma; and NMDAR-Ab for teratoma of the ovary and mediastinum. Other antibodies that are also associated with neurological syndromes but that may or may not have associated cancer include anti-AChR, anti-VGCC, and anti-VGCC.

Detection of these onconeural antibodies may help identify patients with specific clinical syndromes, although certain onconeural antibodies are found in a variety of different PNS and are associated with several different cancers. For example, anti-Hu-Ab, associated with SCLC, can present with sensory neuronopathy, encephalomyelitis, chronic gastrointestinal pseudo-obstruction, cerebellar ataxia, or limbic encephalitis. Anti-Yo antibody presenting with cerebellar ataxia may occur in ovarian, breast, or uterine cancers.

Diagnostic Criteria Diagnostic criteria of PNS include the following: (1) the presence of a classical syndrome and cancer that develops within 5 years of the diagnosis of the neurological disorder; (2) a nonclassical syndrome that resolves or significantly improves after cancer treatment; or (3) a classical or nonclassical syndrome with well-characterized onconeural antibodies even in the absence of cancer. The list of criteria is presented in Table 14.8.

Paraneoplastic Peripheral Nervous System Disorders

Paraneoplastic peripheral nervous system disorders (PPNS) are widely considered the most common paraneoplastic syndrome.[60] While most of the PPNS can also occur on an immunological basis without associated cancer, certain features should raise suspicion of the presence of a paraneoplastic syndrome.[61] The onset of PPNS tends to be acute, with rapid progression of clinical symptoms and signs over weeks to months. The EMG changes tend to evolve rapidly as well.

Common cancers associated with paraneoplastic syndromes include small cell carcinoma, breast cancer, and thymoma. Finally, certain antibodies are characteristically associated with paraneoplastic syndromes (onconeural antibodies) and are summarized in Table 14.9. However, it should be noted that antibody studies may be negative in many patients with PPNS, and the whole clinical picture should be taken into account.

While PPNS are rare and difficult to diagnose, with their incidence among patients with cancer estimated to be less than 1%, prompt identification of PPNS is important for two reasons. First, in a large number of cases, the paraneoplastic syndrome manifests years before the diagnosis of cancer becomes apparent, and prompt identification of occult cancer can lead to proved clinical outcomes. Second, in the majority of PPNS, treatment of the primary tumor can lead to regression of the paraneoplastic syndrome.

Anatomical localization of the origin of PPNS may include the cell body (sensory or motor neuron), the peripheral nerve (sensory—small or large fiber, motor, autonomic fibers), the neuromuscular junction (presynaptic or postsynaptic), or the muscle (inflammatory myopathies; Figure 14.1). Among the various

Table 14-9. Common Onconeural Antibodies Associated with Paraneoplastic Syndromes

ANTIBODY	USUAL TUMOR	COMMONLY ASSOCIATED SYNDROMES
ANNA-1 (anti-Hu)	SCLC	Limbic encephalitis, ataxia, sensory neuronopathy, autonomic and sensorimotor neuropathies
Anti-Yo	Gynecological, breast	Cerebellar degeneration
CRMP-5 (anti-CV2)	SCLC or thymoma	Encephalomyelitis, chorea, neuropathy, optic neuritis
Amphiphysin	Lung or breast cancer	Encephalomyelitis, neuropathy, stiff person syndrome
ANNA-2 (anti-Ri)	Lung or breast cancer	Ataxia, opsoclonus-myoclonus, neuropathy
Anti-Tr	Hodgkin's lymphoma	Cerebellar degeneration
Anti-Ma protein	Testicular germ cell tumors	Limbic encephalitis
Anti-NMDAR	Teratoma of the ovary or mediastinum	Encephalitis with psychiatric symptoms
Anti-VGKC[a]	Thymoma, SCLC	Neuromyotonia, limbic encephalitis
Anti-AChR[a] (muscle)	Thymoma	Myasthenia gravis
Anti-AChR (ganglionic)[a]	SCLC	Autonomic neuropathy
N-type calcium channel antibodies[a]	Lung or breast cancer	Lambert-Eaton myasthenic syndrome

[a]These antibodies are not markers of PNS since the neurological syndromes may occur with or without cancer.

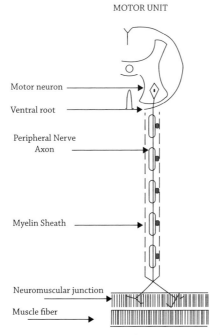

MOTOR UNIT

Motor neuron

Ventral root

Peripheral Nerve Axon

Myelin Sheath

Neuromuscular junction

Muscle fiber

Neuronopathies
 – Stiff person syndrome
 – Subacute sen sory neuronopathy
 – Motor neuronopathy

Neuropathies
 – Sensorimotor PN
 – Sensory neuropathy
 – Motor neuropathy
 – Autonomic neuropathy

Neuromuscular Junction
 – Myasthenia Gravis
 – Lambert-Eaton Myasthenic syndrome
 – Acquired Neuromyotonia

Myopathies
 – Dermatomyositis
 – Polymyositis
 – Acute necrotizing myopathy
 – Carcinomatous neuromyopathy

FIGURE 14.1   Paraneoplastic syndromes associated with the peripheral nervous system.

Table 14-10. List of PNS Primarily Associated with Neuropathic Pain Syndromes[a]

1. Subacute sensory neuronopathy
2. Chronic sensorimotor neuropathies including neuropathy associated with malignant monoclonal gammopathies[b]
3. Acute sensorimotor neuropathy (Guillain-Barré syndrome, plexitis)
4. Autonomic neuropathy
5. Stiff person syndrome
6. Vasculitis of the nerve and muscle
7. Neuromyotonia

[a]The table lists the major PNS associated with neuropathic pain syndromes and is not meant to be an exhaustive list.
[b]Covered elsewhere in this book.

central and peripheral PNS, we shall discuss the clinical features, laboratory findings, and management of those major PNS primarily associated with neuropathic pain syndromes as outlined in Table 14.10. Neuropathies associated with monoclonal gammopathies and amyloid neuropathies are covered elsewhere in this book (Chapters 13 and 16) and will not be discussed here even though they may be considered to be PNS.

SUBACUTE SENSORY NEURONOPATHY

Epidemiology

Subacute sensory paraneoplastic neuropathy, also referred to as *pure sensory neuropathy*, *sensory ganglionopathy*, or *sensory neuronopathy*, is the most common PPNS.[59,62] It is estimated that about 20% of cases of sensory neuropathy are due to paraneoplastic sensory neuronopathy, with the remainder being associated with human immunodeficiency virus (HIV).[63] systemic autoimmune disease, notably Sjögren syndrome[64] or toxin exposure such as cisplatin chemotherapy and pyridoxine toxicity,[65] or are idiopathic. The onset of sensory paraneoplastic neuropathy tends to be more rapid, evolving over weeks or months, compared to other causes, especially Sjögren syndrome-associated neuronopathy.

Sensory paraneoplastic neuropathy is typically associated with small cell carcinoma of the lung (70%–80% of cases).[66] However, it has also been associated with many other cancers, including breast cancer, ovarian cancer, prostate cancer, gallbladder cancer, Hodgkin's lymphoma, and thymoma.[67,68]

Clinical Features

Sensory paraneoplastic neuropathy typically presents as a subacute sensory neuropathy (SSN) and has certain distinct clinical features.[69,70] The onset is subacute, and then the neuropathy rapidly evolves over weeks, leading to marked debility in a significant number of patients. Symptoms, such as numbness and paresthesias, usually start in the distal upper or lower extremity and then can involve other parts of the body. Painful paresthesias and dysesthesias are frequently noted even though sensory ataxia is a common associated neurological finding. The distribution is frequently asymmetrical and almost always involves the upper limbs. Among the various sensory fibers the large fibers are typically involved, leading to marked loss of proprioception and gait unsteadiness (sensory ataxia). Romberg's sign is typically positive. Severe proprioceptive loss leading to improper coordination of muscles may lead to the wrong conclusion of weakness. Typically, if the patients can watch their muscles, strength appears to be normal, but if they are not looking, weakness may be perceived. Subacute sensory neuropathy frequently occurs in conjunction with autonomic neuropathy (see below), particularly gastrointestinal dysmotility.

Neurological symptoms typically precede the diagnosis of cancer in up to 80% of patients, with a median duration of about 5 months.[71] The diagnosis of cancer may be difficult because the cancers are often small and cannot be detected by routine radiological investigations such as CT. However, if the CT scan is negative, a PET scan should be considered in appropriate cases, such as in a smoker with unexplained weight loss. If the initial cancer screening is negative, repeat studies at close intervals, such as every 3 months, are appropriate. Bronchoscopy is usually not helpful for the diagnosis of occult SCLC. Despite intensive surveillance, it is not uncommon for the detection of cancer to be delayed by over a year.

Laboratory Findings

The cerebrospinal fluid (CSF) examination is nonspecific and usually shows increased CSF protein, white cells, and oligoclonal bands, suggesting that SSN is an immunologically mediated disease. Nerve conduction studies demonstrate a marked decrease in sensory nerve potential amplitudes in a non-length-dependent fashion.[72] For example, the radial sensory response may be absent, while the sural sensory response is only mildly reduced. Since the sensory paraneoplastic neuropathy is due to injury to the cell bodies of the sensory nerve cells in the dorsal nerve root ganglia, the nerve conduction findings are not typical of a distal stocking-glove axonopathy usually observed in garden variety peripheral neuropathies. Motor nerve action potentials may be normal or only mildly affected. Several pathological studies have confirmed an inflammatory degeneration of the dorsal root ganglion cells (ganglionitis), presumably on an immune basis. While routine skin biopsy for diagnosis of SSN is not useful, it should be considered in individual cases to rule out other differential causes, such as toxin exposure or autoimmune disease.[73]

As no clinical features or routine laboratory findings are specific for the diagnosis of SSN, there has been a lot of interest in identification of the onconeural antibody associated with SSN. The characteristic antibody associated with SSN is the anti-Hu-Ab (ANNA-1) antibody, which can be found in both the CSF and the serum.[74] Anti-Hu-Ab is most commonly seen with SSN associated with small cell carcinoma of the lung, and it is estimated that this cancer is found in more than 80% of patients who are seropositive for anti-Hu.[72,75] Anti-Hu-Ab recognizes a family of 35 to 40 kDa neuronal nuclear RNA-binding proteins and labels the nuclei (and, to a lesser extent, the cytoplasm) of all neurons, including peripheral neurons in dorsal root ganglia and autonomic ganglia.

Anti-Hu-Ab is estimated to have a sensitivity of about 80% and a specificity of almost 100% for the diagnosis of SSN. In other words, for 20% of SSNs the anti-Hu-A will be negative and thus cannot be used exclusively for the diagnosis of SSN. A recent case-control study by Camdessanché et al. (2009)[75a] suggested that presence of the following may accurately distinguish SSN from other sensory neuropathies with greater than 90% sensitivity and specificity: ataxia in the lower or upper limbs, asymmetrical distribution, sensory loss not restricted to the lower limbs, at least one sensory action potential absent or three sensory action potentials <30% of the lower limit of normal in the upper limbs, and one nerve with an abnormal motor nerve conduction study in the lower limbs.

Treatment

As with other PNS, prompt identification and treatment of the primary tumor can lead to improvement in SSN and is perhaps the only treatment with good results. While a number of immunosuppressive therapies, including intravenous immunoglobulins, plasma exchange, corticosteroids, and cyclophosphamide, have been tried, there has been only a modest benefit, if any.[76,77] (Recently, given the impressive results of rituximab, an anti-CD20 monoclonal antibody, in the treatment of B-cell lymphomas and many autoimmune disorders, researchers tried treating SSN with rituximab, but with limited success. Shams'ili et al. treated nine patients with anti-Hu or anti-Yo-associated PNS with a maximum of four monthly intravenous (IV) infusions of rituximab (375 mg/m²) and reported that three patients improved with the therapy.[78] This is likely due to the fact that the underlying pathology of SSN involves destruction of the sensory neurons.

CHRONIC SENSORIMOTOR NEUROPATHY

Epidemiology

Chronic sensory or sensorimotor neuropathy is classically associated with monoclonal gammopathies, including monoclonal gammopathy of undetermined significance (MGUS), multiple myeloma, Waldenström's macroglobulinemia, and primary amyloidosis. This is important to recognize because about 25% of patients with MGUS and neuropathy have an underlying myeloma or lymphoma, particularly those with

M-protein levels >1 g/L, progressive neuropathy, or weight loss.[78a] Peripheral neuropathies associated with monoclonal gammopathies are discussed in Chapter 16 and will be briefly reviewed here. Other cancers associated with chronic sensorimotor neuropathy include SCLC, breast cancer, and lymphoma.[79]

Clinical Features

Chronic sensory or sensorimotor neuropathy typically presents as a distal, symmetric, predominantly sensory or sensorimotor peripheral neuropathy with a male predominance. The symptoms progress slowly and are usually not debilitating. Sensory symptoms usually occur first with paresthesias, which can be painful, involving the feet and gradually ascending to above the ankle and involving the hands. Gradually, motor dysfunction occurs with predominantly distal weakness, and with the lower limbs being affected more than the upper limbs. Examination shows distal sensory loss to pinprick, temperature, and vibration in a stocking-glove distribution. Mild distal weakness and loss of distal reflexes (ankle jerks) can be found. The differential diagnosis includes toxic (cisplatin, taxol, vincristine, thalidomide, bortezomib) neuropathies, metabolic (steroid-induced diabetes), and nutritional deficiency neuropathies. Entrapment neuropathies (such as carpal tunnel syndrome) and direct infiltration of the nerve roots by malignant cells need to be considered as well.

Laboratory Features

Electromyography usually shows a sensorimotor length-dependent loss of sensory and motor amplitudes with preserved velocities. A few neuropathies associated with immunoglobulin M (IgM) monoclonal gammopathies may show demyelination with prolonged distal motor latencies and reduced conduction velocities. Spinal fluid analysis, primarily to evaluate for the presence of malignant cells, is often needed. Approximately 50% of patients with neuropathy and IgM gammopathy have IgM autoantibodies to myelin-associated glycoprotein (MAG). A positive anti-MAG assay confirmed by Western blot is strongly suggestive of an immune-mediated peripheral neuropathy,

usually associated with an IgM paraprotein. Anti-MAG autoantibodies often cross-react with other peripheral nerve glycolipids, including 3-sulfated glucuronyl paragloboside and sulfated glucuronyl lactosaminylparagloboside, which share an antigenic carbohydrate determinant with MAG.

Another group of onconeural antibodies associated with sensorimotor neuropathy are the anti-CV2-Abs. The typical manifestations of patients with anti-CV2-Abs include cerebellar degeneration, uveitis, and sensorimotor peripheral neuropathy.[80] Unlike anti-Hu-Abs, anti-CV2-Abs react with the peripheral nerve antigen CV2, a 66 kD protein belonging to the family of Ulip/CRMP proteins that are involved in the control of neuronal development and axonal transport.[80]

Treatment

Treatment of the malignancy can result in improvement of the neuropathy in approximately two-thirds of cases.[78a] However, immunosuppressive therapies alone are generally not effective.

ACUTE SENSORIMOTOR NEUROPATHY

Epidemiology

Acute sensorimotor neuropathy, also referred to as *acute inflammatory demyelinating polyradiculopathy* (AIDP) or *Guillain-Barré syndrome* (GBS), has been reported as a paraneoplastic syndrome. It is classically seen with Hodgkin's lymphoma, where it is postulated that the tumor antigens trigger an immune response against molecularly identical antigens in the PNS resulting in GBS.[81,82] Other cancers associated with GBS include non-SCLC, kidney cancer, esophageal cancer, and chronic lymphocytic leukemia.[83] In about 50% of patients GBS occurs concomitantly with the diagnosis of cancer, while in others the diagnosis of cancer usually becomes apparent in a few months.

It should be noted that acute sensorimotor paraneoplastic neuropathy can also present as acute brachial plexopathies other than GBS. In these syndromes, patients develop pain, weakness, and numbness in the distribution of one or more components of the brachial plexus as a result of an immune mechanism in association with a malignancy but not due to direct tumor infiltration. Clearly, PNS is not the most frequent diagnosis in a patient with brachial plexopathy and cancer. Direct malignant infiltration by tumor or metastasis and side effects of radiation therapy are more likely. However, a few patients with Hodgkin's lymphoma and PNS brachial plexopathy have been reported, and PNS should be kept in mind in the differential diagnosis of a brachial plexopathy.

Clinical Features

The clinical features of paraneoplastic acute sensorimotor neuropathy are similar to those of classical GBS, with distal sensory loss, rapidly progressive ascending weakness, and diffuse areflexia. Sensory symptoms are seen frequently and often precede the onset of weakness. Numbness and paresthesia in an acral distribution are frequently reported by patients with GBS. Pain is seen frequently in these patients; it occurs in the back and is often experienced as a tight band-like sensation around the trunk. Some patients may have a pure motor neuropathy. The patients describe progressive muscles weakness that usually begins in a symmetric fashion involving the distal muscles before the proximal ones and the lower limbs before the upper ones but rapidly becomes generalized, involving proximal and distal muscles equally (ascending paralysis). Difficulty walking or unsteady gait, falling, requiring assistance to walk, and reduced dexterity can all be initial manifestations of the weakness. The onset is usually acute, with a time to nadir of <4 weeks, although most cases peak within 5–7 days.[83] Cranial nerve involvement, particularly facial nerve involvement, diaphragmatic involvement, and autonomic dysfunction may occur.

Laboratory Findings

Nerve conduction studies show a demyelinating neuropathy with prolonged distal motor latencies, reduced conduction velocities, prolonged F-waves, and conduction block or temporal dispersion. A mixed axonal and demyelinating pattern[83] may also be observed. No specific onconeural antibodies have been reported. Spinal fluid protein is elevated, but no abnormal cells are found (albuminocytological dissociation).

Treatment

Besides treatment of the underlying malignancy, the treatment is similar to GBS therapy with plasmapheresis and IV immunoglobulin. However, the response is not as dramatic, and despite treatment, the mortality of patients with GBS and cancer is about four times higher than that of patients with nonmalignancy-related GBS.[83]

PARANEOPLASTIC AUTONOMIC NEUROPATHY

Epidemiology

Autonomic neuropathy can be present in up to 30% of patients with PNS and is the predominant symptom at presentation in about 10% of patients with PPNS.[72] It usually coexists with other PNS such as sensory neuronopathy, limbic and brainstem encephalitis, encephalomyelitis, cerebellar degeneration, and myasthenia gravis.[84] The presence of subacute autonomic dysfunction along with another neurological syndrome should raise the suspicion of a PNS.

Like sensory neuronopathy, autonomic neuropathy is most commonly associated with SCLC.[72,85] Other tumors that have been associated with autonomic neuropathy include thymoma, Hodgkin's lymphoma, bladder cancer, pancreatic cancer, and rectal cancer, among others.[72,86]

Clinical Features

Paraneoplastic autonomic neuropathy usually presents as a subacute panautonomic neuropathy with symptoms preceding the diagnosis of cancer. However, acute or chronic neuropathy can also occur. The clinical features are secondary to autonomic dysfunction and include clinical features of sympathetic dysfunction such as orthostatic hypotension and anhidrosis (dry skin and/or heat intolerance), as well as clinical features of parasympathetic dysfunction such as impaired cardiovagal function (cardiac dysrhythmias), erectile dysfunction, pupillary dysfunction, dry eyes, dry mouth, sphincteric dysfunction, and gastrointestinal problems. The last symptom is very common, usually consisting of severe constipation, gastroparesis, or intestinal pseudo-obstruction. Sometimes, localized presentations may also occur, such as gastrointestinal dysmotility without other autonomic features, a condition referred to as *paraneoplastic enteric neuropathy*. Abdominal pain (from gastrointestinal autonomic dysfunction) is common, and peripheral neuropathic pain can be part of this PNS. The presence of pupillary abnormalities and prominent gastrointestinal symptoms can help distinguish autoimmune and paraneoplastic autonomic neuropathies from degenerative autonomic disorders. Paraneoplastic neurological syndrome autonomic dysfunction may also be a part of other PNS such as encephalomyelitis or Lambert-Eaton myasthenic syndrome (LEMS).

Laboratory Features

Autonomic tests of parasympathetic as well as sympathetic function are generally abnormal in paraneoplastic autonomic neuropathies. Tests for parasympathetic function include tests for cardiovagal regulation such as heart rate analysis during standing, heart rate variation with deep breathing, and the Valsalva ratio. Tests of sympathetic adrenergic vascular regulation include blood pressure analysis while standing, the Valsalva maneuver, sustained handgrip, mental stress, and the cold water immersion test, and tests of sympathetic cholinergic function include the sympathetic skin response, quantitative sudomotor axon reflex testing, sweat box testing, quantification of sweat imprints, and tests of pupil function tested pharmacologically. Gastrointestinal motility tests and genitourinary tests can also be done at specialized institutions.

The onconeural antibody most commonly associated with paraneoplastic autonomic neuropathy is the anti-Hu (ANNA-1) antibody. Anti-Hu antibody also occurs in other paraneoplastic syndromes such as sensory neuropathy and brainstem encephalitis, both of which have been reported to occur concomitantly with paraneoplastic autonomic neuropathy.[87].

Another antibody that is associated with paraneoplastic autonomic neuropathy is the antibody to ganglionic acetylcholine receptors (AchR). Vernino et al.[88] reported the presence of autoantibodies to ganglionic receptors in 41% of patients with idiopathic or paraneoplastic autonomic neuropathy. The clinical feature that most reliably predicted seropositivity for the ganglionic receptor-binding antibody was the presence of an impaired pupillary response. Higher levels of the binding antibodies have been correlated with more severe autonomic dysfunction, and a decrease in levels correlated with clinical improvement as well, suggesting that these antibodies might have a pathogenic role in paraneoplastic autonomic neuropathy.[89]

Treatment

Treatment of paraneoplastic autonomic neuropathy generally consists of supportive treatments to alleviate the troublesome symptoms, such as midodrine and fludocortisone for orthostatic hypotension and pyridostigmine for gastrointestinal pseudo-obstruction.[90] Immune suppression with steroids, mycophenylate, IV immunoglobulins, and plasma exchange has been anecdotally reported to be successful, particularly as a combination therapy.[91-93] Nevertheless, as with other PPNS, every effort should be made to locate and treat the underlying malignancy. In many cases, autonomic function improves once the malignancy is effectively treated, but in others, even with prompt diagnosis and appropriate treatment, patients are left with some degree of residual autonomic deficits.

STIFF-PERSON SYNDROME

Epidemiology

Stiff person syndrome (SPS) is very rare, with a prevalence of 1 in 1 million.[94] Women are slightly more affected than men. The majority of SPS patients have an autoimmune etiology, without any associated malignancy, and have anti-GAD (glutamic acid decarboxylase) antibodies (60%) detectable in the serum. A minority of SPS, however, is paraneoplastic and associated with breast and lung cancers. In patients with cancer, antiamphiphysin antibodies (onconeural antibodies) are often detected.

It is thought that failed modulation of the spinal cord reflexes is responsible for the stiffness, spasms, and pain of SPS. Gamma-aminobutyric acid (GABA) is the neurotransmitter responsible for these spinal cord reflexes. It is produced by GAD, against which 60%–70% of the patients have been found to have antibodies. Impairment of GABAergic inhibition is the presumed mechanism of the stiffness and spasms. Amiphysin-Ab-associated SPS may work through similar effect on GABA signaling.

Clinical Features

Strictly speaking, SPS is a central nervous system disorder that presents with peripheral manifestations. Patients, typically between the ages of 30 and 50, present with stiffness and rigidity in truncal and proximal limb muscles.[94] Abdominal and thoracolumbar paraspinals are prominently affected. Intermittent intensely painful spasms, precipitated by volitional movement, tactile stimuli, noise, and emotional upset, can be extremely debilitating, resulting in difficult ambulation or falls. Although cancer and noncancer-associated SPS may be indistinguishable clinically, recent studies suggest that PNS stiffness involves the arms and neck. The stiffness and rigidity disappear during sleep.

Laboratory Findings

An EMG evaluation shows continuous contractions of agonist and antagonist muscles. Antibodies against ampiphysin may be detected in the serum and CSF. Some patients with associated encephalomyelitis may have anti-Ri-Ab as well. In patients without cancer, anti-GAD-Ab are detected along with type 1 diabetes. These antibodies (anti-GAD and antiampiphysin) are against spinal cord inhibitory interneuron antigens. Perivascular lymphocytic infiltration has been documented in the anterior horn cells of the spinal cord.

Treatment

Gamma-aminobutyric acid agonist drugs such as diazepam, clonazepam, baclofren,

and gabapentin are often helpful symptomatically. However, treatment of the underlying tumor along with immunotherapy is the more concrete treatment approach.[95] In contrast to GAD-Ab-associated SPS, which responds to intravenous immune globulin (IVIG), ampiphysin-Ab- associated SPS responds to plasma exchange with steroids and removal of the underlying cancer.

VASCULITIS OF THE NERVE AND MUSCLE

Epidemiology

Vasculitic mononeuropathy is a rare nonsystemic multiplex disorder associated with SCLC and lymphoma. Vincent et al. reported a series of 50 cases, 7 of which were associated with malignancy.[96] Lung and prostate cancer and Hodgkin's lymphoma are the reported cancers associated with this PNS. In the few case reports, there is a predilection for older men, as expected in the types of cancer reported. In addition to SCLC and lymphoma, renal cell carcinoma, gastric cancer, bile duct cancer, and prostate cancer have been reported.[97]

Clinical Features

Painful asymmetric sensorimotor neuropathy, mononeuropathy multiplex, or symmetric peripheral neuropathy are the presenting forms of this neuropathy. Systemic and constitutional symptoms are generally lacking.

Laboratory Features

Nerve conduction and EMG studies show asymmetric sensory and motor axonal loss. The erythrocyte sedimentation rate and CSF protein may be elevated. Nerve biopsy shows intraneural and perivascular inflammatory infiltrates, although necrotizing vasculitis is usually not seen.

Treatment

Treatment of the tumor, use of corticosteroids, and cyclophosphamide are often needed before a response is seen.

NEUROMYOTONIA

Neuromyotonia, also called *Isaac's syndrome*, *syndrome of peripheral nerve hyperexcitability*, and *Armadillo syndrome*, is characterized by spontaneous and continuous muscle fiber activity.

Clinical Features

Patients present with muscle cramps, paresthesias including pain, muscle twitching, and excessive sweating. Pain is often the presenting symptom.[98] Muscles may show worm-like contractions (myokymia) and, due to continuous contractions, become hypertrophic. One-quarter of the patients with neuromyotonia have central nervous system dysfunction including mood irritability, hallucinations, delusions, and sleep dysfunction.

Laboratory Features

Electromyography shows fibrillations, fasciculations, myokymia, and doublet, triplet, or multiple single discharges that have a high burst frequency. Antibodies to voltage-gated potassium channels associated with lung cancer and thymoma are often noted in approximately 40% of the patients. The antibodies against the potassium channel result in prolongation of the action potential and an increase in the release of acetylcholine-containing vesicles.[99]

Treatment

Symptomatic treatment with antiepileptic drugs such as phenytoin and carbamazpine, removal of the tumor, and immune therapies with plasma exchange and IVIG have been the modalities used for treatment.

REFERENCES

1. Wolf S, Barton D, Kottschade L, Grothey A, Loprinzi C. Chemotherapy-induced peripheral neuropathy: prevention and treatment strategies [review]. *Eur J Cancer*. 2008;44(11):1507–1515.
2. van der Hoop RG, van der Burg ME, ten Bokkel Huinink WW, van Houwelingen C, Neijt JP. Incidence of neuropathy in 395 patients with ovarian cancer treated with or without cisplatin. *Cancer*. 1990;66(8):1697–1702.
3. Von Schlippe M, Fowler CJ, Harland SJ. Cisplatin neurotoxicity in the treatment of metastatic germ cell tumour: time course and prognosis. *Br J Cancer*. 2001;85(6):823–826.
4. Albers J, Chaudhry V, Cavaletti G, Donehower R. Interventions for preventing neuropathy caused by cisplatin and related compounds. *Cochrane Database Syst Rev*. 2007;(1):CD005228.
5. Pace A, Giannarelli D, Galiè E, Savarese A, Carpano S, Della Giulia M, Pozzi A, Silvani A, Gaviani P, Scaioli V, Jandolo B, Bove L, Cognetti F. Vitamin E neuroprotection for cisplatin neuropathy: a randomized, placebo-controlled trial. *Neurology*. 2010;74(9):762–766.
6. Pasetto LM, D'Andrea MR, Rossi E, Monfardini S. Oxaliplatin-related neurotoxicity: how and why [review]? *Crit Rev Oncol Hematol*. 2006;59(2):159–168.
7. Grolleau F, Gamelin L, Boisdron-Celle M, Lapied B, Pelhate M, Gamelin E. A possible explanation for a neurotoxic effect of the anticancer agent oxaliplatin on neuronal voltage-gated sodium channels. *J Neurophysiol*. 2001;85(5):2293–2297.
8. Wilson RH, Lehky T, Thomas RR, Quinn MG, Floeter MK, Grem JL. Acute oxaliplatin-induced peripheral nerve hyperexcitability. *J Clin Oncol*. 2002;20(7): 1767–1774.
9. Park SB, Goldstein D, Lin CS, Krishnan AV, Friedlander ML, Kiernan MC. Acute abnormalities of sensory nerve function associated with oxaliplatin-induced neurotoxicity. *J Clin Oncol*. 2009;27(8):1243–1249.
10. Petrioli R, Pascucci A, Francini E, Marsili S, Sciandivasci A, Tassi R, Civitelli S, Tanzini G, Lorenzi M, Francini G. Neurotoxicity of FOLFOX-4 as adjuvant treatment for patients with colon and gastric cancer: a randomized study of two different schedules of oxaliplatin. *Cancer Chemother Pharmacol*. 2008;61(1): 105–111.
11. Andre T, Boni C, Navarro M, Tabernero J, Hickish T, Topham C, Bonetti A, Clingan P, Bridgewater J, Rivera F, de Gramont A. Improved overall survival with oxaliplatin, fluorouracil, and leucovorin as adjuvant treatment in stage II or III colon cancer in the MOSAIC Trial. *J Clin Oncol*. 2009;27(19):3109–3116.
12. Gamelin L, Boisdron-Celle M, Delva R, Guerin-Meyer V, Ifrah N, Morel A, Gamelin E. Prevention of oxaliplatin-related neurotoxicity by calcium and magnesium infusions: a retrospective study of 161 patients receiving oxaliplatin combined with 5-fluorouracil and leucovorin

for advanced colorectal cancer. *Clin Cancer Res.* 2004;10(12 pt 1):4055–4061.

13. Grothey A, Hart LL, Rowland KM, Rowland KM, Ansari RH, Alberts SR, Chowhan NM, Shpilsky A, Hochster HS. Intermittent oxaliplatin administration and time to treatment failure in metastatic colorectal cancer: final results of the phase III CONcePT trial [abstract]. *J Clin Oncol.* 2008;26:180s.

14. Swain SM, Arezzo JC. Neuropathy associated with microtubule inhibitors: diagnosis, incidence, and management [review]. *Clin Adv Hematol Oncol.* 2008;6(6):455–467.

15. Canta A, Chiorazzi A, Cavaletti G. Tubulin: a target for antineoplastic drugs into the cancer cells but also in the peripheral nervous system [review]. *Curr Med Chem.* 2009;16(11):1315–1324.

16. Lee JJ, Swain SM. Peripheral neuropathy induced by microtubule-stabilizing agents [review]. *J Clin Oncol.* 2006;24(10):1633–1642.

17. Freilich RJ, Balmaceda C, Seidman AD, Rubin M, DeAngelis LM. Motor neuropathy due to docetaxel and paclitaxel. *Neurology.* 1996;47(1):115–118.

18. Gelmon K, Eisenhauer E, Bryce C, Tolcher A, Mayer L, Tomlinson E, Zee B, Blackstein M, Tomiak E, Yau J, Batist G, Fisher B, Iglesias J. Randomized phase II study of high-dose paclitaxel with or without amifostine in patients with metastatic breast cancer. *J Clin Oncol.* 1999;17(10):3038–3047.

19. Henderson IC, Bhatia V. Nab-paclitaxel for breast cancer: a new formulation with an improved safety profile and greater efficacy [review]. *Expert Rev Anticancer Ther.* 2007;7(7):919–943.

20. Sarris AH, Hagemeister F, Romaguera J, Rodriguez MA, McLaughlin P, Tsimberidou AM, Medeiros LJ, Samuels B, Pate O, Oholendt M, Kantarjian H, Burge C, Cabanillas F. Liposomal vincristine in relapsed non-Hodgkin's lymphomas: early results of an ongoing phase II trial. *Ann Oncol.* 2000;11:69–72.

21. Kanbayashi Y, Hosokawa T, Okamoto K, Konishi H, Otsuji E, Yoshikawa T, Takagi T, Taniwaki M. Statistical identification of predictors for peripheral neuropathy associated with administration of bortezomib, taxanes, oxaliplatin or vincristine using ordered logistic regression analysis. *Anticancer Drugs.* 201021(9):877–881.

22. Mahajan SL, Ikeda Y, Myers TJ, Baldini MG. Acute acoustic nerve palsy associated with vincristine therapy. *Cancer.* 1981;47(10):2404–2406.

23. Verstappen CC, Koeppen S, Heimans JJ, Verstappen CC, Koeppen S, Heimans JJ, Huijgens PC, Scheulen ME, Strumberg D, Kiburg B, Postma TJ. Dose-related vincristine-induced peripheral neuropathy with unexpected off-therapy worsening. *Neurology.* 2005;64:1076–1077.

24. Ozyurek H, Turker H, Akbalik M, Bayrak AO, Ince H, Duru F. Pyridoxine and pyridostigmine treatment in vincristine-induced neuropathy. *Pediatr Hematol Oncol.* 2007;24(6):447–452.

25. Sørensen JB, Frank H, Palshof T. Cisplatin and vinorelbine first-line chemotherapy in nonresectable malignant pleural mesothelioma. *Br J Cancer.* 2008;99(1):44–50.

26. Singhal S, Mehta J, Desikan R, Ayers D, Roberson P, Eddlemon P, Munshi N, Anaissie E, Wilson C, Dhodapkar M, Zeddis J, Barlogie B. Antitumor activity of thalidomide in refractory multiple myeloma. *N Engl J Med.* 1999;341(21):1565–1571.

27. Barlogie B, Tricot G, Anaissie E, Shaughnessy J, Rasmussen E, van Rhee F, Mateos MV, Oriol A, Martínez-López J, Gutiérrez N, Teruel AI, de Paz R, García-Laraña J, Bengoechea E, Martín A, Mediavilla JD, Palomera L, de Arriba F, González Y, Hernández JM, Sureda A, Bello JL, Bargay J, Peñalver FJ, Ribera JM, Martín-Mateos ML, García-Sanz R, Cibeira MT, Ramos ML, Vidriales MB, Paiva B, Montalbán MA, Lahuerta JJ, Bladé J, Miguel JF. Thalidomide and hematopoietic-cell transplantation for multiple myeloma. *N Engl J Med.* 2006;354(10):1021–1030.

28. Mateos MV, Oriol A, Martínez-López J, Gutiérrez N, Teruel AI, de Paz R, García-Laraña J, Bengoechea E, Martín A, Mediavilla JD, Palomera L, de Arriba F, González Y, Hernández JM, Sureda A, Bello JL, Bargay J, Peñalver FJ, Ribera JM, Martín-Mateos ML, García-Sanz R, Cibeira MT, Ramos ML, Vidriales MB, Paiva B, Montalbán MA, Lahuerta JJ, Bladé J, Miguel JF. Bortezomib, melphalan, and prednisone versus bortezomib, thalidomide, and prednisone as induction therapy followed by maintenance treatment with bortezomib and thalidomide versus bortezomib and prednisone in elderly patients with untreated multiple myeloma: a randomised trial. *Lancet Oncol.* 2010;11(10):934–941.

29. Mileshkin L, Prince HM. The troublesome toxicity of peripheral neuropathy with thalidomide. *Leuk Lymphoma.* 2006;47(11):2276–2279.

30. Glasmacher A, Hahn C, Hoffmann F, Naumann R, Goldschmidt H, von Lilienfeld-Toal M, Glasmacher A, Hahn C, Hoffmann F, Naumann R, Goldschmidt H, von Lilienfeld-Toal M, Orlopp K, Schmidt-Wolf I, Gorschlüter M. A systematic review of phase-II trials of thalidomide monotherapy in patients with relapsed

or refractory multiple myeloma. *Br J Haematol.* 2006;132(5):584–593.

31. Mohty B, El-Cheikh J, Yakoub-Agha I, Moreau P, Harousseau JL, Mohty M. Peripheral neuropathy and new treatments for multiple myeloma: background and practical recommendations [review]. *Haematologica.* 2010;95(2):311–319.

32. Chaudhry V, Cornblath DR, Polydefkis M, Ferguson A, Borrello I. Characteristics of bortezomib- and thalidomide-induced peripheral neuropathy. *J Peripher Nerv Syst.* 2008;13(4): 275–282.

33. Richardson PG, Barlogie B, Berenson J, Singhal S, Jagannath S, Irwin D, Rajkumar SV, Srkalovic G, Alsina M, Alexanian R, Siegel D, Orlowski RZ, Kuter D, Limentani SA, Lee S, Hideshima T, Esseltine DL, Kauffman M, Adams J, Schenkein DP, Anderson KC. A phase 2 study of bortezomib in relapsed, refractory myeloma. *N Engl J Med.* 2003;348(26):2609–2617.

34. San Miguel JF, Schlag R, Khuageva NK, Dimopoulos MA, Shpilberg O, Kropff M, Spicka I, Petrucci MT, Palumbo A, Samoilova OS, Dmoszynska A, Abdulkadyrov KM, Schots R, Jiang B, Mateos MV, Anderson KC, Esseltine DL, Liu K, Cakana A, van de Velde H, Richardson PG. Bortezomib plus melphalan and prednisone for initial treatment of multiple myeloma. *N Engl J Med.* 2008;359(9):906–917.

35. Richardson PG, Briemberg H, Jagannath S, Wen PY, Barlogie B, Berenson J, Singhal S, Siegel DS, Irwin D, Schuster M, Srkalovic G, Alexanian R, Rajkumar SV, Limentani S, Alsina M, Orlowski RZ, Najarian K, Esseltine D, Anderson KC, Amato AA. Frequency, characteristics, and reversibility of peripheral neuropathy during treatment of advanced multiple myeloma with bortezomib. *J Clin Oncol.* 2006;24(19):3113–3120.

36. Badros A, Goloubeva O, Dalal JS, Can I, Thompson J, Rapoport AP, Heyman M, Akpek G, Fenton RG. Neurotoxicity of bortezomib therapy in multiple myeloma: a single-center experience and review of the literature [review]. *Cancer.* 2007;110(5):1042–1049.

37. Lanzani F, Mattavelli L, Frigeni B, Rossini F, Cammarota S, Petrò D, Jann S, Cavaletti G. Role of a pre-existing neuropathy on the course of bortezomib-induced peripheral neurotoxicity. *J Peripher Nerv Syst.* 2008;13(4):267–274.

38. Richardson PG, Xie W, Mitsiades C, Chanan-Khan AA, Lonial S, Hassoun H, Avigan DE, Oaklander AL, Kuter DJ, Wen PY, Kesari S, Briemberg HR, Schlossman RL, Munshi NC, Heffner LT, Doss D, Esseltine DL, Weller E, Anderson KC, Amato AA. Single-agent bortezomib in previously untreated multiple myeloma: efficacy, characterization of peripheral neuropathy, and molecular correlations with response and neuropathy. *J Clin Oncol.* 2009;27(21):3518–3525.

39. El-Cheikh J, Stoppa AM, Bouabdallah R, de Lavallade H, Coso D, de Collela JM, Auran-`Schleinitz T, Gastaut JA, Blaise D, Mohty M. Features and risk factors of peripheral neuropathy during treatment with bortezomib for advanced multiple myeloma. *Clin Lymphoma Myeloma.* 2008;8(3):146–152.

40. Richardson PG, Sonneveld P, Schuster MW, Stadtmauer EA, Facon T, Harousseau JL, Ben-Yehuda D, Lonial S, Goldschmidt H, Reece D, Bladé J, Boccadoro M, Cavenagh JD, Boral AL, Esseltine DL, Wen PY, Amato AA, Anderson KC, San Miguel J. Reversibility of symptomatic peripheral neuropathy with bortezomib in the phase III APEX trial in relapsed multiple myeloma: impact of a dose-modification guideline. *Br J Haematol.* 2009;144(6):895–903.

41. Colvin LA, Johnson PR, Mitchell R, Colvin LA, Johnson PR, Mitchell R, Fleetwood-Walker SM, Fallon M. From bench to bedside: a case of rapid reversal of bortezomib-induced neuropathic pain by the TRPM8 activator, menthol. *J Clin Oncol.* 2008;26:4519.

42. Lee FY, Borzilleri R, Fairchild CR, et al. BMS-247550: a novel epithilone analog with a mode of action similar to paclitaxel but possessing superior antitumor efficacy. *Clin Cancer Res.* 2001;7:1429–1437.

43. Cortes J, Baselga J. Targeting the microtubules in breast cancer beyond taxanes: the epithilones [review]. *Oncologist.* 2007;12(3):271–280.

44. Morris PG, Fornier MN. Novel anti-tubulin cytotoxic agents for breast cancer [review]. *Expert Rev Anticancer Ther.* 2009;9(2):175–185.

45. Thomas E, Gomez HL, Li RK, Thomas ES, Gomez HL, Li RK, Chung HC, Fein LE, Chan VF, Jassem J, Pivot XB, Klimovsky JV, de Mendoza FH, Xu B, Campone M, Lerzo GL, Peck RA, Mukhopadhyay P, Vahdat LT, Roché HH. Ixabepilone plus capecitabine for metastatic breast cancer progressing after anthracycline and taxane treatment. *J Clin Oncol.* 2007;25:5210–5217.

46. Baselga J, Zambetti M, Llombart-Cussac A, Manikhas G, Kubista E, Steger GG, Makhson A, Tjulandin S, Ludwig H, Verrill M, Ciruelos E, Egyhazi S, Xu LA, Zerba KE, Lee H, Clark E, Galbraith S. Phase II genomics study of ixabepilone as neoadjuvant treatment for breast cancer. *J Clin Oncol.* 2009;27(4):526–534.

47. Sparano JA, Vrdoljak E, Rixe O, Xu B, Manikhas A, Medina C, Da Costa SC, Ro J, Rubio G, Rondinon

M, Perez Manga G, Peck R, Poulart V, Conte P. Randomized phase III trial of ixabepilone plus capecitabine versus capecitabine in patients with metastatic breast cancer previously treated with an anthracycline and a taxane. *J Clin Oncol.* 2010;28(20):3256–3263.

48. Hensley ML, Hagerty KL, Kewalramani T, Green DM, Meropol NJ, Wasserman TH, Cohen GI, Emami B, Gradishar WJ, Mitchell RB, Thigpen JT, Trotti A 3rd, von Hoff D, Schuchter LM. American Society of Clinical Oncology 2008 clinical practice guideline update: use of chemotherapy and radiation therapy protectants. *J Clin Oncol.* 2009;27(1):127–145.

49. Dropcho EJ. Neurotoxicity of radiation therapy [review]. *Neurol Clin.* 2010;28(1):217–234.

50. Gałecki J, Hicer-Grzenkowicz J, Grudzień-Kowalska M, Michalska T, Załucki W. Radiation-induced brachial plexopathy and hypofractionated regimens in adjuvant irradiation of patients with breast cancer—a review. *Acta Oncol.* 2006; 45(3):280–284.

51. Harper CM Jr, Thomas JE, Cascino TL, Litchy WJ. Distinction between neoplastic and radiation-induced brachial plexopathy, with emphasis on the role of EMG. *Neurology.* 1989;39(4): 502–506.

52. Jaeckle KA Neurologic manifestations of neoplastic and radiation-induced plexopathies. *Semin Neurol.* 2010;30(3):254–262.

53. Hoeller U, Rolofs K, Bajrovic A, Berger J, Heesen C, Pfeiffer G, Alberti W. A patient questionnaire for radiation-induced brachial plexopathy. *Am J Clin Oncol.* 2004;27(1):1–7.

54. Du R, Auguste KI, Chin CT, Engstrom JW, Weinstein PR. Magnetic resonance neurography for the evaluation of peripheral nerve, brachial plexus, and nerve root disorders. *J Neurosurg.* 2010;112(2):362–371.

55. Killer HE, Hess K. Natural history of radiation-induced brachial plexopathy compared with surgically treated patients. *J Neurol.* 1990;237(4): 247–250.

56. Glantz MJ, Burger PC, Friedman AH, Radtke RA, Massey EW, Schold SC Jr. Treatment of radiation-induced nervous system injury with heparin and warfarin. *Neurology.* 1994;44(11): 2020–2027.

57. Delanian S, Balla-Mekias S, Lefaix JL. Striking regression of chronic radiotherapy damage in a clinical trial of combined pentoxifylline and tocopherol. *J Clin Oncol.* 1999;17: 3283–3290.

58. Posner JB. Paraneoplastic syndromes. *Curr Opin Neurol.* 1997;10:471–476.

59. Graus F, Delattre JY, Antoine JC, et al. Recommended diagnostic criteria for paraneoplastic neurological syndromes. *J Neurol Neurosurg Psychiatry.* 2004;75:1135–1140.

60. Grisold W, Drlicek M. Paraneoplastic neuropathy [review]. *Curr Opin Neurol.* 1999;12(5):617–625.

61. Sghirlanzoni A, Pareyson D, Lauria G. Sensory neuron diseases. *Lancet Neurol.* 2005;4:349–361.

62. Croft PB, Urich H, Wilkinson M. Peripheral neuropathy of sensorimotor type associated with malignant disease. *Brain.* 1967;90:31–66.

63. Esiri MM, Morris CS, Millard PR. Sensory and sympathetic ganglia in HIV-1 infection: immunocytochemical demonstration of HIV-1 viral antigens, increased MHC class II antigen expression and mild reactive inflammation. *J Neurol Sci.* 1993;114:178–187.

64. Griffin JW, Cornblath DR, Alexander E, Campbell J, Low PA, Bird S, Griffin JW, Cornblath DR, Alexander E, Campbell J, Low PA, Bird S, Feldman EL. Ataxic sensory neuropathy and dorsal root ganglionitis associated with Sjogren's syndrome. *Ann Neurol.* 1990;27:304–315.

65. Krarup-Hansen A, Helweg-Larsen S, Schmalbruch H, Rorth M, Krarup C. Neuronal involvement in cisplatin neuropathy: prospective clinical and neurophysiological studies. *Brain.* 2007;130:1076–1088.

66. Ansari J, Nagabhushan N, Syed R, Bomanji J, Bacon CM, Lee SM. Small cell lung cancer associated with anti-Hu paraneoplastic sensory neuropathy and peripheral nerve microvasculitis: case report and literature review. *Clin Oncol (R Coll Radiol).* 2004;16(1):71–76.

67. Baird AD, Cornford PA, Helliwell T, Woolfenden KA. Small cell prostate cancer with anti-Hu positive peripheral neuropathy. *J Urol.* 2002;168(1):192.

68. Uribe-Uribe NO, Jimenez-Garduño AM, Henson DE, Albores-Saavedra J. Paraneoplastic sensory neuropathy associated with small cell carcinoma of the gallbladder. *Ann Diagn Pathol.* 2009;13(2):124–126.

69. Chalk CH, Windebank AJ, Kimmel DW, McManis PG. The distinctive clinical features of paraneoplastic sensory neuronopathy. *Can J Neurol Sci.* 1992;19:346–351.

70. Kuntzer T, Antoine JC, Steck AJ. Clinical features and pathophysiological basis of sensory neuronopathies (ganglionopathies). *Muscle Nerve.* 2004;30:255–268.

71. Graus F, Keime-Guibert F, Reñe R, et al. Anti-Hu-associated paraneoplastic encephalomyelitis: analysis of 200 patients. *Brain.* 2001;124: 1138–1148.

72. Camdessanche JP, Antoine JC, Honnorat J, Vial C, Petiot P, Convers P, Camdessanché JP, Antoine JC, Honnorat J, Vial C, Petiot P, Convers P, Michel D. Paraneoplastic peripheral neuropathy associated with anti-Hu antibodies. A clinical and electrophysiological study of 20 patients. *Brain.* 2002;125:166–175.

73. Sommer C, Lauria G. Skin biopsy in the management of peripheral neuropathy [review]. *Lancet Neurol.* 2007;6(7):632–642.

74. Dalmau J, Furneaux HM, Rosenblum MK, Graus F, Posner JB. Detection of the anti-Hu antibody in specific regions of the nervous system and tumor from patients with paraneoplastic encephalomyelitis/sensory neuronopathy. *Neurology.* 1991;41:1757–1764.

75. Lucchinetti CF, Kimmel DW, Lennon VA. Paraneoplastic and oncologic profiles of patients seropositive for type 1 antineuronal nuclear autoantibodies. *Neurology.* 1998;50(3):652–657.

75a. Camdessanché JP, Jousserand G, Ferraud K, Vial C, Petiot P, Honnorat J, Antoine JC. The pattern and diagnostic criteria of sensory neuronopathy: a case-control study. *Brain.* 2009;132 (Pt 7):1723–1733.

76. Widdes-Walsh P, Tavee JO, Schuele S, Stevens GH. Response to intravenous immunoglobulin in anti-Yo associated paraneoplastic cerebellar degeneration: case report and review of the literature [review]. *J Neuro-oncol.* 2003;63(2):187–190.

77. Vernino S, O'Neill BP, Marks RS, O'Fallon JR, Kimmel DW. Immunomodulatory treatment trial for paraneoplastic neurological disorders. *Neuro-Oncology.* 2004;6:55–62.

78. Shams'ili S, de Beukelaar J, Gratama JW, Shams'ili S, de Beukelaar J, Gratama JW, Hooijkaas H, van den Bent M, van 't Veer M, Sillevis Smitt P. An uncontrolled trial of rituximab for antibody associated paraneoplastic neurological syndromes. *J Neurol.* 2006;253:16–20.

78a. Eurelings M, Ang CW, Notermans NC, Van Doorn PA, Jacobs BC, Van den Berg LH. Anti-ganglioside antibodies in polyneuropathy associated with monoclonal gammopathy. *Neurology.* 2001;57(10):1909–1912.

79. Stern BV, Baehring JM, Kleopa KA, Hochberg FH. Multifocal motor neuropathy with conduction block associated with metastatic lymphoma of the nervous system. *J Neurooncol.* 2006;78(1):81–84.

80. Antoine JC, Honnorat J, Camdessanché JP, Magistris M, Absi L, Mosnier JF, Petiot P, Kopp N, Michel D. Paraneoplastic anti-CV2 antibodies react with peripheral nerve and are associated with a mixed axonal and demyelinating peripheral neuropathy. *Ann Neurol.* 2001;49(2):214–221.

81. Lisak RP, Mitchell M, Zweiman B, Orrechio E, Asbury AK. Guillain-Barré syndrome and Hodgkin's disease: three cases with immunological studies. *Ann Neurol.* 1977;1:72–78.

82. Lahrmann H, Albrecht G, Drlicek M, Oberndorfer S, Urbanits S, Wanschitz J, Zifko UA, Grisold W. Acquired neuromyotonia and peripheral neuropathy in a patient with Hodgkin's disease. *Muscle Nerve.* 2001;24(6):834–838.

83. Vigliani MC, Magistrello M, Polo P, Mutani R, Chiò A, Piemonte and Valle d'Aosta Register for Guillain-Barré Syndrome. Risk of Cancer in patients with Guillain-Barré Syndrome (GBS). A population-based study. *J Neurol.* 2004;251(3):321–326.

84. Vernino S, Cheshire WP, Lennon VA. Myasthenia gravis with autoimmune autonomic neuropathy. *Auton Neurosci.* 2001;88(3):187–192.

85. Lennon VA, Sas DF, Busk MF, Lennon VA, Sas DF, Busk MF, Scheithauer B, Malagelada JR, Camilleri M, Miller LJ. Enteric neuronal autoantibodies in pseudoobstruction with small-cell lung carcinoma. *Gastroenterology.* 1991;100:137–142.

86. Vernino S, Lennon VA. Autoantibody profiles and neurological correlations of thymoma. *Clin Cancer Res.* 2004;10(21):7270–7275.

87. Saiz A, Bruna J, Stourac P, Vigliani MC, Giometto B, Grisold W, Honnorat J, Psimaras D, Voltz R, Graus F. Anti-Hu-associated brainstem encephalitis. *J Neurol Neurosurg Psychiatry.* 2009;80(4):404–407.

88. Vernino S, Adamski J, Kryzer TJ, Fealey RD, Lennon VA. Neuronal nicotinic ACh receptor antibody in subacute autonomic neuropathy and cancer-related syndromes. *Neurology.* 1998;50:1806–1813.

89. Gibbons CH, Freeman R. Antibody titers predict clinical features of autoimmune autonomic ganglionopathy. *Auton Neurosci.* 2009;146(1–2):8–12.

90. Anderson NE, Hutchinson DO, Nicholson GJ, Aitcheson F, Nixon JM. Intestinal pseudoobstruction, myasthenia gravis, and thymoma. *Neurology.* 1996;47:985–987.

91. Bohnen NI, Cheshire WP, Lennon VA, Van Den Berg CJ. Plasma exchange improves function in a patient with ANNA-1 seropositive paraneoplastic autonomic neuropathy [abstract]. *Neurology.* 1997;48(suppl):A131-A131.

92. Gibbons CH, Vernino SA, Freeman R. Combined immunomodulatory therapy in autoimmune autonomic ganglionopathy. *Arch Neurol.* 2008;65(2):213–217.

93. Iodice V, Kimpinski K, Vernino S, Sandroni P, Fealey RD, Low PA. Efficacy of immunotherapy in seropositive and seronegative putative autoimmune autonomic ganglionopathy. *Neurology*. 2009;72(23):2002–2008.

94. Duddy ME, Baker MR. Stiff person syndrome [review]. *Front Neurol Neurosci*. 2009;26:147–165.

95. Donofrio PD, Berger A, Brannagan TH 3rd, Bromberg MB, Howard JF, Latov N, Quick A, Tandan R. Consensus statement: the use of intravenous immunoglobulin in the treatment of neuromuscular conditions report of the AANEM Ad Hoc Committee. *Muscle Nerve*. 2009;40(5):890–900.

96. Vincent D, Dubas F, Hauw JJ, Godeau P, Lhermitte F, Buge A, Castaigne P. Nerve and muscle microvasculitis in peripheral neuropathy: a remote effect of cancer? *J Neurol Neurosurg Psychiatry*. 1986;49(9):1007–1010.

97. Oh S. Paraneoplastic vasculitis. *Neurol Clin*. 1997;15(4):849–863.

98. Maddison P. Neuromyotonia. *Clin Neurophysiol*. 2006;117(10):2118–2127.

99. Arimura K, Sonoda Y, Watanabe O, Nagado T, Kurono A, Tomimitsu H, Otsuka R, Kameyama M, Osame M. Isaacs' syndrome as a potassium channelopathy of the nerve [review]. *Muscle Nerve*. 2002;(suppl 11):S55–S58.

15

Herpes Zoster and Postherpetic Neuralgia

CHRISTINA JENSEN-DAHM, KARIN L. PETERSEN, AND MICHAEL C. ROWBOTHAM

THE VARICELLA ZOSTER VIRUS AND THE PATHOGENESIS OF HERPES ZOSTER

THE VARICELLA ZOSTER virus (VZV) is the smallest of the double-stranded DNA herpesviruses and the only one capable of producing two different diseases, varicella (chickenpox) and herpes zoster (HZ, shingles).[1] Varicella is primarily a disease of childhood; its morbidity and mortality are high in the few adults who remain susceptible to primary infection. Prior to the introduction of the live attenuated VZV vaccine (OKA strain), the annual incidence of varicella in the United States was as high as 4 million cases per year with approximately 100 deaths.[2,3] Varicella remains a significant public health problem, but vaccination programs for children and susceptible adults are becoming more widespread.

Nasopharyngeal replication of VZV begins immediately after primary infection.[4,5] Infection of the abundant memory CD4+ T cells in nearby tonsillar lymphoid tissue results in delivery of virus to cutaneous epithelia within several days. Eventually, cell-to-cell spread of virus overcomes innate defenses and results in vesicles containing cell-free virus able to infect sensory nerve endings in epithelia. Virus migration along sensory axons reaches the dorsal root ganglia (DRG), and latency is established.

How latency and reactivation are controlled remain poorly understood, but much has been learned from a guinea pig model. Latently infected human ganglia show restricted expression of only six genes, none of which code for glycoproteins. In postmortem studies of persons without recent HZ, latent VZV DNA sequences were detectable via polymerase chain reaction (PCR) in multiple ganglia along the neuraxis.[6] In situ hybridization studies have shown that the latent genome can be localized to 1%–7% of sensory ganglion neurons with fewer than 10 copies per cell. One hypothesis of how latency is maintained is that phosphorylation of one immediate-early protein prevents translocation from the cytoplasm to the nucleus, thereby interrupting the cascade of viral transcription and replication that accompanies lytic infection.[5] Other work has emphasized viral strategies for evading the immune system.[7]

More than 45 years ago, Hope-Simpson proposed that immunity to VZV plays a pivotal role in the pathogenesis of herpes zoster (HZ).[8] Subsequent observations have supported his thesis that cell-mediated immunity (CMI) to VZV, not circulating antibodies, is the major determinant of the risk of developing HZ and its severity. Whereas levels of antibody to VZV remain relatively constant with increasing age, the increased incidence and severity of HZ and postherpetic neuralgia (PHN) among older adults is linked to a progressive age-related decline in CMI to VZV.[2] Reexposure to VZV has been shown to boost VZV CMI in people who have previously had the virus,[9] such as mothers of children with varicella and adults with frequent contact with children,[10,11] which may help maintain adequate immunity. A small percentage of asymptomatic adults of all ages will have detectable viremia, suggesting that subclinical reactivations (defined as viral replication without pain, neurological deficit, or rash) are common but do not evolve into an episode of HZ because CMI quickly contains the event.[12]

EPIDEMIOLOGY OF HZ IN ADULTS

The incidence of HZ is strongly age-dependent. Herpes zoster is not rare among younger individuals, but the median age of patients with HZ is 64 years compared to a median age of 46 for the U.S. population as a whole. In immunocompetent individuals, the incidence is between 1.2 and 3.4 cases per 1000 person-years. At age 65 and above, the incidence rises to 3.9–11.8 cases per 1000 person-years. By age 80, the yearly risk is nearly 1%.[1] There are an estimated 300,000 to 1 million new cases of HZ each year in the United States. No major insult to the immune system precedes VZV reactivation in the majority of cases, and the old practice of engaging in a lengthy workup for cryptic malignancy in seemingly healthy older persons with HZ has fallen by the wayside. A careful history remains important, as almost any drug or medical disease that impairs CMI can be sufficient to allow VZV reactivation, even brief oral corticosteroid therapy. Stressful life events, such as the death of a spouse or loss of a job, are also risk factors for HZ.

Despite the reduction in childhood varicella through immunization programs, the incidence of HZ is actually increasing. The aging of the population, especially in the developed world, only partially explains the increase. The remainder of the explanation for the increase may be that more patients of all ages are receiving immunosuppressant drugs. For example, the number of patients receiving solid-organ transplants in the United States doubled between 1988 and 2003, and all of them receive long-term immunosuppressant medication. The steady increase in the range of immunosuppressant drugs available, and their increasing use in situations other than organ transplantation, will only add to this trend. Paradoxically, the spread of childhood vaccination programs may also be a contributing factor. As fewer children have symptomatic varicella, the opportunities for subclinical boosting of immunity in adults declines as well.[13] Although susceptible individuals are far more likely to acquire infection after exposure to a patient with varicella than to one with HZ (20% vs. 0.1%), widespread childhood immunization programs have reduced the exposure of susceptible adults and children to children with varicella to the point where a large percentage of new varicella cases are arising from contact with acute zoster patients. Reducing the occurrence of HZ is therefore crucial to eliminating transmission of VZV. The OKA vaccine virus does establish neuronal latency, and appears to reactivate and cause HZ less frequently than wild-type VZV.[14] It has been projected that the incidence of HZ will rise for approximately 20 years after initiation of childhood vaccination programs and remain increased for another 20 years before declining.[3,15] Future generations may see major reductions in both VZV and HZ,[13] but conclusive recent evidence supporting these projections is still awaited.[15]

PREVENTION OF HZ

There is no better way to prevent PHN than prevention of the antecedent disease, HZ. It has long been known that multiple episodes of HZ are rare among immunocompetent persons, presumably because the first episode of HZ boosts immunity to VZV, effectively "immunizing" against a subsequent episode. Work in the early 1990s by Myron Levin and colleagues translated this clinical knowledge into an important new therapy by demonstrating that vaccination increased CMI in older adults and reduced the likelihood of HZ in bone marrow transplant recipients.[16-18] The hypothesis that HZ can be prevented by boosting CMI in healthy older adults through vaccination was definitively proven in the Shingles Prevention Study, a landmark randomized, placebo-controlled study of the live attenuated OKA/Merck vaccine in 38,546 healthy adults over the age of 60.[19] In this extraordinary study, led by Michael Oxman at the University of California at San Diego, more than 95% of the subjects continued in the study to its completion, resulting in a median of 3.12 years of surveillance for HZ after vaccination. Reactions at the injection site were more frequent among vaccine recipients compared to those receiving placebo but were generally mild. A total of 957 cases of HZ were confirmed (315 among vaccine recipients and 642 among placebo recipients). The zoster vaccine was highly effective, reducing the incidence of HZ by 51.3% (from 11.1 per 1000 person-years in the placebo group to 5.4 per 1000 person-years in the vaccine group). Although still effective in persons over the age of 70, the vaccine was significantly better in preventing HZ in those aged 60–69 at the time of vaccination (a 38% reduction vs. 64%; $P < .001$). There was no sex difference in vaccine efficacy.

The Zoster Brief Pain Inventory (ZBPI; a modification of the Brief Pain Inventory) was used to measure the daily burden of illness due to HZ.[20] The burden of illness was reduced by 61% in vaccine recipients. The 957 HZ cases resulted in 107 cases of PHN. Again, the vaccine was highly effective, as only 27 of 315 HZ cases in vaccine recipients resulted in PHN compared to 80 of 642 HZ cases in placebo recipients,

a reduction of 66.5%. There is no proven benefit to vaccinating otherwise healthy persons between the ages of 50 and 59 (or younger). Unless contraindicated, all persons aged 60 and older should receive the HZ vaccine.[5] The recent review by Oxman summarizes data collected since the Shingles Prevention Study was completed.[21]

CLINICAL ASPECTS OF HZ

Once reactivated, VZV initially replicates within the DRG and spreads along the sensory nerves to the skin. During HZ, viral replication can be demonstrated in the affected skin, in blood mononuclear cells, and often in the cerebrospinal fluid.[22] The ensuing inflammation can be intense enough to produce a wide variety of injuries to neural, vascular, and other tissues, especially during trigeminal zoster.[23] The DRG may show acute hemorrhagic necrosis, neuronal loss, and eosinophilic inclusion bodies in satellite cells.[1,24,25] Peripheral nerve axons, both large and small, may show signs of focal demyelination. In the skin, intraepidermal vesicles, ballooning of the epithelial cells, and multinucleated giant cells with eosinophilic intranuclear inclusion bodies are found. A typical zoster rash is shown in Figure 15.1. Recent studies of HZ have provided evidence that despite the unilateral nature of the rash in nearly every case, there is insult to the nervous system on the contralateral side. A relatively high incidence of bilateral injury to segmental motor nerves (which may be clinically inapparent) has been demonstrated by electromyography (EMG).[26,27]

SPECTRUM OF ZOSTER-ASSOCIATED PAIN

Zoster sine herpete, the acute zoster syndrome without the associated skin rash, is uncommon but has been proven to account for some cases of transverse myelitis, cranial and peripheral polyneuritis, chronic radicular pain, and aseptic meningitis.[23] Preherpetic neuralgia is the prodromal radicular pain, along with pruritis and paresthesias produced by inflammation and viral replication in the DRG and peripheral

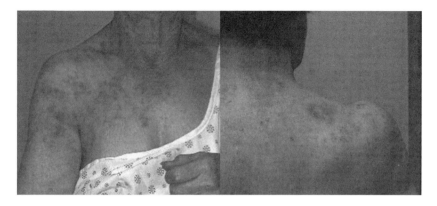

FIGURE 15.1 Anterior and posterior views of a typical zoster rash at about 4 weeks. Which dermatome is affected? (See Figure 15.2 for the answer.)

nerve apparatus before the appearance of the first skin lesions; PHN occurs in 70%–80% of all HZ patients. When prodromal symptoms are prolonged, a fruitless but intensive diagnostic evaluation for diseases characterized by unilateral localized pain, such as cholecystitis, myocardial infarction, glaucoma, nephrolithiasis, and spinal nerve compression, may ensue. A few cases of preherpetic neuralgia lasting for 3 or more months have been documented.[28] The appearance of skin lesions (usually within 4 days) marks the transition to clinically evident HZ.

Many studies (mostly of antiviral therapy) have used a simple outcome measure of the number of days of zoster-associated pain (ZAP), beginning with rash onset and ending when pain disappears entirely or reaches a predefined minimum. Studies employing days of ZAP as an outcome measure typically use survival analysis techniques to compare therapies. Use of the ZBPI in the large vaccine trial to measure the burden of zoster pain and disability is an important improvement upon the ZAP concept.

The transition from HZ to PHN is typically defined as occurring when pain in the area affected by HZ persists for 3 months or more after crusting of the skin lesions, but definitions vary from as short as 1 month to as long as 6 months after lesion crusting; some authors describe a subacute HZ period lasting for 6 weeks to 4 months.[29,30] Postherpetic neuralgia is considered any pain >0 on a pain scale, but pain scores of only 1 or 2 on a 0–10 scale typically involve little or no disability. Hence, some recent studies have employed the term *clinically meaningful PHN* (CM-PHN, defined as maximum pain VAS (Visual Analog Scale) of ≥30/100 despite treatment), which may better identify patients with pain severe enough to affect daily living and require treatment.[20,31] At this time, we recommend that longitudinal studies report the incidence of both PHN and CM-PHN.

MECHANISMS OF HZ PAIN AND RISK FACTORS FOR DEVELOPMENT OF PHN

Most patients report pain of at least moderate severity during HZ, with components of deep aching, superficial burning and itching, lancinating or electrical shock-like pains, and allodynia to gentle touch.[27,31,32] Allodynia to light mechanical touch on clinical exam has been reported in up to 80% of patients with HZ, with varying degrees of loss of sensory function to warm, cold, and mechanical stimulation as well as heat and mechanical hyperalgesia in affected skin. The tissue inflammation and destruction, activation of nociceptor fibers in the nervi nervorum, abnormal impulse generation from acutely injured or dying neurons, and neural injury that occurs during HZ produce a sufficiently intense nociceptive barrage to account for the acute pain and allodynia.[27,33]

In all published studies, older age and greater severity of initial zoster pain are each found to increase the risk of developing PHN.[34,35] Although the overall incidence of PHN after

HZ is about 10%, the incidence is nearly 80% after the age of 80. Pain severity during acute HZ may predict PHN in two ways.[36] First, severe zoster pain is believed to correlate with a more severe outbreak, that is, more severe inflammation of the nerve trunk and possibly greater injury to primary afferent nerve fibers. An acute injury to the nervous system produces prolonged and/or intense noxious stimuli, which may initiate prolonged changes in both the peripheral and central nervous systems. Deafferentation and increased peripheral input due to phenomena like primary afferent sensitization and ectopic activity of damaged primary afferents increase the excitability of central pain-transmitting neurons and promote longer-term neural processes, such as changes in gene expression, protein synthesis, and neural connectivity. Second, because greater pain produces greater initial disability and immobility, the elderly may have a difficult time recovering their prior level of function. This is particularly important, as psychosocial factors (living alone, disease conviction, anxiety, and depression) also promote the development of PHN. Loss of thermal sensory function in one study, and touch-evoked allodynia and pinprick hypoesthesia in another, were reported to predict the development of PHN, but the total number of patients who developed PHN was small in both studies.[27,37]

In the most comprehensive study of the natural history of HZ pain to date, a cohort of 94 subjects at elevated risk for PHN were followed at regular intervals until 6 months after the onset of the HZ rash.[31,36,38] Psychosocial factors, sensory testing, the capsaicin response test, and serial skin biopsy of HZ-affected, mirror-image, and distant control skin comprised the battery of measures. Subjects were considered at elevated risk of PHN by virtue of being over the age of 50 and still having average daily pain ≥2/10 severity (despite medication use) when enrolled between 2 and 6 weeks after rash onset. Responses on the Short Form McGill Pain Questionnaire (SF-MPQ) and the Multidimension Pain Inventory (MPI) at study entry were similar to those of a historical control group of chronic severe PHN patients who participated in a large controlled trial of gabapentin during the 1990s.[39] Although

32% still had pain >0/100 at 6 months and met the definition of PHN, pain and disability in the group at this time point were quite mild, with only four subjects still experiencing maximum daily pain ≥30/100 (CM-PHN) despite medication use. At study entry, SF-MPQ, the Ways of Coping Checklist, the Life Events Checklist, and MPI responses all failed to predict PHN, with the exception that "pain severity" and "affective distress" scores on the MPI were higher in eventual PHN patients, as were overall SF-MPQ scores. Slopes analysis showed that the rate of improvement was the same in subjects whose pain resolved fully and those who eventually developed PHN; it was only pain severity at study entry that differed between the two groups. Still, high pain ratings at study entry did not preclude full recovery; even a subject with an average daily pain rating of 98/100 at study entry recovered fully by 6 months.

The sensory testing and skin biopsy aspects of the natural history study were designed to test two hypotheses. The first hypothesis was that PHN develops because of a severe initial neural injury and/or a failure to recover normal neural function.[31] At study entry, eventual PHN subjects had significantly more impairment in detecting warmth and cold, as well as a larger area of altered sensation, a larger area of allodynia, and more severe allodynia. The second hypothesis, that PHN develops because of a failure to recover normal neural function, was not well supported. Sensory recovery by 6 months in HZ skin was limited and selective; sensory symptoms persisted in many pain-free subjects, and slopes analysis showed no recovery in warmth and heat pain detection thresholds in either group. For those aspects of sensory function in HZ skin that did improve (allodynia area and severity, hyperalgesia to von Frey hair, cold detection threshold), PHN and pain-free subjects recovered at the same rate. By virtue of having more severe sensory dysfunction at the beginning of their illness, recovery was less complete in subjects with PHN at 6 months.

The capsaicin response test was used in the zoster natural history study as a selective 60-minute probe of primary afferents and their interaction with central pain processing pathways.[40] The capsaicin receptor, TRPV1, an important molecular integrator of inflammatory pain,[41–43] is upregulated after nerve injury.[44] In patients with long-standing severe PHN, capsaicin application increases pain and allodynia, sometimes dramatically.[40,45] At 6–8 weeks after rash onset, applying 0.075% capsaicin cream on an area of HZ skin only 9 cm^2 in size significantly aggravated HZ pain and sensory symptoms in nearly two-thirds of the subjects. At 6 months, most pain-free subjects no longer experienced pain or allodynia from capsaicin application. In the PHN group, nearly half had significantly aggravated pain and sensory symptoms and the allodynia area expanded by 70 cm^2, suggesting persistent sensitization and/or TRPV1 upregulation.

Three additional factors have been invoked as important contributors to HZ pain and the risk of PHN: sympathetically mediated pain, ongoing inflammation and tissue destruction, and underlying large-fiber neuropathy. Although it has long been recognized that some cases of zoster are complicated by the development of a complex regional pain syndrome, the influence of the sympathetic nervous system on HZ pain and PHN is uncertain.[46] Some authors have described improvement in HZ pain affecting the limbs and torso with sympathetic blocks, but closer inspection of the studies show that the technique used was conventional epidural local anesthetic blockade (with or without steroids).[47] Epidural blockade with local anesthetic is not fiber-type specific, meaning that both sympathetic and unmyelinated afferents are affected. Treatment of cranial/facial HZ with sympathetic blockade of the stellate ganglion is more selective for sympathetics, but it is still confounded by the fact that the systemic local anesthetic blood levels produced are similar to those produced by intravenous lidocaine infusion—a procedure that sometimes dramatically (and briefly) relieves neuropathic pain. Stellate ganglion blockade for trigeminal zoster has not been examined in a large, well-controlled trial.

In a few cases of HZ, later complications (especially ocular) may be due to persistent viral replication and inflammation.[23] Persistent viral replication appears to be very uncommon, and few PHN patients have reproducible pain

relief with additional courses of antivirals. For ophthalmic HZ, ongoing inflammation and progressive tissue damage are not unusual and provide continuing sources of pain.

It has long been thought that large-fiber peripheral neuropathy increases the risk of PHN, with diabetics being especially susceptible. McCulloch and colleagues reported that 129 of 1017 diabetics had a history of shingles and were more likely to develop PHN.[48] More recently, Whitton and colleagues found impaired vibratory sense in 45 PHN patients compared with 45 age-matched healthy controls.[49] Baron and colleagues prospectively followed a group of nondiabetics with severe acute HZ infection.[50] During acute HZ, quantitative vibratory sense testing, histamine response testing, and tests of parasympathetic cardiac innervation were performed. At 6 months, the 17 patients with PHN were age-matched with 17 HZ patients from the group who had become pain-free. Comparing each parameter individually, the authors reported that the only significant difference between the PHN patients and pain-free controls was impaired vibratory threshold, a measure of large-fiber function. In the natural history study described in detail earlier, no relationship between vibratory sensation and the risk of persistent pain could be found in the cohort, which included 10 diabetics but excluded subjects with symptomatic peripheral neuropathy to prevent confounding.[36]

PREVENTION OF PHN VIA AGGRESSIVE TREATMENT OF ACUTE ZOSTER

Herpes zoster is almost always a once-in-a-lifetime event, but the costs of PHN in terms of personal suffering, impact on caregivers, and impact on the health care system are large.[34,35,51] Antiviral therapy of HZ significantly reduces the number of days of ZAP and reduces the proportion of patients with PHN at 6 months.[52,53] Adding oral corticosteroids to antivirals reduces acute pain but does not significantly reduce the incidence of PHN.[54]

Numerous uncontrolled case series have suggested that nerve blocks relieve HZ pain and reduce the incidence of PHN. Pasqualucci and colleagues reported the results of a randomized study of 600 patients over the age of 55 with severe HZ pain comparing continuous administration (for up to 21 days) of bupivacaine plus periodic administration of steroids via epidural catheter compared to intravenous (i.v.) acyclovir plus high-dose i.v. and oral steroids.[55] By 1 month posttreatment, significantly fewer patients in the epidural group reported pain (7.6% vs. 40.5%). At 1 year posttreatment, only 6% in the epidural group described either pain or abnormal sensations compared to 34% in the acyclovir + steroids group. The treatment regimen described by Pasqualucci et al. would be quite expensive and entails risks that would be considered unacceptable in the United States for most physicians. The recent Prevention by epidural Injection of postherpetic Neuralgia in the Elderly (PINE) study of epidural steroids, which was a superior study methodologically, showed a modest reduction in pain in the first month after rash onset, with no effect in preventing PHN, primarily because few patients in either group had persistent pain.[56] Ji et al. found a significant decrease in ZAP and allodynia at 1, 3, 6, and 12 months in a large randomized study of adding 1 week of repetitive paravertebral injections of bupivacaine and prednisolone to oral antivirals plus as-needed oral nonsteroidal anti-inflammatory drugs (NSAIDs).[57]

In a placebo-controlled but methodologically quite limited study, Bowsher reported that low doses of the tricyclic antidepressant amitriptyline prevented PHN when given during HZ infection.[58] Berry and Petersen showed an acute effect of single large doses of gabapentin on zoster pain and allodynia using a placebo-controlled, two-session crossover design.[59] A recent longer-term prospective study showed that opioids were probably the best oral medication choice for treatment of acute zoster pain, while gabapentin was ineffective.[60] Despite the lack of firm evidence, use of tricyclics or the anticonvulsants gabapentin or pregabalin is now relatively common for zoster pain that persists for more than a few weeks. Prospective studies have not determined when treatment with oral medications other than opioids and NSAIDs should begin or which patients are most likely to benefit.

PATHOLOGY OF PHN

Pathological studies of acute zoster and PHN have had an important influence on our understanding of the peripheral nervous system and neuropathic pain. Head and Campbell published the first dermatome chart in 1900 (Figure 15.2) based on a series of asylum patients with acute zoster who were subsequently examined postmortem to confirm which DRG was the origin of the HZ outbreak.[24] Few postmortem examinations that included both the central and peripheral nervous systems have appeared since, with nearly all coming from Peter Watson and colleagues.[25,61] At time periods of up to 1 year after HZ, some excised DRGs and peripheral nerves are still infiltrated with chronic inflammatory cells. In late cases, DRGs may have "ghosts" of sensory neurons or extensive collagen replacement or may even be grossly cystic. Peripheral nerves may show thinning of the myelin sheath in many axons, and in distal branches nearly complete transformation into collagen has been documented. In four PHN cases reported by Watson and coworkers, shrinkage of the ipsilateral dorsal horn over several segments was combined with loss of DRG neurons and peripheral axons, especially of the large myelinated type. However, one case *without* PHN showed ipsilateral subacute myelopathy combined with extensive loss of myelinated axons indistinguishable from long-standing PHN.

Early electron microscopy and reduced-silver staining studies of peripheral nerves and skin following HZ described a reduction in the total number of fibers, possibly greater for large fibers compared to small fibers.[62–65] Obtaining pathological specimens by surgically excising the affected DRG or the affected peripheral nerve (including thoracic intercostal nerves) does not provide consistent clinical benefit.[66] With the advent of immunofluorescence microscopy, skin punch biopsy became a straightforward and practical technique for studying innervation of the dermis and epidermis. Nearly all work on the pathology of HZ and PHN in the past few decades has relied on biopsy specimens from affected skin. In normal skin, virtually all of the epidermal innervation is supplied by unmyelinated fibers, with a small proportion being

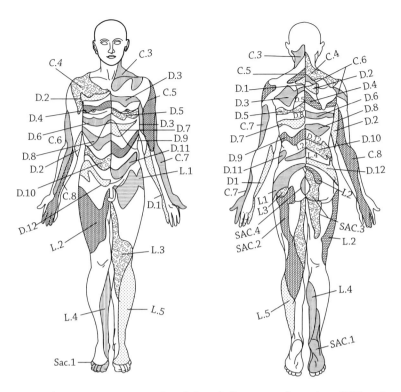

FIGURE 15.2   First dermatome map: Head and Campbell examined a series of HZ patients in an asylum. At postmortem, only a single DRG was affected. For some dermatomes, especially on the arm, they did not have a corresponding HZ case.

Source: Redrawn from Head H, Campbell AW. The pathology of herpes zoster and its bearing on sensory localization. *Brain*. 1900;23:353–523.

thin-caliber, lightly myelinated Aδ fibers.[67] Skin biopsy studies of chronic severe PHN have consistently shown reduced epidermal nerve fiber density compared to that of mirror-image and distant control skin.[40,45,68–70] A subgroup of patients have relatively preserved cutaneous innervation. As illustrated in Figures 15.3 and 15.4, using single- and double-labeling immunofluorescence microscopy to analyze a large skin sample from a man with severe PHN of 8 years' duration, complex abnormalities in cutaneous nerve morphology and immunochemistry were found.[45] In PHN skin, there was a marked reduction in the density of epidermal nerve fibers and a nearly complete dropout of the subepidermal nerve plexus. Furthermore, some patients have patches of skin with severe cutaneous fiber loss adjoining areas with preserved innervation.[40,71]

Acute HZ, a unilateral disease, has bilateral effects. In a longitudinal study of 113 patients

with HZ, Haanpaa et al. demonstrated EMG changes in 53 % of the patients, which were bilateral in 53% of them and more frequent in the patients who developed PHN.[22] In 56% of the patients, magnetic resonance imaging (MRI) lesions attributable to HZ were seen in the brainstem and cervical cord. Leukocytosis in cerebrospinal fluid was demonstrated in 10/14 HZ patients 1–30 days after onset.[22] A clinical MRI study of a patient with an HZ rash located at the L1 level showed an initial contrast enhancement below T10, which was later limited to L1;this led the authors to conclude that the inflammation was widely spread from the primarily affected segment.[72] Watson et al. found inflammatory infiltrates at left T6 and T8 and right T6 and T7 in a patient with a left-sided rash in the T6-T7 dermatome.[61] Skin biopsy studies have not consistently shown bilateral nerve fiber loss. Oaklander and colleagues collected a single set of punch

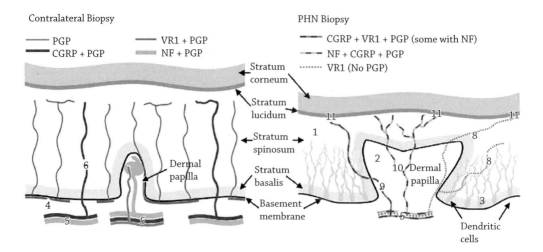

FIGURE 15.3 Schematic summary of the immunochemistry and morphology of cutaneous innervation in PHN skin and contralateral skin. In PHN skin, the epidermis was thinner (1), dermal papillae were larger and irregular (2), dendritic cells were frequent (3), and PGP9.5-labeled innervation was reduced. In PHN skin, most epidermal endings had long oblique trajectories (11) compared to the T-shaped endings in contralateral skin (6).

Source: Petersen KL, Rice F, Suess F, Berro M, Rowbotham MC. Relief of post-herpetic neuralgia by surgical removal of painful skin. *Pain.* 2002;98:119–226. This figure has been reproduced with permission of the International Association for the Study of Pain (IASP®). The figure may not be reproduced for any other purpose without permission.

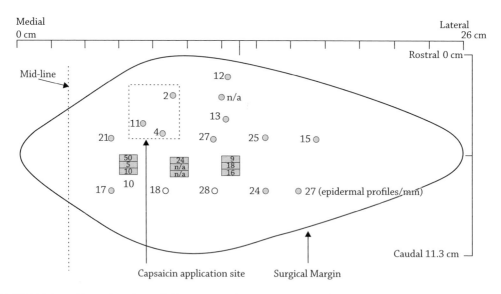

FIGURE 15.4 Map of epidermal fiber counts from 3 mm punch biopsies and 10 mm strip biopsies from a 294 cm² area of resected PHN skin. Note the variability of fiber counts. Allodynia was severe throughout the specimen. Contralateral nonpainful skin had a fiber count of 25 fibers, and PHN skin had a mean fiber count of 16 fibers. (See ref. 45 for more information on study methodology.)

biopsy specimens from pain-free HZ patients and chronic severe PHN patients long after the HZ rash (pain-free average 127 months, PHN average 56 months).[69,70] Her group reported that subjects with PHN had significantly lower epidermal fiber densities in both HZ-affected and mirror-image skin than pain-free post-zoster subjects. In contrast, the zoster natural history showed no deafferentation in contralateral mirror-image skin compared to a distant control site.[38]

Skin biopsy has been used to document nerve regeneration after experimental denervation using capsaicin and has been proposed as an outcome measure in clinical trials of regenerative therapies.[73] Conventional EMG assessment of denervation and reinnervation is insensitive to changes in small-fiber function and is not feasible for the majority of patients with HZ because the rash is located on the torso. Quantitative thermal sensory testing addresses this insensitivity, but it is indirect compared to anatomical visualization of nerve fibers. At present, it is unknown how innervation of post-HZ skin would respond to either experimental focal capsaicin denervation or therapies in development designed to foster nerve regeneration. Death of some DRG neurons during HZ would only partially explain impaired reinnervation, and the extent of scarring and degeneration of Schwann cells more proximally in the nerve trunk after zoster is unknown. The single-visit study by Oaklander and colleagues many years after acute HZ could not assess how the PHN and pain-free groups might have differed initially and whether they had different rates of recovery, but the finding of fewer intraepidermal fibers in HZ skin 10 years later suggests that full reinnervation is uncommon.[70] In the natural history of HZ pain study, there was no evidence of reinnervation of HZ skin by 6 months, even in those subjects without pain.[38] A failure of reinnervation is not surprising in light of studies by Polydefkis and colleagues showing severely impaired regeneration after experimental cutaneous nerve injury in diabetics compared to healthy controls.[73]

IMPLICATIONS OF PATHOLOGICAL STUDIES FOR UNDERSTANDING THE PATHOPHYSIOLOGY OF PHN PAIN

Noordenbos, in 1959, combined sensory and pathological examinations to propose that PHN pain was due to c-nociceptor fiber input into the spinal cord no longer restrained by the inhibitory influence of large myelinated afferents.[63] Later studies by other authors emphasized deafferentation as the cause of the pain. Using bedside tests, Watson et al. reported sensory loss in nearly all of the 208 PHN patients in their series.[74] Nurmikko and Bowsher used quantitative methods to compare PHN patients with pain-free post-HZ patients; 93% of the PHN group and 10% of the non-PHN group had sensory loss.[37] More recent sensory testing studies have included ophthalmic PHN.[75]

The results of a series of studies using clinical examination supplemented by techniques as diverse as infrared thermography, allodynia mapping, quantitative thermal sensory testing, lidocaine injection, epinephrine injection, capsaicin application, and skin punch biopsy analysis of cutaneous innervation have led our group to suggest that PHN is not a homogeneous disorder.[40,68,76–79] Instead, the neural dysfunction observed in PHN patients spans a spectrum that includes (1) irritable nociceptors characterized by minimal deafferentation and allodynia due to peripheral nociceptor input, (2) deafferentation with both sensory loss and allodynia, and (3) deafferentation characterized by marked sensory loss without allodynia. *Irritable nociceptors* refers to preserved, and possibly sensitized, primary afferent nociceptors that remain connected to their peripheral cutaneous and central targets. Abnormal function and probable spontaneous activity in these nociceptors provide sufficient ongoing input to maintain the central nervous system in a state of chronic sensitization. Further increasing c-nociceptor input by application of topical 0.075% capsaicin to a small area of PHN skin (the capsaicin response test) dramatically increases pain and enlarges the area of allodynia. The combination of deafferentation and allodynia may reflect deafferentation-induced rewiring of the dorsal horn in which large-diameter terminals sprout to occupy synaptic spaces left vacant when c-nociceptors die during acute HZ. The allodynia observed reflects the newfound ability of the remaining touch fibers to directly excite second-order pain-transmitting neurons. Alternatively, a sensory deficit and allodynia could be present if many nociceptors, unable to reinnervate the skin, are spontaneously active. Alternatively, spontaneous activity could be present in neurons that are not directly damaged but are in proximity to damaged fibers. The spontaneously active nociceptors maintain the central nervous system in a state of chronic sensitization similar to that of irritable nociceptors. The minority of PHN patients with severe sensory loss but no allodynia are hypothesized to have deafferentation-induced alterations in central nervous system structure and function without spontaneous activity or chronic sensitization. In this scenario, peripheral manipulations do not alter pain, and skin biopsies show few, if any, fibers remaining in the upper dermis and epidermis.

In summary, age and severity of acute HZ pain are the strongest predictors of pain persistence after HZ. Although peripheral nerve damage increases the likelihood of pain persistence, many HZ patients become pain free despite risk factors of age >50, severe acute HZ pain, and evidence of sensory impairment and loss of cutaneous innervation.

CURRENT TREATMENT OF PHN PAIN

Treatment of PHN has improved greatly in the past two decades. Oral medication therapies proven effective by prospective controlled trials now include multiple antidepressants, the anticonvulsants gabapentin and pregabalin, opioids, and topical lidocaine patches.[39,80–84] A few studies have directly compared therapies for PHN, such as the three-period crossover trial performed by Raja and colleagues, in which amitriptyline and an opioid were compared, the four-period crossover study comparing an opioid alone and in combination with gabapentin, and with gabapentin alone and placebo, and a nortriptyline-gabapentin combination crossover study.[85–87] Taking into account

differences in clinical trial methodology and data analysis scheme, these treatments provide at least partial relief in about 50%–60% of PHN patients. About 10% achieve complete relief with a single therapy, making polypharmacy commonplace in the management of PHN.

A large number of reviews of assessment and treatment of zoster and PHN are available, some of which are quite recent and provide guidelines for all types of neuropathic pain.[88–93] Treatment of neuropathic pain is the focus of other chapters in this volume, and the reader is referred to those chapters.

Among the invasive therapies, repetitive peripheral nerve and sympathetic blocks have few advocates once PHN is fully established. The study by Kotani and colleagues in Japan deserves special mention as one that initially appeared promising but then fell from favor. They performed a prospective, controlled trial comparing intrathecal methylprednisolone plus lidocaine with intrathecal lidocaine alone and no-treatment in more than 270 subjects with nontrigeminal PHN of more than 1 year's duration.[94] Subjects received up to four injections at weekly intervals and were followed for 2 years by clinical exam and serial MRI scans to assess the duration of pain reduction and late adverse effects such as arachnoiditis. The mean reduction in pain intensity was approximately 70% in the group receiving steroids, far higher than in any trials of oral medications, and was sustained for the full 2 years. This study was never replicated, and many practitioners consider the protocol too risky, especially in the United States, where labeling of steroids specifically warns against intrathecal administration.

A great variety of destructive surgical therapies have come and gone for PHN pain over the past 100 years; the consensus that has emerged is that destructive procedures like nerve sectioning, dorsal root entry zone lesions, cordotomy, and so on cannot be recommended.[66] One of the most recent variations on this theme involved resecting the skin encompassing the entire area of greatest PHN pain (294 cm²) in a patient with long-standing severe PHN. The initial report presented evidence of benefit in the form of reduced pain, elimination of allodynia, and reduced medication consumption during the first postoperative year.[45] Thereafter, unfortunately, pain steadily increased and eventually exceeded presurgery levels despite increased medication use.[95]

Topical approaches have found broad acceptance for PHN. Lidocaine patches have few systemic side effects and show efficacy after the first few applications.[71,83] They were specifically approved by the U.S. Food and Drug Administration for PHN in 2000. Approval by regional authorities was granted more recently in Germany and elsewhere in the European Union. Topical capsaicin is occasionally used for PHN, but clinical trials have obvious difficulties with blinding. At the 0.075% (nonprescription) strength, burning during the first weeks of treatment is unacceptably severe in a significant proportion of patients and cannot be fully prevented with topical local anesthetics.[96] A study of one application of a high-concentration capsaicin patch (8%) in patients with PHN showed an overall significant decrease in pain after 12 weeks. The patch was well tolerated and was not associated with adverse systemic effects, but only 40% of patients responded to the treatment with a 30% decrease in pain.[97] Another recently published trial showed similar results,[98] and this therapy was approved for the treatment of PHN in 2009. Compounding pharmacies can prepare topical formulations containing various combinations of aspirin, NSAIDs, gabapentin, opioids, and numerous other medications, but these are insufficiently validated, not widely available, and not approved by regulatory authorities.[88] A large number of completed and ongoing trials of topicals for PHN can be found on the clinicaltrials.gov website.

CONCLUSION

Progress is being made on all fronts: vaccination to prevent primary infection, new treatments to supplement antivirals for preventing PHN, and a growing list of therapies for PHN. Vaccination of previously exposed elderly persons may lower the future incidence of HZ and alter its clinical features to reduce the risk of PHN. Advances in understanding the spectrum of neural dysfunction in PHN may lead to mechanism-based treatment of PHN. As monotherapy of PHN frequently fails, more trials evaluating the safety and efficacy of combined treatment strategies will hopefully be performed.

REFERENCES

1. Liesegang TJ. Varicella zoster viral disease. *Mayo Clin Proc.* 1999;74:983–998.
2. Mueller NH, Gilden DH, Cohrs RJ, Mahalingam R, Nagel MA. Varicella zoster virus infection: clinical features, molecular pathogenesis of disease, and latency. *Neurol Clin.* 2008;26:675–697, viii.
3. Edmunds WJ, Brisson M. The effect of vaccination on the epidemiology of varicella zoster virus. *J Infect.* 2002;44:211–219.
4. Gnann JW Jr, Whitley RJ. Clinical practice. Herpes zoster. *N Engl J Med.* 2002;347:340–346.
5. Dworkin RH, Johnson RW, Breuer J, Gnann JW, Levin MJ, Backonja M, Betts RF, Gershon AA, Haanpää ML, McKendrick MW, Nurmikko TJ, Oaklander AL, Oxman MN, Pavan-Langston D, Petersen KL, Rowbotham MC, Schmader KE, Stacey BR, Tyring SK, van Wijck AJM, Wallace MS, Wassilew SW, Whitley RJ. Recommendations for the management of herpes zoster. *Clin Infect Dis.* 2007;44:S1–S26.
6. Mahalingam R, Wellish M, Wolf W, Dueland AN, Cohrs R, Vafai A, Gilden D. Latent varicella-zoster viral DNA in human trigeminal and thoracic ganglia. *N Engl J Med.* 1990;323:627–631.
7. Abendroth A, Kinchington PR, Slobedman B. Varicella zoster virus immune evasion strategies. *Curr Top Microbiol Immunol.* 2010;342:155–171.
8. Hope-Simpson RE. The nature of herpes zoster: a long term study and a new hypothesis. *Proc R Soc Med.* 1965;58:9–20.
9. Vossen MT, Gent MR, Weel JF, de Jong MD, van Lier RA, Kuijpers TW. Development of virus-specific CD4+ T cells on reexposure to varicella-zoster virus. *J Infect Dis.* 2004;190:72–82.
10. Brisson M, Gay NJ, Edmunds WJ, Andrews NJ. Exposure to varicella boosts immunity to herpes-zoster: implications for mass vaccination against chickenpox. *Vaccine.* 2002;20:2500–2507.
11. Thomas SL, Wheeler JG, Hall AJ. Contacts with varicella or with children and protection against herpes zoster in adults: a case-control study. *Lancet.* 2002;360:678–682.
12. Schunemann S, Mainka C, Wolff MH. Subclinical reactivation of varicella-zoster virus in immunocompromised and immunocompetent individuals. *Intervirology.* 1998;41:98–102
13. Levin MJ, Gershon AA, Dworkin RH, Brisson M, Stanberry L. Prevention strategies for herpes zoster and post-herpetic neuralgia. *J Clin Virol.* 2010;48(suppl 1):S14–S19.

14. Hambleton S, Steinberg SP, Larussa PS, Shapiro ED, Gershon AA. Risk of herpes zoster in adults immunized with varicella vaccine. *J Infect Dis.* 2008;197(suppl 2):S196–S199.

15. Reynolds MA, Chaves SS, Harpaz R, Lopez AS, Seward JF. The impact of the varicella vaccination program on herpes zoster epidemiology in the United States: a review. *J Infect Dis.* 2008;197(suppl 2):S224–S227.

16. Levin MJ, Murray M, Rotbart HA, Zerbe GO, White CJ, Hayward AR. Immune response of elderly individuals to a live attenuated varicella vaccine. *J Infect Dis.* 1992;166(2):253–259.

17. Oxman M. Immunization to reduce the frequency and severity of herpes zoster and its complications. *Neurology.* 1995;45(suppl 8):S41–S46.

18. Redman, RL, Nader S, Zerboni L, Liu C, Wong RM, Brown BW, Arvin AM. Early reconstitution of immunity and decreased severity of herpes zoster in bone marrow transplant recipients immunized with inactivated varicella vaccine. *J Infect Dis.* 1997;176(3):578–585.

19. Oxman MN, Levin MJ, Johnson GR, Schmader KE, Straus SE, Gelb LD, Arbeit RD, Simberkoff MS, Gershon AA, Davis LE, Weinberg A, Boardman KD, Williams HM, Zhang JH, Peduzzi PN, Beisel CE, Morrison VA, Guatelli JC, Brooks PA, Kauffman CA, Pachucki CT, Neuzil KM, Betts RF, Wright PF, Griffin MR, Brunell P, Soto NE, Marques AR, Keay SK, Goodman RP, Cotton DJ, Gnann JW, Jr., Loutit J, Holodniy M, Keitel WA, Crawford GE, Yeh SS, Lobo Z, Toney JF, Greenberg RN, Keller PM, Harbecke R, Hayward AR, Irwin MR, Kyriakides TC, Chan CY, Chan IS, Wang WW, Annunziato PW, Silber JL. A vaccine to prevent herpes zoster and postherpetic neuralgia in older adults. N Engl J Med. 2005;352(22):2271–2284.

20. Coplan PM, Schmader K, Nikas A, Chan IS, Choo P, Levin MJ, Johnson G, Bauer M, Williams HM, Kaplan KM, Guess HA, Oxman MN. Development of a measure of the burden of pain due to herpes zoster and postherpetic neuralgia for prevention trials: adaptation of the Brief Pain Inventory. *J Pain.* 2004;5:344–356.

21. Oxman MN. Zoster vaccine: current status and future prospects. *Clin Infect Dis.* 2010;51(2): 197–213.

22. Haanpää M, Dastidar P, Weinber A, Levin M, Miettinen A, Lapinlampi A, Laippala P, Nurmikko T. CSF and MRI findings in patients with acute herpes zoster. *Neurology.* 1998;51:1405–1411.

23. Gilden DH, Kleinschmidt-DeMasters BK, LaGuardia JJ, Mahalingam R, Cohrs RJ. Neurologic complications of the reactivation of varicella-zoster virus. *N Engl J Med.* 2000;342: 635–645.

24. Head H, Campbell AW. The pathology of herpes zoster and its bearing on sensory localization. *Brain.* 1900;23:353–523.

25. Watson CPN, Deck JH. The neuropathology of herpes zoster with particular reference to postherpetic neuralgia and its pathogenesis. In: Watson CPN, ed. *Herpes Zoster and Post-Herpetic Neuralgia.* Amsterdam: Elsevier; 1993: 139–158.

26. Mondelli M, Romano C, Della Porta P, Rossi A. Electrophysiological findings in peripheral fibres of subjects with and without post-herpetic neuralgia. *Electroencephalogr Clin Neurophysiol.* 1996;101:185–191.

27. Haanpää M, Laippala P, Nurmikko T. Pain and somatosensory dysfunction in acute herpes zoster. *Clin J Pain.* 1999;15:78–84.

28. Gilden DH, Dueland AN, Cohrs R, Martin JR, Kleinschmidt-DeMasters BK, Mahalingam R. Preherpetic neuralgia. *Neurology.* 1991;41: 1215–1218.

29. Dworkin R, Schmader K. (2001). The epidemiology and natural history of herpes zoster and postherpetic neuralgia. In: Watson CPN, Gershon A, eds. *Herpes Zoster and Post-Herpetic Neuralgia.* 2nd ed. Amsterdam: Elsevier; 2001:39–64.

30. Desmond RA, Weiss HL, Arani RB, Soong SJ, Wood MJ, Fiddian PA, Gnann JW, Whitley RJ. Clinical applications for change-point analysis of herpes zoster pain. *J Pain Symptom Manage.* 2002;23(6):510–516.

31. Thyregod HG, Rowbotham MC, Peters M, Possehn J, Berro M, Petersen KL. Natural history of pain following herpes zoster. *Pain.* 2007;128:148–156.

32. Nurmikko TJ, Räsänen A, Häkkinen V. Clinical and neurophysiological observations on acute herpes zoster. *Clin J Pain.* 1990;6:284–290.

33. Bennett GJ. Hypotheses on the pathogenesis of herpes zoster-associated pain. *Ann Neurol.* 1994;35:S38–S41.

34. Dworkin RH. Prevention of postherpetic neuralgia. *Lancet.* 1999;353:1636–1637.

35. Johnson RW. Herpes zoster—predicting and minimizing the impact of post-herpetic neuralgia. *J Antimicrob Chemother.* 2001;47:1–8.

36. Petersen KL, Rowbotham MC. Natural history of sensory function after herpes zoster. *Pain.* 2010;150:83–92.

37. Nurmikko, T. and Bowsher, D., Somatosensory findings in postherpetic neuralgia, *Journal of Neurology, Neurosurgery and Psychiatry*, 53 (1990) 135–41.37.

38. Petersen KL, Rice FL, Farhadi M, Reda H, Rowbotham MC. Natural history of cutaneous innervation following herpes zoster. *Pain*. 2010;150:75–82.

39. Rowbotham M, Harden N, Stacey B, Bernstein P, Magnus-Miller L. Gabapentin for the treatment of postherpetic neuralgia: a randomized controlled trial. *JAMA*. 1998;280:1837–1842.

40. Petersen KL, Fields HL, Brennum J, Sandroni P, Rowbotham MC. Capsaicin activation of "irritable" nociceptors in post-herpetic neuralgia. *Pain*. 2000;88:125–133.

41. Tominaga M, Caterina MJ, Malmberg AB, Rosen TA, Gilbert H, Skinner K, Raumann BE, Basbaum AI, Julius D. The cloned capsaicin receptor integrates multiple pain-producing stimuli. *Neuron*. 1998;21(3):531–543.

42. Caterina MJ, Leffler A, Malmberg AB, Martin WJ, Trafton J, Petersen-Zeitz KR, Koltzenburg M, Basbaum AI, Julius D. Impaired nociception and pain sensation in mice lacking the capsaicin receptor. *Science*. 2000;288(5464):306–313.

43. Szallasi A, Cortright DN, Blum CA, Eid SR. The vanilloid receptor TRPV1: 10 years from channel cloning to antagonist proof-of-concept. *Nat Rev Drug Discov*. 2007;6(5):357–372.

44. Ma W, Zhang Y, Bantel C, Eisenach JC. Medium and large injured dorsal root ganglion cells increase TRPV-1, accompanied by increased alpha2C-adrenoceptor co-expression and functional inhibition by clonidine. *Pain*. 2005;113(3):386–394.

45. Petersen KL, Rice F, Suess F, Berro M, Rowbotham MC. Relief of post-herpetic neuralgia by surgical removal of painful skin. *Pain*. 2002;98:119–226.

46. Berry JD, Rowbotham MC, Petersen KL. Complex regional pain syndrome-like symptoms during herpes zoster. *Pain*. 2004;110:e1–e12.

47. Colding A. Treatment of pain: organization of a pain clinic: treatment of acute herpes zoster. *Proc R Soc Med*. 1973;66(6):541–543.

48. McCulloch DK, Fraser DM, Duncan LP. Shingles in diabetes mellitus. *Practitioner*. 1982;226:531–532.

49. Whitton TL, Johnson RW, Lovell AT. Use of the Rydel-Seiffer graduated tuning fork in the assessment of vibration threshold in postherpetic neuralgia patients and healthy controls. *Eur J Pain*. 2005;9:167–171.

50. Baron R, Haendler G, Schulte H. Afferent large fiber polyneuropathy predicts the development of postherpetic neuralgia. *Pain*. 1997;73:231–238.

51. Dworkin RH, White R, O'Connor AB, Hawkins K. Health care expenditure burden of persisting herpes zoster pain. *Pain Med*. 2008;9(3):348–353.

52. Wood MJ, Kay R, Dworkin RH, Soong SJ, Whitley RJ. Oral acyclovir therapy accelerates pain resolution in patients with herpes zoster: a meta-analysis of placebo-controlled trials. *Clin Infect Dis*. 1996;22:341–347.

53. Jackson JL, Gibbons R, Meyer G, Inouye L. The effect of treating herpes zoster with oral acyclovir in preventing postherpetic neuralgia. A meta-analysis. *Arch Intern Med*. 1997;157:909–912.

54. Whitley RJ, Weiss H, Gnann JW Jr, Tyring S, Mertz GJ, Pappas PG, Schleupner CJ, Hayden F, Wolf J, Soong SJ. Acyclovir with and without prednisone for the treatment of herpes zoster. A randomized, placebo-controlled trial. The National Institute of Allergy and Infectious Diseases Collaborative Antiviral Study Group. *Ann Intern Med*.1996;125:376–383.

55. Pasqualucci A, Pasqualucci V, Galla F, De Angelis V, Marzocchi V, Colussi R, Paoletti F, Girardis M, Lugano M, Del Sindaco F. Prevention of postherpetic neuralgia: acyclovir and prednisolone versus epidural local anesthetic and methylprednisolone. *Acta Anesthesiol Scand*. 2000;44:910–918.

56. van Wijck AJ, Opstelten W, Moons KG, van Essen GA, Stolker RJ, Kalkman CJ, Verheij TJ. The PINE study of epidural steroids and local anaesthetics to prevent postherpetic neuralgia: a randomised controlled trial. *Lancet*. 2006;367:219–224.

57. Ji G, Niu J, Shi Y, Hou L, Lu Y, Xiong L. The effectiveness of repetitive paravertebral injections with local anesthetics and steroids for the prevention of postherpetic neuralgia in patients with acute herpes zoster. *Anesth Analg*. 2009;109:1651–1655.

58. Bowsher D. The effects of pre-emptive treatment of postherpetic neuralgia with amitriptyline: a randomized, double-blind, placebo-controlled trial. *J Pain Symptom Manage*. 1997;13(6):327–331.

59. Berry JD, Petersen KL. A single dose of gabapentin reduces acute pain and allodynia in patients with herpes zoster. *Neurology*. 2005;65(3):444–447.

60. Dworkin RH, Barbano RL, Tyring SK, Betts RF, McDermott MP, Pennella-Vaughan J, Bennett GJ, Berber E, Gnann JW, Irvine C, Kamp C, Kieburtz K, Max MB, Schmader KE. A randomized, placebo-controlled trial of oxycodone and of gabapentin for acute pain in herpes zoster. *Pain*. 2009;142:209–217.

61. Watson CP, Deck JH, Morshead C, Van der Kooy D, Evans RJ. Post-herpetic neuralgia: further

post-mortem studies of cases with and without pain. *Pain*. 1991;44(2):105–117.

62. Ebert M. Histologic changes in sensory nerves of the skin in herpes zoster. *Arch Dermatol*. 1949;60:641–648.

63. Noordenbos W. *Pain*. Amsterdam: Elsevier; 1959:68–80.

64. Zacks SI, Langfitt TW, Elliot FA. Herpetic neuritis: a light and electron microscopic study. *Neurology*. 1964;14:744–750.

65. Muller S, Winkelmann R Cutaneous nerve changes in zoster. *J Invest Dermatol*. 1969;52:71–77.

66. Loeser J. Surgery for post-herpetic neuralgia. In: Watson CPN, Gershon A, eds. *Herpes Zoster and Post-Herpetic Neuralgia*. 2nd ed. Elsevier, Amsterdam: Elsevier; 2001:255–264.

67. Pare M, Albrecht PJ, Noto CJ, Bodkin NL, Pittenger GL, Schreyer DJ, Tigno XT, Hansen BC, Rice FL. Differential hypertrophy and atrophy among all types of cutaneous innervation in the glabrous skin of the monkey hand during aging and naturally occurring type 2 diabetes. *J Comp Neurol*. 2007;501(4):543–567.

68. Rowbotham MC, Yosipovitch G, Connolly MK, Finlay D, Forde G, Fields HL. Cutaneous innervation density in the allodynic form of postherpetic neuralgia. *Neurobiol Dis*. 1996;3:205–214.

69. Oaklander AL, Romans K, Horasek S, Stocks A, Hauer P, Meyer RA. Unilateral postherpetic neuralgia is associated with bilateral sensory neuron damage. *Ann Neurol*. 1998;44:789–795.

70. Oaklander A.L. The density of remaining nerve endings in human skin with and without postherpetic neuralgia after shingles. *Pain*. 2001;92(1–2):139–145.

71. Rowbotham MC, Davies PS, Verkempinck CV, Galer BS. Lidocaine patch: double-blind controlled study of a new treatment method for post-herpetic neuralgia. *Pain*. 1996;65:39–44.

72. Hanakawa T, Hashimoto S, Kawamura J, Nakamura M, Suenaga T, Matsuo M. Magnetic resonance imaging in a patient with segmental zoster paresis. *Neurology*. 1997;49(2):631–632.

73. Polydefkis M, Hauer P, Sheth S, Sirdofsky M, Griffin JW, McArthur JC. The time course of epidermal nerve fibre regeneration: studies in normal controls and in people with diabetes, with and without neuropathy. *Brain*. 2004;127 (pt 7):1606–1615.

74. Watson CP, Evans RJ, Watt VR, Birkett N. Post-herpetic neuralgia: 208 cases. *Pain*. 1988;35:289–97.

75. Truini A, Galeotti F, Haanpaa M, Zucchi R, Albanesi A, Biasiotta A, Gatti A, Cruccu G. Pathophysiology of pain in postherpetic neuralgia: a clinical and neurophysiological study. *Pain*. 2008;140(3):405–410.

76. Rowbotham MC, Fields HL. Post-herpetic neuralgia: the relation of pain complaint, sensory disturbance, and skin temperature. *Pain*. 1989;39:129–144.

77. Rowbotham MC, Fields HL. The relationship of pain, allodynia and thermal sensation in postherpetic neuralgia. *Brain*. 1996;119:347–354.

78. Fields HL, Rowbotham M, Baron R. Postherpetic neuralgia: irritable nociceptors and deafferentation. *Neurobiol Dis*. 1998;5:209–227.

79. Rowbotham MC, Petersen KL, Fields HL. Postherpetic neuralgia: more than one disorder? *Pain Forum*. 1998;7:231–237.

80. Watson CP, Evans RJ, Reed K, Merskey H, Goldsmith L, Warsh J. Amitriptyline versus placebo in postherpetic neuralgia. *Neurology*. 1982;32:671–673.

81. Rowbotham MC, Reisner-Keller LA, Fields HL. Both intravenous lidocaine and morphine reduce the pain of postherpetic neuralgia. *Neurology*. 1991;41:1024–1028.

82. Watson CP, Babul N. Efficacy of oxycodone in neuropathic pain: a randomized trial in postherpetic neuralgia. *Neurology*. 1998;50:1837–1841.

83. Galer BS, Rowbotham MC, Perander J, Friedman E. Topical lidocaine patch relieves postherpetic neuralgia more effectively than a vehicle topical patch: results of an enriched enrollment study. *Pain*. 1999;80:533–538.

84. Dworkin RH, Corbin AE, Young JP, Sharma U, LaMoreaux L, Bockbrader H, Garofalo EA, Poole RM. Pregabalin for the treatment of postherpetic neuralgia: a randomized, placebo-controlled trial. *Neurology*. 2003;60:1274–1283.

85. Raja SN, Haythornthwaite JA, Pappagallo M, Clark MR, Travison TG, Sabeen S, Royall RM, Max MB. Opioids versus antidepressants in postherpetic neuralgia: a randomized, placebo-controlled trial. *Neurology*. 2002;59:1015–1021.

86. Gilron I, Bailey JM, Tu D, Holden RR, Weaver DF, Houlden RL. Morphine, gabapentin, or their combination for neuropathic pain. *N Engl J Med*. 2005;352(13):1324–1334.

87. Gilron I, Bailey JM, Tu D, Holden RR, Jackson AC, Houlden RL. Nortriptyline and gabapentin, alone and in combination for neuropathic pain: a double-blind, randomised controlled crossover trial. *Lancet*. 2009;374(9697):1252–1261.

88. Hempenstall K, Nurmikko TJ, Johnson RW, A'Hern RP, Rice AS. Analgesic therapy in postherpetic neuralgia: a quantitative systematic review. *PLoS Med*. 2005;2:e164.

89. Dworkin RH, O'Connor AB, Backonja M, Farrar JT, Finnerup NB, Jensen TS, Kalso EA, Loeser JD, Miaskowski C, Nurmikko TJ, Portenoy RK, Rice AS, Stacey BR, Treede RD, Turk DC, Wallace MS. Pharmacologic management of neuropathic pain: evidence-based recommendations. *Pain.* 2007;132(3):237–251.

90. Whitley RJ, Volpi A, McKendrick M, Wijck A, Oaklander AL. Management of herpes zoster and post-herpetic neuralgia now and in the future. *J Clin Virol.* 2010;48(suppl 1):S20–S28.

91. Cruccu G, Sommer C, Anand P, Attal N, Baron R, Garcia-Larrea L, Haanpaa M, Jensen TS, Serra J, Treede RD. EFNS guidelines on neuropathic pain assessment: revised 2009. *Eur J Neurol.* 2010;17(8):1010–1018.

92. Haanpaa M, Attal N, Backonja M, Baron R, Bennett M, Bouhassira D, Cruccu G, Hansson P, Haythornthwaite JA, Iannetti GD, Jensen TS, Kauppila T, Nurmikko TJ, Rice AS, Rowbotham M, Serra J, Sommer C, Smith BH, Treede RD. NeuPSIG guidelines on neuropathic pain assessment. *Pain.* 2011;152(1):14–27.

93. Finnerup NB, Sindrup SH, Jensen TS. The evidence for pharmacological treatment of neuropathic pain. *Pain.* 2010;150:573–581.

94. Kotani N, Kushikata T, Hashimoto H, Kimura F, Muraoka M, Yodono M, Asai M, Matsuki A. Intrathecal methylprednisolone for intractable postherpetic neuralgia. *N Engl J Med.* 2000;343:1514–1519.

95. Petersen KL, Rowbotham MC. Relief of postherpetic neuralgia by surgical removal of painful skin: 5 years later. *Pain.* 2007;131:214–218.

96. Watson CP, Tyler KL, Bickers DR, Millikan LE, Smith S, Coleman E. A randomized vehicle-controlled trial of topical capsaicin in the treatment of postherpetic neuralgia. *Clin Ther.* 1993;15:510–526.

97. Backonja M, Wallace MS, Blonsky ER, Cutler BJ, Malan P, Jr, Rauck R, Tobias J. NGX-4010, a high-concentration capsaicin patch, for the treatment of postherpetic neuralgia: a randomised, double-blind study. *Lancet Neurol.* 2008;7:1106–1112.

98. Webster LR, Malan TP, Tuchman MM, Mollen MD, Tobias JK, Vanhove GF. A multicenter, randomized, double-blind, controlled dose finding study of NGX-4010, a high-concentration capsaicin patch, for the treatment of postherpetic neuralgia. *J Pain.* 2010;11(10): 972–982.

16

Immune-Mediated Neuropathies

W. DAVID ARNOLD AND JOHN T. KISSEL

INTRODUCTION

THE IMMUNE-MEDIATED OR inflammatory neuropathies are a diverse group of nerve disorders that have historically been classified on the basis of time course, underlying pathophysiology, fiber type, and distribution of nerve involvement. As is true of inflammatory damage to most tissues, pain is a relatively common feature of the immune-mediated neuropathies, although it is an aspect of these conditions that has received relatively little attention. This is somewhat surprising, since pain is often the heralding feature of the inflammatory neuropathies and the symptom that first brings the patient to medical attention.

Traditionally, pain has been considered to be directly related to the rate and kind of nerve fiber loss, with acute nerve injury generally associated with more pain.[1] In this chapter, the immune-mediated neuropathies will therefore be discussed from the

perspective of time course and distribution of involvement, as these features are often tightly correlated with symptoms of pain (Table 16.1).

NEURALGIC AMYOTROPHY

Although first reported in 1887, neuralgic amyotrophy was described in detail as a distinct syndrome in 1948 by Parsonage and Turner; hence, the syndrome is also referred to as *Parsonage-Turner syndrome*.[2,3] The approximate incidence is 2–3 per 100,000 population.[4,5] Traditionally classified as a brachial plexopathy (and sometimes referred to as *idiopathic brachial plexopathy*), neuralgic amyotrophy typically follows a patchy distribution more consistent with one or more peripheral mononeuropathies of the brachial plexus rather than a lesion of the plexus itself. The distribution of weakness can vary from focal

Table 16-1. Spectrum of Immune-Mediated Neuropathy

ACUTE TIME COURSE

Asymmetric/Focal	Neuralgic amyotrophy (Parsonage-Turner syndrome)
Generalized	Guillain-Barré syndrome (motor dysfunction prominent)
	Acute inflammatory demyelinating polyradiculoneuropathy
	Acute motor axonal neuropathy
	Acute motor and sensory axonal neuropathy
	GBS variants (motor dysfunction not prominent)
	Miller-Fisher syndrome
	Pure sensory GBS
	Pan dysautonomia

CHRONIC TIME COURSE

Asymmetric/Generalized	Vasculitis
	Primary systemic vasculitis
	Secondary systemic vasculitis
	Nonsystemic/localized vasculitis
Generalized	Chronic immune-mediated neuropathies
	Chronic inflammatory demyelinating polyradiculoneuropathy
	CIDP associated with other medical conditions
	CIDP variants
	Distal acquired demyelinating sensory
	Multifocal motor neuropathy
	Multifocal acquired demyelinating motor and sensory
	Multifocal acquired motor axonal

to diffuse and from unilateral to bilateral. In approximately a third of cases, both upper limbs are involved, and subclinical involvement is frequently noted.[3,6,7] Weakness is normally found in the distribution of terminal nerve branches of the upper limb, and occasionally individual fascicles of particular nerves are affected in isolation. Eventual development of significant atrophy is typical (see Figure 16.1). Nerves from the upper portion of the brachial plexus are more likely to be involved, but occasional patients present with involvement of nerves from predominantly the lower portion of the brachial plexus. Sensory disturbance is usually less prominent and can be patchy and not in agreement with the motor findings. Nerves proximal to the brachial plexus such as the long thoracic or phrenic nerves, and more rarely the cranial nerves, can be involved.[8]

In most cases, a characteristic prodrome of upper limb pain is the heralding feature of the disorder (see below) and provides a significant clue to the diagnosis, particularly in atypical cases.[9,10] Weakness can begin within hours and is usually noticed within the first week after the onset of pain. It is unusual for weakness to continue to progress once recognized. Traditionally, NA has been considered to have a good prognosis, but recent studies suggest that most patients have some persistent impairment, with only one-third having nearly complete recovery.[7,11] In about 20% of cases there may be a recurrent episode of pain and weakness, sometimes years after the initial onset of symptoms.

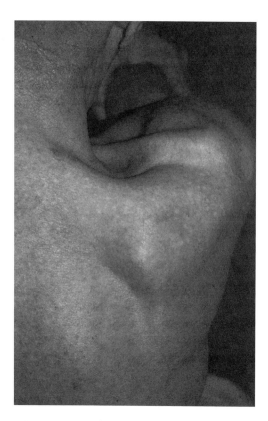

FIGURE 16.1 Shoulder girdle muscle atrophy with scapular winging in a patient with NA.

Pain in Neuralgic Amyotrophy

Pain is quite prominent in neuralgic amyotrophy and usually lasts for days to weeks. It is the presenting symptom in at least 90% of cases, so the absence of pain argues strongly against the diagnosis.[7,12] The pain usually begins abruptly, building over a matter of hours. Pain may last for periods ranging from a few days to a month, but in about one-third of patients it can persist.[6,11] The severity of the pain does not correlate with the severity of subsequent weakness. Most patients present with one or both of two principal pain syndromes. The most prominent and severe pain is usually described as a deep stabbing or aching pain that is in the distribution of the shoulder or forearm. This pain is provoked with movement of the symptomatic limb, so a rotator cuff or another orthopedic injury is initially suspected. The second type of pain that is frequently present is a more typical neuropathic or burning pain that can radiate in a peripheral nerve distribution and is often less intense. Many, if not most, patients present with overlapping features of deep aching pain and superficial burning or neuropathic pain. Weakness may occur immediately at the onset of pain, but often there is a delay in symptoms of weakness. Use of the symptomatic limb may be limited due to pain, causing the weakness to initially go unnoticed because the involved limb is favored.[7]

Diagnosis

The classic presentation of neuralgic amyotrophy is easily recognized by clinicians familiar with the disorder, but the diagnosis is often delayed due to limited awareness.[13] The presentation of transient upper limb pain followed by weakness is quite specific, but neurological disorders such as radiculopathy, entrapment neuropathy, mononeuritis multiplex, spinal cord disorders, herpes zoster infection, traumatic or neoplastic invasion injury of the brachial plexus, or sporadic and infectious motor neuron disease may mimic this disorder. One disorder in the differential diagnosis that deserves specific attention is hereditary neuralgic amyotrophy, a rare autosomal dominant disorder that presents with episodic and sometime recurrent painful attacks associated with multifocal motor and sensory deficits primarily affecting the nerves of the brachial plexus. In 20% of patients with hereditary neuralgic amyotrophy there is an associated mutation of the *SEFT9* gene localized to chromosome 17q25.3.[14,15] Hereditary neuralgic amyotrophy presents in a very similar fashion to neuralgic amyotrophy, and in the absence of a clear family history, it can be difficult to distinguish between the two conditions on a clinical basis[7] (Table 16.2). Musculoskeletal disorders such as rotator cuff tears should also be considered in the differential diagnosis, but incidental findings of rotator cuff tears or degenerative changes of the cervical spine may mislead the clinician to attribute the symptoms to an incorrect etiology.[16] Pain with cervical disk disease can be differentiated from neuralgic amyotrophy, as cervical disc pain is usually exacerbated with extension of the neck, Valsalva maneuver, cough, or provocative tests such as Spurling's maneuver.[17]

Table 16-2. Comparison of Neuralgic Amyotrophy (NA) and Hereditary Neuralgic Amyotrophy (HNA)[7]

	NA	HNA
Median age of onset (years)	41	28
Recurrence	25%	75%
Nearly complete motor recovery	34%	33%
Long-term pain (>3 years after attack)	60%	80%
Preceding event	Infection, surgery, parturition, heavy exercise, immunizations	Similar
Etiology	Unknown, presumed to be immune-mediated	Mutation in *SEPT9* on chromosome 17q25 in approximately 20%
Associated features	Lack of a family history, less frequent complete paralysis of involved muscles	Frequent involvement of nerves outside the brachial plexus, stereotypical physical features (i.e., hypotelorism, short stature, and facial asymmetry), family history (variably present)

Electrodiagnostic studies are invaluable in the evaluation of the patient with possible neuralgic amyotrophy. Electromyography and nerve conduction studies can help characterize the distribution of involvement, underlying pathophysiology, and severity of the condition while excluding other underlying disorders. The characteristic electrodiagnostic finding is motor axonal loss greatly out of proportion to sensory axonal loss, typically in a patchy distribution of a single or multiple peripheral nerves of the arm, shoulder girdle, and, rarely, cranial nerves. Rare cases present without pain, and painless neuralgic amyotrophy is recognized only by the findings of patchy axonal loss of abrupt onset. While sensory symptoms are common, occurring in 80% of patients, sensory nerve conduction is relatively spared, with only about 60% of patients having at least one abnormal sensory nerve response.[18] This is in contrast to traumatic brachial plexopathy, where sensory axons are more sensitive to injury, and sensory axon loss may be the only finding in a mild to moderate traumatic brachial plexopathy.[19] If involved, sensory amplitudes are reduced, with relative sparing of the conduction velocity and distal latencies. Motor conduction studies of involved nerves may demonstrate reduced compound motor action potential amplitude with relatively preserved conduction velocity. Proximal motor conduction studies with needle stimulation of the cervical nerve roots, although not frequently used clinically, have demonstrated motor axon conduction block in some cases.[20]

Treatment

Although the cause is unknown, the underlying pathogenesis of neuralgic amyotrophy is presumed to be immune-mediated. The predominantly monophasic course and associated good prognosis have resulted in limited nerve biopsy data, but brachial plexus biopsies have demonstrated perivascular, epineurial, and endoneurial inflammatory cell infiltrates.[21] While immune mechanisms are presumed, treatment for most patients is predominantly supportive. In general, there is a prolonged delay between onset and arrival at a diagnosis, so many patients' pain and weakness are stable or actually resolving by the time the diagnosis is made. In occasional patients diagnosed early in the course (i.e., within the first month of symptom onset), immunomodulatory treatment and, in particular, short pulses of intravenous or oral steroids may reduce the pain and perhaps even hasten strength recovery. Several retrospective studies have demonstrated a shorter mean duration of pain symptoms and improved functional outcomes in patients treated with oral pulses of prednisone, but there have been no randomized clinical trials of this approach.[22,23] Anecdotal case reports have also suggested that intravenous immunoglobulin treatment may modify the disease course.[24,25] Due to the rarity and the nonspecific presentation of neuralgic amyotrophy, often the diagnosis is not suspected or determined until the patient's symptoms are resolving. Once the pain has resolved, treatment is usually not indicated, as the monophasic nerve injury has occurred and treatment would not be expected to be of benefit. Some patients experience worsening of pain with initiation of rehabilitation, but rehabilitation prescriptions to address joint mobility, limit the effects of deconditioning, maintain normal joint mechanics, and modify activities of daily life for maximum functioning help improve the long-term outcome.[17] Long-term pain in neuralgic amyotrophy is frequently related to dysfunction of the scapulothoracic and glenohumeral joints of the shoulder due to muscle imbalance. Therapy should address these muscular imbalances to help reduce long-term joint irritation and damage.[11]

There are no well-designed studies that have investigated symptomatic pain control in neuralgic amyotrophy. Acutely, pain is usually treated symptomatically with opiates combined with a nonsteroidal anti-inflammatory drug. Many patients experience a dramatic reduction in pain within a month of onset, but in most patients there is persistent pain. Management of the chronic pain usually includes antiepileptic medications or antidepressants including the tricyclic antidepressants and serotonin-norephinephrine reuptake inhibitors. Superficial symptoms of burning pain can be localized and are often well controlled with topical agents such as lidocaine.

GUILLAIN-BARRÉ SYNDROME

The term *Guillain-Barré syndrome* (GBS) applies to a group of generalized acute immune-mediated neuropathies usually associated with flaccid weakness and often proceeded by or associated with an antecedent infection or trigger.[26,27] The classic clinical presentation was originally described as acute ascending weakness by Landry in 1859, and today GBS is clearly the most common cause of acute flaccid paralysis, with an approximate incidence of 1–4 per 100,000.[28,29] Annual direct and indirect costs related to GBS in the United States have been estimated at $1.7 billion.[30]

The classic form of GBS presents with weakness, loss of muscle stretch reflexes, and sensory disturbance progressing over a matter of days to 4 weeks. The full spectrum of GBS includes clinical and pathophysiological variants with and without associated weakness (Table 16.3).

The most common type of GBS is a demyelinating polyradiculoneuropathy, termed *acute inflammatory demyelinating polyradiculopathy*, responsible for the overwhelming majority of GBS cases in the United States.[31] Two similar syndromes characterized by immune attack directed against axons, with resultant axonal loss rather than primary demyelination, have been described. Acute motor axonal neuropathy can occur at any age and presents with acute onset of generalized but (usually) distal predominant weakness.[32] Reduced, normal, or even mildly brisk reflexes have been described.[33,34] Sensory symptoms and signs are absent, but autonomic signs can occur.[35] Acute motor and sensory axonal neuropathy is an acute axonal sensory and motor neuropathy clinically similar to acute demyelinating polyradiculopathy with a less favorable prognosis and often incomplete recovery.[36]

Additional GBS variants have been described in which weakness is absent or, if present, is not the predominant symptom. Miller-Fisher syndrome (MFS) presents with a classic triad of ataxia, areflexia, and ophthalmoplegia.[37] Some patients develop limb weakness, and overlap syndromes with features of typical GBS and MFS occur in 25% of patients.[38,39] Other less common variants of GBS, together comprising fewer than 5% of all cases, include pure sensory, pure autonomic, predominantly small-fiber, brainstem, and central nervous system variants. What links these disorders together under the GBS rubric are several common features including

Table 16-3. Acute Immune-Mediated Neuropathies: Onset of 4 Weeks or Less

	CLINICAL FEATURES	LABORATORY FEATURES	EMG/NCS	IMMUNOMODULATORY TREATMENT
Acute inflammatory demyelinating polyradiculoneuropathy (AIDP)	Symmetric, proximal and distal weakness with sensory loss and reduced or absent reflexes	Elevated CSF protein with no pleocytosis	Sensory and motor demyelinating neuropathy with or without findings of temporal dispersion or conduction block	IVIG and plasma exchange
Acute motor axonal neuropathy (AMAN)	Symmetric, distal > proximal weakness with reduced or occasionally increased reflexes	Elevated CSF protein with no pleocytosis; Frequent GM1 and GD1a autoantibodies	Motor neuropathy with findings of axonal loss	IVIG and plasma exchange
Acute motor and sensory neuropathy (AMSAN)	Symmetric, proximal and distal weakness with sensory loss and reduced or absent reflexes	Elevated CSF protein with no pleocytosis; Frequent GM1 autoantibodies	Sensory and motor neuropathy with axonal loss	IVIG and plasma exchange
Miller-Fisher syndrome (MFS)	Ataxia, areflexia, and ophthalmoplegia with occasional sensory disturbance and weakness	Elevated CSF protein with no pleocytosis	Usually mild sensory > motor axonal neuropathy, but occasional patients show severe sensory and motor axonal neuropathy	IVIG and plasma exchange
Predominantly small fiber	Sensory loss of predominantly small-fiber modalities (pinprick and temperature) usually associated with pain	Elevated CSF protein with no pleocytosis	Standard EMG/NCS normal; Autonomic tests such as the quantitative sudomotor axon reflex test (QSART) may be abnormal	IVIG?
Pure sensory	Asymmetric weakness in the distribution of individual nerves	Elevated CSF protein with no pleocytosis	Sensory axonal neuropathy with normal motor responses	IVIG and plasma exchange?
Pure autonomic	Autonomic failure with variably present sensory disturbance and pain	CSF protein usually elevated with no pleocytosis; Occasional ganglionic acetylcholine receptor autoantibodies	Standard EMG/NCS usually normal; Autonomic test is abnormal	IVIG; Plasma exchange is less favorable due to potentially labile blood pressure

CSF, cerebrospinal fluid; EMG/NCS, electromyography/nerve conduction study; GD1a, GD1a ganglioside; GM1, GM1 ganglioside; IVIG, intravenous immune globulin.

a tendency to develop after infections, a self-limited course with spontaneous resolution without treatment, albuminocytologic dissociation on spinal fluid examination, and the occurrence of multiple overlap variants with features of more typical motor-predominant GBS.[38,40,41]

Pain in GBS

The presence of prominent pain in patients with GBS was emphasized even in the original descriptions of the disorder.[26,42] The most common type of pain in GBS occurs at onset and is typically a moderate to severe throbbing or aching pain in the back and legs. It is present in 50%–80% of patients irrespective of disease severity.[43] The pain is frequently exacerbated with the straight leg raise maneuver, suggesting an underlying process of nerve root irritation. This can be such a striking finding that the clinician is misled into thinking that there is a structural lesion causing the pain and weakness. Imaging studies often reveal contrast enhancement of nerve roots in patients with GBS, and this is more common in patients who present with symptoms of back, leg, or radicular pain.[44,45] Dysesthetic limb pain, often described as burning, tingling, or shock-like, is the second most common pain syndrome at presentation. This typically involves the legs, with occasional upper limb involvement; it is usually not as prominent as the back pain, but often it is more persistent. Other pain patterns or syndromes include myalgia, visceral pain, pressure palsies due to prolonged immobility, and headache[43] (Table 16.4). The severity of pain in GBS does not correlate with the severity of weakness or

with the disease prognosis. The characteristics and prevalence of acute pain within the subtypes of GBS are unclear. Pure motor variants and MFS are not typically associated with pain. Sensory and autonomic variants frequently present with diffuse, severe dysesthetic pain.

While it is generally accepted that acute pain is a common sign in GBS, the frequency, character, and extent of chronic pain are less clear. By comparison with healthy controls, patients with remote GBS experience significantly more pain in association with persistent impairment of function.[46] Pain has been reported in 33%–69% of individuals with remote GBS compared to 11% in controls.[47,48] The persistent or chronic pain is usually dysesthetic in quality and is in the distribution of the distal legs more often than in the arms. Some patients also complain of achy or cramp-like muscle discomfort with joint stiffness. The prevalence of chronic pain within the different subtypes of GBS is not clear, but patients with predominantly sensory and/or autonomic (i.e., small-fiber) involvement often present with severe pain that may be persistent despite treatment. Less severe or absent pain is typical of pure motor variants of GBS.[49]

Diagnosis

The diagnosis of GBS is based on clinical findings, with specific laboratory and electrodiagnostic features helpful in confirming the diagnosis and excluding alternative diagnoses. The differential diagnosis of GBS includes other acute neuropathies as well as diseases of the muscle, spinal cord, motor neuron, and neuromuscular junction. The classic finding of

Table 16-4. Spectrum of Acute Pain in Guillain-Barré Syndrome

Back and leg pain (deep ache often worsened with straight leg raise)	62%
Dysesthetic extremity pain (burning, tingling, shock-like)	49%
Myalgic-rheumatic (muscle or joint pain with range of motion)	35%
Visceral pain (pressure or bloated sensation)	20%
Pressure palsy (related to immobility)	2%
Headache	2%

Source: Reprinted with permission from Moulin DE, Hagen N, Feasby TE, et al. Pain in Guillain-Barré syndrome. *Neurology*. 1997; 48:328–331.

albuminocytological dissociation with elevated spinal fluid protein and few or no mononuclear cells is present in more than 80% of patients 2 weeks after onset of symptoms but is absent in a third of patients during the first week.[26] Spinal fluid pleocytosis greater than 50/mm² should suggest other possible etiologies such as human immune deficiency virus (HIV), sarcoidosis, or Lyme disease.[50,51]

Electrodiagnostic studies are usually helpful in the evaluation of patients with GBS. Early in the disease, these studies may be normal in up to 15% of patients, with abnormalities being absent in some patients for several weeks.[52] A definite diagnosis is possible in 50% of patients 5 days after onset if multiple nerves are studied.[52,53] Proximal conduction studies such as F-wave or H-reflex studies increase the sensitivity of the evaluation.[53] Decreased recruitment on the needle electrode examination is an early finding in the course of the disease when weakness is present. The percentage of patients with demyelinating changes on electrodiagnostic studies varies with the criteria employed, but at least 85% of patients have changes suggestive of demyelination on nerve conduction studies during the course of their disease.[54]

Treatment

The etiology of GBS is presumed to result from immune-mediated processes. Approximately two-third of the cases follow upper respiratory and gastrointestinal infections; cytomegalovirus, Epstein-Barr virus, *Campylobacter jejuni*, and *Mycoplasma pneumoniae* are commonly associated pathogens.[55,56] Immunomodulatory treatments are focused on reducing cumulative nerve damage, but a large percentage of patients are left with persistent deficits. Supportive strategies for managing the acute and chronic sequelae of nerve injury remain of the utmost importance. Acute treatment involves intravenous immunoglobulin (IVIG; 2.0 g/kg over 4–5 days) or plasma exchange (five single-volume infusions over 3–5 days), which are equally effective in shortening the duration of symptoms and lessening the eventual neurological deficits.[57–59] It is not clear whether immunomodulatory treatment with IVIG or plasma exchange modifies the short- and long-term

symptoms of pain, which usually require independent management. Corticosteroids have deleterious effects that may be related to inhibitory effects on macrophages or harmful effects on denervated muscle.[60]

Supportive care remains a vital component in the acute phase to prevent medical complications directly and indirectly related to the underlying disease process. Care in the intensive care unit of a tertiary care center is most appropriate for severely affected individuals. Severe weakness necessitates ventilator support in about one-third of patients. Predictors of respiratory failure include neck flexor weakness, presentation within 7 days following onset of symptoms, inability to cough, and vital capacity less than 60% of the predicted value.[61] Frequent monitoring of pulmonary parameters such as vital capacity and negative inspiratory force is important to help assess the adequacy of diaphragmatic strength. As vital capacity falls below 15 mL/kg intubation and mechanical ventilation should be considered. Immobilization is an independent risk factor for thromboembolic disease, and subcutaneous unfractionated or fractionated heparin and compression stockings are recommended for nonambulatory adults until ambulation is achieved.[62] Autonomic involvement is a frequent occurrence, particularly in severely affected individuals, and can lead to death.[63] Nearly 20% of patients have persistent disability, and death occurs in approximately 5% despite aggressive therapeutic and supportive treatment.[64]

Strategies for management of acute pain in GBS usually involve the judicious short-term use of oral or intravenous opioids, but antiepileptics, specifically gabapentin, have been demonstrated to be effective acutely as well.[65] Epidural opioids have been used in rare cases with severe pain nonresponsive to other interventions.[66,67] In patients with persistent pain, management includes antiepileptic medications or antidepressants including the tricyclic antidepressants and serotonin-norephinephrine reuptake inhibitors.

VASCULITIC NEUROPATHY

The vasculitides are a large, heterogeneous group of disorders bound by the common pathological feature of inflammation and secondary structural damage to blood vessel walls leading to ischemic, hemorrhagic, and thrombotic damage to the tissues or organs supported by these blood vessels. While no universally accepted classification exists, many schemes have been proposed on the basis of etiology, size of involved vessels, histopathology, organ involvement, and other clinical features (see below). Peripheral nerve involvement is a common feature of vasculitides affecting small or medium-sized vessels. Vasculitic neuropathy usually occurs with other features of systemic involvement, but a minority of patients present with an isolated vasculitic neuropathy termed *nonsystemic vasculitis*.[68] Accurate epidemiological studies of vasculitic neuropathy are lacking, but its incidence has been estimated at approximately 10 cases per 1,000,000 population.[69] While vasculitis can occur at any age, it is much more common in older patients; in patients under age 20, it is uncommon.

The clinical presentation of the patient with vasculitic neuropathy depends on the distribution and severity of vessel involvement. Classically, three patterns of peripheral nerve involvement have been characterized: multiple mononeuropathies, overlapping mononeuropathies, and distal symmetric polyneuropathy. The most common presentation is that of overlapping mononeuropathies with asymmetric weakness and sensory loss but not clearly following the pattern of distinct nerves. The classic pattern of multiple mononeuropathies is by far the easiest one to recognize, but it is present only in a minority of patients.[70] Patients with diabetic or nondiabetic radiculoplexus neuropathy typically present with acute pain followed by weakness and atrophy that typically affect the thigh muscles. The largest series of patients with nonsystemic vasculitic neuropathy described an asymmetric polyneuropathy as the most common pattern of deficit, occurring in 77%, followed by multifocal neuropathies in 13%, asymmetric radiculoplexus neuropathies in 8%, and a distal symmetric polyneuropathy in 2%.[70]

Multiple classification schemes have been used to characterize vasculitis. In 1990 the American College of Rheumatology proposed research criteria to distinguish among seven types of systemic vasculitis, but these criteria are of limited diagnostic utility for diagnosis of the individual patient. In 1994 the Chapel Hill Consensus Conference on the Nomenclature of Systemic Vasculitis proposed updated criteria of the vasculitic syndromes on the basis of vessel involvement size and pathology.[71] Recently, a working classification of vasculitis with neuropathy was proposed by a Peripheral Nerve Society task force using merged criteria and expert opinion.[72] This classification proposes three main groups of vasculitis associated with neuropathy: primary systemic, secondary systemic, and nonsystemic (Table 16.5). Primary systemic vasculitis includes disorders affecting small, medium-sized, and large vessels; neuropathy is common, with small artery and arteriole involvement. Secondary systemic vasculitis involves immune-mediated vessel injury in the setting of a preexisting inflammatory condition. Secondary systemic vasculitis can be seen in association with connective tissue diseases, infections, and medications. Nonsystemic vasculitis neuropathy (NSVN) is a condition in which vasculitic involvement is confined to the blood supply of the peripheral nervous system. It is the second most common cause of vasculitis associated with peripheral nerve involvement, accounting for approximately 25% of cases. Localized variants of vasculitic neuropathy, known as *diabetic* and *nondiabetic radiculoplexus neuropathy*, are included in the category of NSVN, as several studies have documented an associated true necrotizing vasculitis.[73–76]

Pain in Vasculitic Neuropathy

The presenting symptoms of patients with vasculitic neuropathy, whether due to NSVN or a primary systemic vasculitic neuropathy, are motor and sensory loss in the distribution of affected nerves associated with burning, dysesthetic pain at the site of nerve injury and in the distribution of the affected nerves.[77] Neuropathic pain appears to be more common in vasculitic neuropathy than in any other type of neuropathy, with some series reporting pain in up to 96% of NSVN patients.[70,78] The frequency of this pain appears to be related to the sudden axon loss related to nerve ischemia. The onset of pain is frequently abrupt, with some

Table 16-5. Peripheral Nerve Society Classification of the Vasculitides Associated with Neuropathy

I. Primary systemic vasculitides
    1. Predominantly small vessel vasculitis
        a. Microscopic polyangiitis[a]
        b. Churg-Strauss syndrome[a]
        c. Wegener's granulomatosis[a]
        d. Essential mixed cryoglobulinemia (non-HCV)
        e. Henoch-Schönlein purpura
    2. Predominantly medium vessel vasculitis
        a. Polyarteritis nodosa (PAN)
    3. Predominantly large vessel vasculitis
        a. Giant cell arteritis
II. Secondary systemic vasculitides associated with one of the following
    1. Connective tissue diseases
        a. Rheumatoid arthritis
        b. Systemic lupus erythematosus
        c. Sjögren's syndrome
        d. Systemic sclerosis
        e. Dermatomyositis
        f. Mixed connective tissue disease
    2. Sarcoidosis
    3. Behcet's disease
    4. Infection (such as HBV, HCV, HIV, CMV, leprosy, Lyme disease, HTLV-I)
    5. Drugs
    6. Malignancy
    7. Inflammatory bowel disease
    8. Hypocomplementemic urticarial vasculitis syndrome
III. Nonsystemic/localized vasculitis
    1. Nonsystemic vasculitic neuropathy
        a. Includes non-diabetic radiculoplexus neuropathy
        b. Includes some cases of Wartenberg's migrant sensory neuritis (provisional)
    2. Diabetic radiculoplexus neuropathy
    3. Localized cutaneous/neuropathic vasculitis
        a. Cutaneous PAN
        b. Others

[a]Anti-neutrophil cytoplasmic antibody (ANCA)-associated vasculitides.

CMV = cytomegalovirus; HBV = hepatitis B virus; HCV = hepatitis C virus; HIV = human immunodeficiency virus; HTLV = human T-lymphotropic virus; PAN = polyarteritis nodosa.

Source: Reprinted with permission from Collins M, Dyck P, Gronseth G, et al. Peripheral Nerve Society Guideline on the classification, diagnosis, and investigation of nonsystemic vasculitic neuropathy. *J Peripher Nerv Syst.* 2010;15(3):176–184.

patients able to recall the exact time of onset of their symptoms. With immunosuppressive treatment, this pain, which is often excruciating, usually abates. Some pain persists chronically in approximately 60% of patients and occasionally can be of ferocious intensity.[70] Asymmetric limb pain, more prominent distally, often in the distribution of individual nerve branches, is characteristic of acute-subacute vasculitic neuropathy. In chronic or long-standing vasculitic neuropathy the pain typically has a length-dependent symmetric pattern rather than the usual presentation of asymmetric pain.

Diagnosis

A thorough history and physical examination, selected laboratory tests to identify or exclude coexistent or associated disorders, nerve biopsy, and electrodiagnostic testing are important in the workup of possible vasculitic neuropathy. Laboratory evaluation should include testing for systemic conditions suggested by the history and examination. The routine laboratory evaluation includes a complete blood count with differential, renal and hepatic panels, urinalysis, C-reactive protein, erythrocyte sedimentation rate, rheumatoid factor, antinuclear antibody, antineutrophil cytoplasmic antibody, hepatitis B surface antigens and hepatitis C antibodies, complement, serum electrophoresis with immunofixation, glucose tolerance testing, and cryoglobulins. Electrodiagnostic studies are extremely valuable in characterizing the distribution and underlying neuropathophysiology (i.e., axonal loss versus demyelination). An asymmetrical axonal neuropathy or multiple axonal mononeuropathies on electrodiagnostic studies support the possibility of an underlying vasculitic neuropathy. Nerve conduction studies usually demonstrate reduced sensory and motor amplitudes signifying axonal loss with normal or mildly reduced conduction velocity. The needle electrode examination demonstrates evidence of denervation, which may be acute and/or chronic, depending on the patient's presentation. Rarely, pseudoconduction block may be seen in the acute phase with ongoing nerve ischemia.[79] Findings of reduced conduction velocity or other signs suggesting demyelination, such as temporal dispersion or persistent conduction block, should prompt the clinician to look for an alternative etiology underlying the patient's symptoms.

Nerve biopsy, although rarely indicated in the evaluation of most neuropathies, is absolutely critical in the evaluation of atypical inflammatory or vasculitic neuropathies, and a histological diagnosis should always be sought to support the potential need for long-term immunomodulatory treatment with toxic side effects. The sural, superficial peroneal, and superficial radial nerves are most commonly biopsied, but the clinical examination and electrodiagnostic evaluation should help determine the biopsy site. A normal examination and nerve conduction response lessen the chance of abnormal findings and reduce the diagnostic yield. A combined nerve and muscle biopsy slightly increases the diagnostic sensitivity. A nerve that is clinically involved should be selected, keeping in mind the morbidity associated with nerve biopsy, which may include persistent numbness and, rarely, pain and dysesthesia. A definite histological diagnosis requires endoneurial or epineurial vessel wall infarction in association with perivascular or transmural infiltration by inflammatory cells (Figure 16.2). Probable vasculitis is supported

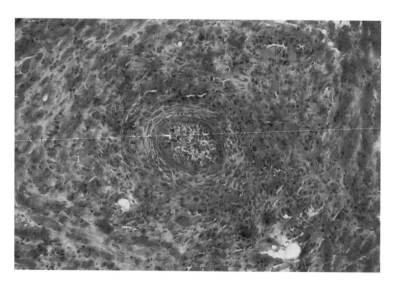

FIGURE 16.2   Epineurial blood vessel showing transmural inflammation in a patient with nonsystemic vasculitis who presented with a painful left foot drop.

by the findings of transmural or perivascular inflammation without vessel wall infarction but is associated with at least one of the following: chronic thrombosis, hemosiderin deposition, asymmetric nerve fiber loss, or prominent Wallerian degeneration.

Treatment

While understanding of the factors initiating vasculitic neuropathy remains incomplete, an immune-mediated process is assumed. Hypersensitivity vasculitis is associated with infection, cancer, and medications. In these cases, antigen removal through treatment of the primary underlying process is an important therapeutic strategy. Otherwise, the vasculitic destruction of blood vessels leading to ischemic damage to tissues including peripheral nerves is believed to be due to both immune complex deposition and cell-mediated mechanisms.[80] Nonspecific immunomodulation must be considered in most patients, and corticosteroids remain the primary modality. Prednisone is usually initiated at 1.5 mg/kg/day as a single morning dose. Some patients show continued disease progression despite high-dose corticosteroid management and require combination therapy. In mild NSVN, high-dose steroids used alone may be sufficient. Aggressive disease, usually defined by the presence of rapidly progressive weakness or multiorgan involvement, should prompt consideration of combination therapy with cytotoxic agents. Cyclophosphamide at 1.5–2.5 mg/kg/day is a cytotoxic medication frequently used for combination therapy. Combination therapy should be started with caution by clinicians familiar with prescribing precautions after carefully weighing the risks and benefits. Other, less well studied agents have been used for disease modification with variable success, including methotrexate, cyclosporine, tacrolimus, chlorambucil, azathioprine, and mycophenolate mofetil.

Neuropathic pain can be severe and debilitating, and usually requires antiepileptic medications or antidepressants including the tricyclic antidepressants and serotonin-norephinephrine reuptake inhibitors in addition to opiates. The pain associated with vasculitis, while severe during disease activity, typically responds dramatically to immunomodulation. Typically, once the disease process is treated, symptomatic pain management can be reduced or even discontinued. In patients with vasculitic neuropathy with no evidence of ongoing vasculitis, worsening pain is often the initial indicator of reemerging disease activity.

CHRONIC INFLAMMATORY DEMYELINATING POLYRADICULONEUROPATHY

Chronic inflammatory demyelinating polyradiculoneuropathy (CIDP) is a chronic acquired neuropathy of presumed immune-mediated origin. Austin originally described two patients with a chronic relapsing neuropathy that was glucocorticoid-responsive in 1958,[81] but it was not until 1975 that Dyck and coworkers clearly defined the clinical disorder now known as CIDP.[82] Whether or not CIDP is a disease or a syndrome remains to be determined, and as in GBS, there are multiple variants within the spectrum of the chronic immune-mediated neuropathies. Variations of the classic CIDP syndrome include those with predominantly motor or sensory symptoms, predominantly distal involvement, primary axonal loss rather than demyelination, and multifocal or asymmetric distributions.

Specific related but seemingly distinct disorders within the spectrum of chronic immune-mediated neuropathies include multifocal acquired demyelinating sensory and motor neuropathy, distal acquired demyelinating symmetric neuropathy with or without anti-myelin-associated glycoprotein antibodies, multifocal motor neuropathy, polyneuropathy, organomegaly, endocrinopathy, monoclonal gammopathy syndrome, and CIDP associated with concurrent systemic disorders such as monoclonal gammopathy of undetermined significance (MGUS), hepatitis B or C, lymphoma, and collagen vascular disorders (Table 16.6). Steroid-responsive chronic axonal neuropathies have also been described, but the clinical limits and features of this entity are still unknown and somewhat controversial.[83,84] The overall prevalence of CIDP is approximately 1–2 cases per 100,000 adult population.[85–87] CIDP is described in all age groups but appears to have

Table 16-6. Chronic Immune-Mediated Neuropathies: Onset of 8 Weeks or More

	CLINICAL FEATURES	LABORATORY FEATURES	EMG/NCS	TREATMENT
Chronic inflammatory demyelinating polyradiculoneuropathy (CIDP)	Symmetric, proximal and distal weakness with sensory loss and reduced or absent reflexes	Elevated CSF protein with no pleocytosis	Sensory and motor demyelinating neuropathy with or without findings of temporal dispersion or conduction block	Steroids, IVIG, and plasma exchange Others include azathioprine, cyclosporine, cyclophosphamide, and methotrexate
CIDP with concurrent medical conditions	Similar to CIDP	Elevated CSF protein with no pleocytosis with other laboratory findings specific to associated condition	Similar to CIDP	Similar to CIDP
Distal acquired demyelinating sensory neuropathy (DADS)	Symmetric, predominantly distal sensory loss > motor weakness, with reduced or absent reflexes	Monoclonal gammopathy in two-thirds (usually IgM kappa), 50% with anti-myelin- associated glycoprotein antibodies	Predominantly distal demyelinating sensory and motor neuropathy, with prolonged distal latencies > reduced conduction velocities Temporal dispersion and conduction block less frequently seen	Rituximab Short-term response to plasma exchange
Multifocal motor neuropathy (MMN)	Predominantly distal, upper limb > lower limb weakness, in the distribution of individual named nerves, with depressed or absent reflexes and relatively preserved muscle bulk	CSF protein usually normal; up to 80% of patients may have IgM ganglioside antibodies (GM1, asialo-GM1, or GM2)	Multifocal demyelinating motor neuropathy, usually with conduction block	IVIG, rituximab, and cyclophosphamide Does not respond to steroids or plasma exchange
Multifocal acquired demyelinating sensory and motor (MADSAM)	Asymmetric weakness and sensory loss in the distribution of individual nerves with predilection for upper limb involvement	CSF protein usually elevated with no pleocytosis	Multifocal demyelinating sensory and motor neuropathy with conduction block	Similar to CIDP
Multifocal acquired motor axonopathy (MAMA)	Asymmetric weakness in the distribution of individual nerves.	Normal CSF studies Most lack ganglioside antibodies	Multifocal axonal motor neuropathy (in the distribution of individual nerves) with no demyelination or conduction block	IVIG? Close observation for signs of motor neuron disease

a slight predilection for middle-aged and older adults.

Presentation/Natural History of Classic CIDP

The most common presentation of CIDP is slowly progressive weakness in a symmetric distribution with distal sensory loss and absent or reduced muscle stretch reflexes. By definition, the onset of symptoms progresses over at least 8 weeks, helping to distinguish CIDP from acute immune neuropathy (GBS).[88] The course of the disease can be slowly progressive, stepwise progressive, or relapsing and remitting even in the absence of disease-modifying treatment. Occasionally, patients present with acute weakness mimicking GBS but have persistent, chronic progression following the acute course, and a third group of patients, with a condition labeled *subacute inflammatory demyelinating polyneuropathy*, fall between the continuum of GBS and CIDP, with progression occurring over 4–8 weeks.[89,90] Distal and proximal weakness are typically present due to the polyradicular pattern of nerve involvement. In approximately 10% of cases, facial weakness is present and

other cranial nerves may be affected.[88,91] Rarely, patients present with weakness confined to the legs, and even more rarely, patients have weakness confined to the arms. Sensory symptoms are common, with most patients demonstrating sensory loss and paresthesias in the feet, distal legs, and hands.

Pain in CIDP

The full spectrum of pain in CIDP is the least well studied in all of the immune-mediated neuropathies and remains unclear. Not surprisingly, pain is less common in CIDP than in other, more quickly progressive neuropathies such as GBS and NSVN. Approximately 20% of CIDP patients complain of moderate to severe pain, and in these patients this may be the presenting complaint.[88,92] Severe low back pain with or without radicular symptoms is also frequently seen in patients at presentation with a more rapidly progressing or acute disease. In these patients, magnetic resonance imaging may demonstrate hypertrophic nerve roots and sometimes true spinal stenosis (Figure 16.3).[93,94] The acute low back and radicular pains are typically transient with or without

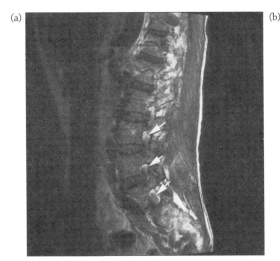 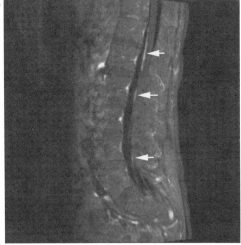

FIGURE 16.3 This magnetic resonance imaging was obtained in a 47-year-old man who presented with severe low back pain and weakness in the setting of chronic inflammatory demyelinating polyradiculoneuropathy. (A) This T2-weighted sagittal image demonstrates enlargement of traversing and exiting nerve roots in the lower lumbar spine, particularly S1. (B) This T1-weighted sagittal postcontrast image demonstrates enhancement of the nerve roots.

treatment. In patients with particularly aggressive disease and significant secondary axonal loss, there may be persistent distal dysesthetic pain described as burning or an uncomfortable tingling.

Diagnosis

The diagnosis of CIDP depends on the clinical findings, laboratory findings of elevated cerebrospinal fluid (CSF) protein, and electrodiagnostic findings suggestive of acquired demyelination. Multiple clinical criteria for the diagnosis of CIDP have been proposed, with varying degrees of sensitivity and specificity.[88,95–101] It is important to remember that some patients who do not meet any established criteria will respond to immunomodulation. Continued work is needed to determine more sensitive criteria with retained specificity.

The clinical hallmark of CIDP is the presence of not only length-dependent or distal weakness but also of prominent proximal weakness suggesting a polyradicular distribution of immune-mediated attack. The clinical findings of symmetric distal and proximal weakness with progression over at least 2 months, with laboratory findings of elevated CSF protein and electrodiagnostic evidence of demyelination, are crucial to the diagnosis.[81,88]

In addition to clinical criteria, electrophysiological and laboratory data are used to support the clinical findings. The main laboratory finding supporting an acquired inflammatory demyelinating neuropathy is elevation of CSF protein in the absence of pleocytosis found in 95% of patients.[88] This finding, while supportive of the diagnosis, is not specific, as it can also be seen in other dysmyelination disorders such as hereditary neuropathies.[102–104] Fasting glucose or glucose tolerance testing and serum electrophoresis with immunofixation should be performed in all patients to exclude coexistent diabetes mellitus and paraprotein. Although several small studies have demonstrated a strong association between diabetes mellitus and CIDP, a recent population-based study did not support this observation.[85,105–109]

Approximately 10% of patients diagnosed with neuropathy have an associated monoclonal protein, and this finding is seen in approximately 10%–20% of patients with CIDP.[88,91,97,110] In the presence of a monoclonal protein, an underlying lymphoproliferative disorder should be excluded. Approximately one-third of patients with a monoclonal gammopathy have an underlying hematological malignancy such as multiple myeloma, Waldenström's macroglobinemia, or plasmacytoma, but the majority of patients have MGUS. These cases are usually designated CIDP with a concurrent condition or CIDP-MGUS.[111] Other laboratory testing may include renal function testing, liver function tests, thyroid stimulating hormone, HIV antibody, hepatitis C and B profiles, antinuclear and extractable antibodies, and angiotensin converting enzyme to help exclude associated or mimicking conditions. In some instances, this association may be purely coincidental; in others, there may be pathogenic significance with prognostic and therapeutic implications.

Electrodiagnostic studies are the most important part of the diagnostic evaluation of a patient with suspected CIDP. Classically, patients have prolongation of distal latency and reduced conduction velocities out of proportion to loss of amplitude on motor nerve conduction studies. Findings of conduction block and temporal dispersion are indicative of a multifocal process and are suggestive of an acquired process. There are multiple existing electrodiagnostic criteria for primary demyelination.[88,95–101] While these criteria are helpful, many are overly restrictive and exclusive, relying strictly on motor nerve function. Approximately two-thirds of patients do not meet the criteria for primary demyelination.[97,112] Occasional patients present with significant weakness and essentially normal nerve conduction studies due to predominantly proximal polyradicular involvement. The needle electrode examination shows reduced recruitment in weak muscles; with severe demyelination, secondary axonal loss can be demonstrated, which suggests a worse prognosis if it is prominent.[113–115]

Nerve biopsy is rarely indicated in the evaluation of possible CIDP, and its sensitivity is poor due to the multifocal distribution of the disease.[116] The classic finding of demyelination with thinly myelinated fibers and onion bulbs occurs in about 70% of cases.[88] Histological examination of an active lesion demonstrates macrophage-associated demyelination, remyelination, and endoneurial inflammatory cell infiltrates with T cells, fiber loss, and formation of onion bulbs.[115,117]

Treatment

CIDP is presumed to be secondary to an immune attack, probably including both humoral and cellular components, directed against a peripheral nerve antigen.[118] The factors that trigger this response remain unknown, necessitating nonspecific rescue and chronic immunomodulatory treatments. Although prednisone remains a mainstay of treatment due to its efficacy, ease of use, familiarity, cost effectiveness, and relatively rapid onset, IVIG is increasingly replacing prednisone as the drug of choice for initial treatment of CIDP.[119–121] Intravenous immunoglobulin is a favored treatment for its demonstrated efficacy and tolerability. Specific IVIG treatment regimens vary among groups and among different studies. The most appropriate dosage and the timing of dosages are unclear. Several randomized trials have demonstrated the efficacy of plasma exchange, and in a direct comparison with IVIG, plasma exchange was equally effective, with slightly increased minor side effects.[122] There is variability among patients in their response to individual treatments, and a percentage of patients respond better to one of the primary treatments (IVIG, prednisone, or plasma exchange) for unknown reasons.[123] Recent work suggests that IVIG responsiveness may be related to underlying genetic determinants, but continued work is needed to help predict an individual patient's response to particular treatments.[124] Other treatment agents with less supportive evidence include azathioprine, cyclosporine, cyclophosphamide, methotrexate, entanercept, mycophenolate mofetil, and rituximab.

In retrospective reports, approximately 60%–90% of patients respond to initial treatment.[88,123,125] The majority of patients require ongoing immunomodulation, as remission without medications is achieved in only about one-third.[88] Immunomodulation is by far the most important component of treatment, but a comprehensive treatment plan including occupational and physical therapy is important. Therapy prescriptions should focus on strengthening and endurance exercises to limit disuse and to promote maximum function. Adaptation of activities of daily living as necessary with the help of occupational therapy should be considered to encourage independent functioning. Treatment of pain in CIDP is largely focused on immunomodulatory treatment of the underlying inflammatory process. In the majority of patients, the pain associated with CIDP responds well to steroids. Strategies for management of acute pain in CIDP are similar to those for GBS and usually involve oral or intravenous opioids. In patients with persistent or chronic pain, management includes antiepileptic medications or antidepressants including the tricyclic antidepressants and serotonin-norepinephrine reuptake inhibitors.

CONCLUSIONS

For most of the immune-mediated neuropathies, the quality, distribution, severity, and duration of pain symptoms usually correlate with the type of nerve injury. Pain in the acute immune-mediated neuropathies begins abruptly over a matter of hours to days and usually improves as nerve injury ceases, while in the chronic immune-mediated neuropathies the pain presents insidiously and is often more persistent in parallel with chronic ongoing nerve loss. These generalizations, while useful clinically, are, however, not always true. Disorders like GBS not uncommonly result in persistent dysesthetic limb pain, while more chronic disorders such as vasculitic neuropathy or CIDP may present acutely with severe disabling pain. During the course of treatment, the symptoms of pain can be helpful in disease monitoring; worsening pain can signal worsening or recurrent disease prior to the appearance of other clinical signs or symptoms.

The treatment of pain associated with the immune-mediated neuropathies requires a comprehensive approach. The primary goal is treatment of the underlying disease process, and in many immune disorders, immunomodulation is the most effective treatment of the painful symptoms. Symptomatic management with pain medications is often necessary acutely and, in many cases, on a chronic basis. In some disorders, for instance GBS, it is unclear whether immuno-modulation with either IVIG or plasma exchange has a direct effect on the severity or duration of the symptoms of pain. In these instances, symptomatic management is the primary goal in the treatment of pain. Continued work is needed to define optimal treatment strategies and the full spectrum of pain associated with the immune-mediated neuropathies.

REFERENCES

1. Dyck PJ, Lambert EH, O'Brien PC. Pain in peripheral neuropathy related to rate and kind of fiber degeneration. *Neurology*. 1976;26:466–471.
2. Dreschfeld J. On some of the rarer forms of muscular atrophies. *Brain*. 1887;9:187–189.
3. Parsonage M, Turner JWA. Neuralgic amyotrophy: the shoulder girdle syndrome. *Lancet*. 1948;1:973–978.
4. Beghi E, Kurland LT, Mulder DW, et al. Brachial plexus neuropathy in the population of Rochester, Minnesota, 1970–1981. *Ann Neurol*. 1985;18:320–323.
5. MacDonald BK, Cockerell OC, Sander JW, et al. The incidence and lifetime prevalence of neurological disorders in a prospective community-based study in the UK [see comment]. *Brain*. 2000;123:665–676.
6. Tsairis P, Dyck PJ, Mulder DW. Natural history of brachial plexus neuropathy. Report on 99 patients. *Arch Neurol*. 1972;27:109–117.
7. van Alfen N, van Engelen BG, van Alfen N, et al. The clinical spectrum of neuralgic amyotrophy in 246 cases. *Brain*. 2006;129:438–450.
8. Guinard S, Huchot E, Couturaud F, et al. [A bilateral diaphragmatic paralysis due to Parsonage and Turner syndrome—its evolution over eight years]. *Rev Pneumol Clin*. 2008;64:137–140.
9. Dinsmore WW, Irvine AK, Callender ME. Recurrent neuralgic amyotrophy with vagus and phrenic nerve involvement. *Clin Neurol Neurosurg*. 1985;87:39–40.
10. Chen YM, Hu GC, Cheng SJ, et al. Bilateral neuralgic amyotrophy presenting with left vocal cord and phrenic nerve paralysis. *J Formosan Med Assoc*. 2007;106:680–684.
11. van Alfen N, van der Werf SP, van Engelen BG, et al. Long-term pain, fatigue, and impairment in neuralgic amyotrophy. *Arch Phys Med Rehabil*. 2009;90:435–439.
12. Schott GD. A chronic and painless form of idiopathic brachial plexus neuropathy. *J Neurol Neurosurg Psychiatry*. 1983;46:555–557.
13. Chisholm K, Scala S, Srinivasan J. Delay in diagnosis of neuralgic amyotrophy in patients initially evaluated by non-neurologists. *Eur J Neurol*. 2008;15:e18.
14. Pellegrino JE, Rebbeck TR, Brown MJ, et al. Mapping of hereditary neuralgic amyotrophy (familial brachial plexus neuropathy) to distal chromosome 17q. *Neurology*. 1996;46:1128–1132.
15. Hannibal MC, Ruzzo EK, Miller LR, et al. SEPT9 gene sequencing analysis reveals recurrent mutations in hereditary neuralgic amyotrophy. *Neurology*. 2009;72:1755–1759.
16. Sahin E, Senocak O, Bacakoglu AK, et al. [Neuralgic amyotrophy as the primary cause of shoulder pain in a patient with rotator cuff tear]. *Acta Orthop Traumatol Turc*. 2009;43:190–192.
17. McCarty EC, Tsairis P, Warren RF. Brachial neuritis. *Clin Orthop Relat Res*. 1999;368: 37–43.
18. van Alfen N, Huisman WJ, Overeem S, et al. Sensory nerve conduction studies in neuralgic amyotrophy. *Am J Phys Med Rehabil*. 2009;88:941–946.
19. Ferrante MA, Wilbourn AJ. The utility of various sensory nerve conduction responses in assessing brachial plexopathies. *Muscle Nerve*. 1995;18:879–889.
20. Lo YL, Mills KR. Motor root conduction in neuralgic amyotrophy: evidence of proximal conduction block. *J Neurol Neurosurg Psychiatry*. 1999;66:586–590.
21. Suarez GA, Giannini C, Bosch EP, et al. Immune brachial plexus neuropathy: suggestive evidence for an inflammatory-immune pathogenesis. *Neurology*. 1996;46:559–561.
22. van Eijk JJ, van Alfen N, Berrevoets M, et al. Evaluation of prednisolone treatment in the acute phase of neuralgic amyotrophy: an observational study. *J Neurol Neurosurg Psychiatry*. 2009;80:1120–1124.
23. van Alfen N, van Engelen BG, Hughes RA, et al. Treatment for idiopathic and hereditary neuralgic amyotrophy (brachial neuritis). *Cochrane Database Syst Rev*. 2009;3:CD006976.
24. Tsao BE, Avery R, Shields RW, et al. Neuralgic amyotrophy precipitated by Epstein-Barr virus. *Neurology*. 2004;62:1234–1235.
25. Nakajima M, Fujioka S, Ohno H, et al. Partial but rapid recovery from paralysis after immunomodulation during early stage of neuralgic amyotrophy. *Eur Neurol*. 2006;55:227–229.
26. Ropper AH, Wijdicks EFM, Truax BT. *Guillain-Barré Syndrome*. Philadelphia: F.A Davis; 1991.
27. Ropper AH. The Guillain-Barré syndrome. *N Engl J Med*. 1992;326:1130–1136.

28. Chio A, Cocito D, Leone M, et al. Guillain-Barre syndrome: a prospective, population-based incidence and outcome survey. *Neurology*. 2003;60:1146–1150.

29. McGrogan A, Madle GC, Seaman HE, et al. The epidemiology of Guillain-Barre syndrome worldwide. A systematic literature review. *Neuroepidemiology*. 2009;32:150–163.

30. Frenzen PD. Economic cost of Guillain-Barré syndrome in the United States. *Neurology*. 2008;71:21–27.

31. Hadden RD, Cornblath DR, Hughes RA, et al. Electrophysiological classification of Guillain-Barré syndrome: clinical associations and outcome. Plasma Exchange/Sandoglobulin Guillain-Barré Syndrome Trial Group. *Ann Neurol*. 1998;44:780–788.

32. Feasby TE, Gilbert JJ, Brown WF, et al. An acute axonal form of Guillain-Barré polyneuropathy. *Brain*. 1986;109:1115–1126.

33. Kuwabara S, Ogawara K, Koga M, et al. Hyperreflexia in Guillain-Barré syndrome: relation with acute motor axonal neuropathy and anti-GM1 antibody. *J Neurol Neurosurg Psychiatry*. 1999;67:180–184.

34. Loffel NB, Rossi LN, Mumenthaler M, et al. The Landry-Guillain-Barré syndrome. Complications, prognosis and natural history in 123 cases. *J Neurol Sci*. 1977;33:71–79.

35. Asahina M, Kuwabara S, Suzuki A, et al. Autonomic function in demyelinating and axonal subtypes of Guillain-Barré syndrome. *Acta Neurol Scand*. 2002;105:44–50.

36. Griffin JW, Li CY, Ho TW, et al. Pathology of the motor-sensory axonal Guillain-Barré syndrome [see comment]. *Ann Neurol*. 1996;39:17–28.

37. Fisher C. An usual variant of acute idiopathic polyneuritis (syndrome of ophthalmoplegia, ataxia, and areflexia). *N Engl J Med*. 1956;255(2):57–65.

38. Yuki N, Wakabayashi K, Yamada M, et al. Overlap of Guillain-Barré syndrome and Bickerstaff's brainstem encephalitis. *J Neurol Sci*. 1997;145:119–121.

39. Ito M, Kuwabara S, Odaka M, et al. Bickerstaff's brainstem encephalitis and Fisher syndrome form a continuous spectrum: clinical analysis of 581 cases. J Neurol. 2008;255:674–682.

40. Oh SJ, LaGanke C, Claussen GC. Sensory Guillain-Barré syndrome. *Neurology*. 2001;56:82–86.

41. Seneviratne U, Gunasekera S. Acute small fibre sensory neuropathy: another variant of Guillain-Barré syndrome? *J Neurol Neurosurg Psychiatry*. 2002;72:540–542.

42. Landry O. Note sur la paralysie ascendante aigue. *Gazette Hebdomadaire*. 1859;6:472–474.

43. Moulin DE, Hagen N, Feasby TE, et al. Pain in Guillain-Barreé syndrome [see comment]. *Neurology*. 1997;48:328–331.

44. Wilmshurst JM, Thomas NH, Robinson RO, et al. Lower limb and back pain in Guillain-Barré syndrome and associated contrast enhancement in MRI of the cauda equina. *Acta Paediatr*. 2001;90:691–694.

45. Gorson KC, Ropper AH, Muriello MA, et al. Prospective evaluation of MRI lumbosacral nerve root enhancement in acute Guillain-Barré syndrome [see comment]. *Neurology*. 1996;47:813–817.

46. Rudolph T, Larsen JP, Farbu E. The long-term functional status in patients with Guillain-Barré syndrome. *Eur J Neurol*. 2008;15:1332–1337.

47. Rekand T, Gramstad A, Vedeler CA, et al. Fatigue, pain and muscle weakness are frequent after Guillain-Barré syndrome and poliomyelitis. *J Neurol*. 2009;256:349–354.

48. Forsberg A, Press R, Einarsson U, et al. Impairment in Guillain-Barré syndrome during the first 2 years after onset: a prospective study. *J Neurol Sci*. 2004;227:131–138.

49. Bernsen RA, Jager AE, Schmitz PI, et al. Long-term sensory deficit after Guillain-Barré syndrome. *J Neurol*. 2001;248:483–486.

50. Rauschka H, Jellinger K, Lassmann H, et al. Guillain-Barré syndrome with marked pleocytosis or a significant proportion of polymorphonuclear granulocytes in the cerebrospinal fluid: neuropathological investigation of five cases and review of differential diagnoses [see comment]. *Eur J Neurol*. 2003;10:479–486.

51. Asbury AK, Arnason AB, Karp HR, McFarlin DE. Criteria for diagnosis of Guillain-Barré syndrome. *Ann Neurol*. 1978;3:565–566.

52. Albers JW, Donofrio PD, McGonagle TK. Sequential electrodiagnostic abnormalities in acute inflammatory demyelinating polyradiculoneuropathy. *Muscle Nerve*. 1985;8:528–539.

53. Gordon PH, Wilbourn AJ. Early electrodiagnostic findings in Guillain-Barré syndrome. *Arch Neurol*. 2001;58:913–917.

54. Meulstee J, van der Meche FG. Electrodiagnostic criteria for polyneuropathy and demyelination: application in 135 patients with Guillain-Barré syndrome. Dutch Guillain-Barré Study Group. *J Neurol Neurosurg Psychiatry*. 1995;59:482–486.

55. Winer JB, Gray IA, Gregson NA, et al. A prospective study of acute idiopathic neuropathy. III. Immunological studies. *J Neurol Neurosurg Psychiatry*. 1988;51:619–625.

56. Winer JB, Hughes RA, Anderson MJ, et al. A prospective study of acute idiopathic neuropathy. II.

Antecedent events. *J Neurol Neurosurg Psychiatry*. 1988;51:613–618.

57. Bril V, Ilse WK, Pearce R, et al. Pilot trial of immunoglobulin versus plasma exchange in patients with Guillain-Barré syndrome. *Neurology*. 1996;46:100–103.

58. Diener HC, Haupt WF, Kloss TM, et al. A preliminary, randomized, multicenter study comparing intravenous immunoglobulin, plasma exchange, and immune adsorption in Guillain-Barré syndrome. *Eur Neurol*. 2001;46:107–109.

59. Anonymous. Randomised trial of plasma exchange, intravenous immunoglobulin, and combined treatments in Guillain-Barré syndrome. Plasma Exchange/Sandoglobulin Guillain-Barré Syndrome Trial Group [see comment]. *Lancet*. 1997;349:225–230.

60. Hughes RA, Swan AV, Raphael JC, et al. Immunotherapy for Guillain-Barré syndrome: a systematic review. *Brain*. 2007;130:2245–2257.

61. Sharshar T, Chevret S, Bourdain F, et al. Early predictors of mechanical ventilation in Guillain-Barré syndrome. *Crit Care Med*. 2003;31:278–283.

62. Hughes RA, Wijdicks EF, Benson E, et al. Supportive care for patients with Guillain-Barré syndrome. *Arch Neurol*. 2005;62:1194–1198.

63. Lichtenfeld P. Autonomic dysfunction in the Guillain-Barré syndrome. *Am J Med*. 1971;50:772–780.

64. Hughes RA, Hadden RD, Rees JH, et al. The Italian Guillain-Barré Study Group. The prognosis and main prognostic indicators of Guillain-Barré syndrome: a multicentre prospective study of 297 patients [see comment]. *Brain*. 1998;121:767–769.

65. Pandey CK, Bose N, Garg G, et al. Gabapentin for the treatment of pain in Guillain-Barré syndrome: a double-blinded, placebo-controlled, crossover study. *Anesth Analg*. 2002;95:1719–1723.

66. Rosenfeld B, Borel C, Hanley D. Epidural morphine treatment of pain in Guillain-Barré syndrome. *Arch Neurol*. 1986;43:1194–1196.

67. Connelly M, Shagrin J, Warfield C. Epidural opioids for the management of pain in a patient with the Guillain-Barré syndrome. *Anesthesiology*. 1990;72:381–383.

68. Dyck PJ, Benstead TJ, Conn DL, et al. Nonsystemic vasculitic neuropathy. *Brain*. 1987;110:843–853.

69. Mendell JR, Kissel JT, Cornblath DR. *Diagnosis and Management of Peripheral Nerve Disorders*. New York: Oxford University Press; 2001.

70. Collins MP, Periquet MI, Mendell JR, et al. Nonsystemic vasculitic neuropathy: insights from a clinical cohort. *Neurology*. 2003;61:623–630.

71. Jennette JC, Falk RJ, Andrassy K, et al. Nomenclature of systemic vasculitides. Proposal of an international consensus conference. *Arthritis Rheum*. 1994;37:187–192.

72. Collins M, Dyck P, Gronseth G, et al. Peripheral Nerve Society Guideline on the classification, diagnosis, and investigation of nonsystemic vasculitic neuropathy. *J Peripher Nerv Syst*. 2010;15(3):176–184.

73. Dyck PJ, Norell JE. Microvasculitis and ischemia in diabetic lumbosacral radiculoplexus neuropathy. *Neurology*. 1999;53:2113–2121.

74. Said G, Lacroix C, Lozeron P, et al. Inflammatory vasculopathy in multifocal diabetic neuropathy. *Brain*. 2003;126:376–385.

75. Dyck PJ, Norell JE. Non-diabetic lumbosacral radiculoplexus neuropathy: natural history, outcome and comparison with the diabetic variety. *Brain*. 2001;124:1197–1207.

76. Dyck PJ, Engelstad J, Norell J. Microvasculitis in non-diabetic lumbosacral radiculoplexus neuropathy (LSRPN): similarity to the diabetic variety (DLSRPN). J Neuropathol Exp Neurol. 2000;59:525–538.

77. Lovshin LaK, J. Peripheral neuritis in periarteritis nodosa. *Arch Intern Med*. 1948;82:321–338.

78. Kissel JT, Slivka AP, Warmolts JR, et al. The clinical spectrum of necrotizing angiopathy of the peripheral nervous system. *Ann Neurol*. 1985;18:251–257.

79. McCluskey L, Feinberg D, Cantor C, et al. "Pseudo-conduction block" in vasculitic neuropathy. *Muscle Nerve*. 1999;22:1361–1366.

80. Kissel JT, Riethman JL, Omerza J, et al. Peripheral nerve vasculitis: immune characterization of the vascular lesions [see comment]. *Ann Neurol*. 1989;25:291–297.

81. Austin JH. Recurrent polyneuropathies and their corticosteroid treatment; with five-year observations of a placebo-controlled case treated with corticotrophin, cortisone, and prednisone. *Brain*. 1958;81:157–192.

82. Dyck PJ, Lais AC, Ohta M, et al. Chronic inflammatory polyradiculoneuropathy. *Mayo Clin Proc*. 1975;50:621–637.

83. Uncini A, Sabatelli M, Mignogna T, et al. Chronic progressive steroid responsive axonal polyneuropathy: a CIDP vaariant or a primary axonal disorder? [see comment]. *Muscle Nerve*. 1996;19:365–371.

84. Gorson KC, Ropper AH, Adelman LS, et al. Chronic motor axonal neuropathy: pathological evidence of inflammatory polyradiculoneuropathy. *Muscle Nerve*. 1999;22:266–270.

85. Laughlin RS, Dyck PJ, Melton LJ 3rd, et al. Incidence and prevalence of CIDP and the association of diabetes mellitus. *Neurology*. 2009;73:39–45.

86. McLeod JG, Pollard JD, Macaskill P, et al. Prevalence of chronic inflammatory demyelinating polyneuropathy in New South Wales, Australia. *Ann Neurol*. 1999;46:910–913.

87. Lunn MP, Manji H, Choudhary PP, et al. Chronic inflammatory demyelinating polyradiculoneuropathy: a prevalence study in southeast England. *J Neurol Neurosurg Psychiatry*. 1999;66:677–680.

88. Barohn RJ, Kissel JT, Warmolts JR, et al. Chronic inflammatory demyelinating polyradiculoneuropathy. Clinical characteristics, course, and recommendations for diagnostic criteria. *Arch Neurol*. 1989;46:878–884.

89. Oh SJ. Subacute demyelinating polyneuropathy responding to corticosteroid treatment. *Arch Neurol*. 1978;35:509–516.

90. Oh SJ, Kurokawa K, de Almeida DF, et al. Subacute inflammatory demyelinating polyneuropathy. *Neurology*. 2003;61:1507–1512.

91. Rotta FT, Sussman AT, Bradley WG, et al. The spectrum of chronic inflammatory demyelinating polyneuropathy. *J Neurol Sci*. 2000;173:129–139.

92. Boukhris S, Magy L, Khalil M, et al. Pain as the presenting symptom of chronic inflammatory demyelinating polyradiculoneuropathy (CIDP). *J Neurol Sci*. 2007;254:33–38.

93. Ginsberg L, Platts AD, Thomas PK. Chronic inflammatory demyelinating polyneuropathy mimicking a lumbar spinal stenosis syndrome. *J Neurol Neurosurg Psychiatry*. 1995;59:189–191.

94. Tazawa K, Matsuda M, Yoshida T, et al. Spinal nerve root hypertrophy on MRI: clinical significance in the diagnosis of chronic inflammatory demyelinating polyradiculoneuropathy. *Intern Med*. 2008;47:2019–2024.

95. Hughes R, Bensa S, Willison H, et al. Randomized controlled trial of intravenous immunoglobulin versus oral prednisolone in chronic inflammatory demyelinating polyradiculoneuropathy. *Ann Neurol*. 2001;50:195–201.

96. Nicolas G, Maisonobe T, Le Forestier N, et al. Proposed revised electrophysiological criteria for chronic inflammatory demyelinating polyradiculoneuropathy. *Muscle Nerve*. 2002;25:26–30.

97. Saperstein DS, Katz JS, Amato AA, et al. Clinical spectrum of chronic acquired demyelinating polyneuropathies. *Muscle Nerve*. 2001;24:311–324.

98. Thaisetthawatkul P, Logigian EL, Herrmann DN, et al. Dispersion of the distal compound muscle action potential as a diagnostic criterion for chronic inflammatory demyelinating polyneuropathy. *Neurology*. 2002;59:1526–1532.

99. Hughes RA, Bouche P, Cornblath DR, et al. European Federation of Neurological Societies/Peripheral Nerve Society guideline on management of chronic inflammatory demyelinating polyradiculoneuropathy: report of a joint task force of the European Federation of Neurological Societies and the Peripheral Nerve Society. *Eur J Neurol*. 2006;13:326–332.

100. Anonymous. Research criteria for diagnosis of chronic inflammatory demyelinating polyneuropathy (CIDP). Report from an Ad Hoc Subcommittee of the American Academy of Neurology AIDS Task Force. *Neurology*. 1991;41:617–618.

101. Van Asseldonk JT, Van den Berg LH, Kalmijn S, et al. Criteria for demyelination based on the maximum slowing due to axonal degeneration, determined after warming in water at 37 degrees C: diagnostic yield in chronic inflammatory demyelinating polyneuropathy. *Brain*. 2005;128:880–891.

102. Ishigami N, Kondo M, Nakagawa M, et al. [Case of Charcot-Marie-Tooth disease type 1A with increased cerebrospinal fluid proteins and nerve root hypertrophy]. *Rinsho Shinkeigaku—Clin Neurol*. 2008;48:419–421.

103. Pareyson D, Testa D, Morbin M, et al. Does CMT1A homozygosity cause more severe disease with root hypertrophy and higher CSF proteins? *Neurology*. 2003;60:1721–1722.

104. Dyck PJ, Swanson CJ, Low PA, et al. Prednisone-responsive hereditary motor and sensory neuropathy. *Mayo Clin Proc*. 1982;57:239–246.

105. Gorson KC, Ropper AH, Adelman LS, et al. Influence of diabetes mellitus on chronic inflammatory demyelinating polyneuropathy. *Muscle Nerve*. 2000;23:37–43.

106. Ayyar DR, Sharma KR, Ayyar DR, et al. Chronic inflammatory demyelinating polyradiculoneuropathy in diabetes mellitus. *Curr Diabetes Rep*. 2004;4:409–412.

107. Sharma KR, Cross J, Farronay O, et al. Demyelinating neuropathy in diabetes mellitus. *Arch Neurol*. 2002;59:758–765.

108. Stewart JD, McKelvey R, Durcan L, et al. Chronic inflammatory demyelinating polyneuropathy (CIDP) in diabetics. *J Neurol Sci*. 1996;142:59–64.

109. Uncini A, De Angelis MV, Di Muzio A, et al. Chronic inflammatory demyelinating polyneuropathy in diabetics: motor conductions are important in the differential diagnosis with diabetic polyneuropathy. *Clin Neurophysiol*. 1999;110:705–711.

110. Katz JS, Saperstein DS, Gronseth G, et al. Distal acquired demyelinating symmetric neuropathy. *Neurology*. 2000;54:615–620.

111. Sander HW, Latov N, Sander HW, et al. Research criteria for defining patients with CIDP. *Neurology*. 2003;60:S8–S15.

112. Bromberg MB. Comparison of electrodiagnostic criteria for primary demyelination in chronic polyneuropathy. *Muscle Nerve*. 1991;14:968–976.

113. Iijima M, Yamamoto M, Hirayama M, et al. Clinical and electrophysiologic correlates of IVIG responsiveness in CIDP. *Neurology*. 2005;64:1471–1475.

114. Vucic S, Black K, Baldassari LE, et al. Long-term effects of intravenous immunoglobulin in CIDP. *Clin Neurophysiol*. 2007;118:1980–1984.

115. Bouchard C, Lacroix C, Plante V, et al. Clinico-pathologic findings and prognosis of chronic inflammatory demyelinating polyneuropathy. *Neurology*. 1999;52:498–503.

116. Vallat JM, Tabaraud F, Magy L, et al. Diagnostic value of nerve biopsy for atypical chronic inflammatory demyelinating polyneuropathy: evaluation of eight cases. *Muscle Nerve*. 2003;27:478–485.

117. Sommer C, Koch S, Lammens M, et al. Macrophage clustering as a diagnostic marker in sural nerve biopsies of patients with CIDP. *Neurology*. 2005;65:1924–1929.

118. Hughes RA, Allen D, Makowska A, et al. Pathogenesis of chronic inflammatory demyelinating polyradiculoneuropathy. *J Peripher Nerv Syst*. 2006;11:30–46.

119. Dyck PJ, O'Brien PC, Oviatt KF, et al. Prednisone improves chronic inflammatory demyelinating polyradiculoneuropathy more than no treatment. *Ann Neurol*. 1982;11:136–141.

120. Merkies IS, Bril V, Dalakas MC, et al. Health-related quality-of-life improvements in CIDP with immune globulin IV 10%: the ICE Study. *Neurology*. 2009;72:1337–1344.

121. Hughes RA, Donofrio P, Bril V, et al. Intravenous immune globulin (10% caprylate-chromatography purified) for the treatment of chronic inflammatory demyelinating polyradiculoneuropathy (ICE study): a randomised placebo-controlled trial [see comment; erratum appears in *Lancet Neurol*. 2008;7(9):771]. *Lancet Neurol*. 2008;7(9):136–144.

122. Dyck PJ, Litchy WJ, Kratz KM, et al. A plasma exchange versus immune globulin infusion trial in chronic inflammatory demyelinating polyradiculoneuropathy. *Ann. Neurol*. 1994;36:838–845.

123. Gorson KC, Allam G, Ropper AH. Chronic inflammatory demyelinating polyneuropathy: clinical features and response to treatment in 67 consecutive patients with and without a monoclonal gammopathy. *Neurology*. 1997;48:321–328.

124. Iijima M, Tomita M, Morozumi S, et al. Single nucleotide polymorphism of TAG-1 influences IVIG responsiveness of Japanese patients with CIDP. *Neurology*. 2009;73:1348–1352.

125. Kuwabara S, Misawa S, Mori M, et al. Long term prognosis of chronic inflammatory demyelinating polyneuropathy: a five year follow up of 38 cases. *J Neurol Neurosurg Psychiatry*. 2006;77:66–70.

17

Entrapment Syndromes

SPENCER HEATON, JUSTIN C. MCARTHUR, AND PAUL J. CHRISTO

INTRODUCTION

THIS CHAPTER WILL review the more common nerve entrapment syndromes, specifically their clinical features and differential diagnosis. The syndromes covered include common nerve entrapments in the upper limb (thoracic outlet syndrome, ulnar/median and radial nerve entrapments) and in the lower limb (inguinal entrapment, lateral cutaneous nerve entrapment, and peroneal/tibial entrapments). The reader is referred to more comprehensive texts for more detailed anatomical and clinical discussions.[1] Typically, nerve entrapment develops when focally increased pressure is applied to the nerve as it traverses an enclosed space. This may be a bony tunnel (e.g., the cubital tunnel) or one bounded by ligaments (e.g., the anterior interosseous membrane in the forearm through which the anterior interosseous nerve passes). The mechanisms of nerve injury from compression usually include neuropraxia

with demyelination (i.e., no interruption of axonal integrity). Wallerian degeneration does not occur with neuropraxia, so recovery requires only remyelination and not regenerative regrowth (see Figure 17.1). Motor nerve fibers are more affected than sensory nerve fibers, and autonomic function is usually retained. More extensive injuries may produce axonotmesis (more extensive trauma produces axonal interruption, without disruption of the endoneurium) or even neuronotmesis (axonal interruption with disruption of the endoneurium).

The pathology includes variable components of focal edema, impaired axonal transport, and ischemia. Two important contributing principles to the severity of entrapment neuropathies are (1) superimposed systemic causes of neuropathy, such as diabetes mellitus or chemotherapy, and (2) more proximal causes of nerve injury producing a vulnerability to more distal entrapment—sometimes called

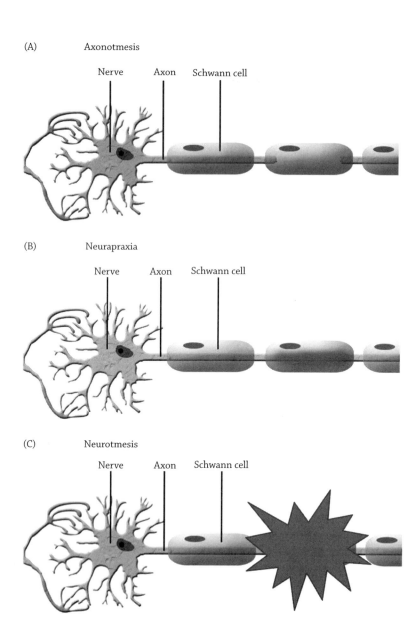

(A)   Axonotmesis

Nerve   Axon   Schwann cell

(B)   Neurapraxia

Nerve   Axon   Schwann cell

(C)   Neurotmesis

Nerve   Axon   Schwann cell

FIGURE 17.1   (A) Neuropraxia. (B) Axonotomesis. (C) Neuronotmesis.

the *double-crush* phenomenon. There are rare genetic causes with a susceptibility to entrapment syndromes such as hereditary pressure-sensitive neuropathy, tomaculous neuropathy, and hereditary neuropathy with liability to pressure palsies (HNPP). The identified gene defect in HNPP is the loss of a single copy of the *PMP22* gene or alterations within the gene. *PMP22* encodes for peripheral myelin protein 22, which is a major component of peripheral nerve myelin. While the consequences of *PMP22* mutations are not clearly known, it is most likely that these mutations render myelin unstable, leading to increased sensitivity to pressure on the nerves.

Nerve entrapment syndromes can, of course, also occur within the spine canal, at the skull base, or within neural foramina, but these are outside the purview of this review. In addition, nerve tumors and neurofibromatosis will not be covered in this review.

Further details on the use of pain-modifying agents are provided in Chapter 9 of this volume and will only be summarized in this review.

Surgical treatments are reviewed briefly, and the surgical release of multiple nerve entrapments is not covered. This technique has been promoted by the Dellon Institutes for Peripheral Nerve Surgery for multiple release procedures at the common entrapment sites. This technique is frequently used not only for entrapment neuropathies but also for diabetic polyneuropathy, toxic neuropathies, and other neuropathies. Despite numerous claims of providing effective relief of symptoms, no definitive trial of this surgical technique has been completed.

MEDIAN NERVE: CARPAL TUNNEL SYNDROME

Epidemiology (Incidence, Prevalence, and Risk Factors)

The epidemiology of entrapment syndromes is quite comprehensive for specific entrapment syndromes such as median nerve entrapment at the wrist (carpal tunnel syndrome [CTS]). For most of the entrapment syndromes, however, epidemiological details are sparse or incomplete.

Epidemiological studies of CTS have been conducted because of the occupational importance of CTS and its high prevalence. Hirata[2] summarizes these studies to indicate that the lifetime risk of acquiring CTS is 10%, the annual incidence is 0.1% among adults, and the prevalence is 2.7% among the general population. The most common cause is idiopathic inflammation of the flexor tendon sheath induced by activities involving repetitive wrist movement. A recent review[3] stresses the importance of rigor in identifying CTS because of the pitfalls in using self-reported symptoms or even physical examination to define the entrapment. As an example, a frequently cited cross-sectional study by Silverstein et al.[4] found a strongly positive association (odds ratio = 15; $P < .001$) between high repetition/high-hand grip force and the prevalence of CTS among 652 active workers. However, the diagnosis of CTS was established only on the basis of patient-volunteered symptoms and physical examination, without confirmation by nerve conduction velocity (NCV) studies. Despite the application of more accurate diagnostic techniques, including NCV studies, it remains uncertain whether repetitive injury related to occupation is in fact causative for CTS. Divergent results have been reported, with some identifying an occupational risk for CTS (see refs. 5 and 9) and others showing no relationship (see refs. 7, 8, and 10), even in industries such as meat processing that have traditionally been thought to be associated with high rates of CTS. This paradoxical and perhaps surprising conclusion defies some of the clinical observations that most neurologists encounter frequently.[5-10]

Predisposing factors for CTS have also been extensively reviewed. These include HNPP, contributions from generalized neuropathies related to diabetes or chemotherapy, pregnancy, degenerative changes to bones and ligaments impinging on the carpal tunnel, and congenital stenosis. Rheumatoid arthritis, hypothyroidism, and uremia are other common contributors and should be searched for. Tenosynovitis is not thought to be a common precipitant of CTS.[1]

Clinical and Diagnostic Features

PATHOPHYSIOLOGY

The carpal tunnel is bounded by the transverse carpal ligament, a heavy band of fibers that runs between the hamate and pisiform bones medially to the scaphoid and trapezium bones laterally. The transverse carpal ligament forms a fibrous sheath that contains the carpal tunnel anteriorly within a fibro-osseous tunnel. The carpal contains the median nerve finger flexor tendons (to the flexor digitorum superficialis, flexor digitorum profundus, and flexor pollicis longus). The motor branch of the median nerve arises under or just distal to the flexor retinaculum, and then winds around the distal border of the flexor retinaculum to reach the thenar muscles and the lateral two lumbricals. Numerous anatomical variations in the branching patterns have been described. The sensory branches innervate the lateral three and a half digits and the palm of the hand. Carpal tunnel syndrome is thought to develop because of chronically sustained (or episodic) pressure within the carpal tunnel with damage to the median nerve, either from kinking against the transverse carpal ligament or from direct pressure on the median nerve within the carpal tunnel.

CLINICAL FEATURES

Symptoms   Most patients with CTS present with pain or paresthesias in the hand, usually initially affecting the fingertips. Despite the anatomical distribution of the median nerve, the actual description of the distribution of the sensory symptoms can be variable. Some patients may describe paresthesias only in the tips of the thumb, index, and middle fingers. In other patients, by contrast, pain occurs in a pattern radiating up into the forearm or even the upper arm. One characteristic is that the pain is often worse in the dominant hand, after exertion, or upon wakening, and the patient typically attempts to relieve the pain by shaking or "flicking" the hand vigorously. A scale to quantify the severity of symptoms has been developed, known as the Boston CTS Questionnaire.[11]

Examination   The clinical signs of CTS relate to weakness in muscles and sensory deficits in skin innervated by the median nerve (with the derivation of this supply occurring in or distal to the carpal tunnel). There is substantial variability in the anatomy of the median nerve in the arm, and common anomalies can affect the interpretation of the examination. For example, the most common anomaly is the Martin-Gruber anastomosis, in which nerve fibers (usually destined to innervate the hand intrinsic) cross over from the median nerve in the forearm to the ulnar. A less common anomaly is the Riche-Carnieu anastomosis between the deep motor branch of the ulnar nerve and the median nerve, which also produces anomalous innervation of the hand. Another important anatomical point is that the palmar cutaneous nerve arises *above* the wrist and does not traverse the carpal tunnel. Finally, the recurrent motor branch of the median nerve, which is one of two terminal branches, if compressed, can result in exclusively motor symptoms, with no sensory deficit. The motor examination is summarized in Figure 17.2, along with important differential points to help distinguish CTS from mimickers. Sensory testing is best performed with light touch, although some feel that two-point discrimination and von Frey monofilament testing increase sensitivity.

Differential Diagnosis   Several conditions can mimic CTS, and the clinical features are summarized in Figure 17.2. Where symptoms

Carpal tunnel: pain/paresthesias in hand (digits I-IV, splitting ring finger); weakness of APB, OP; + Tinel's and Phalen's signs

Acute brachial neuropathy: pain/paresthesias in shoulder, arm and hand; weakness of ant. Interosseous and pronator teres

Pronator teres syndrome: pain in forearm after exertion with +Tinel's in forearm; minimal weakness

Pronator teres syndrome: pain in forearm after exertion with +Tinel's in forearm; minimal weakness

Anterior interosseous syndrome: pain in forearm after exertion with prominent weakness of thumb/finger pinching; no sensory component

Neurogenic thoracic outlet syndrome: pain in inner aspect of arm/forearm/V digit with wasting of median-innervated muscles

FIGURE 17.2   Carpal tunnel differential.

and signs are not typical, electrophysiological confirmation is usually required.

Provocative Tests for CTS   Several provocative tests for CTS have been proposed. All rely on producing additional pressure on the trapped median nerve within the carpal tunnel and eliciting or inducing increased symptoms. The wrist-flexion test (Phalen's test) has been demonstrated to be the most sensitive, while the nerve percussion test (Tinel's test) has been found to be less sensitive but most specific.[12] The tourniquet test is believed to be both insensitive and nonspecific and has fallen out of use. Similarly, the direct carpal compression test is rarely used.

Phalen's test: The patient rests the elbows on a flat surface, holds the forearms vertically, and actively places the wrists in complete and forced flexion for at least 1 minute Typically, patients describe reproduction of their typical pain or paresthesias.

Tinel's sign: Light percussion over the median nerve as it passes under the transverse carpal ligament may elicit a shock-like sensation that radiates into the median field of the hand. Percussion should begin distally and progress proximally.

Electrophysiological Testing for CTS   Electrophysiological testing remains the gold standard for diagnosis. Case series have been reported with clinical features of CTS but normal NCVs.[13] Median nerve conduction testing shows slowed NCVs and reduced compound muscle action potentials (CMAPs) across the wrist. Electromyography (EMG) may show fibrillations and positive sharp waves in median-innervated muscles, which, if present, indicate some degree of axonal degeneration. Practice guidelines have been established for the correct performance and interpretation of electrophysiological tests for suspected CTS (American Academy of Orthopaedic Surgeons, May 2007).

Other Diagnostic Tests for CTS   Given the importance of certain underlying medical conditions, a screen for diabetes mellitus (hemoglobin A1C), for hypothyroidism, and, where clinically suspected, serological testing for rheumatoid arthritis are reasonable. The need for other diagnostic studies is relatively unusual, but plain X-rays may be useful where there has been previous injury, severe arthritis, or recently broken or dislocated bones. Ultrasound permits examination of the size of the median nerve and the carpal tunnel, as do computed tomography (CT) scans. Systematic comparisons of ultrasonography and NCV testing suggest that the latter is more sensitive.[14] If a nerve tumor, neurofibroma, or infection is suspected, then magnetic resonance imaging (MRI) with gadolinium contrast should be performed. Figure 17.3 illustrates CTS as demonstrated by MRI.

Treatment

Treatment should be guided by the severity of symptoms, using questionnaires such as the Boston CTS Questionnaire, and the degree of electrophysiological damage. The first step is to prescribe the use of a wrist splint, which ideally would be worn at night and as much as possible during the day. The purpose of the splint is to prevent excessive flexion at the wrist and permit remyelination of the injured nerve.

INTERVENTIONAL INJECTION THERAPY

Injection of a local anesthetic and a corticosteroid is often advocated as an option for the long-term relief of symptoms. However, systemic reviews suggest that even though steroid injections reduce symptoms for 1 to 3 months, compared to both oral steroids and placebo injections, they do not provide long-term benefit or reduce the risk of surgery.[15-17] The optimal dose of an injected steroid is unknown, but a trend toward longer-lasting results with 60 mg methylprednisolone compared to 20 mg and 40 mg has been reported.[18] There is no evidence to support lasting benefit from a series of injections compared to a single injection.[19] Both proximal and distal sites of injection yield good results with needle entry between the flexor carpi radialis and palmaris longus muscles, through the flexor carpi radialis tendon or medial to the palmaris longus muscle with the tip directed laterally.[20,21]

A recent cost analysis of surgical versus nonsurgical treatments of CTS suggests that

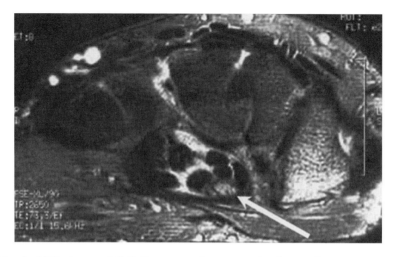

FIGURE 17.3 An MRI picture of CTS. Fast spin-echo T2-weighted MRI illustrates more pronounced increased signal within the median nerve (arrow). Note the small amount of fluid within the carpal tunnel, a secondary sign of inflammation. Slightly less optimal fat saturation is noted than on other images, which is a common occurrence.

From Norvell JG, Steele M. Carpal Tunnel Syndrome in Emergency Medicine Workup. Medscape from WebMD 2009. Image reprinted with permission from Medscape.com, 2011. Available at: http://emedicine.medscape.com/article/822792-overview

surgery, rather than medical treatments, should be the first-line form of treatment when patients are diagnosed with CTS that is confirmed by NCVs, as this provides a very cost-effective approach to promote the resolution of symptoms.[22]

ULNAR NERVE: ENTRAPMENT AT THE ELBOW

Epidemiology

The epidemiology of ulnar nerve entrapment is much less clearly delineated than that of CTS. Nonetheless, clinical experience suggests that ulnar nerve entrapment at the elbow is very common, perhaps even more common than CTS. It is also often underrecognized.

ANATOMY AND PATHOPHYSIOLOGY

The ulnar nerve is derived from the C8 and T1 spinal roots, with an inconsistent contribution from C7. Arising from the brachial plexus's lower trunk and medial cord, the nerve then travels down the arm, passes into the ulnar (condylar) groove behind the medial epicondyle, and then passes under the aponeurotic arch of the flexor carpi ulnaris. This arch has a variable thickness. The nerve then traverses the cubital tunnel, composed of the aponeurotic arch and flexor carpi ulnaris muscle fibers. As with the median nerve in the forearm, there may be anatomical anomalies that are of clinical relevance. For example, the anconeus epitrochlearis muscle arises from the triceps and can compress the ulnar nerve in the condylar groove. There may also be compressive fibrous bands or bony spurs.

The term *cubital tunnel syndrome* is widely misused to indicate entrapment of the ulnar nerve at the elbow. In reality, it is often impossible to determine whether the nerve injury is in the condylar groove or in the tunnel itself. Injury is frequently provoked by repetitive movements because the nerve is stretched with elbow flexion. Activities commonly associated with ulnar nerve injuries include elbow leaning, weight lifting, and painting. Worldwide, leprosy is probably the most common cause of neuropathy predisposing to ulnar nerve injury. Diabetes mellitus is not a common accompaniment.

Clinical and Diagnostic Features

SYMPTOMS AND SIGNS

Entrapment of the nerve at the elbow typically produces pain around the elbow, often provoked by elbow flexion. Sometimes a spontaneous Tinel's sign is described by patients, either with radiating paresthesias or dysesthesias, or a sensation "like hitting the funny bone." There is variable weakness in muscles innervated by the ulnar nerve, depending on the site of injury. In the forearm, the muscular branches of the ulnar nerve supply the flexor carpi ulnaris and flexor digitorum profundus (medial half). In the hand, the deep branch of the ulnar nerve supplies the hypothenar muscles (opponens digiti minimi, abductor digiti minimi, and flexor digiti minimi brevis), as well as the adductor pollicis, third and fourth lumbrical muscles, dorsal interossei, palmar interossei, and the deep head of the flexor pollicis brevis. In the hand, the superficial branch of the ulnar nerve supplies the palmaris brevis muscle.

Sensory disturbance can be quite variable because differential fascicular involvement is common, so there may only be partial, or even very restricted, sensory loss. Tinel's sign is usually floridly positive over the condylar groove or cubital tunnel (see Figure 17.4 for differential diagnosis).

DIAGNOSTIC TESTING

Electrophysiological testing is useful for confirmation, as with median nerve entrapment.

Typically, there is NCV slowing across the elbow, with dispersion of CMAPs. Some have advocated an "inching" technique to identify more precisely the site of entrapment. Imaging is rarely used but can indicate the site of entrapment (Figure 17.5).

Treatment

The most important aspect of management is to identify the activity that is causing the injury and counsel the patient accordingly. Elbow pads should be used during the day for protection. The use of a long arm splint at night for 6–8 weeks may be effective for entrapments without a significant motor component, but if there is denervation on EMG, surgery should be considered. Unlike therapy for median nerve entrapment, local injections are *not* used for ulnar entrapment. The most commonly recommended surgical techniques include simple (in situ) decompression by cutting the aponeurosis, decompression with medial epicondylectomy, anterior subcutaneous transposition, and anterior submuscular transposition of the ulnar nerve.[23] It is unclear whether the transposition surgeries, which typically require months of recovery time, are more effective than simple decompression.

ULNAR NERVE ENTRAPMENT AT THE WRIST

Ulnar nerve entrapment at the wrist is less common than CTS or ulnar nerve entrapment at the elbow, but it can cause confusion clinically.

Ulnar entrapment at elbow: pain/paresthesisas in foream and hand (IV/V digits); weakness of ADM and intrinsics

Cervical spondylotic radiculopathy: pain/paresthesias radiating from shoulder into hand; increased triceps reflex; weakness of triceps and hand muscles

Brachial plexus lesion (lower trunk/medial cord): pain/paresthesias radiating from shoulder; weakness of median and radial-innervated muscles

Ulnar entrapment at wrist: pain/paresthesias in hand (IV/V digits, dependent on sensory branch affected); weakness of ADM and intrinsics

FIGURE 17.4   Cubital tunnel differential.

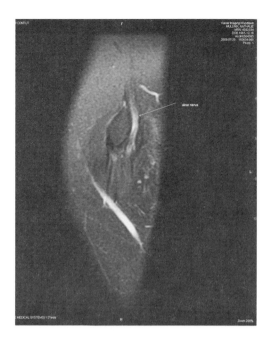

FIGURE 17.5   An MRI view of the cubital tunnel.

At the wrist, the nerve passes through Guyon's canal (formed from the fusion of the transverse carpal ligament and the pisohamate ligament) and can be compressed by degenerative changes, tenosynovitis in rheumatoid arthritis, or excessive use. The clinical features of entrapment at this site include pain and paresthesias in the hand (affecting the IV/V digits, but dependent on the sensory branch affected) and weakness of the abductor digiti minimi and the hand intrinsic. Tinel's sign may be positive at the wrist over Guyon's canal. Electrophysiology can confirm the site of the entrapment.

RADIAL NERVE ENTRAPMENT

Of the entrapment syndromes associated with the three major nerves in the arm, radial nerve entrapment is the least frequent. Obvious causes of injury and entrapment include fracture of the humerus, especially in the middle third or at the junction of the middle and distal thirds. The nerve may be compressed by the lateral intermuscular septum. Nerve injury may occur acutely at the time of the humerus injury, secondary to fracture manipulation, or from a healing callus. Other less common causes of

radial nerve palsy in the arm include compression at the fibrous arch of the lateral head of the triceps muscle and compression by an accessory subscapularis-teres-latissimus muscle. A so-called "Saturday night" palsy results from compression of the radial nerve in the humeral groove from prolonged pressure, usually during an intoxicated state (involving alcohol or other drugs of abuse).

The clinical presentation includes weakness of all extensors of the wrist and fingers, as well as of the forearm supinators. The triceps may be weak if the lesion is proximal. Sensory loss is seen in the dorsoradial aspect of the hand and the dorsal aspect of the radial three and a half digits. An important clinical point is that sensation over the distal and lateral forearm is supplied by the lateral antebrachial cutaneous nerve and is therefore preserved. Recovery is to be expected over 4–8 weeks since the lesion is usually neuropraxia with focal demyelination rather than axonotmesis.

Radial Tunnel Syndrome

The radial tunnel syndrome is thought to be an overuse syndrome, possibly an early posterior interosseous nerve syndrome. Clinical features include pain over the anterolateral proximal forearm in the region of the radial neck (see Figure 17.6 for differential). This syndrome is common in individuals whose work requires repetitive elbow extension or forearm rotation.

Pronator Teres Syndrome

The pronator teres syndrome is a controversial entity in the sense that a consensus has not formed on the frequency or even the clinical features of this syndrome. Compression of or injury to the median nerve at the elbow or in the proximal part of the forearm can cause pain or sensory disturbance in the distribution of the distal median nerve. Weakness of the muscles innervated by the anterior interosseous nerve—the flexor pollicis longus, the flexor digitorum profundus of the index finger, and the pronator quadratus—can also be found with careful examination. Table 17.1 presents

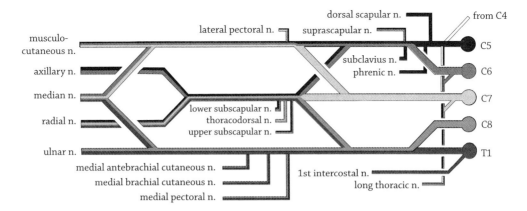

FIGURE 17.6   Brachial plexus.

some of the criteria that have been proposed for this syndrome.[24]

THORACIC OUTLET SYNDROME

Epidemiology and Risk Factors

The *true thoracic outlet* refers to the superior thoracic aperture through which the trachea, esophagus, nerves, and vessels emerge from the thorax to the lower neck and upper extremities. Although the term *thoracic outlet syndrome* (TOS) implies a thoracic location, emerging nerves and vessels actually become obstructed exterior to the aperture of the root of the neck in the region more aptly termed the *thoracic inlet*.[24,25]

Peet et al. coined the term *thoracic outlet syndrome* in 1956 to describe compression of one or several neurovascular structures (brachial plexus, subclavian artery or vein) that cross the thoracic outlet.[26] The brachial plexus and subclavian vessels are vulnerable to compression as they cross three distinct areas in the cervicoaxillary canal: the interscalene triangle, costoclavicular triangle, and subcoracoid space.[27] The scalene triangle is a critical anatomical space in the thoracic outlet and is composed of the anterior and middle scalene muscles, which form the sides of the triangle, as well as the first rib, which forms the base (Figure 17.7).

The five nerve roots of the brachial plexus, subclavian artery, and subclavian vein all pass through this narrow space. Neurovascular structures can become compressed by repetitive motion or trauma of the scalene muscles, resulting in hypertrophy or fibrosis.

Three basic forms of TOS exist—neurogenic (brachial plexus compression), arterial (subclavian artery compression), and venous (subclavian

Table 17-1. Criteria Proposed by Johnson and Spinner for Diagnosis of the Pronator Teres Syndrome

Pronator teres tenderness/firmness to palpation

Positive Tinel's sign over pronator teres

Increased paresthesias of radial three and a half digits with weak compression of pronator

Variable weakness of median nerve-innervated muscles

Absence of night symptoms

Reproduction of symptoms with provocative test

Abnormal electrophysiological study

Muscle spasm/cramping with repetitive pinch-type exercise

Reproduction of symptoms with use of blood pressure cuff

Source: Adapted from Johnson RK, Spinner M, Shrewsbury MM. Median nerve entrapment syndrome in the proximal forearm. *J Hand Surg (Am)*. 1979;4(1):48–51.

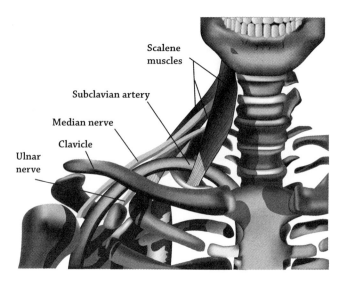

FIGURE 17.7   Scalene triangle.

vein compression)[28]—but 95% of cases are considered neurogenic.[28] A subclassification of neurogenic TOS includes nonspecific neurogenic TOS (common TOS with chronic pain symptoms suggestive of brachial plexus compromise),[29,30] and this type represents 99% of neurogenic cases.[28] In this chapter, we will highlight the clinical aspects of neurogenic TOS.

Both congenital anomalies and acquired environmental factors may cause the array of symptoms seen in TOS. For instance, cervical ribs can lead to all three forms of TOS, have an incidence of 1% in the general population, and occur bilaterally 50% of the time.[31,32] Less frequently, a bifid first rib or a long C7 transverse process may lead to TOS. In patients with neurogenic thoracic outlet syndrome (NTOS), anomalous fibromuscular bands may compress or irritate the brachial plexus, but they rarely affect the subclavian vessels.[33,34] Some have considered anatomical variations in the size and insertion points of the scalene muscles to be etiologies for NTOS.[35]

Many patients with NTOS report neck trauma, often from auto accidents or repetitive stress injuries at work.[36,37] Vulnerable patients include those involved in occupations requiring repetitive motion, such as assembly line workers, data entry personnel, flautists, and violinists.[38] Further, repetitive athletic activity ranging from swimming to weight lifting or even suboptimal posture may predispose to TOS.[35] Symptoms usually occur in young and middle-aged persons and present three times more frequently in women than in men.[38] Persons with neurogenic and nonspecific neurogenic types of TOS compose the majority of patients seeking treatment. The apparent prevalence of TOS seems to vary according to the experience of the particular specialist. For instance, vascular surgeons tend to make the diagnosis of TOS much more frequently than neurologists, perhaps in part because this syndrome is not emphasized during clinical training in neurology.[39]

Clinical and Diagnostic Features

CLINICAL FEATURES

Symptoms associated with NTOS are due to compression or irritation of the roots of the brachial plexus and may mimic symptoms of other entrapment neuropathies. Pain is a prime symptom among patients with TOS. It can present as throbbing, dull, burning, stabbing, or achy with associated paresthesias.[40] Commonly, patients experience point tenderness in the neck, shoulder, occipital, or mastoid regions and may complain of headaches. Further, pain often leads to the avoidance of certain movements or postures involving the upper quarter of the body such as typing, lifting, painting, working overhead, doing housework, or washing windows. Patients may need to limit their daily activities, work-related functions, or social engagements due to the pain. Years of discomfort, a missed diagnosis, and ineffective treatments can lead to a poor quality of life and dramatic functional limitations.

DIAGNOSTIC FEATURES

Thoracic outlet syndrome remains a controversial entity without standardized methods or uniform criteria for diagnosis, treatment, patient selection for surgery, indications for surgery, or treatment approaches.[41–46] Some argue that the lack of specific objective diagnostic tests for recognition of the compressed structures exemplifies the real controversy.[29,44,47] No definitive test exists for TOS; electrodiagnostics, radiographs, and MRI cannot establish the diagnosis definitively.[38] In fact, some argue that subtle neurological changes representative of the disease are not detectable by objective electrodiagnostic measures; therefore, TOS may in fact be relatively underdiagnosed.[48] Yet, electrodiagnostics are important to exclude other neurological abnormalities such as radiculopathy, CTS, cubital tunnel syndrome, polyneuropathy, and motor neuron disease.[28]

Clinically, patients often demonstrate tenderness over the scalene muscles, and reproduction of symptoms by the elevated arm stress test can greatly assist the diagnosis.[36] In one sample, 94% of patients with NTOS demonstrated symptom reproduction with this provocative maneuver,[49] and in another sample, 100% of patients showed concordance of symptoms.[36] Classic NTOS presents with substantial atrophy of the abductor pollicis brevis, involvement of the interossei and hypothenar muscles, sensory loss in the ulnar part of the hand and forearm, and dull and aching pain in the lateral neck, shoulder, axilla, scapula, and inner arm and forearm.[29,50] Among the forms of TOS, there seems to be agreement that classic NTOS is rare (comprising less than 1% of all NTOS cases)[28] and is caused by a cervical rib or band compressing the lower trunk.[39] This neurogenic form may be relatively painless and may display significant electrodiagnostic and neurological findings. In contrast, nonspecific NTOS often presents with diffuse, nondermatomal pain associated with paresthesias and located in the ulnar forearm and arm most often.[29]

The anterior scalene muscle derives from the anterior tubercles of the transverse processes of the C3-C6 vertebrae and attaches to the first rib. Functionally, the anterior scalene acts as an accessory muscle of respiration by raising the first rib and slightly bending and rotating the neck.[51] Anterior scalene block may serve as a reliable diagnostic test by temporarily blocking or paralyzing the muscle in spasm and reducing symptoms of TOS. This technique was first described in 1939[52] and may be one of the more effective tests to confirm a diagnosis of NTOS.[28] For instance, a positive response to the block correlates well with good surgical outcomes for NTOS.[42,53–55] The test can be performed either with[53,56] or without[54,55,57] EMG guidance and may incorporate the use of lidocaine[52–56,58,59] or, more recently, bupivicaine.[57]

Treatment

NONSURGICAL INTERVENTIONS

The management of TOS ranges from lifestyle changes to surgical decompression. Patients benefit from modifying their environment to minimize or avoid repetitive activities or overhead work. A healthy posture can lead to relaxation of the cervical musculature, thus decompressing the thoracic outlet. Pharmacological therapies such as nonsteroidal anti-inflammatory agents, muscle relaxants, anticonvulsants, and tricyclic antidepressants should be considered as analgesics and to facilitate physical therapy.[57a] Physical therapy can be of great value as a single method of treatment and/or during a patient's postoperative course. Symptomatic relief can be achieved with strengthening, stretching, postural realignment, exercise, and enhanced flexibility. A 3-month course of physical therapy prior to surgery may reduce pain and improve function in patients with NTOS and should be implemented before proceeding with surgical decompression.

Botulinum toxin type A injection into more than one scalene muscle, as well as into upper thoracic or chest wall muscles, has been effective in reducing the symptoms of NTOS.[58–60]

Studies have used electrophysiologically, fluoroscopically, or ultrasonographically guided botulinum toxin injections of both the anterior scalene muscle and surrounding muscles.[58-60] A recent investigation by Christo et al. suggested that a single, low-dose CT injection of botulinum toxin into the anterior scalene muscle may offer an effective, minimally invasive treatment for NTOS.[57] Statistically significant pain reduction was noted for 3 months after botulinum toxin injection on both sensory and visual analog scale scores. Hence, selected botulinum toxin injections may be of value to nonsurgical candidates who wish to add to a conservative approach to therapy or who are interested in bridge therapy to surgical intervention.

SURGICAL INTERVENTION

Surgical decompression is considered if pain and disability dominate a patient's life to the extent that activities of daily living and the quality of life are compromised. Moreover, patients who do not benefit from more conservative measures (e.g., medications, physical therapy, botulinum toxin injections) should view surgery as an option. Surgical success rates as high as 90% with complications as low as 1% have been reported for (nonspecific) NTOS[48]; however, persistent disability in 60% of patients 1 year following surgery with a complication rate exceeding 30% has also been described.[61] Nevertheless, improvement in the quality of life has been demonstrated with surgical decompression for appropriately selected patients with NTOS.[62]

There are several surgical approaches; the most common include transaxillary rib resection with anterior scalenectomy and supraclavicular scalenectomy with or without first rib resection. The former approach offers relatively easy access to the anterior scalene muscle and first rib without significant manipulation of the neurovascular structures. Cervical ribs can be removed using this technique, and recovery is generally reasonably rapid. The latter approach provides good exposure to the thoracic outlet, and cervical ribs can be removed easily; however, there is greater risk of injury to the neurovascular structures as well as to the long thoracic and phrenic nerves.

ENTRAPMENT SYNDROME OF THE LOWER LEG

There are numerous syndromes, of variable frequency and severity in which nerves in the lower leg can be injured or compressed. This review does not cover all of them in detail. For a more comprehensive review, the reader is referred to the eMedicine online resource, Nerve Entrapment Syndromes of the Lower Extremity.[63] Figure 17.8 illustrates some of the common syndromes that may produce neuropathic pain in the lower extremities.

LATERAL FEMORAL CUTANEOUS NERVE

Epidemiology and Risk Factors

Injury or entrapment of the lateral femoral cutaneous nerve (LFCN) is also known as *meralgia paresthetica*, a term derived from the Greek *meros*, meaning "thigh," and *algo*, meaning "pain." The syndrome includes paresthesia and pain in the lateral and anterolateral thigh, and is relatively easy to detect and diagnose. The LFCN is derived from the ventral primary rami of L2-L4. The dorsal portions fuse to form the lateral femoral cutaneous nerve in the midpelvic region of the psoas major muscle. The nerve then courses over the iliacus toward the anterior superior iliac spine (ASIS). The nerve travels posterior to the inguinal ligament and superior to the sartorius muscle at the iliac crest region and then divides into anterior and posterior branches. The anterior branch arises about 10 cm distal to the inguinal ligament in line with the ASIS and then provides cutaneous sensation to the lateral thigh.

The nerve is most susceptible to entrapment at the point of exit from the pelvis to the lower extremity, resulting in the clinical condition of meralgia paresthetica.[64] The incidence rate of meralgia paresthetica in the general population is estimated to be 4/10,000 person-years, although among patients with a complaint of leg pain, the prevalence can be as high as 6.7%–35%.[65,66] Mechanical risk factors are numerous but are unified by a common mechanism of nerve insult as the pelvic LFCN transitions to the femoral LFCN with

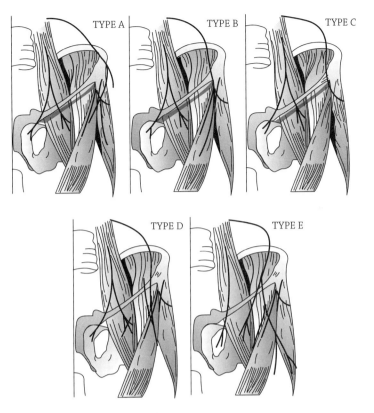

FIGURE 17.8　Lower extremities differential.

a 100 degree angle where the inguinal ligament meets the ASIS.[67] Reported risk factors include tight clothing, utility belts, obesity, medication-induced weight gain, pregnancy, seat belts, direct trauma, prone positioning for spine surgery, iliac crest bone harvesting, abdominal and pelvic surgery, bariatric surgery, pelvic masses, malignancy, and femoral vascular catheterization.[68–82] Cadaveric dissections of the LFCN have also suggested five anatomical course variants, three of which predispose to nerve entrapment.[64] Metabolic risk factors include lead poisoning, ethanol, diabetes mellitus, leprosy, and hypothyroidism.[66,83] Despite a multitude of risk factors, 39%–79% of cases are idiopathic.[65,74]

Clinical and Diagnostic Features

SYMPTOMS

Patients present with dysesthesias, hyperalgesia, or anesthesia in the lateral thigh, not extending below the knee, with symptoms described as numbness and tingling with superficial or deep burning and aching pain.[84] The sensation is often so disturbing that an area of local hair loss may be found due to persistent rubbing of the affected area.[66] Symptoms are aggravated by activities requiring hip extension, such as standing or walking.[85] Bilateral symptoms are reported in 10%–50% of patients.[71,86,87]

This syndrome can occur in people of all ages and is typically associated with weight loss or gain, wearing tight pants, or localized trauma. Extended periods of standing or walking can also trigger entrapment by increasing pressure within the inguinal ligament. Laparoscopic approaches to herniorraphy have been associated with meralgia paresthetica.

EXAMINATION

Clinical evaluation relies on the patient's accurate description of the distribution of the pain within the anatomical boundaries of the nerve. Careful mapping of the hypesthesia or allodynia using a light touch technique will define the boundaries and permit diagnosis. It is sometimes possible to elicit a Tinel's sign over the inguinal ligament. On physical exam, there may be diminished sensation over the lateral thigh to all sensory modalities, as well as tenderness or a positive Tinel's sign over the LFCN near the ASIS, while elements of the motor and reflex examinations are unchanged.[74,83] Provocative testing for radicular pain symptoms, including a straight leg raise test (for lumbar radiculopathy), should be performed and found to be negative. Recently, a novel examination maneuver, termed the *pelvic compression test*, has been described in which direct pressure over the iliac crest in a patient in the lateral position with the affected side up will result in relief of symptoms attributed to entrapment of the LFCN (see Figure 17.9 for an illustration of test).[88]

DIFFERENTIAL DIAGNOSIS

Common conditions that mimic meralgia paresthetica include lumbar spinal stenosis, lumbar disc herniation with L2 or L3 nerve root compression, or intrapelvic masses compressing the lumbar plexus.[89] These conditions usually manifest with both sensory and motor deficits, a distinguishing feature from meralgia paresthetica. Nevertheless, a misdiagnosis rate of 61% has been reported in patients with lateral thigh pain.[87]

DIAGNOSTIC TESTING

While the site of LFCN entrapment usually cannot be identified through radiological studies, a complete workup including MRI is indicated to rule out lumbar spine pathology as well as retroperitoneal compression of the LFCN by malignancy.[90] Electrophysiology or punch skin biopsy for denervation changes is not usually required, but in difficult cases either can be helpful in solidifying an unclear but suspected diagnosis. Sensory nerve conduction testing in affected nerves will show decreases in conduction velocity and action potential amplitudes. This is arguably the most useful electrodiagnostic test despite some reports of high false-positive ratings.[87,91,92] In obese patients, in whom NCVs cannot always be reliably recorded, somatosensory evoked potentials (SSEP) may be useful despite their low sensitivity (52%) and specificity (76%).[93] A proposed method of diagnosis based on ratios of SSEP latency between LFCN and ipsilateral posterior tibial nerve recordings has shown promise, with a sensitivity of 85.7% and a specificity of 82.4%.[94] Selective blockade of the LFCN with injected local anesthetic is a valuable diagnostic tool and has the advantage of also providing therapeutic benefit.[75,89]

Natural History and Management

NATURAL HISTORY

Many patients suffer for prolonged periods prior to being diagnosed and receiving therapy.

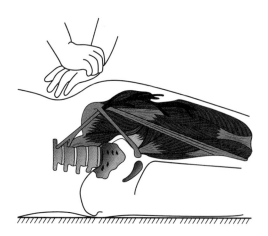
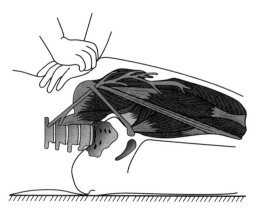

FIGURE 17.9   Pelvic compression test.

Spontaneous remission occurs in idiopathic cases as well as in cases in which predisposing risk factors resolve without medical intervention. Overall remission occurs in 25%–91% of patients at 2 years.[95]

PHARMACOLOGICAL AND BEHAVIORAL THERAPY

Initial treatment consists of rest and avoidance of aggravating activities. Some patients may experience complete recovery from simply correcting risk factors such as tight clothing or obesity. It is estimated that one in four patients will have complete relief from conservative behavioral and medication therapy with a combination of nonsteroidal anti-inflammatory drugs (NSAIDs), tricyclic antidepressants, pain-modifying anticonvulsants, antiarrhythmics, topical application of capsaicin or local anesthetics, and transcutaneous electrical nerve stimulation.[66,75,83,84,89] In meralgia paresthetica in a pregnant woman, the proper course is reassurance that the symptoms will likely resolve spontaneously within a few months after delivery and that the condition poses no harm to the infant.[76,96]

INTERVENTIONAL INJECTION THERAPY

Incomplete relief with medication management should be followed by injection of a local anesthetic and a corticosteroid around the LFCN. Complete relief of symptoms is achieved in 74%–100% of patients at 1-year follow-up after a series of three injections.[66,84,89] Conventionally, the location of the LFCN is identified for injection by anatomical landmarks, relying on the close proximity of the LFCN to the ASIS.[67] However, interpatient anatomical variability in the setting of a "blind" injection technique yields success rates as low as 40%.[97,98] Improved success rates as high as 100% have been described using ultrasound guidance or nerve-stimulating needles.[99,100] Case reports of long-term relief following pulsed radiofrequency therapy of the LFCN via sheathed conducting needles are promising and may represent an alternative to conventional injection therapy.[101]

SURGICAL TREATMENT

For those patients in whom conservative and injection therapies provide insufficient relief, surgical options have been shown to be effective. Neurolysis with or without nerve transposition consists of surgically releasing the LFCN from perineural adhesions or anatomical sites of compression.[66,102] In addition, complete nerve transection is advocated by some as providing more reliable symptom relief.[95] Overall, long-term success rates of 60%–95% are attainable through surgery.[79,88]

ILIOINGUINAL NERVE

Epidemiology and Risk Factors

The ilioinguinal nerve originates from the lumbar plexus with contributions from the L1 and L2 nerve roots. After emerging from the lateral border of the psoas muscle, it travels along the inner abdominal wall until it pierces the transversus abdominis muscle near the ASIS, after which its course is approximately parallel to that of the inguinal ligament at a distance of 1 cm cephalad. At the level of the inguinal ligament, the ilioinguinal nerve moves superficially and travels between the internal oblique and external oblique muscles, where it is most susceptible to entrapment due to variations in musculoaponeurotic connections.[103] Spontaneous ilioinguinal entrapment is exceptionally rare, and most cases are attributable to either blunt trauma or previous abdominopelvic surgery, with a postoperative prevalence of moderate to severe pain at 1 year after inguinal hernia repair or chronic pain after a Pfannenstiel incision estimated to be 3.7%–12%.[104-107] Although there are numerous etiologies of postsurgical chronic pain, 81% of patients with chronic pain after inguinal hernia repair were found on reoperation to have entrapment of the ilioinguinal nerve, which can be attributed to sutures, staples, adhesions, or surgical mesh.[108-110]

Clinical and Diagnostic Features

SYMPTOMS AND EXAMINATION

Patients commonly present with a clinical triad of symptoms: (1) burning or lancinating pain over the lower abdomen and inguinal region that radiates to the upper medial thigh and involves the anterior scrotum in men and the labia majora in women. The pain is aggravated by activities requiring hip extension, such as standing or walking, and by increased intra-abdominal pressure such as occurs with coughing, sneezing, and the Valsalva maneuver; (2) hyperesthesia, dysesthesia, or other sensory abnormalities along the same distribution as the pain; and (3) tenderness or a positive Tinel's sign with palpation 2–3 cm medial and inferior to the ASIS.[109,111,112] Despite muscular innervations of the transversus abdominis and internal oblique, there is no reliable component of motor examination suggestive of ilioinguinal entrapment; notably, the cremasteric reflex is intact.[113,114]

DIFFERENTIAL DIAGNOSIS

Myriad conditions resulting in groin pain can mimic ilioinguinal entrapment, including inguinal hernia, tumor, varicocele, hydrocele, spermatocele, transient testicular or ovarian torsion, myofascial injury, and entrapment of the iliohypogastric or genitofemoral nerves.[112,114]

DIAGNOSTIC TESTING

Abdominopelvic imaging including CT, MRI, or ultrasound to rule out other etiologies for groin pain is recommended but will not confirm a diagnosis of ilioinguinal entrapment.[115] Magnetic resonance neurograms can rarely demonstrate nerve entrapment and rely greatly on technical expertise. Nerve conduction studies show increased latency and decreased amplitude in affected nerves.[116,117] Definitive diagnosis is reliably obtained through ilioinguinal nerve blockade with a local anesthetic and a corticosteroid, which also offers the advantage of providing pain relief.[109,112] In cases of suspected entrapment within the pelvis, a diagnosis of ilioinguinal entrapment can be suggested by pain relief following selective nerve root blocks at T12, L1, and L2.[118]

Management

PHARMACOLOGICAL AND BEHAVIORAL THERAPY

Medications intended for the treatment of neuropathic pain are first-line agents including antiepileptics (such as gabapentin, pregabalin, or carbamazepine) and tricyclic antidepressants.[106,107,114] Standard management also includes NSAIDs, oral steroids, mild narcotics, and topical local anesthetics as well as transcutaneous electrical nerve stimulation and physical therapy.[112,119]

INTERVENTIONAL INJECTION THERAPY

Incomplete relief with medication management should be followed by injection of a local anesthetic and a corticosteroid around the ilioinguinal nerve. Temporary relief is readily achieved in any patient with ilioinguinal entrapment outside the pelvis, and complete long-term relief of symptoms is reported in 56% of patients after a series of one to three injections.[107,111,115,120,121] Conventionally, the injection site is determined by anatomical landmarks, relying on the close proximity of the ilioinguinal nerve to the ASIS and the inguinal ligament.[109] However, the final needle position in relation to the nerve is difficult to ascertain since a tactile "pop" as the needle passes through fascial planes is the only indicator of needle depth.[122,123] Ultrasound techniques with visualization of abdominal muscle layers and the ilioinguinal nerve itself have been described with successful nerve block achieved using smaller volumes of injectate.[124] Case reports of long-term relief following pulsed radiofrequency of the ilioinguinal nerve or nerve roots via sheathed conducting needles and reports of cryoanalgesic therapy of the ilioinguinal nerve are promising and may represent alternatives to conventional injection therapy.[118,119,125] In addition, implanted peripheral nerve stimulation devices with leads running along the course of the ilioinguinal nerve have potential as an emerging therapy.[126]

SURGICAL TREATMENT

Since most patients with ilioinguinal neuralgia have previously had abdominopelvic surgery, the nerve entrapment is often a result of surgical mesh, adhesions, sutures, or staples and may be refractory to medication or injection therapies. In such cases, effective relief can usually be attained through removal of surgical foreign bodies, scar revision, or surgical neurolysis, nerve transposition, or complete neurectomy.[108,109,112,115,119,127]

PERONEAL NERVE

Epidemiology and Risk Factors

The peroneal nerve is the lateral component of the sciatic nerve with contributions arising from the L4, L5, S1, and S2 nerve roots. It separates from the tibial component of the sciatic nerve immediately superior to the popliteal fossa, after which it courses laterally between the insertion site of the biceps femoris muscle and the lateral head of the gastrocnemius muscle. As it enters the lower leg, and shortly before dividing into the deep peroneal nerve and the superficial peroneal nerve, the peroneal nerve passes between the peroneus longus muscle and the fibula in a fibrous tunnel (referred to as the *fibular tunnel*), which is the most common site of entrapment.[128–130] Peroneal nerve entrapment is the most common nerve entrapment of the lower extremity, comprising an estimated 15% of all peripheral nerve injuries. As the peroneal nerve enters the fibular tunnel, its superficial location and proximity to bone predispose it to compression and entrapment; common risk factors typically lead to nerve entrapment as a result of increased external pressure or tethering of the nerve in the fibular tunnel.[129] Risk factors include fibular fracture, ankle sprain, prolonged squatting, competitive sports, leg crossing, immobility (e.g., due to alcoholism, coma, or stroke), weight loss, anorexia, lower extremity casting, knee injury or surgery, blunt trauma, malignancy,

and chronic compartment syndrome.[131–137] In addition, systemic risk factors and less common causes of peroneal nerve compression in the popliteal fossa include HNPP, diabetes mellitus, vascular aneurysm, ganglion cysts, and popliteal fossa masses.[138–140]

Clinical and Diagnostic Features

SYMPTOMS

Patients typically present with a variable combination of sensory and motor deficits in the distribution of one or both of the deep peroneal and superficial peroneal nerves. Bilateral symptoms are present in 10% of patients.[141] Pain, numbness, and dysesthesias in the lateral calf and dorsum of the foot that worsen with exercise are common and are attributed to the superficial peroneal nerve, as is weakness with foot eversion (peroneus longus and peroneus brevis muscles).[132] Sensory deficit complaints related to the deep peroneal nerve are less noticeable since sensory innervation only involves the web space between the great and second toes; however, weakness with ankle dorsiflexion (tibialis anterior muscle) and toe extension (extensor digitorum longus and brevis and extensor hallucis longus) result in significant gait dysfunction commonly referred to as *foot drop*.[142–144]

EXAMINATION

On physical examination there may be decreased sensation to all modalities along the lateral calf and dorsum of the foot, including the web space between the great and second toes. Weakness with ankle dorsiflexion, toe extension, and foot eversion may be present, but many patients demonstrate only sensory deficits.[145] A detailed motor examination is critical to distinguish peroneal nerve entrapment from L5 radiculopathy, which manifests with weakness of foot inversion. Since strength testing of foot inversion is best achieved with ankle dorsiflexion, it may be necessary to passively dorsiflex the foot of patients with foot drop during this portion of the exam to avoid a false diagnosis of L5 radiculopathy.[146] Provocative maneuvers include eliciting Tinel's sign with palpation over the superior fibula as well as reproduction of pain with palpation along the fibular tunnel with the foot in positions that stretch the peroneal nerve (passive plantar flexion with foot inversion).[133,147]

DIFFERENTIAL DIAGNOSIS

Common conditions that mimic peroneal nerve entrapment include sciatic mononeuropathy, L5 radiculopathy, motor neuron disease, lumbosacral plexopathy, and anterior compartment syndrome.[130,141,148,149] See Figure 17.10 for the differential diagnosis.

DIAGNOSTIC TESTING

In contrast to other lower extremity nerve entrapment syndromes, peroneal nerve entrapment can be suggested with MRI and ultrasound, both of which allow direct visualization of the nerve in the fibular tunnel as well as surrounding structures.[148,150–152] Electrodiagnostic studies are valuable in confirming the location of the injury and determining the severity and chronicity of nerve injury.[144] Nerve conduction studies provide more reliable information than EMG and may show decreased amplitude, increased latency, and focal slowing or conduction block near the fibular tunnel in affected nerves.[128,130,148,153,154]

Natural History and Management

NATURAL HISTORY

Recovery depends on the inciting event and the severity of nerve injury and is difficult to predict.[135] Spontaneous recovery is typically incomplete and occurs over a period of 18–24 months.[155]

PHARMACOLOGICAL AND BEHAVIORAL THERAPY

For patients with dynamic peroneal nerve entrapment related to leg position, behavioral changes such as reducing habitual leg crossing or squatting may provide complete relief of symptoms.[148] Physical therapy, massage, galvanic

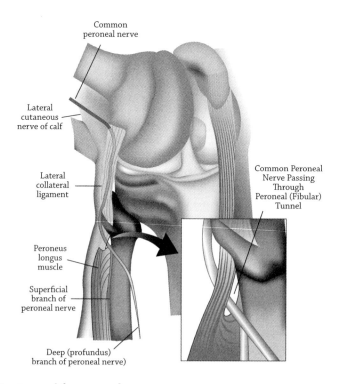

Common peroneal nerve

Lateral cutaneous nerve of calf

Lateral collateral ligament

Peroneus longus muscle

Superficial branch of peroneal nerve

Deep (profundus) branch of peroneal nerve)

Common Peroneal Nerve Passing Through Peroneal (Fibular) Tunnel

FIGURE 17.10   Anatomy of the peroneal nerve.

stimulation, splinting, and conservative medication management with NSAIDs are commonly recommended; however, success with such measures is limited.[142,145,154]

INTERVENTIONAL INJECTION THERAPY

There is little evidence to support the routine use of local anesthetic or steroid injections in the treatment of classic peroneal nerve entrapment. However, in cases resulting from entrapment in the popliteal fossa with involvement primarily of the lateral cutaneous nerve of the calf, local anesthetic injections at the point of maximal tenderness are effective.[156]

SURGICAL TREATMENT

Definitive therapy for typical peroneal nerve entrapment often involves surgical decompression of the nerve in the fibular tunnel, resulting in excellent long-term symptom relief.[128,132,135,137,142,145,147,154] For less common causes of nerve entrapment, a variety of procedures to free the nerve from entrapment by local masses have been described.[140,143,152]

TARSAL TUNNEL SYNDROME

Anatomy and Pathophysiology

The most common nerve entrapment syndrome in the foot is the tarsal tunnel syndrome (TTS), with entrapment of the posterior tibial nerve. The posterior tibial nerve is derived from the sciatic nerve. The tarsal tunnel is a fibroosseous canal formed by the laciniate ligament as it extends from the medial malleolus down onto the calcaneus (See Figure 17.11 for anatomy). Compression of the posterior tibial nerve as it traverses this canal may cause focal injury and entrapment. The most common causes of TTS include trauma, varicosities, heel varus, fibrosis, and heel valgus. Tendonitis within the tunnel can cause entrapment of the posterior tibial nerve due to the decreased space, and tethering at the abductor hallucis can cause a stretch injury at the branches of the tibial nerve within the tunnel.

Clinical Features

Typically, the pain and sensory features of TTS radiate to the sole of the foot rather than the dorsal aspect of the foot. This is a helpful point of differentiation from length-dependent neuropathies. Another symptom is the relationship to activity, including standing or exercising, or wearing particular types of shoes. Usually symptoms are worse after exertion, especially if the provoking factor is excessive exercise. The branch to the calcaneus is spared, so pain does not involve the heel. The most common provocative maneuver is direct pressure over the tarsal tunnel or elicitation of a positive Tinel's sign. Weakness of toe intrinsics is difficult to

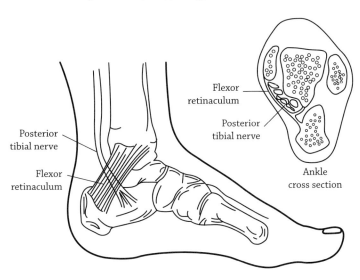

FIGURE 17.11   Tarsal tunnel.

determine clinically. A newly described provocative test may add specificity.[157] In this test, the ankle is passively everted maximally and dorsiflexed while all of the metatarsophalangeal joints are maximally dorsiflexed and held in this position for 5 to 10 seconds.

Treatment

As with ulnar nerve entrapment at the elbow, identification and avoidance of the provoking activities is key to successful treatment. This is frequently adequate to attenuate symptoms.

INTERVENTIONAL INJECTION THERAPY

Case reports and anecdotal evidence suggest that local anesthetic and corticosteroid injections in the tarsal tunnel are useful for symptom relief; however, there are no data to suggest a reduction in the ultimate need for surgical intervention.[158–162] The injection is typically performed using the palpable posterior tibial artery and the medial malleolus as landmarks. Many practitioners also recommend ultrasound guidance to increase successful block rates and decrease injectate volumes.[163] Pulsed radiofrequency is another alternative. The technique is similar to thermocoagulation radiofrequency ablation but differs in that a lower level of heat is produced. This does not actually destroy the nerve tissue.

SURGICAL TREATMENT

Surgery is rarely needed, especially when symptoms progress or activities are substantially limited by pain. The most common surgical technique is decompression. There have been relatively few reported series of surgical treatment, with success rates varying from 40% to 60%.[164] One study suggests only about a 44% success rate and concludes that "unless there is an associated lesion near or within the tarsal tunnel preoperatively, decompression of the posterior tibial nerve should be considered with caution."[165,]

REFERENCES

1. Stewart JD. *Focal Peripheral Neuropathies*. 2nd ed. New York: Raven Press; 1993:522.

2. Hirata H. [Carpal tunnel syndrome and cubital tunnel syndrome]. *Rinsho Shinkeigaku*. 2007; 47(11):761–765.

3. Kao SY. Carpal tunnel syndrome as an occupational disease. *J Am Board Fam Pract*. 2003;16(6):533–542.

4. Silverstein BA, Fine LJ, Armstrong TJ. Occupational factors and carpal tunnel syndrome. *Am J Ind Med*. 1987;11(3):343–358.

5. Stetson DS et al. Median sensory distal amplitude and latency: comparisons between nonexposed managerial/professional employees and industrial workers. *Am J Ind Med*. 1993;24(2): 175–189.

6. Nathan PA, Meadows KD, Doyle LS. Occupation as a risk factor for impaired sensory conduction of the median nerve at the carpal tunnel. *J Hand Surg (Br)*. 1988;13(2):167–170.

7. Nathan PA et al. Longitudinal study of median nerve sensory conduction in industry: relationship to age, gender, hand dominance, occupational hand use, and clinical diagnosis. *J Hand Surg (Am)*. 1992;17(5):850–857.

8. Schottland JR et al. Median nerve latencies in poultry processing workers: an approach to resolving the role of industrial "cumulative trauma" in the development of carpal tunnel syndrome. *J Occup Med*. 1991;33(5): 627–631.

9. Osorio AM et al. Carpal tunnel syndrome among grocery store workers. *Am J Ind Med*. 1994;25(2):229–245.

10. Moore JS, Garg A. Upper extremity disorders in a pork processing plant: relationships between job risk factors and morbidity. *Am Ind Hyg Assoc J*. 1994;55(8):703–715.

11. Levine DW et al. A self-administered questionnaire for the assessment of severity of symptoms and functional status in carpal tunnel syndrome. *J Bone Joint Surg (Am)*. 1993. 75(11): p. 1585–92.

12. Gellman H et al. Carpal tunnel syndrome. An evaluation of the provocative diagnostic tests. *J Bone Joint Surg (Am)*. 1986;68(5):735–737.

13. Witt JC, Hentz JG, Stevens JC. Carpal tunnel syndrome with normal nerve conduction studies. *Muscle Nerve*. 2004;29(4):515–522.

14. Kaymak B et al. A comparison of the benefits of sonography and electrophysiologic measurements as predictors of symptom severity and functional status in patients with carpal tunnel syndrome. *Arch Phys Med Rehabil*. 2008;89(4):743–748.

15. Hamamoto Filho PT et al. A systematic review of anti-inflammatories for mild to moderate

carpal tunnel syndrome. *J Clin Neuromusc Dis.* 2009;11(1):22–30.

16. Marshall S, Tardif G, Ashworth N. Local corticosteroid injection for carpal tunnel syndrome. *Cochrane Database Syst Rev.* 2007(2):CD001554.

17. Management of carpal tunnel syndrome. *Drug Ther Bull.* 2009;47(8):86–89.

18. Dammers JW et al. Injection with methylprednisolone in patients with the carpal tunnel syndrome: a randomised double blind trial testing three different doses. *J Neurol.* 2006;253(5):574–577.

19. Wong SM et al. Single vs. two steroid injections for carpal tunnel syndrome: a randomised clinical trial. *Int J Clin Pract.* 2005;59(12):1417–1421.

20. Ozturk K et al. Comparison of carpal tunnel injection techniques: a cadaver study. *Scand J Plast Reconstr Surg Hand Surg.* 2008;42(6): 300–304.

21. Racasan O, Dubert T. The safest location for steroid injection in the treatment of carpal tunnel syndrome. *J Hand Surg (Br).* 2005;30(4): 412–414.

22. Pomerance J, Zurakowski D, Fine I. The cost-effectiveness of nonsurgical versus surgical treatment for carpal tunnel syndrome. *J Hand Surg (Am).* 2009;34(7):1193–1200.

23. Gellman H. Compression of the ulnar nerve at the elbow: cubital tunnel syndrome. *Instr Course Lect.* 2008;57:187–197.

24. Moore KL, Dalley AF, Agur AMR. *Clinically Oriented Anatomy.* 5th ed. Baltimore: Lippincott Williams & Wilkins; 2006:85.

25. Davies DV, Davies F. *Gray's Anatomy.* 33rd ed. London: Longmans, Green; 1962.

26. Peet RM et al. Thoracic-outlet syndrome: evaluation of a therapeutic exercise program. *Proc Staff Meet Mayo Clin.* 1956;31(9):281–287.

27. Urschel JD, Hameed SM, Grewal RP. Neurogenic thoracic outlet syndromes. *Postgrad Med J.* 1994;70:785–789.

28. Sanders RJ, Hammond SL, Rao NM. Thoracic outlet syndrome. A review. *The Neurologist.* 2008;14(6):365–373.

29. Huang JH, Zager EL. *Thoracic outlet syndrome. Neurosurgery.* 2004;55(4):897–902.

30. Wilbourn A. *The thoracic outlet syndrome is overdiagnosed. Arch Neurol.* 1990;47:328–330.

31. Adson W. Surgical treatments for symptoms produced by cervical ribs and the scalenus anticus muscle. *Surg Gynecol Obstet.* 1947;85:687–700.

32. Leffert, R. *Thoracic outlet syndromes. Hand Clin.* 1992;8:285–297.

33. Thomas GI, Jones TW, Stavney LS, Manhas DR. The middle scalene muscle and its contribution to the thoracic outlet syndrome. J Am Dent Assoc. 1993;145:589–592.

34. Roos D. *Congenital anomalies associated with thoracic outlet syndrome. Am J Surg.* 1976;132: 771–778.

35. Fugate MW, Rotellini-Coltvet L, Freischlag JA. *Current management of thoracic outlet syndrome. Curr Treat Options Cardiovasc Med.* 2009;11(2): 176–183.

36. Sanders RJ, Hammond SL, Rao NM. *Diagnosis of thoracic outlet sydndrome. J Vasc Surg.* 2007;46: 601–604.

37. Kai Y, Oyama M, Kurose S, et al. Neurogenic thoracic outlet syndrome in whiplash injury. *J Spinal Disord.* 2001;14:487–493.

38. Brantigan CO, Roos DB. Diagnosing thoracic outlet syndrome. *Hand Clin.* 2004;20(1): 27–36.

39. Campbell WW, Landau ME. *Controversial entrapment neuropathies. Neurosurg Clin North Am.* 2008;19:597–608.

40. Crotti FM et al. TOS pathophysiology and clinical features. *Acta Neurochir.* 2005;92:7–12.

41. Sheth RN, Belzberg AJ. *Diagnosis and treatment of thoracic outlet syndrome. Neurosurg Clin North Am.* 2001;12(2):295–309.

42. Atasoy E. Thoracic outlet compression syndrome. *Orthop Clin North Am.* 1996;27(2):265–303.

43. Landry GJ et al. Long-term functional outcome of neurogenic thoracic outlet syndrome in surgically and conservatively treated patients. *J Vasc Surg.* 2001;33:312–319.

44. Mackinnon SE, Novak CB. *Thoracic outlet syndrome. Curr Prob Surg.* 2002;39:1070–1145.

45. Pang D, Wessel HB. Thoracic outlet syndrome. *Neurosurgery.* 1988;22(1 pt 1):105–121.

46. Urschel HC, Razzuk MA. Neurovascular compression in the thoracic outlet: changing management over 50 years. *Ann Surg.* 1998;228: 609–617.

47. Remy-Jardin M et al. Functional anatomy of the thoracic outlet: evaluation with spiral CT. *Radiology.* 1997;205(3):843–851.

48. Roos DB. Thoracic outlet syndrome is underdiagnosed. *Muscle Nerve.* 1999;22:126–129; discussion 136–137.

49. Sanders RJ, Haug CE. *Thoracic Outlet Syndrome: A Common Sequela of Neck Injuries.* Philadelphia: Lippincott;1991:77.

50. Gilliatt RW et al. Wasting of the hand associated with a cervical rib or band. *J Neurol Neurosurg Psychiatry.* 1970;33(5):615–624.

51. Atasoy E. Thoracic outlet syndrome: anatomy. *Hand Clin.* 2004;20(1):7–14.

52. Gage M. Scalenus anticus syndrome: a diagnostic and confirmatory test. *Surgery*. 1939;5:599–601.

53. Jordan SE, Machleder HI. Diagnosis of thoracic outlet syndrome using electrophysiologically guided anterior scalene blocks. *Ann Vasc Surg*. 1998;12:260–264.

54. Sanders RJ, Pearce WH. The treatment of thoracic outlet syndrome: a comparison of different operations. *J Vasc Surg*. 1989;10:626–634.

55. Sanders RJ et al. Scalenectomy versus first rib resection for treatment of the thoracic outlet syndrome. *Surgery*. 1979;85:109–121.

56. Braun RM, Sahadevan DC. Feinstein J. Confimatory needle placement technique for scalene muscle block in the diagnosis of thoracic outlet syndrome. *Tech Hand Up Extrem Surg*. 2006;10:173–176.

57. Christo PJ et al. Single CT-guided chemodenervation of the anterior scalene muscle with botulinum toxin for neurogenic thoracic outlet syndrome. *Pain Med*. 2010;11(4): 504–511.

57a. Christo PJ, McGreevy K. Updated Perspectives on Neurogenic Thoracic Outlet Syndrome. Anesthetic Techniques in Pain Management. Current Pain and Headache Reports, Philadelphia, PA., 15 (1): 14-21; DOI 10.1007/s11916-010-0163-1 (2011).

58. Jordan SE, Ahn SS, Freischlag JA, Gelabert HA, Machleder HI. Selective botulinum chemodenervation of the scalene muscles for treatment of neurogenic thoracic outlet syndrome. *Ann Vasc Surg*. 2000;14:365–369.

59. Jordan SE, Ahn SS, Gelabert HA. Combining ultrasonography and electromyography for botulinum chemodenervation treatment of thoracic outlet syndrome: comparison with fluoroscopy and electromyography guidance. *Pain Physician*. 2007;10:541–546.

60. Monsivais JJ, Monsivais DB. Botulinum toxin in painful syndromes. *Hand Clin*. 1996;12: 787–789.

61. Franklin GM et al. Outcome of surgery for thoracic outlet syndrome in Washington state worker's compensation. *Neurology*. 2000;54:1252–1257.

62. Chang DC et al. Surgical intervention for thoracic outlet syndrome improves patient's quality of life. *J Vasc Surg*. 2009;49(3):630–635; discussion 635–637.

63. Hollis MH, Lemay DE. (2009) *Nerve entrapment syndromes of the lower extremity*. Emedicine. 2009. http://emedicine.medscape.com/article/1234809-overview. Accessed 29 January, 2012.

64. Aszmann OC, Dellon ES, Dellon AL. Anatomical course of the lateral femoral cutaneous nerve and its susceptibility to compression and injury. *Plast Reconstr Surg*. 1997;100(3):600–604.

65. van Slobbe AM et al. Incidence rates and determinants in meralgia paresthetica in general practice. *J Neurol*. 2004;251(3):294–297.

66. Grossman MG et al. Meralgia paresthetica: diagnosis and treatment. *J Am Acad Orthop Surg*. 2001;9(5):336–344.

67. Dias Filho LC et al. Lateral femoral cutaneous neuralgia: an anatomical insight. *Clin Anat*. 2003;16(4):309–316.

68. Mirovsky Y, Neuwirth M. Injuries to the lateral femoral cutaneous nerve during spine surgery. *Spine* (Philadelphia, 1976). 2000;25(10): 1266–1269.

69. Boyce JR. Meralgia paresthetica and tight trousers. *JAMA*. 1984;251(12):1553.

70. Deal CL, Canoso JJ. Meralgia paresthetica and large abdomens. *Ann Intern Med*. 1982;96 (6 pt 1):787–788.

71. Ecker AD, Woltman HW. Meralgia paresthetica—a report of one hundred fifty cases. *J Am Med Assoc*. 1938;110(20):1650–1652.

72. Butler R, Webster MW. Meralgia paresthetica: an unusual complication of cardiac catheterization via the femoral artery. *Catheter Cardiovasc Intervent*. 2002;56(1):69–71.

73. Cho KT, Lee HJ. Prone position-related meralgia paresthetica after lumbar spinal surgery: a case report and review of the literature. *J Korean Neurosurg Soc*. 2008;44(6):392–395.

74. Ducic I, Dellon AL, Taylor NS. Decompression of the lateral femoral cutaneous nerve in the treatment of meralgia paresthetica. *J Reconstr Microsurg*. 2006;22(2):113–118.

75. Erbay H. Meralgia paresthetica in differential diagnosis of low-back pain. *Clin J Pain*. 2002; 18(2):132–135.

76. Sax TW, Rosenbaum RB. Neuromuscular disorders in pregnancy. *Muscle Nerve*. 2006;34(5): 559–571.

77. Yang SH, Wu CC, Chen PQ. Postoperative meralgia paresthetica after posterior spine surgery: incidence, risk factors, and clinical outcomes. *Spine* (Philadelphia, 1976). 2005;30(18):E547–E550.

78. Mondelli M, Rossi S, Romano C. Body mass index in meralgia paresthetica: a case-control study. *Acta Neurol Scand*. 2007;116(2):118–123.

79. Siu TL, Chandran KN. Neurolysis for meralgia paresthetica: an operative series of 45 cases. *Surg Neurol*. 2005;63(1):19–23; discussion 23.

80. Tharion G, Bhattacharji S. Malignant secondary deposit in the iliac crest masquerading as meralgia paresthetica. *Arch Phys Med Rehabil*. 1997;78(9):1010–1011.

81. Chlebowski S, Bashyal S, Schwartz TL. Meralgia paresthetica: another complication of antipsychotic-induced weight gain. *Obes Rev.* 2009;10(6):700–702.

82. Koffman BM et al. Neurologic complications after surgery for obesity. *Muscle Nerve.* 2006; 33(2):166–176.

83. Harney D, Patijn J. Meralgia paresthetica: diagnosis and management strategies. *Pain Med.* 2007;8(8):669–677.

84. Dureja GP et al. Management of meralgia paresthetica: a multimodality regimen. *Anesth Analg.* 1995;80(5):1060–1061.

85. Stookey B. Meralgia paresthetica: etiology and surgical treatment. *J Am Med Assoc.* 1928;90(21): 1705–1707:.

86. Ivins GK. Meralgia paresthetica, the elusive diagnosis: clinical experience with 14 adult patients. *Ann Surg.* 2000;232(2):281–286.

87. Seror P, Seror R. Meralgia paresthetica: clinical and electrophysiological diagnosis in 120 cases. *Muscle Nerve.* 2006;33(5):650–654.

88. Nouraei SA et al. A novel approach to the diagnosis and management of meralgia paresthetica. *Neurosurgery.* 2007;60(4):696–700; discussion 700.

89. Haim A et al. Meralgia paresthetica: a retrospective analysis of 79 patients evaluated and treated according to a standard algorithm. *Acta Orthop.* 2006;77(3):482–486.

90. Trummer M et al. Lumbar disc herniation mimicking meralgia paresthetica: case report. *Surg Neurol.* 2000;54(1):80–81.

91. Seror P. Lateral femoral cutaneous nerve conduction vs somatosensory evoked potentials for electrodiagnosis of meralgia paresthetica. *Am J Phys Med Rehabil.* 1999;78(4):313–316.

92. Cordato DJ et al. Evoked potentials elicited by stimulation of the lateral and anterior femoral cutaneous nerves in meralgia paresthetica. *Muscle Nerve.* 2004;29(1):139–142.

93. Seror P. Somatosensory evoked potentials for the electrodiagnosis of meralgia paresthetica. *Muscle Nerve.* 2004;29(2):309–312.

94. Caramelli R et al. Proposal of a new criterion for electrodiagnosis of meralgia paresthetica by evoked potentials. *J Clin Neurophysiol.* 2006; 23(5):482–485.

95. van Eerten PV, Polder TW, Broere CW. Operative treatment of meralgia paresthetica: transection versus neurolysis. *Neurosurgery.* 1995;37(1): 63–65.

96. Van Diver T, Camann W. Meralgia paresthetica in the parturient. *Int J Obstet Anesth.* 1995;4(2): 109–112.

97. Shannon J et al. Lateral femoral cutaneous nerve block revisited. A nerve stimulator technique. *Reg Anesth.* 1995;20(2):100–104.

98. Carai A et al. Anatomical variability of the lateral femoral cutaneous nerve: findings from a surgical series. *Clin Anat.* 2009;22(3): 365–370.

99. Bodner G et al. Ultrasound of the lateral femoral cutaneous nerve: normal findings in a cadaver and in volunteers. *Reg Anesth Pain Med.* 2009;34(3):265–268.

100. Hurdle MF et al. Ultrasound-guided blockade of the lateral femoral cutaneous nerve: technical description and review of 10 cases. Arch Phys Med *Rehabil.* 2007;88(10):1362–1364.

101. Philip CN et al. Successful treatment of meralgia paresthetica with pulsed radiofrequency of the lateral femoral cutaneous nerve. *Pain Physician.* 2009;12(5):881–885.

102. Williams PH, Trzil KP. Management of meralgia paresthetica. *J Neurosurg.* 1991;74(1):76–80.

103. Ndiaye A et al. Anatomical basis of neuropathies and damage to the ilioinguinal nerve during repairs of groin hernias. (about 100 dissections). *Surg Radiol Anat.* 2007;29(8):675–681.

104. Cunningham J et al. Cooperative hernia study. Pain in the postrepair patient. *Ann Surg.* 1996;224(5):598–602.

105. Luijendijk RW et al. The low transverse Pfannenstiel incision and the prevalence of incisional hernia and nerve entrapment. *Ann Surg.* 1997;225(4):365–369.

106. Zacest AC et al. Long-term outcome following ilioinguinal neurectomy for chronic pain. *J Neurosurg.* 2009;112(4):784–789.

107. Suresh S et al. Ultrasound-guided serial ilioinguinal nerve blocks for management of chronic groin pain secondary to ilioinguinal neuralgia in adolescents. *Paediatr Anaesth.* 2008;18(8):775–778.

108. Vuilleumier H, Hubner M, Demartines N. Neuropathy after herniorraphy: indication for surgical treatment and outcome. *World J Surg.* 2009;33(4):841–845.

109. Choi PD, Nath R, Mackinnon SE. Iatrogenic injury to the ilioinguinal and iliohypogastric nerves in the groin: a case report, diagnosis, and management. *Ann Plast Surg.* 1996;37(1):60–65.

110. Starling JR, Harms BA. Diagnosis and treatment of genitofemoral and ilioinguinal neuralgia. *World J Surg.* 1989;13(5):586–591.

111. Mitra R, Zeighami A, Mackey S. Pulsed radiofrequency for the treatment of chronic ilioinguinal neuropathy. *Hernia.* 2007;11(4):369–371.

112. Kim DH et al. Surgical management of 33 ilioinguinal and iliohypogastric neuralgias at Louisiana State University Health Sciences Center. *Neurosurgery*. 2005;56(5):1013–1020.

113. McCrory P, Bell S. Nerve entrapment syndromes as a cause of pain in the hip, groin and buttock. *Sports Med*. 1999;27(4):261–274.

114. ter Meulen BC et al. Acute scrotal pain from idiopathic ilioinguinal neuropathy: diagnosis and treatment with EMG-guided nerve block. *Clin Neurol Neurosurg*. 2007;109(6):535–537.

115. Loos MJ, Scheltinga MR, Roumen RM. Surgical management of inguinal neuralgia after a low transverse Pfannenstiel incision. *Ann Surg*. 2008;248(5):880–885.

116. Benito-Leon J et al. Gabapentin therapy for genitofemoral and ilioinguinal neuralgia. *J Neurol*. 2001;248(10):907–908.

117. Monga M, Ghoniem GM. Ilioinguinal nerve entrapment following needle bladder suspension procedures. *Urology*. 1994;44(3):447–450.

118. Rozen D, Parvez U. Pulsed radiofrequency of lumbar nerve roots for treatment of chronic inguinal herniorraphy pain. *Pain Physician*. 2006;9(2):153–156.

119. Fanelli RD et al. Cryoanalgesic ablation for the treatment of chronic postherniorraphy neuropathic pain. *Surg Endosc*. 2003;17(2):196–200.

120. Sippo WC, Burghardt A, Gomez AC. Nerve entrapment after Pfannenstiel incision. *Am J Obstet Gynecol*. 1987;157(2):420–421.

121. Aroori S, Spence RA. Chronic pain after hernia surgery—an informed consent issue. *Ulster Med J*. 2007;76(3):136–140.

122. Hu P, Harmon D, Frizelle H. Ultrasound guidance for ilioinguinal/iliohypogastric nerve block: a pilot study. *Ir J Med Sci*. 2007;176(2):111–115.

123. Peng PW, Tumber PS. Ultrasound-guided interventional procedures for patients with chronic pelvic pain—a description of techniques and review of literature. *Pain Physician*. 2008;11(2):215–224.

124. Eichenberger U et al. Ultrasound-guided blocks of the ilioinguinal and iliohypogastric nerve: accuracy of a selective new technique confirmed by anatomical dissection. *Br J Anaesth*. 2006;97(2):238–243.

125. Rozen D, Ahn J. Pulsed radiofrequency for the treatment of ilioinguinal neuralgia after inguinal herniorrhaphy. *Mt Sinai J Med*. 2006;73(4):716–718.

126. Rauchwerger JJ et al. On the therapeutic viability of peripheral nerve stimulation for ilioinguinal neuralgia: putative mechanisms and possible utility. *Pain Pract*. 2008;8(2):138–143.

127. Tosun K et al. Treatment of severe bilateral nerve pain after Pfannenstiel incision. *Urology*. 2006;67(3):623.e5–623.e6.

128. Mitra A et al. Peroneal nerve entrapment in athletes. *Ann Plast Surg*. 1995;35(4):366–368.

129. Ryan W et al. Relationship of the common peroneal nerve and its branches to the head and neck of the fibula. *Clin Anat*. 2003;16(6):501–505.

130. Masakado Y et al. Clinical neurophysiology in the diagnosis of peroneal nerve palsy. *Keio J Med*. 2008;57(2):84–89.

131. Shahar E, Landau E, Genizi J. Adolescence peroneal neuropathy associated with rapid marked weight reduction: case report and literature review. *Eur J Paediatr Neurol*. 2007;11(1):50–54.

132. Yang LJ, Gala VC, McGillicuddy JE. Superficial peroneal nerve syndrome: an unusual nerve entrapment. Case report. *J Neurosurg*. 2006;104(5):820–823.

133. Styf J. Entrapment of the superficial peroneal nerve. Diagnosis and results of decompression. *J Bone Joint Surg (Br)*. 1989;71(1):131–135.

134. Kabayel L et al. Development of entrapment neuropathies in acute stroke patients. *Acta Neurol Scand*. 2009;120(1):53–58.

135. Kim DH, Kline DG. Management and results of peroneal nerve lesions. *Neurosurgery*. 1996;39(2):312–319; discussion 319–320.

136. Meals RA. Peroneal-nerve palsy complicating ankle sprain. Report of two cases and review of the literature. *J Bone Joint Surg (Am)*. 1977;59(7):966–968.

137. Sevinc TT et al. Bilateral superficial peroneal nerve entrapment secondary to anorexia nervosa: a case report. *J Brachial Plex Peripher Nerve Inj*. 2008;3(1):12.

138. Rawal A et al. Compression neuropathy of common peroneal nerve caused by an extraneural ganglion: a report of two cases. *Microsurgery*. 2004;24(1):63–66.

139. Yoo JH et al. A case of extension loss of great toe due to peroneal nerve compression by an osteochondroma of the proximal fibula. *Arch Orthop Trauma Surg*. 2010;130(9):1071–1075.

140. Rawlings CE 3rd, Bullard DE, Caldwell DS. Peripheral nerve entrapment due to steroid-induced lipomatosis of the popliteal fossa. *Case report*. *J Neurosurg*. 1986;64(4):666–668.

141. Katirji B. Peroneal neuropathy. *Neurol Clin*. 1999;17(3):567–591.

142. Anselmi SJ. Common peroneal nerve compression. *J Am Podiatr Med Assoc*. 2006;96(5):413–417.

143. Jang SH, Lee H, Han SH. Common peroneal nerve compression by a popliteal venous aneurysm. *Am J Phys Med Rehabil*. 2009;88(11): 947–950.

144. Levin KH. Common focal mononeuropathies and their electrodiagnosis. *J Clin Neurophysiol*. 1993;10(2):181–189.

145. Fabre T et al. Peroneal nerve entrapment. *J Bone Joint Surg* (*Am*). 1998;80(1):47–53.

146. Katirji MB, Wilbourn AJ. Common peroneal mononeuropathy: a clinical and electrophysiologic study of 116 lesions. *Neurology*. 1988;38(11):1723–1728.

147. Styf J, Morberg P. The superficial peroneal tunnel syndrome. Results of treatment by decompression. *J Bone Joint Surg* (*Br*). 1997;79(5):801–803.

148. Campbell WW. Diagnosis and management of common compression and entrapment neuropathies. *Neurol Clin*. 1997;15(3):549–567.

149. Saal JA et al. The pseudoradicular syndrome. Lower extremity peripheral nerve entrapment masquerading as lumbar radiculopathy. *Spine* (Philadelphia, 1976). 1988;13(8):926–930.

150. Loredo R et al. MRI of the common peroneal nerve: normal anatomy and evaluation of masses associated with nerve entrapment. *J Comput Assist Tomogr*. 1998;22(6):925–931.

151. Martinoli C et al. US of nerve entrapments in osteofibrous tunnels of the upper and lower limbs. *Radiographics*. 2000;20 spec no:S199–S213; discussion S213–S217.

152. Ramelli GP et al. Ganglion cyst of the peroneal nerve: a differential diagnosis of peroneal nerve entrapment neuropathy. Eur Neurol. 1999;41(1):56–58.

153. Marciniak C et al. Practice parameter: utility of electrodiagnostic techniques in evaluating patients with suspected peroneal neuropathy: an evidence-based review. *Muscle Nerve*. 2005;31(4):520–527.

154. McCrory P, Bell S, Bradshaw C. Nerve entrapments of the lower leg, ankle and foot in sport. *Sports Med*. 2002;32(6):371–391.

155. Vastamaki M. Decompression for peroneal nerve entrapment. *Acta Orthop Scand*. 1986; 57(6):551–554.

156. Haimovici H. Peroneal sensory neuropathy entrapment syndrome. *Arch Surg*. 1972;105(4): 586–590.

157. Kinoshita M et al. The dorsiflexion-eversion test for diagnosis of tarsal tunnel syndrome. *J Bone Joint Surg* (*Am*). 2001;83A(12): 1835–1839.

158. Mondelli M, Giannini F, Reale F. Clinical and electrophysiological findings and follow-up in tarsal tunnel syndrome. *Electroencephalogr Clin Neurophysiol*. 1998;109(5):418–425.

159. Diers DJ. Medial calcaneal nerve entrapment as a cause for chronic heel pain. *Physiother Theory Pract*. 2008;24(4):291–298.

160. Antoniadis G, Scheglmann K. Posterior tarsal tunnel syndrome: diagnosis and treatment. *Dtsch Arztebl Int*. 2008;105(45):776–781.

161. DiStefano V et al. Tarsal-tunnel syndrome. Review of the literature and two case reports. *Clin Orthop Relat Res*. 1972;88:76–79.

162. Lloyd K, Agarwal A. Tarsal-tunnel syndrome, a presenting feature of rheumatoid arthritis. *Br Med J*. 1970;3(5713):32.

163. Redborg KE et al. Ultrasound improves the success rate of a tibial nerve block at the ankle. *Reg Anesth Pain Med*. 2009;34(3): 256–260.

164. Gondring WH, Shields B, Wenger S. An outcomes analysis of surgical treatment of tarsal tunnel syndrome. *Foot Ankle Int*. 2003;24(7):545–550.

165. Pfeiffer WH, Cracchiolo A 3rd. Clinical results after tarsal tunnel decompression. *J Bone Joint Surg* (*Am*). 1994;76(8):1222–1230.

18

Traumatic Peripheral Nerve Injuries

CRAIG G. CARROLL AND WILLIAM W. CAMPBELL

INTRODUCTION

TRAUMATIC PERIPHERAL NERVE injury (TPNI) is a ubiquitous problem, creating substantial disability both in the civilian sector and in military settings. Roughly 2%–3% of patients admitted to Level I trauma centers have peripheral nerve injuries. The incidence increases to about 5% if plexus and root injuries are included.[1] Complicating the evaluation of peripheral nerve injuries is the common association with other injuries. Of the patients with traumatic brain injury admitted to rehabilitation units, 10%–34% have associated peripheral nerve injuries,[2-4] and 60% of patients with peripheral nerve injuries have a concomitant traumatic brain injury (TBI).[1] Aside from associated central nervous system trauma, there may be massive injuries to muscles, blood vessels, or vital organs that often make recognition of the peripheral nerve injury problematic or even overlooked at the time of trauma. In the civilian setting, these injuries are most commonly secondary to motor vehicle accidents and, less commonly, secondary to penetrating trauma, falls, sports-related accidents, or industrial accidents. In a 16-year retrospective study of 456 consecutive patients with 557 peripheral nerve injuries, upper limb injuries occurred in 73.5%.[5] The radial, ulnar, and median nerves are most commonly injured, with the specific incidence rates varying among studies. In the study cited above, the ulnar nerve was most commonly injured. However, in other studies, injury to the radial nerve was most frequent.[6,7] In general, the lower extremity nerves are less commonly injured; the sciatic nerve is injured most frequently, followed by the peroneal nerve. The tibial and femoral nerves are uncommonly injured. In the current wartime conflicts, peripheral nervous system injuries have, unfortunately, become common. Much of our knowledge about peripheral nerve injury, repair, and recovery has come from experience stemming from various wars throughout history.[8-10] In fact, peripheral nerve injuries were first studied systematically during the American Civil War by the neurologist S. Weir Mitchell. In a combat setting, most peripheral nerve injuries were formerly due to shrapnel.[11] However, an increasingly common cause of TPNI during modern combat is blast injury, most often from bombs or improvised explosive devices. These injuries are often complex and cause not only nerve injury, but extensive soft tissue and vascular injury as well. Peripheral nerves may be involved because of the concussive force of blast exposure, shrapnel, or limb ischemia with compartment syndrome.[12] In the current Middle East conflict, given the improvements in body armor, more U.S. and coalition soldiers are surviving wounds that would formerly have been fatal. As a result, the incidence of peripheral nerve injuries is increasing. In order to diagnose and manage peripheral nerve injuries and related pain appropriately, an understanding of the classification, pathophysiology, and electrodiagnosis of these injuries is essential.

CLASSIFICATION OF NERVE INJURIES

In order to understand the somewhat complex classification of nerve injuries, a brief review of basic nerve anatomy is necessary. Understanding the anatomy is critical to grasping the pathophysiological concepts that underlie the clinical management of patients with TPNI. The endoneurium surrounds the individual axons. Fascicles are collections of axons that are surrounded by perineurium. The epifascicular (internal) epineurium lies between the fascicles. The peripheral nerve trunk is a collection of fascicles, and the epineurial (external) epineurium surrounds the nerve trunk proper. Plexuses of microvessels run longitudinally in the epineurium, and send transverse branches that penetrate through the perineurium to form a vascular network consisting primarily of capillaries in the endoneurium.[12]

The two commonly used schemes for classifying nerve injuries are that of Seddon[9] and that of Sunderland.[7,10,13] The Seddon scheme is more commonly cited in the literature;

however, the Sunderland scheme is more useful despite its complexity. Seddon divided injuries into the categories *neurapraxia, axonotmesis, and neurotmesis.* Neurapraxia is the mildest form of injury and is due to segmental demyelination. Compressive injury with mechanical deformation leading to focal demyelination and/or ischemia is the underlying mechanisms of neurapraxic injuries[7] (also see Chapter 17 on entrapment syndromes). In neurapraxia, the nerve is anatomically intact but cannot transmit impulses. The axons are anatomically intact; however, they are nonfunctional. Thus, there is motor and sensory loss in the affected body part due to demyelination, without axonal disruption or Wallerian-type degeneration. Electrophysiologically, the nerve conducts normally distally, but there is conduction block or impaired conduction across the lesion because of the focal demyelination and loss of saltatory conduction. Loss of function persists until remyelination occurs, which translates clinically into a recovery time of a few weeks to a few months. Full spontaneous recovery is expected without the need for intervention by 12 weeks, and often earlier, provided that there is no ongoing compression. Due to the fact that axons may be remyelinated at different rates and to different degrees, function may be regained unevenly.[12] Motor paralysis can last as long as 6 months; however, most lesions resolve by 3 months.[14] Common examples of neurapraxic injuries include the classic "Saturday night" radial palsy and peroneal nerve palsies related to compression of the nerve at the fibula head caused by leg crossing or prolonged bed rest.

• More severe peripheral nerve injury affects more than just the myelin, causing anatomical disruption of axons or of the nerve trunk proper. In axonotmesis, the axon is damaged or destroyed but most of the connective tissue framework is maintained. There is axon discontinuity, but the endoneurium is intact. The surrounding stroma (i.e., the Schwann cell tubes, endoneurium, and perineurium) is at least partially intact. As expected, whenever the axon is disrupted, Wallerian-type degeneration occurs (see below for further discussion of Wallerian degeneration) but subsequent axonal regrowth may proceed along the intact endoneurial Schwann cell tubes. Axonotmesis commonly results from crush injuries and stretch injuries (such as from motor vehicle accidents and falls) as well as percussion injuries (such as from gunshot wounds). The capacity for reinnervation depends on the degree of internal disorganization as well as the distance to the target muscle. In neurotmesis, the nerve trunk is disrupted and is not in anatomical continuity. In other words, the nerve is completely severed, and the ends may actually be separated by some distance. There is a loss of nerve trunk continuity with complete disruption of all supporting elements, including the axon, endoneurium, perineurium, and epineurium. Eventually, the denervated Schwann cells disappear and inhibitory proteoglycans are formed. This situation prevents regenerative regrowth of axons.[15] Without surgery, the prognosis for recovery is extremely poor. Neurotmesis is seen with sharp injuries/lacerations, massive trauma/percussion injuries, severe traction with nerve rupture, or injection of noxious drugs.[7] A penetrating knife wound is a common example of neurotmetic injuries in the civilian setting. In the military setting, considering modern warfare, shrapnel injury is a common example of both axonotmetic and neurotmetic injuries.

The Sunderland classification of nerve injuries uses a more subdivided scheme, with five groups instead of three.[10] Sunderland's first-, second-, and fifth-degree lesions correspond to Seddon's classification of neurapraxia, axonotmesis, and neurotmesis, respectively (see Table 18.1). However, the Sunderland classification adds two useful subclasses of axonotmesis. As already mentioned, a second-degree lesion corresponds to Seddon's axonotmesis and involves disruption of the axon but with completely intact endoneurium and stroma. Therefore, recovery can occur by axonal regrowth along the intact endoneurial tubes. In a third-degree lesion, there is axonotmesis with disruption of not only the axon but also the endoneurial tubes, while the surrounding perineurium remains intact (Figure 18.1). Recovery is variable and much less efficient than in a second-degree injury due to the disruption of the endoneurial tubes. There is variable reinnervation, rarely to more than 60%–80% of normal function.[12] Recovery depends upon how well the regenerating axons can cross the site of the lesion and find endoneurial tubes. In Sunderland's fourth-degree lesion, there is disruption of the axon, endoneurial tubes, and perineurium. The individual nerve fascicles are transected, and nerve continuity is maintained only by the intact epineurium. Although the nerve is grossly intact, the internal scarring prevents regenerating axons

Table 18-1. The Seddon and Sunderland Classifications of Nerve Injury

SEDDON	PROCESS	SUNDERLAND
Neurapraxia	Segmental demyelination	First degree
Axonotmesis	Axon severed but endoneurium intact (optimal circumstances for regeneration)	Second degree
Axonotmesis	Axon discontinuity, endoneurial tube discontinuity, perineurium and fascicular arrangement preserved	Third degree
Axonotmesis	Loss of continuity of axons, endoneurial tubes, perineurium and fasciculi; epineurium intact (neuroma in continuity)	Fourth degree
Neurotmesis	Loss of continuity of entire nerve trunk	Fifth degree

Sunderland subdivided axonotmesis into three types with different degrees of nerve disruption and different capabilities for spontaneous regeneration.

Source: Reprinted from Campbell WW. Evaulation and management of peripheral nerve injury. *Clin Neurophysiol.* 2008;119:1951–1965, with permission from Elsevier.

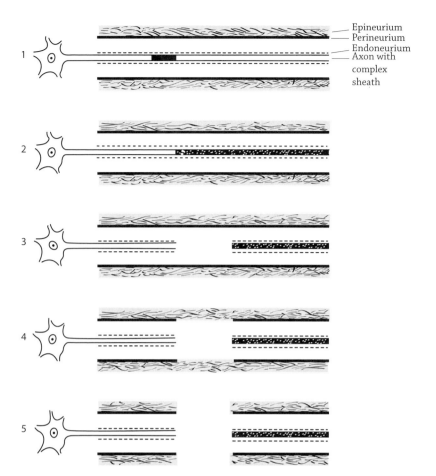

FIGURE 18.1   Diagrammatic representation of the five degrees of nerve injury. (1) Segmental demyelination causing conduction block but no damage to the axon and no Wallerian degeneration. (2) Damage to the axon severe enough to cause Wallerian degeneration and denervation of the target organ, but with an intact endoneurium and good prospects for axon regeneration. (3) Disruption of the axon and its endoneurial sheath inside an intact perineurium; loss of integrity of the endoneurial tubes will limit axon regeneration. (4) Disruption of the fasciculi, with nerve trunk continuity maintained only by epineurial tissue, severe limitation of axon regeneration, and formation of a mass of misdirected axons (neuroma in continuity). (5) Transaction of the entire nerve trunk.

from reaching the distal stump. Thus, the large amount of internal disruption precludes effective reinnervation. As the axon attempts to regenerate, the regenerating sprouts may create a ball or mass of nerve fibers (neuroma in continuity). A fifth-degree lesion is a nerve that is not in continuity. As no reinnervation occurs in fourth- and fifth-degree lesions, the prognosis for spontaneous recovery without surgical intervention is poor. Some authors have also referred to a sixth-degree lesion (a mixed lesion) consisting of some degree of

neurapraxia accompanied by a variable degree of axonal damage.[16] While in clinical practice this type of lesion is probably quite common, this class was not included in Sunderland's original classification.

WALLERIAN DEGENERATION

As alluded to earlier, soon after the axon becomes disrupted (i.e., axonotmetic or neurotmetic injuries), Wallerian-type degeneration occurs.[17,18] This is the process by which the damaged nerve begins preparing for nerve regeneration. During this process, there are changes in both the axon and the cell body. A number of changes take place in the distal axon in the first couple of days. These early changes include leakage of intra-axonal fluid from the injured nerve, swelling of the distal nerve segment, and disappearance of neurofibrils in the distal segment. By the third day, there is fragmentation of both axon and myelin with the beginning of digestion of myelin components.[7] Myelin is transformed into neutral fat and phagocytosed by macrophages. Debris of the axon and the myelin sheath forms ovoids that are gradually digested and disappear (digestion chambers).[19] While this process occurs in a distal-to-proximal fashion, degeneration may extend several centimeters proximal to the lesion.[19a] Degeneration usually stops at the first internode in mild injuries but may extend further proximally in severe injuries. By the eighth day, the axon has been digested and Schwann cells are attempting to bridge the gap between the two nerve segments.[7] In the distal stump, although the axon degenerates and disappears, the connective tissue basement membranes remain, forming endoneurial tubes. Schwann cells proliferate and line the endoneurial tubes in linear arrays known as *bands of Bungner*. These arrays of Schwann cells and processes within the basement membrane provide the pathway and scaffolding for axonal regeneration. The Schwann cells are not permanent, however, and will involute and disappear if axonal regeneration does not occur. The time frame for this process has been mapped in humans using sural nerve transection (for diagnostic purposes) as a model. Typically, Schwann cells disappear within 200 days of the injury.[20] Endoneurial tubes that do not receive a regenerating axon shrink and are eventually obliterated by scar tissue. Wallerian-type degeneration begins within hours and is complete by 6–8 weeks, leaving a distal stump comprised only of endoneurial tubes lined by Schwann cells.[21,22] In addition to the changes in the axon, a complex series of anatomical, biochemical, and physiological reactive changes in the cell body occur, referred collectively as the *retrograde axon reaction*.[23] In many ways, this retrograde axon reaction prepares the cell for

regeneration. Within the first 2 days, the Nissl bodies (the cell's rough endoplasmic reticulum) break apart into fine particles. By 2 to 3 weeks following the injury, the cell's nucleolus becomes eccentrically displaced within the nucleus. These changes may reverse as recovery occurs.[7]

MECHANISMS OF RECOVERY

In contrast to the central nervous system mechanism of recovery of function that occurs by way of plasticity using intact areas to take over the function of damaged areas, the peripheral nervous system is able to repair itself.[24] Repair following peripheral nervous system injury can occur through one of three mechanisms (or a combination thereof): remyelination, collateral sprouting distally from uninjured axons, and regeneration from the site of injury.[25] Remyelination in neurapraxic injuries can occur fairly rapidly. This is the simplest concept to understand. Again, no Wallerian-type degeneration occurs. Resolution of the conduction block resulting from ischemia or demyelination is probably the first mechanism to promote recovery of strength after nerve injury. Remyelination over an injured segment may take up to several months, depending the severity of demyelination and the length of the demyelinated segment.[26] Deficits that persist longer than 8–12 weeks usually indicate that there has been axonal damage. With less severe axonotmetic injuries, the main mechanisms of recovery are collateral sprouting (if it is a partial axon loss injury) and regeneration from the site of injury.[12,25] With more severe axonotmetic injuries involving complete axon loss and neurotmesis (if surgically reconnected), regeneration is the only mechanism for recovery, as collateral sprouting cannot occur without some population of intact axons.

Collateral distal sprouting of motor fibers from intact axons can provide reinnervation in partial nerve injuries in 2 to 6 months. When there are many surviving axons, this may be a very effective mechanism of recovery. With lesions involving less than 20%–30% of the axons, recovery occurs predominantly through this mechanism. Previous observations have shown that within 4 days following nerve injury, sprouts begin to form from intact axons, usually from distal nodes of Ranvier (nodal sprouts) or from nerve terminals (terminal sprouts) near denervated muscle.[7,27] Occasionally, when regeneration occurs simultaneously with distal sprouting, those muscles that have been reinnervated by the collateral sprouts may become dually innervated (by the sprout and the regenerated fiber).[27]

Attempts at regeneration from the injury site, the third mechanism of recovery, also begin soon after injury. This is the main mechanism of recovery when more than 90% of the axons are injured.[12] It has been observed that in the first 1–2 days after injury, axons from the proximal nerve stump start to penetrate the area of injury.[7] However, in more severe injuries, there may be an initial shock phase lasting for several weeks, after which attempts at nerve regeneration begin. The ultimate effectiveness of recovery by this process depends on multiple factors, including the degree of injury, the presence of scar formation, approximation of the two nerve ends, and the age of the patient, as well as, in large part, the distance from the injury site.[7,23] Regeneration and repair processes go on at multiple sites following nerve injury, including the nerve cell body, the segment between the neuron and the injury site (proximal stump), the injury site itself, the segment between the injury site and the end organ (distal stump), and the end organ.[24,28] The repair processes may be disrupted at one or more of these sites. A cascade of events involving cell-signaling molecules and trophic factors occurs after nerve injury that is similar to that seen in the inflammatory response. Neurotrophic factors and the blood-nerve barrier play important roles.[25,29–31] Schwann cells play an indispensable role in promoting regeneration by increasing their synthesis of surface cell adhesion molecules and by elaborating basement membrane-containing extracellular matrix proteins, such as laminin and fibronectin.[32] Schwann cells produce neurotrophic factors that bind to tyrosine kinase receptors and are responsible for a signal that leads to gene activation. Within days of injury, Schwann cells begin to divide and create a pool of dedifferentiated daughter cells. These dedifferentiated Schwann cells upregulate expression of nerve

growth factor (NGF), other neurotrophic factors, cytokines, and other compounds that lead to Schwann cell differentiation in anticipation of the arrival of a regenerating sprout. Nerve growth factor receptors on the Schwann cells lining the endoneurial tubes increase. Nerve growth factor on these Schwann cell receptors stimulates regenerating axonal sprouts.[29] The stimulation effect radiates retrogradely from the periphery to the nerve cell body, producing a stimulus that activates processes in the neuron that foster regeneration. The neuron's ability to sustain regenerative attempts persists for at least 12 months after injury. Regeneration depends on activity at a specialized growth cone at the tip of each axonal sprout.[33,34] The receptivity of the injured tissue to accepting a regenerating axon is also a critical factor. Schwann cells contacted by regenerating sprouts redifferentiate, begin to express normal myelin mRNAs, and begin the process of ensheathing and remyelinating the fresh axon. The growth cone contains multiple filopodia that adhere to the basal lamina of the Schwann cell and use it as a guide. The growth cone produces a protease that helps dissolve material blocking its path. Axons that successfully enter the endoneurial tubes in the distal stump stand a good chance of reaching the end organ. Axonal regeneration is a tenuous and delicate process with intricate maneuvering of the advancing sprout orchestrated by signal transduction.[31,35,36] In relatively minor axonotmetic lesions in which the endoneurial tubes are intact (i.e., Sunderland second-degree injury or a Seddon axonotmetic injury), the axons can traverse the segment of injury in 8 to 15 days and then regenerate along the distal nerve segment at a rate of 1–5 mm/day.[7,10] Clinically, an estimate of 1 mm/day or 1 inch/month is generally used. The variability depends on several factors. Regeneration is better proximally, and in shorter and younger individuals.[23,24] Experimental models of regenerative regrowth suggest that diabetics and human immunodeficiency virus-infected individuals also have impaired repair.[37] Functional recovery is far more common when the lesion is distal rather than proximal. This is likely because the shorter the distance that the regenerating nerve fibers have to navigate in the distal nerve stump, the less likely they are to be misrouted, and hence the more likely they are to reinnervate their target organ. Regeneration after surgical repair is slower than spontaneous regeneration.

The prognosis for spontaneous regrowth in more severe axonotmetic injuries, in which there is distortion of endoneurial tubes with or without perineurial disruption (Sunderland third- and fourth-degree injuries), is much worse. The scaffolding created normally by the Schwann cell tubes is distorted and the environment is less responsive to regenerating axons, leading to decreased regeneration. Incomplete motor recovery after more severe axonotmetic injuries may be due to a number of factors. With severe injuries that disrupt the endoneurial tubes, regenerating sprouts may encounter formidable obstacles. They may "wander" into adjacent tissue or become encased in the scar that invariably forms within the gap between the proximal and distal stumps. Extensive scarring reduces the speed with which regenerating axons can traverse the lesion and, more significantly, reduces the likelihood that they will ever reach their end organs.[7] Sprouts that do not find their way into the distal stump may grow into disorganized swirls and form a neuroma.[23] A scar within the bridging tissue may not only impede regeneration, but may also lead to misdirection and aberrant regeneration into the wrong end organ as axons sprout into functionally unrelated endoneurial tubes. In some cases, especially when a large neuroma is present, surgical intervention is required. In complete neurotmesis (Sunderland fifth-degree injury), axonal regrowth is usually not possible without surgical intervention.[7] The nerve ends must be freed from scar tissue and surgically reapproximated, either directly or using a cable graft. With reapproximation, nerve growth can then occur along the endoneurial tubes of the distal segments. It is important to note that the use of cable grafts simply provides a conduit for axonal regrowth and does not provide axons directly.[7,38]

Another critical factor is the length of the gap between the injury or repair site and the target muscle. Aside from the aforementioned obstacles the regenerating axon must overcome, recovery of motor function also depends on the integrity of the muscle when the axon reaches it. The time after which irreversible muscle changes occur and an operation cannot provide benefit is 18–24 months.[7] After this time, the target muscle will become atrophied and fibrotic, making axon regrowth useless because the muscle is no longer viable. The Schwann cells and the endoneurial tubes also remain viable for 6–24 months after injury. If they do not receive a regenerating axon within this time span, the tubes degenerate. Reinnervation must occur not only before the muscle undergoes irreversible changes, but also before the endoneurial tubes will no longer support nerve growth. Axons that cannot reach the distal stump are essentially wasted. Thus, the time- distance equation has two primary variables: irreversible changes in critical target muscles that occur after 12–18 months and axon regrowth at a rate of 1 mm/day from the site of injury or the site of surgical repair. Axon regeneration is not synonymous with return of function. Even after the axon reaches its target, a maturation process must evolve, including remyelination, axonal enlargement, and the establishment of connections with the end organ before functional recovery can ensue.

The above-described mechanisms of recovery apply to motor axons. Even when good motor recovery occurs, sensory deficits, particularly in proprioception, may impair the functional outcome. While the mechanisms of axonal regeneration for sensory axons are similar, there are some key differences. Firstly, there may be redistribution of sensory function such that intact fibers provide cutaneous sensation to a larger area than it had prior to the injury.[39,40] Secondly, pain and temperature sensibility is subserved through free nerve endings, that is, there are no target organs to degenerate, as occurs in muscle. Therefore, sensory recovery may continue for a longer period of time than motor recovery.

While the mechanisms of recovery for neurapraxic and axonotmetic injuries have been considered separately, it is important to realize that many injuries are mixed.[7] In these situations, the patient often notices two or more phases of recovery. There may be a fairly rapid initial improvement in the first several weeks as the neurapraxic component recovers. This is often followed by a slower phase of axonal recovery involving collateral axonal sprouting and regeneration. Based on the discussion above, the sensory recovery may take even more time.

A physical examination is extremely useful in following patients with peripheral nerve injury. A flicker of movement or some degree of preserved sensation indicates that the lesion is incomplete. Substitute or *trick* movements often make the determination challenging. A trick movement occurs when the patient uses a normal muscle or movement to substitute for a weak muscle. An example of this is the "bartender's sign," referring to a patient with a weak biceps who pulls the elbow backward when the examiner tries to examine the biceps.[41] Elicitation of Tinel's sign is also helpful. The growing tips of nerves are electrically excitable by mechanical distortion, and their percussion may elicit a tingling or electric sensation. This sign was first described by Tinel in a series of crush injuries.[42] With a first-degree lesion, Tinel's sign remains focal over the area of abnormality, and although there may be weakness, muscle atrophy does not occur. With a second-degree lesion atrophy does develop, sometimes rapidly, and Tinel's sign moves distally at a rate of approximately 1 inch/month. With a third- degree lesion there is atrophy, and Tinel's sign does progress distally, but at a slower rate. With fourth-degree (neuroma in continuity) and fifth-degree (neurotmetic) lesions, atrophy is usually severe and rapid, but Tinel's sign never migrates distally. Tinel pointed out in his original writings that a distally migrating "signe du fourmillement" predicted recovery only 50% of the time.[42]

ELECTRODIAGNOSTIC EVALUATION IN DETERMINING THE PROGNOSIS AND GUIDING MANAGEMENT

An electromyogram (EMG) with nerve conduction studies (NCS) is an invaluable part of the evaluation to aid in determining the underlying pathophysiology (i.e., neurapraxia vs. axonotmesis), which, in turn, is helpful in estimating the overall prognosis. Additionally, the electrodiagnostic evaluation may aid in localizing the site of peripheral nerve injury. Although the site of nerve injury may be obvious, in cases with extensive trauma the exact site of injury within this large area of trauma may not be known. Exact localization would be important for any surgical considerations. While a full review of the electrodiagnosis is beyond the scope of this discussion, a few salient points will be made. Localization on electrodiagnostic studies is suggested by one of two methods: (1) detecting conduction block or focal slowing on the NCS and (2) assessing the pattern of denervation (fibrillation potentials) on the needle EMG study (using knowledge of the branching order to various muscles).[7]

As discussed earlier, injuries that are predominantly neurapraxic have an excellent prognosis for recovery within a few months. In neurapraxic injuries, the NCS will essentially remain normal if stimulation is carried out distal to the lesion, as Wallerian degeneration does not occur.[12] Stimulation proximal to the lesion will reveal a partial or complete conduction block, with varying degrees of loss of the compound motor action potential (CMAP) and slowing of the conduction velocity. Electromyographic abnormalities would remain limited to a pattern of decreased recruitment of the muscles supplied distal to the injured nerve.[7,12] While some investigators have suggested that fibrillation potentials can occasionally occur in purely neurapraxic injuries, conventional teaching is that no denervation is seen. In our opinion, the finding of fibrillation potentials in neurapraxic injuries more likely suggests minimal secondary axon loss, since the EMG is more sensitive than NCS in detecting minor degrees of axon loss. Furthermore, from a practical standpoint, some combination of neurapraxia and axonotmesis tends to be the rule rather than the exception. The abnormalities seen in neurapraxic injuries should improve or disappear when remyelination is complete, provided that there is no persistent pressure on the nerve. Some conduction slowing may be permanent because remyelination characteristically leaves shorter, thinner internodes than were present originally, but this does not interfere with function.[12]

The electrodiagnostic findings in axonotmesis and neurotmesis depend on how much time has passed between the injury and the evaluation. A study carried out in the first few days following an axonotmetic or neurotmetic injury will likely show no conduction abnormality except for the inability to conduction an impulse across the lesion on proximal stimulation. In other words, a study carried out in the first couple of days would not be able to distinguish axonotmesis or neurotmesis from a neurapraxic injury, as the NCS findings would be the same. The main utility of obtaining an electrodiagnostic evaluation at this point would be for precise localization of the injury. Once the process of Wallerian degeneration has been completed after 10–14 days, however, the electrodiagnostic findings differ quite substantially. The CMAP and sensory nerve action potentials (SNAP) distal to the injury decrease in amplitude roughly in proportion to the degree of axonal loss. This loss of amplitude is usually complete by day 9 for the motor studies and day 11 for the sensory studies. The earlier loss of the CMAP amplitudes is related to changes in the neuromuscular junction.[12] If there is complete axonal involvement (i.e., electrophysiologically complete), the nerve may even be inexcitable (i.e., SNAPs and CMAPs will be unobtainable). By 2 weeks following injury, the NCS can help estimate the degree of axon loss versus segmental demyelination. The axon loss can be estimated by comparing the ratio of the CMAP amplitude on the injured side to that on the normal side. The amount of segmental demyelination can be estimated by comparing the drop in proximal CMAP amplitude to the distal CMAP amplitude (i.e., conduction block) as well as assessing for focal conduction slowing. In pure axon loss lesions, aside from a decrease in the CMAP amplitudes, there may be generalized slowing throughout the entire nerve (nonlocalizable). Therefore, after Wallerian degeneration has been completed, NCS are no longer helpful for precisely localizing injuries along the involved nerve and the EMG findings must be relied upon. Although precise localization may not be possible, some information regarding localization can still be obtained. For example, important information in determining a preganglionic (proximal to the dorsal root ganglion) location, such as nerve root avulsion, versus a postganglionic (distal to the dorsal root

ganglion) location can still be obtained. Furthermore, brachial plexus versus single-nerve involvement can still be determined in this time frame. Needle EMG findings can indicate axon loss, but they do not quantify the degree of loss except to distinguish between electrophysiologically complete and incomplete lesions. If the lesion is electrophysiologically complete, there will be no motor units under voluntary control in muscles innervated by the injured nerve. The appearance of denervation potentials (fibrillations and positive sharp waves) is time and length dependent. In proximally innervated muscles these potentials appear after 10–14 days, while in distally innervated muscles they occur in 3–4 weeks.[12] As muscle trauma can result in denervation potentials, this is a potential confounding variable that an electromyographer must keep in mind to avoid a false localization.[43]

The time when the electrodiagnostic evaluation should take place depends, in large part, on the question being asked. In general, the greatest amount of information can be obtained by a single study performed about 3–4 weeks after the injury. At this point, Wallerian-type degeneration is complete and enough time has passed to detect fibrillation potentials on the EMG examination. Thus, inferences can be made not only about localization (based on NCS and the pattern of EMG involvement) but also about the degree of neurapraxia versus axonotmesis/neurotmesis and whether or not the lesion is electrophysiologically complete or incomplete. The problem is that precise localization of the lesion along the injured nerve is lost, especially when there is a relatively large area of trauma. The period of time when the distal stump continues to conduct normally (approximately the first week) allows for precise localization, since there will be no conduction across the site of any major injury associated with anatomical disruption. Detection of such axon discontinuity conduction block precisely identifies the site of the responsible lesion. In these cases, an early study performed within the first several days after injury may be helpful. The localization opportunity is lost when Wallerian degeneration occurs and the distal stump ceases to conduct normally (if there is axonal involvement). At 1–2 weeks, while the ability to precisely localize the injury along the nerve in an axonal lesion disappears, neurapraxia (the distal stump conducts normally) versus axonotmesis/neurotmesis (the distal stump no longer conducts normally) can then be determined. However, enough time to detect fibrillation potentials on the EMG has not passed. Thus, unless precise localization is necessary, an initial study performed 3–4 weeks following an injury provides the most information at a single sitting.

Further EMG studies, in conjunction with the clinical exam, may also be helpful in detecting evidence of reinnervation, assisting in the evaluation of the need for surgical exploration. Electromyographic abnormalities correlating with axonal collateral sprouting include changes in the morphology of the existing motor units. Specifically, the amplitude increases, the duration becomes prolonged, and the percentage of polyphasic potentials increases.[7] The earliest EMG finding in axonal regrowth is the presence of small polyphasic, often unstable, potentials, which have been referred to as *nascent potentials*. The EMG is more sensitive than the physical examination for detecting reinnervation; therefore, the return of voluntary motor unit action potentials on the needle examination in the muscles in the injured nerve distribution closest to the injury site is typically the first evidence of reinnervation. In other words, this finding often precedes the onset of clinically evident voluntary movement. These nascent potentials represent the earliest definitive evidence of axonal reinnervation in complete lesions and can occur weeks to months before voluntary contraction is visible.[44] The prognosis for axonotmesis is quite variable. An absolute distinction between milder axonotmesis (Sunderland second- and third-degree injuries), which often recover spontaneously, and more severe axonotmesis (Sunderland fourth-degree injury) and neurotmesis (Sunderland fifth-degree injury), which require surgical exploration, cannot always be made with the initial electrodiagnostic study. Thus, the need for surgical intervention cannot usually be determined on the initial evaluation. Lesions that have spontaneous recovery are usually treated conservatively since surgical repair is unlikely to be better than natural recovery. Lesions with no evidence of axonal regrowth may require operative exploration with possible grafting. One must consider that any surgical exploration must be performed within a specific time frame so that sprouts can reach the target muscle before the irreversible changes previously described occur at 12–18 months. With a regrowth rate of about 1 inch/month, the amount of time during which reinnervation should occur can be estimated. In general, a repeat electrodiagnostic study is recommended in 3–6 months, depending on the clinical recovery, to assess for signs of reinnervation in previously completely denervated muscles; the study will assist the evaluation for possible surgery. Thus, a common approach where nerve continuity is uncertain, or when there has been blunt or massive trauma, is to wait and see if there is clinical or EMG evidence of reinnervation, and then to operate on patients without evidence of reinnervation, usually within 3 months (especially if the lesion is proximal). Proximal nerve injuries, above the elbow and above the knee, are somewhat problematic because the long distance sprouts must travel makes it difficult to reinnervate critical distal muscles before irreversible changes occur.[12] Clinical decision making regarding exploration must occur over a much shorter time frame. Therefore, in these situations, a repeat study closer to 3 months after injury is probably more appropriate. In these cases, exploration with the assistance of intraoperative nerve action potentials is often the best choice.

PATHOPHYSIOLOGY OF PAIN IN NERVE INJURIES

Neuropathic pain, specifically hyperalgesia and allodynia, is common following peripheral nerve injuries (also see Chapters 1 and 2 in this volume). The classic example of such neuropathic pain was first described by Weir Mitchell and colleagues, who coined the term *causalgia* to characterize the burning pain described by American Civil War soldiers with projectile injuries to major peripheral nerves.[45] Much of what we know about the pathophysiology of the development of neuropathic pain following nerve injury stems from animal models as well as pharmacological models. The development of pain following nerve injury appears to have its basis in alterations in afferent function at sites beyond the injury site itself. Peripheral nerve injury unleashes multiple peripheral and central nerve system processes that all contribute to persistent pain and abnormal sensation. These processes include morphological and biochemical changes in the spinal processing of nociceptive information. The powerful effect of local anesthetics suggests that at least a portion of this post-nerve injury pain may arise from ongoing afferent activity in the injured nerve terminal as well as the dorsal root ganglion (DRG).[45] Injury to the peripheral nerve triggers an initial barrage of afferent information. After an interval of days to weeks, persistent spontaneous firing leads to a state of hyperexcitability originating from small afferent fibers at the injury site (neuroma) as well as at the DRG of the injured nerve. This state of hyperexcitability in the primary afferent nociceptors is known as *peripheral sensitization*.[46] In turn, central neurons in the dorsal horn of the spinal cord innervated by these nociceptors undergo dramatic functional changes including the development of a state of hyperexcitability known as *central sensitization*. This spontaneous firing/state of hyperexcitability is not seen in the normal axon and is believed to play a critical role in perpetuating the pain state. Normally, this peripheral and central sensitization subsides as the tissue heals and inflammation ceases. However, occasionally primary afferent function is altered in an enduring way, and these processes may persist and cause refractory pain. It is important to examine the changes at each of these various levels that lead to this alteration in afferent processing.

In order to understand these changes better, one must begin at the level of the neuroma. As discussed in detail above, following axonal injury, Wallerian-type degeneration occurs and the injured axon begins to sprout, sending out its growth cone. This growth cone attempts to regenerate along intact endoneurial tubes. If the integrity of the endoneurial tubes has been disrupted, successful regrowth is interrupted and the growth cones may form a local collection of sprouts known as a *neuroma*. Aside from being composed of regenerating axons, these neuromas are vascularized and develop significant sympathetic innervation.[47] It is also known that these regenerating axons display novel ion channels and receptors not seen in the normal axon.[45] Novel α receptors have been pharmacologically demonstrated in animal models.[45,48] It is known that the regenerating axons have a significant increase in the density of sodium channels.[45,49] Based on pharmacological models, it appears likely that N- or L-type calcium channels may also be present.[45,50,51] Increased ionic conductance, particularly related to the increased density of sodium channels, may result in the increase in spontaneous activity that develops in the sprouting axon. As a result of the ingrowth of sympathetic terminals into the neuroma coupled with the display of novel channels and receptors, these growing tips of the regenerating nerves develop significant chemical sensitivity not possessed by the original axon.[45] As explained earlier, these axonal sprouts also develop mechanical sensitivity, as manifested by the Tinel's sign with percussion at the leading edge of regrowth. In addition to their mechanical and chemical sensitivity, these regenerating sprouts show sensitivity to a number of humoral factors, such as prostaglandins, catecholamines, and cytokines.[45,52] In summary, as a result of these changes at the level of the neuroma, increased spontaneous afferent nociceptive firing with ectopic discharges, as well as increased mechanical and chemical sensitivity, develop that were not seen in the original axon and play a critical role in perpetuating the pain state.

The DRG of an injured axon may also be a source of persistent spontaneous afferent activity, further perpetuating neuropathic pain. Prominent alterations in the function and morphology of the DRG cells are also observed following peripheral nerve injury.[45] Hyperinnervation of type A ganglion cells by sympathetic terminals has been observed.[45,53] This sympathetic hyperinnervation has been shown to exert an excitatory drive on both the neuroma and, independently, the DRG cells. Cross-linkage between A and C fibers also develops.[45,54] In addition, it has been suggested that injury to the peripheral nerve leads to the elaboration of certain neurotrophic factors, which are transported in retrograde fashion to the cell body. Upon arrival, these neurotrophic factors trigger changes that are important to the subsequent development of a pain state.[45]

In addition to changes at the level of the neuroma and the DRG, alterations in central processing in the spinal cord dorsal horn are seen after peripheral nerve injury (central sensitization). In animal models following peripheral nerve injury, dark-staining neurons in the dorsal horn that are believed to presage cell death are seen.[45,55] Many cells in this region contain large amounts of glycine and gamma-aminobutyric acid (GABA), both of which are inhibitory interneuron neurotransmitters.[56] Thus, it is speculated that these darkly stained neurons reflect the cell death of neurons that lead to an important loss of this tonic GABAergic or glycinergic inhibitory tone. Loss of such tone has been shown experimentally to induce an allodynic state. There is little doubt that the spinal release of glutamate and likely aspartate, both excitatory neurotransmitters, contributes significantly to the establishment of the post-nerve injury pain state. Studies have shown that, following sciatic nerve injury, there is significant enhancement in the amount of glutamate in the cerebrospinal fluid. The origins of this increased release are unknown, but it is believed to be secondary to the loss of local inhibition (as a result of loss of GABA and glycine) This glutamate release appears in the context of increased spontaneous activity in the primary afferents as well as loss of spinal interneurons that may ordinarily serve to modulate resting glutamate secretion.[45] Like other neurotransmitters, glutamate is known to act on a variety of different receptors. Specifically, glutamate's action on the N-methyl-D-aspartate (NMDA) receptors appears to be primarily responsible for the long-term damage due to excitotoxicity.[57] Through glutamate's action on NMDA receptors, these receptors appear to play an important role in generating and maintaining this facilitated hyperexcitable state of the spinal nociceptive neurons that is evoked by the repetitive small afferent stimulation.[58,59] Additionally, as a result of the chronic afferent electrical barrage that develops as described above, there is an increase in mRNA for specific neurotransmitters such as substance P, the appearance of immediate early gene products such as c-fos, altered levels of opioid binding sites, and alterations in the relative levels of neuropeptides, many of which have neuromodulatory roles.[45] A significant change in afferent processing also occurs. Normally, the larger (αβ) myelinated afferents penetrate the dorsal horn, travel ventrally, and then terminate in Rexed laminae III and deeper. In contrast, the small unmyelinated afferents penetrate directly and terminate no deeper than lamina II (substantia gelatinosa). Following peripheral nerve injury, it has been shown that there is prominent sprouting of large afferents up from lamina III into laminae I and II.[60] Thus, large afferents that normally encodes low-threshold information now gain access to spinal termination regions that originally received input only from high-threshold (pain) afferents. In other words, in this altered state of processing, low-intensity afferent input (i.e., normal sensory input) is encoded as a noxious event.[45] Therefore, the enhanced glutamate release as a result of a loss of local inhibition, as well as the significant alterations in afferent processing, lead to a facilitated state of processing that is critical in the development of post-nerve injury pain.

In summary, an oversimplified but practical pathophysiological approach in considering the medical therapy of the pain state following nerve injury includes the following: (1) peripheral sensitization-increased primary afferent nociceptive firing or hyperexcitability of the primary afferent nociceptors, in large part resulting from abnormal collections of sodium channels in damaged peripheral nerve fibers; (2) decreased inhibition of neuronal activity in central structures (e.g., due to loss of inhibitory neurons); and (3) central sensitization: as a result of the changes described in peripheral sensitization, central processing becomes altered so that normal sensory input is amplified and sustained.[46]

MEDICAL THERAPY OF POSTTRAUMATIC NERVE PAIN

Further discussion of the use of medical therapies for neuropathic pain can be found in Chapter 6. The control of pain is often the most pressing consideration in the early management of peripheral nerve injury. Pharmacological management is certainly not a cure and should be considered an integral component of a more comprehensive approach to treatment that includes physical therapy and psychological treatments.[46] The pain resulting from peripheral nerve injury, like other neuropathic pain syndromes, may be constant or intermittent. Most patients describe both a spontaneous constant burning and intermittent lancinating "shooting" or "electric shock-like" dysesthesias. Many patients often have prominent allodynia and hyperpathia, sometimes so severe that the patient will not allow the physician or therapist to even touch the affected limb. Therefore, medications specific for neuropathic pain are necessary. Few randomized, double-blind, placebo-controlled trials concerning pain specifically following traumatic peripheral nerve injuries are available, and much of what we know about medical therapies for neuropathic pain in these situations is extrapolated from studies involving other neuropathic pain syndromes, mainly diabetic neuropathy and postherpetic neuralgia. However, as described in detail above, the underlying mechanisms may, in fact, differ. Each mechanism of injury may respond differently to medications with different mechanisms of action. Management often becomes an exercise in trial and error, with medications often used in combination. The main classes of medications will be discussed in turn.

Antidepressants

No randomized, double-blind, placebo-controlled trials exist specifically addressing the antidepressants used in neuropathic pain following TPNI. However, although specific trials in peripheral nerve injury-related pain are lacking, the analgesic effects of the tricyclic antidepressants (TCAs) in other neuropathic pain states have been well demonstrated. The most commonly used TCAs include nortriptyline and amytriptyline, followed by desipramine, imipramine, and clomipramine. The analgesic mechanism of the TCAs is not completely known but is likely related to the combined reuptake inhibition of norepinephrine and serotonin, blockade of α1-adrenergic receptors and sodium channels, and reduction of sympathetic efferent activity and NMDA receptor antagonism.[61] The TCAs are usually initiated at low doses (10–25 mg) once a day at bedtime

and then titrated every 3–7 days as tolerated up to 75 to 150 mg/day. The selective serotonin reuptake inhibitors do not appear to be as effective as the tricyclic antidepressants. The newer dual serotonin/norepinephrine reuptake inhibitors, including venlafaxine, duloxetine, and milnacipran (approved for fibromyalgia as Savella®), have shown promise in treating neuropathic pain. These agents presumably work through mechanisms similar to those of the TCAs but appear to have a better side effect profile. Further establishment in clinical trials is necessary.

Anticonvulsants

Like the TCAs, the anticonvulsants have been a mainstay of therapy for neuropathic pain. However, as also is true of the TCAs, few studies specifically addressing the anticonvulsants in TPNI have been conducted. Commonly used anticonvulsants in the treatment of pain following TPNI include carbamazepine, phenytoin, gabapentin, pregabalin, and lamotrogine. While carbamazepine, phenytoin, and lamotrigine appear to act mainly against sodium channels, gabapentin and pregabalin bind to and block the α2-δ subunit of the voltage-sensitive presynaptic Ca^{2+} channels that modulate the release of neurotransmitters from presynaptic terminals.[62] Despite the widespread clinical use of these agents for neuropathic pain, it is important to note that only two recent double-blind, randomized, placebo-controlled studies involving the anticonvulsants in the treatment of TPNI-induced pain have been conducted. One study, a multicenter crossover study involving 120 patients, was conducted to evaluate the efficacy and safety of gabapentin in the treatment of neuropathic pain caused by traumatic nerve injury.[62] This study was the first randomized, controlled study in traumatic nerve injury pain. It did not meet its primary endpoint, which involved demonstrating a significant difference between gabapentin and placebo on the change in the mean pain intensity score from baseline to the last week of treatment. However, using doses up to 2400 mg/day, a number of secondary outcome measures did improve, including several domains of pain relief, quality of life, and sleep interference caused by pain, compared with placebo. More patients had at least a 30% pain reduction, and both patients' and clinicians' global impressions of change indicated a better response with gabapentin compared to placebo. Additionally, a significant difference in the sleep interference score was seen. More recently, a multicenter double-blind, placebo-controlled study of pregabalin involving 254 adult patients with posttraumatic peripheral neuropathic pain was conducted.[63] In this study, patients were randomized to receive flexible-dose pregabalin (150–600 mg/day for 4 weeks of dose optimization), followed by fixed dosing for 4 weeks. The average pregabalin dose was 326 mg/day. The study found that patients treated with pregabalin experienced significantly reduced self-reported pain compared to those receiving placebo. Patients receiving pregabalin had, on average, a pain score that was 0.62 point lower on an 11-point scale compared to those receiving placebo. Additionally, the patients receiving pregabalin reported less pain interference with sleep. These patients had an average self-reported weekly pain-related sleep interference score of 2.73 on an 11-point scale compared to 4.13 for those receiving placebo. Other newer anticonvulsants such as zonisamide and topirimate may also be useful; however, controlled studies are necessary.

Antiarrhythmics

The two antiarrhythmics that are most often utilized for neuropathic pain are lidocaine and its oral analog, mexilitene. The action of systemically administered local anesthetics is especially interesting. Studies have shown that systemic lidocaine can reduce the spontaneous afferent activity in the structures discussed previously, with the order of sensitivity being: dorsal horn > DRG > neuroma > injured terminal >>> axon conduction.[45,64,65] Multiple studies have shown that systemic lidocaine and its oral analog (i.e., mexilitene) are successful in treating neuropathic pain syndromes.[66,67] Controlled studies in peripheral nerve injuries have clearly demonstrated significant short-term analgesia with intravenous lidocaine.[66–68] The effects appear to peak at 1–2 hours postinfusion, with effects lasting for up to 6 hours.[66] Given the

short-acting effect of systemic lidocaine as well as the intravenous route, however, this would not be practical for longer-term management. Several studies have shown that infusion of lidocaine is a useful diagnostic test to identify patients who may potentially benefit from its orally administered analogs.[66,69] A typical dose of lidocaine that has been shown to be effective is a 30-minute constant rate infusion of 5 mg/kg. Mexilitene has been tested in several postherpetic neuralgia trials at dosages between 450 and 750 mg/day. In small controlled studies of peripheral nerve injury patients, the higher dosages have provided effective analgesia.[70] These agents have in common the ability to block sodium channels.[66] Therefore, it may be expected that they act only on that subset of neuropathic symptoms mediated by abnormal activation of sodium channels. Thus, previous investigators have suggested that lidocaine and its oral analogs may have modality-specific analgesic effects. Specifically, it has been shown that lidocaine is more effective in spontaneous pain and mechanical allodynia/hyperalgesia compared to cold or heat allodynia/hyperalgesia.[66] Considering the above discussion, a reasonable clinical approach would be to consider the nature of the patient's pain. If the history and exam reveal prominent mechanical (as opposed to thermal) allodynia/hyperalgesia, a screening test with lidocaine using the above dosing regimen should be considered. If the patient shows a significant analgesic effect with the lidocaine trial, then therapy with mexilitene could be given, starting at 200 mg/day and titrating every week as high as 1000 mg as tolerated for pain relief.

Opiates

While opiates clearly have a role in treating somatic pain, their benefits in neuropathic pain appear to be conflicting. Although they are frequently prescribed for neuropathic pain, much of the data suggest a relatively poor effect of these agents in some neuropathic conditions in humans.[71] In animal models with electrophysiological observations, it has been shown that following brachial plexus lesions, the spontaneous activity in dorsal horn neurons is insensitive to opiates.[72] Several recent studies have suggested efficacy in postherpetic neuralgia and painful diabetic neuropathies. However, there are no controlled studies demonstrating efficacy in TPNI. Therefore, the use of narcotics to treat pain in these situations should generally be considered a last resort.

Topical Agents

Lidocaine transdermal patches have shown efficacy in postherpetic neuralgia; however, no studies examining their benefit in other pain conditions have been conducted. Their excellent safety and tolerability make them an attractive option.[73] However, only anecdotal evidence concerning their use in TPNI exists. The analgesic properties of topical 0.075% capsaicin have been demonstrated in polyneuropathy and postherpetic neuralgia, but no evidence demonstrating its efficacy in treating pain following peripheral nerve injury exists.[73] A higher concentration of capsaicin (~ 8%; Qutenza®) has recently been approved for postherpetic neuralgia, but to date, no studies have been published concerning its use in posttraumatic nerve injuries. These therapies may be reasonable for focal pain but are probably not useful for more widespread pain.

Other Agents

Tramadol is a centrally acting agent with an analgesic effect mediated by the μ-opioid receptor as well as by nonopioid mechanisms including serotonin and noradrenaline reuptake inhibition.[73] In some studies, tramadol has been reported to have efficacy similar to that of antidepressants and antiepileptics for the treatment of neuropathic pain; however, substantiation of this effect in further studies is required. Again, the existing data apply mainly to postherpetic neuralgia and Peripheral diabetic neuropathy (PDN), and data on TPNI pain are lacking. Alpha-2 agonists, such as clonidine (transdermal and oral), have shown efficacy in certain neuropathic pain syndromes. Experimentally, they appear to act presynaptically to reduce sympathetic terminal release, an important mechanism in the establishment of peripheral sensitization.[45] Thus, theoretical benefit exists for a role in treating neuropathic pain

secondary to TPNI; however, to date, no studies have been conducted.

NMDA Receptor Antagonists

As discussed above, the role of NMDA receptor complex activation in the development of posttraumatic neuropathic pain seems well established. The NMDA receptors appear to have an important role in the generation and maintenance of the facilitated state, or central hyperexcitability, in the dorsal horn that is evoked by repetitive afferent stimulation and, therefore, evoked pain to mechanical stimuli.[74] Evidence from available studies suggest that ketamine, an NMDA receptor antagonist, decreases neuropathic pain, including posttraumatic pain.[58,61,75,76] The most significant effect, like that of systemic lidocaine, appears to be on mechanical allodynia and hyperalgesia, with less of an effect on thermal allodynia.[76,77] The dosage strategy of ketamine in the literature ranges from 0.1 to 7 mg/kg, with infusion times ranging from 20 minutes to 8 hours.[78] In one study showing its effectiveness in posttraumatic neuralgia, a bolus dose of 60 μg/kg was followed by a continuous infusion of 6 μg/kg/min for 20 minutes. Unfortunately, the continuous infusion of ketamine is often not feasible because of intolerable side effects, including painful indurations at the infusion site and psychomimetic effects such as sedation, slowed reaction times, hallucinations, and dissociative states.[69] Therefore, despite its theoretical benefit based on mechanistic considerations, this therapy remains impractical. Dextromethorphan is a weak orally administered NMDA antagonist that has shown benefit in neuropathic pain. There is some evidence to suggest that the response to an intravenous ketamine infusion (0.1 mg/kg) may predict the response to dextromethorphan.[79,80] In several small studies, a clinically relevant benefit was seen in diabetic neuropathy at doses of 381–400 mg/day.[6,81] However, no benefit was seen with postherpetic neuralgia. Clinical trials investigating dextromethorphan in TPNI pain are necessary. Memantine is another oral NMDA receptor antagonist that is approved for the treatment of Alzheimer's disease (Namenda®).

However, to date, its effect in treating posttherpetic neuralgia and diabetic neuropathy has been disappointing.[81]

Nerve Blocks

When the above medical therapies fail, pain control with regional anesthetic blocks may be necessary. This may be accomplished by infusion of a local anesthetic using a single-injection peripheral nerve block or by continuous infusions via an indwelling catheter placed close to the peripheral nerve. The obvious limitation of single-injection peripheral nerve blocks is that the effectiveness is limited by the duration of action of the local anesthetic used. The use of continuous peripheral nerve blockade (CPNB) provides the benefits of single-injection techniques, including a decreased incidence of systemic side effects, with the added benefit of providing more prolonged anesthesia. The application of sophisticated regional anesthesia techniques for acute and chronic pain control has grown significantly over the past decade. The introduction and refinements of mechanical and electric pumps for continuous infusion of local anesthetic have made this technique much more efficient and practical and have even allowed for its use in an outpatient environment.[82] The specific technical details are beyond the scope of this discussion. Numerous studies have shown superior efficacy of CPNB for postoperative pain; however, more limited evidence for its use in neuropathic pain exists. Despite the lack of large-scale controlled clinical trials, a large body of anecdotal evidence suggests efficacy in the complex regional pain syndrome.[83] Although no randomized clinical trials for TPNI pain exist, there is a clear theoretical benefit; thus, this technique represents a promising therapy.

Neurostimulation

Although pharmacological measures can often be effective, many patients do not achieve sufficient pain relief with medication alone. Although the best marker of what is considered significant pain reduction remains debatable, using a target of >50% pain relief, only 30%–40% of patients with chronic neuropathic pain

achieve that target with pharmacotherapy.[84,85] Therefore, an increasing a number of nonpharmacological measures have been developed. Neurostimulation therapy is one such nonpharmacological treatment that is increasingly being used as a substitute for surgical lesions in refractory neuropathic pain syndromes. These neurostimulation techniques that are useful in TPNI can be divided into two categories: (1) peripheral stimulation therapies including transcutaneous electrical nerve stimulation (TENS) and peripheral nerve stimulation (PNS) and (2) central stimulation therapies including spinal cord stimulation (SCS) and deep brain stimulation (DBS). The most commonly used and most readily available technique used in TPNI pain is TENS. In this technique, surface electrodes are placed over the painful area or the nerve that innervates it, and the stimulation is delivered at high frequency and low intensity (below the pain threshold) to produce an intense activation of $\alpha\beta$ afferents and to evoke parasthesias that cover the painful area.[86] (Peripheral nerve stimulation involves the same principles. However, in order to provide more stable and efficient stimulation, electrodes can be implanted percutaneously or intraoperatively to contact the nerve and can be connected subcutaneously to a stimulation unit. The mechanism of action appears to be related to disinhibition of neurons within the dorsal horn related to stimulation of the $\alpha\beta$ fibers.[54] Additionally, TENS or PNS activation of the release of endogenous opioids likely also plays a role.[87] Although there are plenty of controlled studies and meta-analyses of TENS in nociceptive pain, its effectiveness in neuropathic pain is disappointing. While numerous controlled studies involving TENS in other neuropathic pain syndromes have been carried out, only a single randomized, double-blind, placebo-controlled trial involving TPNI is available. In this study, 19 patients with hypersensitivity in their hands within or adjacent to the site of injury were examined. The treatment group received daily 20-minute applications of electrical stimulation for 2 weeks. Using validated pain scales, the investigators found significantly lower pain levels in the treatment group compared to the placebo group. No randomized studies using PNS in TPNI-related pain are available. However, one retrospective analysis of 22 posttraumatic neuropathy patients treated by PNS showed that 62% of them experienced adequate pain control for an average of 25 months.[88] If these peripheral neurostimulation techniques provide no benefit, then central stimulation techniques can be considered. Spinal cord stimulators are increasingly being used for the control of neuropathic pain. Spinal cord stimulation appear to exert its effect by modulating the previously discussed hyperexcitability in the dorsal horn with increased release of GABA and, in turn, diminished glutamate activity. This technique consists of inserting electrodes into the posterior epidural space of the thoracic or cervical spine ipsilateral to the pain and at the appropriate rostrocaudal level. While good evidence exists for the effectiveness of SCS in failed back syndrome and complex regional pain syndrome, the available evidence for its effect in TPNI is based only on positive case series evidence.[86] The most extensive data on SCS for use in pain following peripheral nerve injury was reported by Lazorthes et al.[89] In this cooperative retrospective study from two different centers involving 152 patients, 85% showed good or excellent results at >2 years. Confirmatory comparative trials are necessary before the use of SCS can be firmly recommended for therapy in this condition. Although DBS may offer promise as a future therapy, no evidence to date exists regarding its effectiveness in TPNI.

CONCLUSION

Traumatic peripheral nerve injury remains a common and growing problem. By understanding the classification schemes of injury as well as the mechanisms of reinnervation, one can manage these injuries more effectively. Effective management often requires a multidisciplinary approach with a focus on rehabilitation issues, as well as possible surgical interventions depending on the degree of injury and pain control. As with any type of nerve injury, allodynia and hyperalgesia are common clinical problems and are often one of the most pressing management issues. Over the last several decades, the elucidation of the underlying pathophysiological mechanisms of development

of neuropathic pain has allowed expansion of the available therapies. These therapies stand in contrast to the general strategies used for nociceptive pain. While much has been learned regarding many neuropathic pain syndromes, especially postherpetic neuralgia and painful diabetic neuropathy, much remains to be learned regarding specific therapies for TPNI, as the underlying mechanisms may be different. Further randomized, double-blind, placebo-controlled trials specifically examining the aforementioned therapies in this situation are necessary before specific guidelines or recommendations can be made. Until this literature exists, the managing provider must continue to extrapolate information from other neuropathic pain syndromes.

DISCLAIMER

The opinions or assertions contained herein are the private views of the authors and are not to be construed as official or as reflecting the views of the Department of the Army, the Navy, or the Department of Defense.

REFERENCES

1. Noble J, Munro CA, Prasad VS, Midha R. Analysis of upper and lower extremity peripheral nerve injuries in a population of patients with multiple injuries. *J Trauma*. 1998;45(1):116–122.
2. Cosgrove JL, Vargo M, Reidy ME. A prospective study of peripheral nerve lesions occurring in traumatic brain-injured patients. *Am J Phys Med Rehabil*. 1989;68:15–17.
3. Garland DE, Bailey S. Undetected injuries in head-injured adults. *Clin Orthop Relat Res*. 1981;155:162–165.
4. Stone L, Keenan MA. Peripheral nerve injuries in the adult with traumatic brain injury. *Clin Orthop Relat Res*. 1988;233:136–144.
5. Kouyoumdjian JA. Peripheral nerve injuries: a retrospective survery of 456 cases. *Muscle Nerve*. 2006;34:785–788.
6. Nelson KA, Park KM, Robinovitz E, et al. High-dose oral dextromethorphan versus placebo in painful diabetic neuropathy and postherpetic neuralgia. *Neurology*. 1997;48(5):1212–1218.
7. Robinson LR. Traumatic injury to peripheral nerves. *Muscle Nerve*. 2000;23(6):863–873.
8. Haymaker W, Woodhall B. *Peripheral Nerve Injuries*. Philadelphia: W.B. Saunders; 1953:333.

9. Seddon HJ. *Surgical Disorders of the Peripheral Nerves*. 2nd ed. New York: Churchill Livingstone; 1975:21–23.

10. Sunderland S. *Nerves and Nerve Injuries*. 2nd ed. New York: Churchill Livingstone; 1978:133–138.

11. Maricevic A, Erceg M. War injuries to the extremities. *Milit Med*. 1997;162(12):808–811.

12. Campbell WW. Evaulation and management of peripheral nerve injury. *Clin Neurophysiol*. 2008;119:1951–1965.

13. Sunderland S. The anatomy and physiology of nerve injury. *Muscle Nerve*. 1990; 13(9):771–784.

14. Dumitru D, Zwarts MJ, Amato AA. Peripheral nervous system's reaction to injury. In: Dumitru D, Amato AA, Zwarts M, eds. *Electrodiagnostic medicine*. 2nd ed. Philadelphia: Hanley and Belfus; 2001:115–156.

15. Höke A. Mechanisms of Disease: what factors limit the success of peripheral nerve regeneration in humans? *Nat Clin Pract Neurol*. 2006

16. Mackinnon SE, Dellon AL. *Surgery of the Peripheral Nerve*. New York: Thieme; 1988.

17. Koeppen AH. Wallerian degeneration: history and clinical significance. *J Neurol Sci*. 2004;220 (1–2):115–117.

18. Stoll G, Muller W. Nerve injury, axonal degeneration and neural regeneration: basic insights. *Brain Pathol*. 1999;9(2):313–325.

19. Chaudhry V, Glass JD, Griffin JW. Wallerian degeneration in peripheral nerve disease. *Neurol Clin*. 1992;10(3):613–627.

19a. Devor M, Wall PD. Cross-excitation in dorsal root ganglia of nerve injured and intact rats. *J Neurophysiol*. 1990;64:1733–1746.

20. Ebenezer GJ, McArthur JC, Thomas D, Murinson B, Hauer P, Polydefkis M, Griffin JW. Denervation of skin in neuropathies: the sequence of axonal and Schwann cell changes in skin biopsies. *Brain* 2007;130(Pt 10):2703–2714.

21. Hall SM. Regeneration in the peripheral nervous system. *Neuropathol Appl Neurobiol*. 1989; 15(6):513–529.

22. Kang H, Tian L, Thompson W. Terminal Schwann cells guide the reinnervation of muscle after nerve injury. *J Neurocytol*. 2003;32(5–8):975–985.

23. Selzer ME. Nerve regeneration. *Semin Neurol*. 1987;7(1):88–96.

24. Burnett MG, Zager EL. Pathophysiology of peripheral nerve injury: a brief review. *Neurosurg Focus*. 2004;16(5):E1.

25. Zochodne DW, Levy D. Nitric oxide in damage, disease and repair of the peripheral nervous system. *Cell Mol Biol (Noisy -le-grand)*. 005; 51(3):255–267.

26. Fowler TJ, Danta G, Gilliatt RW. Recovery of nerve conduction after a pneumatic tourniquet: observations on the hindlimb of the baboon. *J Neurol Neurosurg Psychiatry*. 1972;35: 638–647.

27. Hoffman H. Local reinnervation in partially denervated muscle: a histophysiological study. *Aust J Exp Biol Med Sci*. 1950;28:383.

28. Seckel BR. Enhancement of peripheral nerve regeneration. *Muscle Nerve*. 1990; 13(9): 785–800.

29. Liuzzi FJ, Tedeschi B. Peripheral nerve regeneration. *Neurosurg Clin North Am*. 1991;2(1): 31–42.

30. Seitz RJ, Reiners K, Himmelmann F, Heininger K, Hartung HP, Toyka KV. The blood-nerve barrier in Wallerian degeneration: a sequential long-term study. *Muscle Nerve*. 1989;12(8):627–635.

31. Zheng M, Kuffler DP. Guidance of regenerating motor axons in vivo by gradients of diffusible peripheral nerve-derived factors. *J Neurobiol*. 2000;42(2):212–219.

32. Fu SY, Gordon T. The cellular and molecular basis of peripheral nerve regeneration. *Mol Neurobiol*. 1997;14:67–116.

33. Chierzi S, Ratto GM, Verma P, Fawcett JW. The ability of axons to regenerate their growth cones depends on axonal type and age, and is regulated by calcium, cAMP and ERK. *Eur J Neurosci*. 2005;21(8):2051–2062.

34. Krystosek A, Seeds NW. Plasminogen activator release at the neuronal growth cone. *Science*. 1981;213(4515):1532–1534.

35. Gallo G, Letourneau P. Axon guidance: proteins turnover in turning growth cones. *Curr Biol*. 2002;12:R560–R562.

36. Kuffler DP. Promoting and directing axonal outgrowth. *Mol Neurobiol*. 1994;9:233–243.

37. Ebenezer GJ, O'Donnell R, Hauer P, Cimino NP, McArthur JC, Polydefkis M. Impaired neurovascular repair in subjects with diabetes following experimental intracutaneous axotomy. *Brain*. 2011 Jun;134(Pt 6): 1853–1863.

38. Seddon HJ. Nerve grafting. *J Bone Joint Surg (Br)*. 1963;45:447–455.

39. Speidel CC. Studies of living nerves: growth adjustments of cutaneous terminal arborization. *J Comp Neurol*. 1942;76:57–73.

40. Weddell G, Glees P. The early stages in the degeneration of cutaneous nerve fibers. *J Anat*. 1941;76:65–93.

41. Campbell WW. *Dejong's the Neurologic Examination*. 6th ed. Philadelphia: Lippincott, Williams & Wilkins; 2005.

42. Tinel J. Nerve wounds: symptomatology of peripheral nerve lesions caused by war wounds. In: Joll CA, ed. Trans. F. Rothwell. New York: William Wood Co.; 1918.

43. Partanen JV, Danner R. Fibrillation potentials after muscle injury in humans. *Muscle Nerve*. 1982;5:S70–S73.

44. Kline DG. Clinical and electrical evaluation. In: Kim DH, Midha R, Murovic JA, Spinner RJ, eds. Kline and Hudson's Nerve Injuries. 2nd ed. Philadelphia: Elsevier; 2008:43–63

45. Yaksh TL, Chaplan SR. Physiology and pharmacology of neuropathic pain. *Anesthesiol Clin North Am*. 1997;15(2):335–352.

46. Dworkin RH, Backonja M, Rowbotham MC, et al. Advances in neuropathic pain: diagnosis, mechanisms and treatment recommendations. *Arch Neurol*. 2003;60:1524–1534.

47. Chung K, Kim HJ, Na HS, et al. Abnormalities of sympathetic innervations in the area of an injured peripheral nerve in a rat model of neuropathic pain. *Neurosci Lett*. 1993;182:85–88.

48. Sato J, Perl ER. Adrenergic excitation of cutaneous pain receptors induced by peripheral nerve injury. *Science*. 1991;251:1608–1610.

49. Devor M, Govrin-Lippmann R, Angelides K. Na⁺ channel immunolocalization in peripheral mammalian axons and changes following nerve injury and neuroma formation. *J Neurosci*. 1993;13:1976–1992.

50. Xiao W, Xie Y. Ca²⁺ channels and the abnormal electrical activity of demyelinated nerve. *Chung Kuo I Hsueh Yuan Hsueh Pao*. 1992;14:59–62

51. Xie YK, Xiao WH, Li HQ. The relationship between new ion channels and ectopic discharges from a region of nerve injury. *Sci China B*. 1993;36:68–74.

52. Devor M. Neuropathic pain and injured nerve-peripheral mechanisms. *Br Med Bull*. 1991;47:619–630.

53. Mclachlan EM, Janig W, Devor M, et al. Peripheral nerve injury triggers noradrenergic sprouting within dorsal root ganglia. *Nature*. 1993;363:543–546.

54. Cheing GLY, Luk MLM. Transcutaneous electrical nerve stimulation for neuropathic pain *J Hand Surg* (British and European Volume). 2005;30B;1:50–55.

55. Garrison CJ, Dougherty PM, Kajander KC, et al. Staining of glial fibrillary acidic protein (GFAP) in lumbar spinal cord increases following a sciatic nerve constriction injury. *Brain Res*. 1991;565:1–7.

56. Todd AJ, Sullivan AC. Light microscope study of the coexistence of GABA-like and glycine-like immunoreactivities in the spinal cord of a rat. *J Comp Neurol*. 1990;296:496–505.

57. Gilman S, Newman SW. *Manter and Gatz's Essentials of Clinical Neuroanatomy and Neurophysiology*. 9th ed. Philadelphia; F.A. Davis; 1996:237–250.

58. Jorum E, Warncke T, Stubbhaug A. Cold allodynia and hyperalgesia in neuropathic pain: the effect of N-methyl-D-aspartate(NMDA) receptor antagonist ketamine—a double-blind, cross-over comparison with alfentanil and placebo. *Pain*. 2003;101:229–235.

59. Leung A, Wallace MS, Ridgeway B, Yaksh T. Concentration-effect relationship of intravenous alfentil and ketamine on peripheral neurosensory thresholds, allodynia and hyperalgesia of neuropathic pain. *Pain*. 2001;91:177–187.

60. Yaksh TL. The spinal pharmacology of facilitation of afferent processing evoked by high-threshold afferent input of the postinjury pain state. *Curr Opin Neurol Neurosurg*. 1993;6:250–256.

61. Max MB, Byas-Smith MG, Gracely RH, Bennett GJ. Intravenous infusion of the NMDA antagonist, ketamine, in chronic posttraumatic pain with allodynia: a double-blind comparison to alfentanil and placebo. *Clin Neuropharmacol*. 1995;18(4):360–368.

62. Gordh T, Stubhaug A, Jensen TS, et al. Gabapentin in traumatic nerve injury pain: a randomized, double-blind, placebo-controlled, cross-over, multi-center study. *Pain*. 2008;138:255–266.

63. Van Seventeer R, Murphy K, Temple J, et al. Pregabalin is effective in the treatment of posttraumatic peripheral neuropathic pain. *J Pain*. 2009;10(4 supp 1):S35.

64. Devor M, Wall PD, Catalan N. Systemic lidocaine silences ectopic neuroma and DRG discharges without blocking nerve conduction. *Pain*. 1992;48:261–268.

65. Tanelian DL, MacIver MB. Analgesic concentrations of lidocaine suppress tonic A-fiber and C-fiber discharges produced by acute injury. *Anesthesiology*. 1991;74:934–936.

66. Attal N, Rouaud J, Brasseur M, Chauvin M, Bouhassira D. Systemic lidocaine in pain due to peripheral nerve injury and predictors of response. *Neurology*. 2004;62:218–225.

67. Mao J, Chen LL. Systemic lidocaine for neuropathic pain. *Pain*. 2000;8:7–17.

68. Marchetiini P, Lacerenza M, Marangoni C, Pellegata G, Sotgiu ML, Smirne S. Lidocaine test in neuralgia. *Pain*. 1992;48:377–382.

69. Kingery WS. A critical review of controlled clinical trials for peripheral neuropathic pain and complex regional pain syndromes. *Pain*. 1997;73:123–129.

70. Chabal C, Jacobson L, Mariano A, Chaney E, Brittell, CW. The use of oral mexilitene for the treatment of pain after peripheral nerve injury. *Anesthesiology*. 1992;76:513–517.

71. Arner S, Meyerson BA. Lack of analgesic effect of opioids on neuropathic and idiopathic forms of pain. *Pain*. 1988;33:11–23.

72. Lombard MC, Besson JM. Attempts to gauge the relative importance of pre- and postsynaptic effects of morphine on the transmission of noxious messages in the dorsal horn of the rat spinal cord. *Pain*. 1989;37:335–345.

73. Zin CS, Nissen LN, Smith MT, et al. An update on the pharmacological management of postherpetic neuralgia and painful diabetic neuropathy. *CNS Drugs*. 2008;22(5):417–442.

74. Woolf CJ, Thompson SWN. The induction and maintenance of central sensitization is dependent on N-methyl-D-aspartate acid receptor activity: implication for the treatment of post-injury pain hypersensitivity. *Pain*. 1991;44:293–299.

75. Backonja M, Arndt G, Gombar KA, Check B, Zimmermann M. Response of chronic neuropathic pain syndromes to ketamine: a preliminary study published erratum. *Pain*. 1994; 56(1):51–57.

76. Eide PK, Jorum E, Stubhaug A, Bremnes J, Breivik H. Relief of postherpetic neuralgia with the N-methyl-D-aspartic acid receptor antagonist ketamine: a double-blind, cross-over comparison with morphine, and placebo. *Pain*. 1994; 58:347–354.

77. Felsby S, Nielsen J, Arendt-Nielsen L, Jensen TS. NMDA receptor blockade in chronic neuropathic pain; a comparison of ketamine and magnesium chloride. *Pain*. 1996;64:283–291.

78. Sunder R, Toshniwal G, Dureja GP. Ketamine as an adjuvant in sympathetic blocks for management of central sensitization following peripheral nerve injury. *J Brachial Plexus Peripher Nerve Inj*. 2008;3:22–28.

79. Cohen SP, Verdolin MH, Change AS, et al. The intravenous ketamine test predicts subsequent response to an oral dextromethorphan treatment regimen in fibromyalgia patients. *J Pain*. 2006;7(6):391–398.

80. Cohen SP, Wang S, Chen L, et al. An intravenous ketamine test as a predictive response tool in opioid-exposed patients with persistent pain. *J Pain Symptom Manage*. 2009;37(4): 698–708.

81. Sang CN, Booher S, Gilron I, et al. Dextromethorphan and memantine in painful diabetic neuropathy and postherpetic neuralgia; efficacy and dose-response trials. *Anesthesiology*. 2002;96(5):1053–10061.

82. Richman JM, Spencer SL, Courpas G, et al. Does continuous peripheral nerve block provide superior pain control to opioids? A meta-analysis. *Reg Anesth*. 2006;102: 248–257.

83. Rho RH, Brewer RP, Lamer TJ, Wilson PR. Complex regional pain syndrome. *Mayo Clin Proc*. 2002;77(2):174–180.

84. Attal N, Cruccu G, Haanpaa M, et al. EFNS guidelines on pharmacological treatment of neuropathic pain. *Eur J Neurol*. 2006;13: 1153–1169.

85. Finnerup NB, Otto M, McQuay HJ, et al. Algorithm for neuropathic pain treatment: an evidence based proposal. *Pain*. 2005;118: 289–305.

86. Cruccu G, Aziz TZ, Garcia-Larrea L, et al. EFNS guidelines on neurostimulation therapy for neruopathic pain. *Eur J Neurol*. 2007;14 :952–970.

87. Fukazawa Y, Maeda T, Hamabe W, et al. Activation of spinal anti-analgesic system following electroacupuncture stimulation in rats. *J Pharmacol Sci*. 2005;99:408–414.

88. Law JD, Swett J, Kirsch WM. Retrospective analysis of 22 patients with chronic pain treated by peripheral nerve stimulation. *J Neurosurg*. 1980;52(4):482–485.

89. Lazorthes Y, Siegfried J, Verdie JC, Casaux J. Chronic spinal cord stimulation in the treatment of neurogenic pain. Cooperative and retrospective study on 20 years of follow-up. *Neurochirurgie*. 1995;41(2):73–86.

19

Chronic Postsurgical Pain

KAYODE A. WILLIAMS, STEVEN P. COHEN, AND SRINIVASA N. RAJA

INTRODUCTION

AS OUR POPULATION has aged, the number of surgeries performed each year has increased both in absolute numbers and on a per capita basis.[1,2] In conjunction with the growing sophistication of these surgeries, morbidity and mortality have continued to decline, mostly as a result of improved anesthetic techniques. These facts have led to increased weight being given to improving secondary outcome measures, such as functional capacity and psychological well-being. This emphasis is seen perhaps most prominently in efforts to prevent and treat chronic postsurgical pain (CPSP).

Most patients who undergo surgery recover uneventfully and resume their normal lives within several weeks. But a substantial number develop debilitating chronic pain that can interfere with their professional, social, and psychological well-being. Similar to the treatment of other pain conditions, a multimodal approach that identifies those patients at risk for CPSP, undertakes rational preemptive measures, minimizes iatrogenic trauma, utilizes aggressive postsurgical analgesic techniques, addresses coexisting psychopathology that can exacerbate or even precipitate neuropathic pain states, and assumes appropriate postprocedure surveillance is imperative to controlling this underappreciated yet burgeoning issue.

DEFINITIONS AND DIAGNOSIS

The definition of CPSP itself is problematic. Extrapolating from definitions for chronic pain, one might logically define it as pain that lasts longer than the temporal course of natural healing associated with the operation[3] or pain persisting for more than 3 months after surgery.[4] No single definition for CPSP is currently accepted, and controversy exists about whether universally acknowledged standard reference criteria are even possible. Hence, the diagnosis is generally one of exclusion. One must first rule out a recurrence of the initial surgical pathology, such as a recurrent hernia (inguinal or abdominal), and then exclude a new pathological condition (e.g., pneumothorax). The pattern and character of the pain can also help increase the index of suspicion that the pain generator is unlikely to be of visceral or somatic origin. In 1999, Macrae[5] proposed a definition for CPSP based on four criteria: (1) development after a surgical procedure; (2) duration ≥2 months; (3) exclusion of other causes; and (4) an attempt to explore and exclude the possibility that the pain persists from a preexisting problem. However, this definition itself is fraught with inherent dilemmas.

For many surgical procedures associated with high prevalence rates of CPSP, such as inguinal herniorrhaphy and laminectomy/spinal arthrodesis, one of the prime indications for the intervention itself is pain. Many patients who undergo spinal decompression, gallbladder removal, or hernia repair present with minimal or ambiguous pathology, which can make distinguishing the preexisting condition from iatrogenic-induced pain extremely challenging. The International Statistical Classification of Diseases and Health Related Problems (ICD-9-CM codes) tabular index attempts to bypass this distinction for certain conditions with diagnostic codes that do not imply an etiology (e.g., 722.8, postlaminectomy syndrome; 576, postcholecystectomy pain). As it is not always possible to discriminate among the different causes of CPSP, for definitional purposes per se, it may be more prudent not to try to distinguish between pain that ensues after surgery and that which preceded it (Table 19.1).

CLINICAL FEATURES

The clinical features of postsurgical pain are a function of the type of surgery that precipitates the symptoms. Regardless of the causative factor, most patients use typical descriptors of neuropathic pain to describe their symptoms, such as "shooting," "burning," and "stabbing." The pain is typically limited to the region of the surgery or around the scar. The patients may complain of associated symptoms, including dysuria or testicular pain after hernia repair, pleuritic pain after thoracotomy, radiation into

Table 19-1. Classification of Different Types of CPSP

PERSISTENT PRESURGICAL PAIN	PAIN 2° INTRAOPERATIVE TRAUMA	PAIN 2° POSTOPERATIVE FACTORS
Incorrect diagnosis	Surgical factors Nerve injury/entrapment Prolonged postoperative pain	Deafferentation (e.g., phantom limb pain)
Wrong operation	Anesthetic factors Neuropraxia from positioning Nerve injury during blocks Ischemic nerve or tissue damage	Recurrence (e.g., herniated disc, cancer)
Technically unsuccessful operation (e.g., pseudoarthrosis, hardware malfunction)		Abnormal tissue growth (heterotopic ossification, adhesive scar tissue, seroma)
Incomplete resolution (e.g., incomplete tumor resection)		Predictable sequelae (e.g., instability after spine decompression, back pain after lower limb amputation, adjacent segment disease after fusion)

the ipsilateral arm after mastectomy, and phantom sensations following limb amputation.

EPIDEMIOLOGY

The prevalence rate of CPSP is likely contingent on multiple factors (Table19.2), though the precise role each plays in the pathogenesis needs to be better elucidated. Because many of the factors affecting the development of CPSP are dynamic (e.g., demographics of surgical patients, breakdown of operations), one should expect the incidence to vary in concert. In addition to changing demographic and clinical factors, both the method and the frequency of surveillance can influence estimates of CPSP.[6] For example, whereas crude early estimates of the incidence of phantom limb pain were routinely less than 5%,[7,8] more recent sophisticated measures have gauged the incidence at between 50% and 80%[9,10]

Nonetheless, several investigators have attempted to quantify the scope of CPSP. Perhaps as a result of variability in definitions and surveillance methods, these estimates vary widely, from less than 0.5%[11] to upward of 10%. In one prospective study, Hayes et al. and Visser estimated the prevalence of neuropathic pain 1 year after surgery to be between 0.5% and 1.5%.; this was corroborated in a subsequent epidemiological review by Visser[12,13] Among patients who seek medical attention at

pain management clinics, surgery is a contributing factor in approximately 20% of cases.[14] Table 19.3 lists the estimated incidence rates of CPSP stratified by type of surgery.

FINANCIAL BURDEN

Although it is generally well accepted that CPSP is associated with substantial socioeconomic consequences,[15,16] there is a glaring absence of literature regarding the economic and psychosocial burdens created by the condition. To appreciate the societal burden of CPSP, one must therefore extrapolate from the few studies that have examined the quality-of-life (QOL) and economic costs of neuropathic pain.

Multiple studies have found that neuropathic pain can negatively impact a broad range of QOL issues and that the effects may be greater than those for chronic nociceptive pain.[17] Indeed, some evidence indicates that pain can actually cause depression and other psychological conditions in addition to impeding functional capacity.[18] Not surprisingly, the degree of

Table 19-2. Factors Affecting the Incidence of CPSP

Genetic background

Younger age

Female gender

Opioid-induced hyperalgesia

Intensity and duration of pain

Presence of coexisting pain disorders

Educational level

Psychosocial factors

Anesthesia regimen

Surgical trauma

Type of surgery and technique (i.e., laparoscopic vs. open)

Table 19-3. Estimated Incidence of Chronic Pain After Surgical Procedures

TYPE OF SURGERY	INCIDENCE OF CHRONIC PAIN
Mastectomy	20%–50%
Thoracotomy	30%–60%
Inguinal hernia repair	5%–35%
Sternotomy	30%–50%
Major limb amputation	30%–80%
Cholecystectomy	10%–40%
Vasectomy	5%–20%
Cesarean section	5%–10%
Craniotomy	10%–25%
Hip or knee arthroplasty	15%–40%
Dental surgery	5%–15%
Radical prostatectomy	10%–25%
Breast augmentation	15%–35%

Source: Visser EJ. Chronic post-surgical pain: epidemiology and clinical implications for acute pain management. Acute Pain. 2006;8:73–81; Macrae WA. Chronic post-surgical pain: 10 years on. Br J Anaesth. 2008;101:77–86; Akkaya T, Ozkan D. Chronic post-surgical pain. Agr.i 2009;21:1–9.

neuropathic pain has been directly correlated with the extent of QOL degradation,[19] and improvement in pain is correspondingly associated with improvement in QOL.[20]

The economic burden of CPSP can be attributed to several different factors, including but not limited to medication costs, physician and other health care visits, missed work days, hospitalizations, and diagnostic and therapeutic interventions. A study by Dworkin et al.[21] estimated the health care expenditures attributed to postherpetic neuralgia to range between $2200 and $5400 per patient during the year after herpes zoster diagnosis. In another retrospective study involving 504 consecutive patients with neuropathic pain treated in pain clinics across Spain, Rodriguez and Garcia[22] estimated the average cost of health care to be 363 euros per month, with the bulk of the expenditures resulting from hospitalizations and medication costs. Finally, the economic burden of acute herpes zoster in the United Kingdom was assessed by prospectively following 186 newly diagnosed patients for 6 months.[23] The investigators found that the average patient missed 4.4 days of work over the study period. Whereas medical expenses comprised the majority of costs for elderly patients, a decreased capacity to work accounted for most of the costs in individuals less than 65 years of age.

RISK FACTORS AND PREDICTORS OF CPSP

In recent years, the predictive factors for persistent pain after surgery have been studied following various surgical procedures. These studies have identified a number of preoperative and host-related factors, as well as surgical, intraoperative, and postoperative risk factors.[24–26] Chronic pain after surgery is commonly neuropathic in nature, and like most neuropathic pain states, it remains a therapeutic challenge. Hence, understanding the risk factors and developing preventive strategies is important.

Several potential risk factors have been associated with an increased likelihood of developing chronic pain. These include the duration of surgery, low-volume surgical units, open versus endoscopic approach, pericostal versus intercostal stitches, conventional hernia repair, and intraoperative nerve damage.[27,28] There is no conclusive evidence of a direct causative relationship between these factors and CPSP, but one common element is the presence of greater surgical trauma and possible intraoperative nerve injury. This acute nerve injury is thought to be associated with changes in the injured nerves, neighboring nerves, and the central nervous system. Evidence from animal studies shows that injury to peripheral nerves results in long-lasting, high-frequency bursts of activity. This activity sensitizes the nociceptive pathways through the N-methyl-D-aspartate receptors in the central nervous system.[29] A rat model for post-laparotomy pain in which a subcostal incision was made to enter the peritoneal cavity revealed a 50% decrease in locomotor activity 24 hours after surgery. This reduction in locomotor activity was reversed by morphine and ketorolac, suggesting behavioral aspects akin to postoperative pain.[30]

Preoperative and Host-Related Factors

PREOPERATIVE PAIN

A consistent patient-related factor associated with CPSP is the presence of pain preoperatively, either as the indication for surgery or at an unrelated site. In a survey examining the presence of CPSP after hysterectomy, a prevalence of 31.9% was observed 1 year after surgery. The risk factors identified by multiple logistic regression were preoperative pelvic pain, pain as an indication for surgery, previous cesarean delivery, and pain problems elsewhere.[31] A subsequent prospective study in patients undergoing hysterectomy also revealed that preoperative pain problems elsewhere were associated with the presence of pain 4 months after hysterectomy.[31] A similar tendency, although not statistically significant, was seen for preoperative pelvic pain.

PSYCHOLOGICAL FACTORS

A number of psychosocial predictors of chronic postsurgical pain and/or disability have been identified.[32–35] These include fear of surgery, traits such as increased preoperative anxiety, introverted personality, catastrophizing, and psychic vulnerability. The effect of presurgical psychological distress and somatic preoccupation in predicting persistent pain after reconstructive surgery postmastectomy was examined prospectively in 295 women. Abdominal and back pains were significantly associated with affective distress, depressive and anxiety symptoms, and somatization. These psychological measures also predicted more severe breast pain 1 year after reconstructive surgery.[36]

GENETIC FACTORS

Studies in experimental animals and human twins suggest a role for genetic factors in the risk of developing chronic pain. The screening of hundreds of genes regulated in the dorsal root ganglia following peripheral nerve injury helped to identify the gene encoding for guanosine triphosphate cyclohydrolase 1 (GCH1). The GCH1 enzyme catalyzes tetrahydrobiopterin (BH4), an essential cofactor for the production of several mediators that are increased in peripheral inflammation and injury (e.g., catecholamine, serotonin, and nitric oxide).[37] In humans, the presence of a haplotype of GCH1 (population frequency 15.4%) was associated with a lower frequency of persistent radiculopathic pain after surgical discectomy.[37] Other genes with identified polymorphisms have also been implicated in chronic pain. These include the genes encoding a serotonin transporter, 5-HTTLPR, and the enzyme COMT (catechol-O-methyltransferase), which inactivates dopamine, epinephrine, and norepinephrine in the nervous system. A future goal is the genotyping of a panel of "pain genes" for patients undergoing surgery with the objective of accurately predicting the patient's risk for postprocedural pain and the response to various analgesics.

Surgicaland Intraoperative Factors

SURGICAL FACTORS

A retrospective study of 243 patients who underwent video-assisted thoracoscopy or thoracotomy suggested that younger age, radiotherapy, pleurectomy, and more extensive surgery were predictive of CPSP. A survey of postmastectomy patients indicated that the surgical site may be a potential risk factor for persistent pain. Women who had undergone right-sided mastectomy were more likely to report the current presence of breast pain, more likely to have experienced phantom breast pain, and more likely to describe themselves as disabled.[38] Pain-related sequelae (e.g., work disability) were also more common following right-sided mastectomy. It is unclear whether other types of surgery show a similar laterality effect.

ANESTHETIC MANAGEMENT

In an epidemiological survey study that examined risk factors for persistent pain after hysterectomy, spinal anesthesia but not epidural anesthesia was associated with a reduced risk of chronic pain 1 year after surgery.[31] This observation is consistent with the finding that spinal anesthesia was associated with a lower frequency of chronic pain 1 year after cesarean delivery than general anesthesia.[39] It is postulated that the more complete blockade of central impulse traffic in spinal anesthesia may exert a protective effect against the development of chronic pain.

Postoperative Factors

ACUTE POSTOPERATIVE PAIN

A reliable predictor of persistent pain after surgery is the intensity of pain in the early postoperative period. The primary predictor of chronic pain 18 months after thoracotomy with a lateral incision was the pain intensity at rest and with movement 24 hours after surgery.[40] A prospective study of hysterectomy patients also revealed that high acute postoperative pain intensity was associated with the presence of pain 4 months after the procedure.[41] Similarly, Taillefer and coworkers showed that patients undergoing cardiac surgery who had greater analgesic needs while hospitalized were more at risk of reporting CPSP up to 3 years after the operation.[42] Studies comparing different analgesic strategies in the postoperative period also have shown that interventions resulting in decreased postoperative pain or a reduced area of hyperalgesia surrounding the wound are associated with decreased CPSP.[43,44]

POSTTRAUMATIC STRESS DISORDER

Recent studies indicate that posttraumatic stress symptoms are associated with CPSP months to years later. Katz and Seltzer prospectively examined the relationship between posttraumatic stress symptoms and CPSP in patients undergoing thoracotomies.[45] They observed incidence rates of 68.1% and 61.1% at 6- and 12-month follow-up visits, respectively. Emotional numbing, but not avoidance symptoms, contributed substantially to the explanation of pain disability at the two follow-up time points. The mechanisms underlying these relationships have yet to be determined.

TYPES OF CPSP

Postmastectomy Pain

Persistent postmastectomy pain is quite common and has been classified into three distinct types: phantom breast pain, scar pain, and other mastectomy-related pain (e.g., in the medial aspect of the arm in the distribution of the intercosto-brachial nerve). In a study conducted at Johns Hopkins University, Baltimore, Maryland USA, 278 women who were, on average, several years postmastectomy completed questionnaires assessing pain, pain-related physical function, and psychosocial distress. The three types of postmastectomy pain were strongly related to one another (i.e., women reporting one type of pain were more likely to report the other types as well). In general, the degree of disability and distress was proportionate to the number of postmastectomy pain categories that a woman reported.[46]

Postthoracotomy Pain

The International Association for the Study of Pain (IASP) defines chronic postthoracotomy pain as "pain that recurs or persists along a thoracotomy incision at least two months following the surgical procedure."[47] Chronic postthoracotomy pain syndrome (PTPS) has been recognized as a chronic pain condition only

within the last six to seven decades. Though the first intercostal thoracotomy was described in 1892, PTPS was first reported in 1944 by U.S. army surgeons, who observed that men who underwent thoracotomy for chest trauma experienced chronic intercostal pain. They also noted the difficulties associated with treatment and return to function. Five decades passed before there was a resurgence of interest in this condition. In a study of 56 patients followed for 5 years postthoracotomy, Dajczman et al. found that 50% of the patients had chronic postthoracotomy pain at 4 years.[48] A subsequent study by Pertunnen et al.[48a] revealed the incidence of PTPS to be 80% at 3 months.

Several, pre-, intra-, and postoperative factors have been suggested as contributing to the development of PTPS. Preoperative factors include the primary etiology (e.g., the presence of an invading intrathoracic tumor), tumor recurrence, and the presence of preoperative pain requiring analgesics.[49] Factors related to surgical technique have also been implicated. The main surgical approaches for thoracotomy include a posterolateral approach, which may be muscle sparing if the latissimus dorsi muscle is retracted and not incised, an auxiliary approach, and an anterior approach, both of which spare the muscle. In a review of the literature, Kehlet Aasvang et al. revealed that there was no difference in the incidence of PTPS with the type of incision (i.e., with or without muscle sparing).[50] (However Normori et al. compared the classical posterolateral approach with the anterior access approach and reported that the anterior access approach was associated with a lower incidence of PTPS.[51]) Video-assisted thoracoscopic surgery (VATS) has been developed recently, after the introduction of a cystoscope into the pleural cavity in 1913, in order to lyse adhesions to treat tuberculosis. The technique has gained increasing popularity over the last 20 years as a means of reducing the morbidity associated with thoracotomies. This novel approach is based on the assumption that multiple small incisions through which the scopes can be manipulated result in less tissue trauma than one longer incision. In their review, Kehlet Aasvang et al. reported that one prospective trial comparing muscle-sparing posterolateral thoracotomy (PLT) and VATS found no difference in the incidence of PTPS; the same conclusion was drawn in a similar study that compared non-muscle-sparing PLT with VATS. However, in the same review, the authors examined a large retrospective study that demonstrated a reduction in the incidence of PTPS in patients who had a VATS procedure compared to those who had the muscle-sparing PLT. The authors concluded that a more detailed prospective study that carefully matched patient populations for pre-, intra-, and postsurgical factors would be necessary to clearly elucidate the impact of the different surgical approaches on the incidence of PTPS. Finally, the influence of the loss of superficial abdominal reflexes as a measure of loss of lower intercostal nerve function following a PLT approach was examined by Benedetti et al.[52] The authors found that both acute and chronic pain reflected nerve damage, and that chronic pain and analgesic consumption increased in the patients with postoperative loss of superficial abdominal reflexes.

Very few randomized, controlled studies have examined the surgical risk factors for PTPS, and even fewer have included all of the pre-, intra-, and postoperative factors that may contribute to the development of PTPS. Thus, the preventive and treatment strategies currently available are limited, and treatment outcomes remain variable. The overall treatment approach will be reviewed later in this chapter.

Postamputation Pain

Postamputation pain syndromes refer to both residual limb (stump) pain and phantom limb pain, two pain conditions usually associated with the loss of an extremity or part of the limb. Pain in the residual body part and phantom pains also have been reported after the loss of other body parts, including the tongue, nose, bladder, and testes. Phantom limb and stump pain were recognized by the French military surgeon Ambrose Pare as early as the mid-sixteenth century. In 1870, S. Weir Mitchell recorded his observations of the magnitude of suffering associated with this type of pain in the U.S. Civil War and is credited with coining the term *phantom limb pain*. Research conducted over the last few decades has provided greater insight into the mechanisms responsible for phantom and residual limb pains.

Phantom Limb Pain

Phantom limb pain is defined as chronic pain perceived in the absent body part. Phantom limb pain occurs in 60%–80% of patients, irrespective of the cause of amputation, and diminishes over time.[53] Although the incidence of phantom limb pain is reported to increase with more proximal amputations, the incidence in the upper and lower extremities varies widely—as high as 72% in the lower extremity and as low as 51% in the upper extremity.[54,55] Phantom limb pain has been reported to begin as early as 1 day and as late as 40 years after the amputation.[56] The intensity of phantom limb pain may decrease over time, and eventually the pain may resolve; however, studies have shown that even at 2 years, up to 60% of patients still experience this type of pain.

The etiology and pathophysiological mechanisms of phantom limb pain have not been clearly elucidated. Peripheral and central neuronal mechanisms have been implicated, but none independently accounts for the characteristics of the condition. Three possibilities are considered important. First, it has been observed that in the periphery, spontaneous and abnormal evoked activity results after mechanical or neurochemical stimulation of neuromas.[57] Increased neurochemical sensitivity in the nerve endings may partly explain the exacerbation of phantom limb pain by stress and other emotional states associated with increased catecholamine release. The increased activity is thought to be related to upregulation of sodium channels[58] and has been demonstrated in the cells of dorsal root ganglia. Second, increased activity in dorsal root ganglia is assumed to be associated with long-term changes in the dorsal horn manifested by increased neuronal activity, elaboration of immediate early genes, and expansion of receptive fields. Increased activity in the NMDA receptor-operated systems may result in central sensitization. This central sensitization has been demonstrated to be reduced by the effects of NMDA receptor antagonists and confirmed in human amputees.[59] Finally, supraspinal and central mechanisms that mimic these processes in the periphery and spinal cord have been suggested as possible mechanisms involved in the perception and maintenance of phantom limb pain. Thalamic stimulation, which is otherwise nonnoxious, has been shown to result in phantom pain in amputees, suggesting that the thalamus is involved in the development of chronic pain.[60] Functional imaging studies have corroborated cortical reorganization after amputation.[61-63]

The clinical presentation of postamputation pain varies with the limb or tissue involved. The areas with the highest cortical representation, such as fingers or toes, are associated with the most intense sensations. Amputees may experience "telescoping" of the limb, a phenomenon in which sensation is lost from the midportion of the amputated limb and persistent in the distal portion of the affected limb. Phantom limb pain is neuropathic in nature.[64] Pain descriptors such as "burning," "deep aching," "throbbing," "sharp," "electric shock-like," and "cramping" typify the neuropathic nature of the pain. The pain is generally intermittent, but in rare circumstances it may be constant. Stump pain differs from phantom limb pain in that the pain is limited to the stump and may be associated with spontaneous movement ranging from myoclonic jerks to severe clonic contractions. Typically, phantom limb pain remains unchanged or decreases over time. Up to 56% of patients show improvement or even complete resolution. However, if the symptoms worsen or change after a period of stability, one should suspect other possible causes. Important differential diagnoses that should be considered include radicular pain from a herniated disc, development or reactivation of postherpetic neuralgia, and possible metastatic disease in a patient whose amputation was performed for malignant disease.[65,66] The treatment options are addressed below.

Postherniorrhaphy Pain

The incidence of chronic pain after inguinal herniorrhaphy has been reported to vary from 0% to 37%.[67] In a recent retrospective study, Aasvang et al. performed a nationwide survey of 1443 patients who underwent inguinal hernia

operations between February and March 1998. Of the 1166 respondents, 335 (28.7%) reported chronic postinguinal hernia pain 1 year after hernia repair. Eleven percent of these respondents reported associated functional impairment. A follow-up study revealed that chronic pain with functional impairment decreased from approximately 11% after 1 year to 6% after 6.5 years.[68] This finding makes chronic pain perhaps one of the more important adverse outcomes of hernia surgery. Yet, to date, the exact neurophysiological changes and pathophysiological mechanisms of postherniorrhaphy pain remain unclear. In a controlled prospective trial that used quantitative sensory testing, Aasvang et al. found that large- and small-fiber dysfunction with evidence of central sensitization was more profoundly evident in postherniorrhaphy patients with pain than in the control group. Because of the correspondence between pain location and sensory disturbance, the authors concluded that the pain was neuropathic in nature; however, no conclusion could be drawn regarding the specific mechanism of nerve injury. Possible mechanisms include direct intraoperative nerve injury or secondary nerve injury resulting from an inflammatory response to the mesh.[69] Magnetic resonance imaging (MRI) has been suggested as a possible diagnostic tool using indicators such as "contrast enhancement in the groin," "edema," and "spermatic cord caliber increase." However, an initial assessment indicates that additional examination is required to identify specific MRI-assessed pathology that would minimize interobserver variation.[70]

PREVENTION OF CPSP

Intuitively, it seems likely that the use of minimally invasive surgical techniques would decrease the incidence of CPSP. However, the evidence to date is limited. Studies suggest that multimodal analgesia—the technique of combining multiple modalities of pain relief—may provide more effective analgesia than any one method, decrease the incidence of adverse effects, and result in a lower incidence of CPSP. For example, a single 1200 mg dose of gabapentin administered 1 hour before mastectomy decreased postoperative morphine consumption and pain during movement.[71] Gabapentin, as part of a multimodal analgesic regimen, also decreased the incidence of CPSP at 10 weeks after breast surgery.[72]

Free radical scavengers, such as vitamin C, N-acetyl-L-cysteine (NAC), and mannitol, are considered to be neuroprotective against excitotoxic insults. Use of vitamin C, initiated 2 days before surgery and continued for 50 days at a daily dose of 500 mg, has been suggested to reduce the prevalence of complex regional pain syndrome (CRPS) after wrist joint arthroplasty.[73] However, a recent study in which mannitol was given to 41 CRPS patients concluded that intravenous administration of 10% mannitol is no more effective than placebo in reducing complaints of CRPS I.[74]

TREATMENT

There is no specific treatment algorithm for CPSP. Postsurgical pain presents mainly as neuropathic pain, and therefore most treatment strategies have included pharmacological neuromodulators such as anticonvulsants, antidepressants, opioids, and, ultimately, neuromodulation if all other conservative treatment modalities fail (Figure 19.1). O'Connor and Dworkin recently published consensus treatment guidelines for neuropathic pain developed under the auspices of the Neuropathic Pain Special Interest Group (NeuPSIG) section of the IASP. Based on randomized, controlled trials, the consensus group recommended as first-line treatments for neuropathic pain antidepressants, including tricyclic antidepressants and dual reuptake inhibitors of both serotonin and norepinephrine; calcium channel $\alpha2\delta$ ligands, such as gabapentin and pregabalin; and topical lidocaine. Second-line agents included opioid analgesics and tramadol. The authors indicate that second-line agents can be used as first-line agents under specific clinical conditions in which the patient requires prompt relief for acute neuropathic pain, with a plan to transition to a recommended first-line agent later. Other medications that are considered third-line agents include other antidepressants and anticonvulsants, including topical

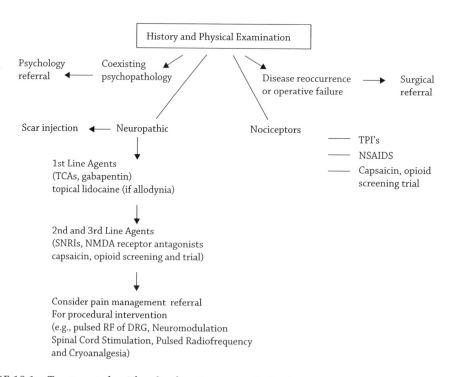

FIGURE 19.1   Treatment algorithm for chronic postsurgical pain.

capsaicin, mexiletine, and NMDA receptor antagonists.[75]

Interventional treatment modalities may be of benefit, particularly with postamputation and postthoracotomy pain. Epidural analgesia, as well as intercostal, ilioinguinal, and genitofemoral nerve blocks, may be performed to address phantom limb, postthoracotomy, and postherniorrhaphy pain. If pharmacological therapy and nerve blocks fail to provide benefit, pulsed radiofrequency of the dorsal root ganglia and spinal cord stimulation are treatment modalities that are becoming increasingly recognized as valuable tools in selected patients with neuropathic pain, including CPSP.[76,77] Pulsed radiofrequency of the dorsal root ganglia is superior to pharmacotherapy or pulsed radiofrequency of the intercostal nerves in the treatment of chronic postsurgical thoracic pain.[77]

Innovative treatment modalities have been developed to address challenging CPSP. One of them is mirror visual feedback therapy for the treatment of phantom limb pain. Mirror visual feedback therapy involves the use of visual imagery utilizing a mirror placed vertically in the sagittal plane; the amputated limb is placed behind the nonreflective side of the mirror, and the intact limb is placed opposite the reflective side. The individual is then required to move the intact limb, which is now reflected as a mirror image of the amputated limb; the individual gets a visual impression of the amputated limb obeying motor commands sent to both limbs. Since the early report of the use of mirror therapy for phantom limb pain by Ramachandran et al., other workers have replicated this work and continue to demonstrate the efficacy of mirror visual feedback therapy, both in primary outcome measures of reduction in activity-related visual analog pain scores and in secondary outcomes measures including motor function assessed by the Wolf motor function test.[78–80]

SUMMARY

Very few studies have clearly defined CPSP. The lack of an operational definition has made epidemiological research, clinical research, and cross-comparison difficult. However, CPSP is reported to occur in up to 10% of patients undergoing surgery. The type, extent, and duration of surgery are factors that affect the risk of postsurgical pain. Based on our current knowledge, avoiding surgery, whenever possible, is the only reliable preventive measure that can be taken. However, when surgery is a necessary treatment option, a high index of suspicion should exist if postoperative pain persists beyond 2–3 months. Considerable research efforts are being focused on developing a predictive risk index, that includes a combination of preoperative, intraoperative, and postoperative factors, to help identify the high risk patients for persistent pain after surgery. The early institution of a neuropathic treatment regimen, including interventional therapies such as nerve blocks, epidural injections, and spinal cord stimulation, provides the best chance of a successful treatment outcome. Innovative noninterventional treatment modalities such as mirror visual feedback therapy may form part of the armamentarium in managing challenging forms of CPSP such as phantom limb pain.

REFERENCES

1. Rutkow IM. Surgical operations in the United States: then (1983) and now (1994). *Arch Surg.* 1997;132:983–990.
2. Hospital episode statistics online, 2003-2010. http://www.hesonline.nhs.uk/Ease/servlet/ContentServer?siteID=1937&categoryID=890. Last accessed on March 2012.
3. Shipton EA, Tait B. Flagging the pain: preventing the burden of chronic pain by identifying and treating risk factors in acute pain. *Eur J Anaesth.* 2005;22(6):405–412.
4. Cohen SP, Argoff CE, Carragee EJ. Management of low back pain. *BMJ.* 2008;337:a2718.
5. Macrae WA, Davies HTO. Chronic postsurgical pain. In: Crombie IK, Linton S, Croft P, Von Korff M, LeResche L, eds. Epidemiology of pain. Seattle, IASP Press, 1999, pp 125-42.
6. Stone AA, Broderick JE, Shiffman SS, Schwartz JE. Understanding recall of weekly pain from a momentary assessment perspective: absolute agreement, between- and within-person consistency, and judged change in weekly pain. *Pain.* 2004;107:61–69.
7. Ewalt JR, Randall GC, Morris H. The phantom limb. *Psychosom Med.* 1947;9:118–123.

8. Henderson WR, Smyth GE. Phantom limbs. J Neurol Neurosurg Psychiatry. 1948;11:88–112.

9. Nikolajsen L, Ilkjær S, Jensen TS. Relationship between mechanical sensitivity and postamputation pain: a prospective study. *Eur J Pain.* 2000;4:327–334.

10. Houghton AD, Nicholls G. Phantom pain: natural history and association with rehabilitation. *Ann R Coll Surg Engl.* 1994;76:22–25.

11. Macrae WA. Chronic post-surgical pain: 10 years on. *Br J Anaesth.* 2008;101:77–86.

12. Hayes C, Browne S, Lantry G, Burstal R. Neuropathic pain in the acute pain service: a prospective survey. *Acute Pain.* 2002;4:45–48.

13. Visser EJ. Chronic post-surgical pain: epidemiology and clinical implications for acute pain management. *Acute Pain.* 2006;8:73–81.

14. Davies HT, Crombie IK, Macrae WA, Rogers KM. *Pain clinic* patients in Northern Britain. *Pain Clin.* 1992;5:129–135.

15. Akkaya T, Ozkan D. Chronic post-surgical pain. *Agri* 2009;21:1–9.

16. Galvez R, Marsal C, Vidal J, Gálvez R, Marsal C, Vidal J, Ruiz M, Rejas J. Cross-sectional evaluation of patient functioning and health-related quality of life in patients with neuropathic pain under standard care conditions. *Eur J Pain.* 2007;11:244–255.

17. Smith BHM, Torrance NM, Bennett MIM, Lee AJM. Health and quality of life associated with chronic pain of predominantly neuropathic origin in the community. *Clin J Pain.* 2007;23:143–149.

18. Jensen MP, Turner JA, Romano JM. Changes after multidisciplinary pain treatment in patient pain beliefs and coping are associated with concurrent changes in patient functioning. *Pain.* 2007;131:38–47.

19. Jensen MP, Chodroff MJ, Dworkin RH. The impact of neuropathic pain on health-related quality of life: review and implications. *Neurology.* 2007;68:1178–1182.

20. Deshpande MA, Holden RR, Gilron I. The impact of therapy on quality of life and mood in neuropathic pain: what is the effect of pain reduction? *Anesth Analg.* 2006;102:1473–1479.

21. Dworkin RH, White R, O'Connor AB, Baser O, Hawkins K. Healthcare costs of acute and chronic pain associated with a diagnosis of herpes zoster. *J Am Geriatr Soc.* 2007;55:1168–1175.

22. Rodriguez MJ, Garcia AJ. A registry of the aetiology and costs of neuropathic pain in pain clinics: results of the registry of aetiologies and costs (REC) in neuropathic pain disorders study. *Clin Drug Invest.* 2007;27:771–782.

23. Scott FT, Johnson RW, Leedham-Green M, Davies E, Edmunds WJ, Breuer J. The burden of herpes zoster: a prospective population based study. *Vaccine.* 2006;24:1308–1314.

24. Burke SN, Shorten GD. When pain after surgery doesn't go away.... *Biochem Soc Trans.* 2009;37(part 1):318–322.

25. Katz J, Seltzer Z. Transition from acute to chronic postsurgical pain: risk factors and protective factors. *Expert Rev Neurother.* 2009;9:723–744.

26. Kehlet H, Jensen TS, Woolf CJ. Persistent postsurgical pain: risk factors and prevention. *Lancet.* 2006;367:1618–1625.

27. Tasmuth T, Blomqvist C, Kalso E. Chronic posttreatment symptoms in patients with breast cancer operated in different surgical units. *Eur J Surg Oncol.* 1999;25: 38–43.

28. Liem MS, van Duyn EB, van der Graaf Y, van Vroonhoven TJ; CoalaTrial Group. Recurrences after conventional anterior and laparoscopic inguinal hernia repair: a randomized comparison. *Ann Surg.* 2003;237:136–141.

29. Seltzer Z, Cohn S, Ginzburg R, Beilin B. Modulation of neuropathic pain behavior in rats by spinal disinhibition and NMDA receptor blockade of injury discharge. *Pain.* 1991;45: 69–75.

30. Martin TJ, Buechler NL, Kahn W, Crews JC, Eisenach JC. Effects of laparotomy on spontaneous exploratory activity and conditioned operant responding in the rat. *Anesthesiology.* 2004;101:191–203.

31. Brandsborg B, Nikolajsen L, Hansen CT, Kehlet H, Jensen TS. Risk factors for chronic pain after hysterectomy: a nationwide questionnaire and database study. *Anesthesiology.* 2007;106:1003–1012.

32. Peters ML, Sommer M, de Rijke JM. Somatic and psychologic predictors of long-term unfavorable outcome after surgical intervention. *Ann Surg.* 2007;245:487–494.

33. Roth RSPH, Lowery JCP, Davis JMHS, Wilkins EGM. Psychological factors predict patient satisfaction with postmastectomy breast reconstruction. *Plast Reconstr Surg.* 2007;119: 2008–2015.

34. Forsythe ME, Dunbar MJ, Hennigar AW, Sullivan MJ, Gross M. Prospective relation between catastrophizing and residual pain following knee arthroplasty: two-year follow-up. *Pain Res Manag.* 2008;13:335–341.

35. Hanley MA, Jensen MP, Ehde DM. Psychosocial predictors of long-term adjustment to lower-limb amputation and phantom limb pain. *Disabil Rehabil.* 2004;26:882–893.

36. Roth RSPH, Lowery JCP, Davis JMHS, Wilkins EGM. Psychological factors predict patient satisfaction with postmastectomy breast reconstruction. *Plast Reconstr Surg*. 2007;119: 2008–2015.

37. Tegeder I, Costigan M, Griffin RS, Abele A, Belfer I, Schmidt H, Ehnert C, Nejim J, Scholz J, Marian C. GTP cyclohydrolase and tetrahydrobiopterin regulate pain sensitivity and persistence. *Nat Med*. 2006;12:1269–1277.

38. Edwards RR, Raja S. The laterality of long-term pain following mastectomy. *J Pain Symptom Manage*. 2006;31:98–99.

39. Nikolajsen L, Sorensen HC, Jensen TS, Kehlet H. Chronic pain following Caesarean section. *Anaesth Scand*. 2004;48:111–116.

40. Katz JP, Jackson MBA, Kavanagh BPM, Sandler ANM. Acute pain after thoracic surgery predicts long-term post-thoracotomy pain. *Clin J Pain*. 1996;12:50–55.

41. Brandsborg BM, Dueholm MP, Nikolajsen LP, Kehlet HM, Jensen TSP. A prospective study of risk factors for pain persisting 4 months after hysterectomy. *Clin J Pain*. 2009;25:263–268.

42. Taillefer MC, Carrier M, Bélisle S, Levesque S, Lanctôt H, Boisvert AM, Choinière M. Prevalence, characteristics, and predictors of chronic nonanginal postoperative pain after a cardiac operation: a cross-sectional study. *J Thorac Cardiovasc Surg*. 2006;131:1274–1280.

43. De Kock M, Lavand'homme P, Waterloos H. The short-lasting analgesia and long-term antihyperalgesic effect of intrathecal clonidine in patients undergoing colonic surgery. *Anesth Anal*. 2005;101:566–572.

44. Iohom G, Abdalla H, O'Brien J, Szarvas S, Larney V, Buckley E, Butler M, Shorten GD. The associations between severity of early postoperative pain, chronic postsurgical pain and plasma concentration of stable nitric oxide products after breast surgery. *Anesth Anal*. 2006;103:995–1000.

45. Katz J, Seltzer Z. Transition from acute to chronic postsurgical pain: risk factors and protective factors. *Expert Rev Neurother*. 2009;9:723–744.

46. Kudel I, Edwards RR, Kozachik S, Block BM, Agarwal S, Heinberg LJ, Haythornthwaite J, Raja SN. Predictors and consequences of multiple persistent postmastectomy pains. *J Pain Symptom Manage*. 2007;34:619–627.

47. Merskey H. Classification of chronic pain: description of chronic pain syndromes and definition of pain terms. *Pain*. 1986;3: S138–S139.

48. Dajczman E, Gordon A, Kreisman H. Long-term postthoracotomy pain. *Chest*. 1991;99:270–274.

48a. Pertunnen K, Tasmuth T, Kalso E. Chronic pain after thoracic surgery: a follow up study. *Acta Anaesthesiol Scand*. 1999;43(5);563–567.

49. Keller SM, Carp NZ, Levy MN, Rosen SM. Chronic postthoracotomy pain. *J Cardiovasc Surg*. 1994;35:161–164.

50. Aasvang EK, Jensen KE, Fiirgaard B, Kehlet H. MRI and pathology in persistent postherniotomy pain. *J Am Coll Surg*. 2009;208:1023–1028.

51. Nomori H, Horio H, Fuyuno G,Kobayashi R,: Non-serratus-sparing antero-axillary thoracotomy with disconnection of anterior rib cartilage. Improvement in postoperative pulmonary function and pain in comparison to posterolateral thoracotomy. *Chest*. 1997;111:572–576.

52. Benedetti F, Amanzio M, Casadio C, Filosso PL, Molinatti M, Oliaro A, Pischedda F, Maggi G. Postoperative pain and superficial abdominal reflexes after posterolateral thoracotomy. *Ann Thorac Surg*. 1997;64:207–210.

53. Nikolajsen L, Ilkjær S, Jensen TS. Relationship between mechanical sensitivity and postamputation pain: a prospective study. *Eur J Pain*. 2000;4:327–334.

54. Ehde DM, Czerniecki JM, Smith DG, Campbell KM, Edwards WT, Jensen MP, Robinson LR. Chronic phantom sensations, phantom pain, residual limb pain, and other regional pain after lower limb amputation. Arch Phys Med Rehabil. 2000;81:1039–1044.

55. Kooijman CM, Dijkstra PU, Geertzen JHB, Elzinga A, van der Schans CP. Phantom pain and phantom sensations in upper limb amputees: an epidemiological study. *Pain*. 2000;87:33–41.

56. Manchikanti L, Singh V. Managing phantom pain. *Pain Physician*. 2004;7:365–375.

57. Wall PD, Gutnick M. Ongoing activity in peripheral nerves: the physiology and pharmacology of impulses originating from a neuroma. *Exp Neurol*. 1974;43:580–593.

58. Novakovic SD, Tzoumaka E, McGivern JG, Haraguchi M, Sangameswaran L, Gogas KR, Eglen RM, Hunter JC. Distribution of the tetrodotoxin-resistant sodium channel PN3 in rat sensory neurons in normal and neuropathic conditions. *J Neurosci*. 1998;18:2174–2187.

59. Nikolajsen L, Hansen CL, Nielsen J, Keller J, Rendt-Nielsen L, Jensen TS. The effect of ketamine on phantom pain: a central neuropathic disorder maintained by peripheral input. *Pain*. 1996;67:69–77.

60. Davis KD, Kiss ZHT, Luo L, Tasker RR, Lozano AM, Dostrovsky JO. Phantom sensations

generated by thalamic microstimulation. *Nature*. 1998;391:385–387.

61. Willoch F, Rosen G, Tolle TR, Oye I, Wester HJ, Berner N, Schwaiger M, Bartenstein P. Phantom limb pain in the human brain: unraveling neural circuitries of phantom limb sensations using positron emission tomography. *Ann Neurol*. 2000;48:842–849.

62. Mackert BMC, Sappok T, Grusser S, Flor H, Curio G. The eloquence of silent cortex: analysis of afferent input to deafferented cortex in arm amputees. *Neuroreport*. 2003;14:409–412.

63. Karl A, Birbaumer N, Lutzenberger W, Cohen LG, Flor H. Reorganization of motor and somatosensory cortex in upper extremity amputees with phantom limb pain. *J Neurosci*. 2001;21:3609–3618.

64. Jensen TS, Krebs BR, Nielsen JR, Rasmussen P. Phantom limb, phantom pain and stump pain in amputees during the first 6 months following limb amputation. *Pain*. 1983;17: 243–256.

65. Finneson BE, Haft H, Krugger EG. Phantom limb syndrome associated with herniated nucleus pulposus. *J Neurosurg*. 1957;14:344–346.

66. Wilson PR, Person JR, Su DW, Wang JK. Herpes zoster reactivation of phantom limb pain. *Mayo Clin Proc*. 1978;53:336–338.

67. Bay-Neilsen M, Perkins FM, Kehlet H. Pain and functional impairment 1 year after inguinal herniorrhaphy: a nationwide questionnaire study. *Ann Surg*. 2001;233:1–7.

68. Aasvang EK, Bay-Neilsen M, Kehlet H. Pain and functional impairment 6 years after inguinal herniorrhaphy. *Hernia*. 2006;10:316–321.

69. Aasvang EK, Brandsborg B, Christensen B, Jensen TS, Kehlet H. Neurophysiological characterization of postherniotomy pain. *Pain*. 2008;137:173–181.

70. Aasvang EK, Jensen KE, Fiirgaard B, Kehlet H. MRI and pathology in persistent postherniotomy pain. *J Am Coll Surg*. 2009;208: 1023–1028.

71. Dirks J, Moiniche S, Hilsted KL, Dahl JB. Mechanisms of postoperative pain: clinical indications for a contribution of central neuronal sensitization. *Anesthesiology*. 2002;97:1591–1596.

72. Iohom G, Abdalla H, O'Brien J, Szarvas S, Larney V, Buckley E, Butler M, Shorten GD. The associations between severity of early postoperative pain, chronic postsurgical pain and plasma concentration of stable nitric oxide products after breast surgery. *Anesth Analg*. 2006;103:995–1000.

73. Zollinger PE, Tuinebreijer WE, Breederveld RS, Kreis RW. Can vitamin C prevent complex regional pain syndrome in patients with wrist fractures? *J Bone Joint Surg*. 2008;89:1424–1431.

74. Perez RS, Pragt E, Geurts J, Zuurmond WW, Patijn J, van Kleef M. Treatment of patients with complex regional pain syndrome type I with mannitol: a prospective, randomized, placebo-controlled, double-blinded study. *J Pain*. 2008;9:678–686.

75. O'Connor AB, Dworkin RH. Treatment of neuropathic pain: an overview of recent guidelines. *Am J Med*. 2009;122:S22–S32.

76. Cruccu G, Aziz TZ, Garcia-Larrea L, Hasson P, Jensen TS, Lefaucheur JP, Simpson BA, Taylor RS EFNS guidelines on neurostimulation therapy for neuropathic pain. *Eur J Neurol*. 2007;14:952–970.

77. Cohen SP, Sireci A, Wu CL, Larkin TM, Williams KA, Hurley RW. Pulsed radiofrequency of the dorsal root ganglia is superior to pharmacotherapy or pulsed radiofrequency of the intercostal nerves in the treatment of chronic postsurgical thoracic pain. *Pain Physician*. 2006;9:227–235.

78. Chan BL, Witt R, Charrow AP, Magee A, Howard R, Pasquina PF, Heilman KM, Tsao JW. Mirror therapy for phantom limb pain. *N Engl J Med*. 2007;357 (21):2206–2207.

79. Ramachandran VS, Rogers-Ramachandran D. Synaesthesia in phantom limbs induced by mirrors. *Proc Biol Soc*. 1996;263:377–386.

80. Ramachandran VS, Altschuler EL. The use of visual feedback, in particular mirror visual feedback, in restoring brain function. *Brain*. 2009;132(pt 7):1693–1710.

81. Visser EJ. Chronic post-surgical pain: epidemiology and clinical implications for acute pain management. *Acute Pain*. 2006;8:73–81.

82. Macrae WA. Chronic post-surgical pain: 10 years on. *Br J Anaesth*. 2008;101:77–86.

20

Central Neuropathic Pain

PER HANSSON AND JÖRGEN BOIVIE

INTRODUCTION

CENTRAL NEUROPATHIC PAIN (CNeP) is pain arising as a direct consequence of a lesion or disease affecting the somatosensory part of the central nervous system (CNS).[1] Results from research, converging with clinical experience, suggest that a lesion of pathways subserving nociception and temperature sensation, that is, the spino (trigemino)-thalamo-cortical pathway, is a prerequisite for the development of such pain.[2,3] Clinically, however, a lesion of these pathways is often present without concomitant pain. Thus, there is a missing link in the understanding of what initiates and maintains CNeP.

Numerous lesions and diseases may lead to CNeP (Table 20.1). The most extensively studied CNeP conditions comprise pain following stroke, multiple sclerosis, and spinal cord injury. There is a paucity of studies in other conditions, and only a few sufficiently large randomized, controlled treatment studies in CNeP have been published. Only recently have systematic data been published regarding pain in patients with Parkinson's disease (PD), indicating that 40%–50% of the patients report pain related to the underlying disease.[4] The prevalence of CNeP in PD is not known.

In this chapter, the most common CNeP conditions will be reviewed to provide the reader with information and concepts relevant for their identification and practical management. Nonneuropathic types of pain are also frequent in individuals with CNS lesions and diseases (e.g., ref. 5), but they will not be reviewed here. From a pain diagnostic perspective, regardless of the diagnostic entity, the reader is referred to the diagnostic flow chart presented in a recently published consensus paper.[1] The authors state that the pain descriptors used by patients should not be part of the foundation on which to base the diagnosis of NeP because pathognomonic descriptors are lacking. Therefore,

Table 20-1. Lesions/Diseases of the CNS That May Be Accompanied by CNeP

Stroke (infarction, hemorrhage)

Multiple sclerosis and other inflammatory diseases

Spinal cord injury

Vascular malformation

Traumatic brain injury

Syringomyelia, syringobulbia

Tumor

Abscess

Epilepsy

Parkinson's disease?

---

such information is not included in this chapter when the clinical characteristics of different conditions are described.

In the diagnostic assessment, it is difficult to determine if pain in a region with sensory disturbances is neuropathic since other pain may also be present in such areas. It seems likely that the pain is neuropathic in areas with somatosensory dysfunction if the pain is experienced in the entire area with sensory alterations, although this is far from the clinical reality in many patients. The location of CNeP, whether even or patchy in distribution, is explained by basic neuroanatomy, that is, the somatotopic organization in sensory pathways, nuclei, and cortical regions.

Due to the scarcity of randomized, controlled treatment trials in CNeP,[6] the recommendations provided rest on a relatively frail foundation. Therefore, at the end of the chapter, a more general discussion on treatment strategies of neuropathic pain in general is provided. This discussion considers treatment modalities that have not been explored in CNeP but that have had successful outcomes in peripheral neuropathic pain (PNeP) conditions. Thus, they may be reasonably adapted as part of the armamentarium for patients with neuropathic pain due to CNS disease or injury.

Given the difficulties of modeling CNeP in animals, few attempts have been made, using different measures to alter the function of the spinal cord (e.g., ref. 7). It is uncertain to what

extent hypersensitivities and other abnormal behaviors correspond to symptoms and signs in patients.[8]

Stroke

Central pain is a well-known though often overlooked consequence of stroke.[9] Dejerine and Roussy's description of thalamic pain is most often cited as the seminal report in the medical literature describing CNeP in association with other symptoms of stroke.[10] However, the term *thalamic syndrome* or *thalamic pain* is misleading in describing pain following a stroke, since lesions at any level of the brainstem and brain that affect nociceptive/temperature pathways may result in CNeP.[11] The thalamus is indirectly involved regardless of the site of the lesion within these pathways, either by injured incoming fibers or fibers projecting toward cortical areas. The term *central poststroke pain* (CPSP) is more appropriate to describe neuropathic pain following the development of a cerebrovascular lesion.[12]

CLINICAL CHARACTERISTICS

A small proportion of stroke patients experience CNeP. In the only existing prospective study, this was found to take place during the first poststroke year in 8% of 207 patients.[13] A higher proportion, 25%, of patients with CNeP has been reported 6 months after lateral medullary infarcts of the brainstem (Wallenberg's syndrome).[14]

Interestingly, pain onset is not infrequently reported with latency after the stroke. Months and even years may go by before the pain problem develops. In a prospective Danish study[13] of 207 patients, 10 reported the presence of CNeP after 1 month, 13 after 6 months, and 16 after a full year, but a latency of up to 33 months has also been reported[12] (Figure 20.1). The "slow progressors" represent a diagnostic challenge, and neurologists and others familiar with CPSP may no longer be caring for these patients when their painful neuropathic symptoms occur.[11]

From the perspective that pain is part of the somatosensory system, the occurrence of negative or positive sensory symptoms and signs

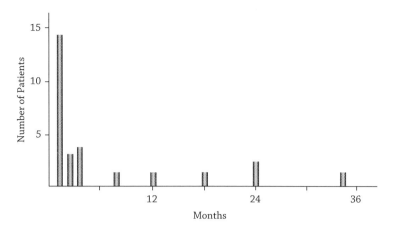

FIGURE 20.1   Time to onset of central neuropathic pain after stroke.

Source: Boivie J. Central pain. In: Wall PD, Melzack R, eds. *Textbook of Pain*, 4th ed., pp .879–914. Copyright Elsevier 1999. Reprinted with permission.

in the same body region[11] is important for the diagnosis but also has an impact on the patient (Figure 20.2). Boivie and coworkers[2] stated that somatosensory abnormalities are the only unifying characteristic in these patients and all patients reported disturbances of temperature or pain sensibility, a finding that has gained support from others.[13] Motor deficiencies did not correlate with the presence of pain.[12] The universal presence of altered temperature sensibility in CPSP is both a useful diagnostic cue and an observation that supports the hypothesis that lesions affecting the spino-thalamo-cortical tract can result in symptoms of CPSP. The overall pattern of somatosensory abnormalities across different somatosensory modalities associated with CPSP is, however, far from uniform among all patients,[11] and clearly many demonstrate these abnormalities without developing CNeP.

DIAGNOSIS

In order to make a diagnosis of CNeP in stroke patients, it is important to delineate the neuro-anatomical distribution of positive and negative symptoms and signs.[15] A pain drawing that has been filled out by the patient can be helpful in surveying the distribution of spontaneous pain and other sensory percepts. As for other CNeP conditions, no pain features have been identified that are pathognomonic for CPSP.[16] Since the

body region exactly corresponding to the location of the stroke is difficult to identify, the distribution of pain and sensory abnormalities is difficult to anticipate in an individual patient. Pain may be reported to be superficial or deep or a combination of both.[12] A comprehensive bedside examination, including probing of somatosensory functions, especially within the pain and temperature domains, should be performed, since the presence of somatosensory abnormalities is a prerequisite for the diagnosis of CPSP. Somatosensory examination will provide information about the status of different sensory pathways and should be explored using an array of instruments, including a camel hair brush or cotton for touch sensation, a cold and a warm metallic roller (the "Lindblom rollers"[17]) for temperature sensations, and a pin for pain experience.[15] Altered sensations such as hypo- or hyperesthesia and hyperalgesia/allodynia to noxious and nonnoxious temperatures are to be expected in patients with CPSP.[2] Before arriving at a diagnosis of neuropathic pain within areas of sensory disturbances, one must also consider the possibility of pain types other than neuropathic pain.

TREATMENT

Randomized controlled trials (RCTs) regarding the treatment of CPSP are few, and only small

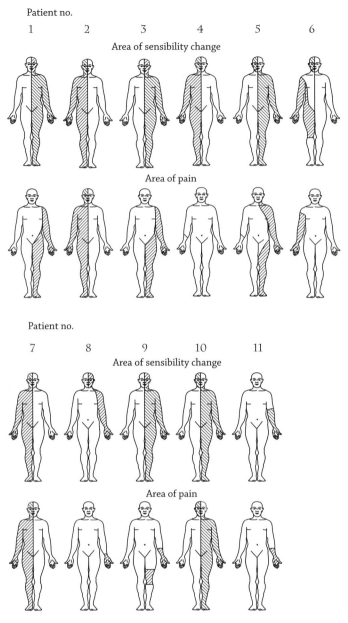

FIGURE 20.2   From patients' pain drawings and physicians' sensibility charts (touch and pinprick testing) in 11 patients with CPSP, it is evident that in the majority of patients (8/11) the area of pain was smaller than the area of sensibility alterations. In three patients, the area of pain and the area of sensory disturbances were identical.

Source: Vestergaard K, Nielsen J, Andersen G, Ingeman-Nielsen M, Arendt-Nielsen L, Jensen TS. Sensory abnormalities in consecutive, unselected patients with central post-stroke pain. *Pain*. May 1995;61(2):177–186. This figure has been reproduced with permission of the International Association for the Study of Pain (IASP®). The figure may not be reproduced for any other purpose without permission.

numbers of patients have been included. Therefore, pharmacological treatment recommendations are not well founded and are limited to positive outcomes of trials with amitriptyline,[18] lamotrigine,[19] and pregabalin.[20] The study of pregabalin included mixed CNeP conditions, and only 19 of 40 subjects had CPSP. There is no information available to guide initial treatment choices based on presenting pain symptoms and signs or other factors, such as lesion site. It seems reasonable, however, to abstain from initial use of lamotrigine since this is a drug with potentially serious skin-related adverse effects (Stevens-Johnsons/Lyells syndrome). The utility of amitriptyline is limited by its well-known and sometimes serious side effects, especially in the more vulnerable older population, including sedation, urinary retention, orthostatic hypotension, and cardiac arrhythmia. A study on mixed central neuropathic pain conditions (involving 6 of 16 CPSP patients)[21] demonstrated that intravenous lidocaine provided relief compared to placebo, but the regimen has not gained popularity.

Electrical stimulation of the motor cortex, in areas corresponding somatotopically to the painful areas, resulted in a reduction of CPSP in subsets of patients,[22] and subsequent studies arrived at the same conclusion.[23,24] Based on case series without a comparator, about 50% of patients with CPSP reported at least 50% pain relief from motor cortex stimulation.[25] In patients with projected pain to the arm and face, application of electrodes on the motor cortex convexity poses fewer problems than in patients with leg pain, in whom the electrodes have to be placed subdurally on the medial aspect of the motor strip. This invasive procedure is suggested as an alternative only in the most treatment-resistant cases. Potentially serious complications include seizures and extradural hematomas.[25]

Transcranial high-frequency magnetic stimulation, a virtually harmless noninvasive technique applied to the motor strip, has been reported to reduce CPSP. However, the effect is short-lasting and modest and cannot be recommended as the sole measure in the treatment of CPSP.[25]

Multiple Sclerosis

Contrary to what has previously been claimed in the literature, several studies from the last two decades have shown that numerous patients with multiple sclerosis (MS) report pain and that pain is a major problem for many of them.[5,26,27] In the early literature, it was accepted that a small minority of MS patients have trigeminal neuralgia (TN), even fewer have painful tonic seizures, and some have pain caused by spasticity, but the last pain is not commonly a problem for MS patients.

CLINICAL CHARACTERISTICS

Recent research demonstrates that 44%–79% of all MS patients report pain.[5,26,27] In a study specifically aiming at surveying CNeP in MS, the prevalence of definite[1] CNeP among 364 MS patients was 27.5%, including 4.9% with TN.[27] These findings compare well with the results of other studies.[28,29] The prevalence of CNeP was reported to increase with age and disease duration, with a peak between 40 and 60 years of age and between 10 and 20 years of disease duration, but was not increased with higher degrees of disability.[27] The prevalence of CNeP was already as high as 31% 10 years after the onset of MS, remained much the same over the next decade and then decreased to about 15%.[27] It thus appears that neither increasing age nor increasing duration of MS raises the risk of developing CNeP. This is in partial contradiction to the results of some previous studies, where it was found that pain prevalence increased with age,[28,30,31] disease duration,[32] and disability.[31] Prospective studies are needed to give more reliable information on these matters.

An extensive body of clinically useful information on CNeP in MS was reported by Österberg et al.[27] Interestingly, a large variety of time intervals between the clinical onset of MS and the onset of CNeP was demonstrated, ranging from 7 years before other symptoms appeared to 25 years after the start of other symptoms. Furthermore, CNeP started within 5 years of onset of the disease in 57% of the patients, and after 10 years the corresponding figure was 73%. Central neuropathic pain preceded other symptoms in 6% of the patients and was one of the initial symptoms in 20% of patients with CNeP, as well as in 5.5% of MS patients in general. Also, more than one-third of the patients with CNeP who were examined by the Swedish researchers[27] experienced such pain in two to four separate loci, often with differing modalities, time of onset, and intensity. The most

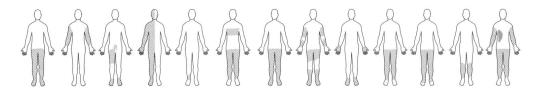

FIGURE 20.3   Pain drawings from 13 patients with CNeP in MS. A majority of subjects reported pain in the lower extremities. Only a subgroup of pain drawings from the 86 patients is shown.

Source: Reprinted from Osterberg A, Boivie J, Thuomas KA. Central pain in multiple sclerosis—prevalence and clinical characteristics. *Eur J Pain.* 2005;9(5):531–542, with permission from Elsevier.

common location of CNeP was in the lower extremities (87%) and the upper extremities (31%; Figure 20.3). Half of the patients experienced their pain as both superficial, in the skin, and in deeper parts of the body.[27] In addition, the pain was usually steady and spontaneously ongoing. Although not systematically studied in MS, it has been noted that many of the patients experienced worsening of pain after physical activity. Some patients with CNeP due to MS also had spasticity, but this was not the cause of their pain, though many patients thought this to be the case,[27] a view shared by many clinicians.

Like other MS symptoms, CNeP can be one of several symptoms occurring during a relapse, or it may be the only symptom.[30] The distribution of the three forms of MS among the patients with CNeP did not differ from that among MS patients in general (relapsing-remitting, secondary progressive, and primary progressive).

One can only speculate about the location of the lesions responsible for the development of CNeP in MS because, as shown with imaging techniques, many patients have disseminated lesions in both the brain and the spinal cord. However, on clinical grounds, it is proposed that much of the CNeP experienced in the lower extremities is due to lesions in the spinal cord. The often bilateral nature of the pain supports this idea. Two paroxysmal CNePs occur in MS: TN and, rarely, painful tonic seizures.[27]

DIAGNOSIS

The most common neurological sign in patients with CNeP in MS is sensory disturbance.[3] With few exceptions, patients report at least one abnormal finding during the sensory examination (at the bedside and when using more sophisticated quantitative techniques), with decreased sensitivity to cold occurring more often than alterations in other modalities.[3] These authors also reported a large variation among patients with regard to the involved modality and the degree of abnormality. From their reported quantitative tests, all patients except two (97%) had abnormal sensitivity to temperature and/or pain. The results of these sensory tests indicate that most, if not all, patients with CNeP in MS have lesions affecting the spino-thalamo-cortical pathways and, to a lesser degree, the medial lemniscal pathways (tactile, position sense, and vibration).[3] As for other CNeP conditions, a lesion of the pathway subserving thermal and nociceptive senses is not the only prerequisite for the development of pain; patients may report such sensory aberrations without concomitant pain.

TREATMENT

As for other CNeP conditions, few RCTs have been published with regard to pharmacological treatment of this type of pain in MS. Two controlled trials on CNeP in MS have been performed, both with a cannabis-based medicine. In the larger study, 66 patients were randomized to canabidiol or placebo oromucosal spray for 5 weeks.[33] In the other study, 24 patients were tested in a 3-week placebo-controlled crossover study with the oral cannabinoid dronabinol.[34] In both studies, significant but partial relief from CNeP was found. An open-label follow-up of the U.K. study indicated virtually no development of tolerance over

2 years.[35] Due to the nature of the drugs studied to date in CNeP in MS they cannot be recommended as first-line treatment and should only be considered in refractory cases.

Among the antiepileptic drugs, carbamazepine and oxcarbazepine are recommended for TN in MS, although no placebo-controlled studies on this specific form of TN have been published.[36] The evidence for the efficacy of carbamazepine is stronger, but safety concerns and drug interactions are less of a concern with oxcarbazepine. There is insufficient evidence to support or refute the effectiveness of surgical management of TN in MS.[36] Only data from small case series have been published regarding common surgical approaches (e.g., gamma knife and microvascular decompression) to TN; such measures tend to have less efficacy in this population of TN patients. Based on a retrospective case series, it was reported that spinal cord stimulation (SCS) provided relief in MS patients with CNeP due to spinal lesions, but the nature of the study precludes any recommendations on its usefulness in this condition.[25] The treatment of MS with interferons and other immunomodulating agents does not appear to relieve CNeP, but this has not been specifically studied.

Spinal Cord Injury

Patients with spinal cord injury (SCI) suffer from loss of ability related to moving, walking, and sexual function, and have diminished ability to control bowel and bladder function. Pain was reported by 65% of SCI patients at follow-up 6 months after injury.[37] A 5-year follow up demonstrated the presence of pain in 81% of subjects.[38] Pain may have varying etiologies including muscle spasm, spasticity, muscle overuse, mechanical instability of the spine, and neuropathic pain related to spinal cord or nerve root injury. A significant proportion of these patients complain of long-term pain, some to the extent that they are willing to trade pain relief for increased loss of function.[39] Experienced pain clinicians state that CNeP related to SCI is among the most treatment-resistant pain conditions in medicine.

Encouragingly, research in this field has given new insights in recent years, providing hope for patients.

CLINICAL CHARACTERISTICS

The two most common types of neuropathic pain that emerge after SCI are at-level and below-level pain[37,40] (Figure 20.4). At-level neuropathic pain (i.e., transitional zone pain), located in a segmental pattern at the level of injury, is one main type of neuropathic pain reported by SCI patients. It may be caused by the spinal cord injury itself, that is, a CNeP condition, or may be due to nerve root injury. Regardless of the etiology, it may present with unilateral or bilateral symptoms and is a diagnostic challenge. Below-level pain is a CNeP caused by the injury to the spinal cord and is usually perceived in a wide distribution bilaterally in regions below the level of injury in areas with total or partial loss of sensibility; it may develop years after the injury. Such pain is commonly unrelated to movement and is present constantly, although with variable intensity.

Syringomyelia should be suspected in SCI patients when there is a delayed onset of pain, amounting to years, and especially if the level of sensory loss moves in a cranial direction.[41] In the cervical region this may result in the central cord syndrome, characterized by pain and weakness of the shoulders and arms.

To what extent visceral pain in SCI could be part of the CNeP after such injury is unknown. No gold standard diagnostic workup is available to classify such pain. It has been suggested that pain from visceral areas should initially be considered as nociceptive/inflammatory. Only after the failure of investigations to find evidence of visceral pathology, and only if treatment has been unsuccessful, should the pain be regarded as an expression of CNeP and treated accordingly.[42]

Epidemiological studies in SCI patients have demonstrated a point prevalence 6 months after injury of about 35% with at-level pain and about 20% with below-level neuropathic pain.[37] At 5 years the corresponding figures are 40% and 35%, respectively.[38]

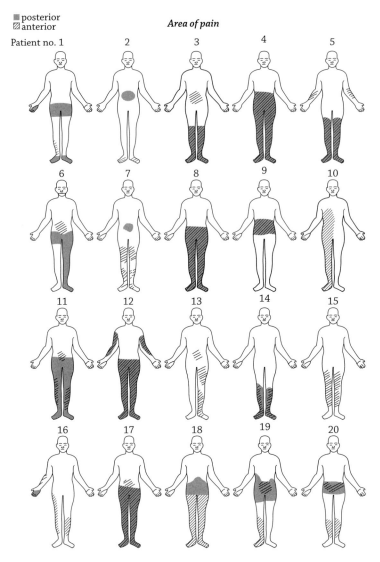

FIGURE 20.4 Pain drawings (spontaneous ongoing pain) from 20 patients with CNeP due to SCI. Patients 1 (neurological injury level at C6), 5 (C4), 10 (C5), 12 (C5), and 16 (C4) reported both at-level and below-level pain.

Source: Reprinted with permission from Finnerup NB, Johannesen IL, Fuglsang-Frederiksen A, Bach FW, Jensen TS. Sensory function in spinal cord injury patients with and without central pain. *Brain* 2003;126(1):57–70.

DIAGNOSIS

As for other neuropathic pains, somatosensory abnormalities should be present in the painful area. In complete and nearly complete injury to the cord, this does not pose a diagnostic problem for below-level pain. In partial and more limited injuries to the spinal cord, the presence of sensory dysfunction in painful areas is the main focus of the examination. At-level pain is usually obviously related to areas of sensory dysfunction.

TREATMENT

There are several available RCTs on successful oral pharmacological treatment of CNeP related to SCI. In a small crossover trial involving 20 patients, gabapentin proved efficacious over an 8 week period compared to placebo.[43] A larger Australian trial demonstrated pregabalin to be significantly more effective than placebo in a parallel group trial on 137 patients.[44] Patients reporting at least 50% pain relief comprised 22% of the group receiving pregabalin compared to 8% of the placebo group (number needed to treat = 7.1). In a trial with mixed CNeP conditions, also including such pain in SCI patients (21/40 patients), pregabalin was reported to be efficacious.[20] A 4 week placebo-controlled study of tramadol indicated a pain-relieving potential compared to placebo.[45] Small trials with intravenous ketamine[46,47] and alfentanil[46] have shown efficacy. In studies on intrathecal drug delivery of baclofen[48] and morfin with clonidine,[49] there was relief of CNeP in SCI patients. Importantly, intravenous and intrathecal drug delivery should be employed in specialized pain centers only.

Neurostimulation techniques have been explored very seldom in this type of pain. Spinal cord stimulation was reported to be efficacious in a retrospective case series, but further studies are needed to be able to assess its usefulness in CNeP in SCI.[25] Dorsal root entry zoon treatment for SCI-related CNeP, particularly at-level pain, has weak scientific support.[50] Surgical approaches to treat syringomyelia include decompression of the arachnoid scar or insertion of a drainage tube connected to the subarachnoid space or the peritoneal cavity. If the CNeP is caused by syringomyelia, the pain is not necessarily relieved by collapsing the syrinx.

GENERAL TREATMENT ASPECTS OF NEUROPATHIC PAIN

Oral Pharmacological Treatment

The majority of treatment studies on neuropathic pain have been performed in peripheral conditions, mostly painful diabetic polyneuropathy and postherpetic neuralgia; few studies have focused on conditions with CNeP.[6] Drugs that are efficacious in peripheral neuropathic pain (PNeP) also would provide relief in patients with CNeP since several drugs have been demonstrated in RCTs to relieve both types of pain, such as amitriptyline (CPSP), gabapentin (CNeP in SCI), and pregabalin (mixed conditions with

CNeP).[51] Clinical empiricism also points to some efficacy in subgroups of patients of such drugs across neuropathic pain conditions. This may reflect the possible underlying pathophysiological mechanisms of the pain condition and an occasional match between the dominant pain mechanism and the mechanism of action of a drug.

Studies on the pathophysiology of peripheral and central neuropathic pain have also indicated shared underlying mechanisms, such as expression of aberrant sodium channels[52,53] and cortical reorganization.[54,55] This gives further credence to the notion that similar therapeutic strategies may be efficacious in both types of pain. In parts of the world where legal or financial restrictions do not prohibit the use of off-label pharmacological treatment strategies across diagnostic entities and do not rely on an evidence-based foundation, any drug with some evidence base in PNeP may also be tried in CNeP conditions. Such an approach would then allow the use of serotonin and noradrenaline reuptake inhibitors such as duloxetine and venlafaxine, and perhaps opioids, in patients with CNeP.[6]

Neurostimulation

In addition to the techniques mentioned above, transcutaneous electrical nerve stimulation (TENS) has been available for decades, but trials including patients with CNeP conditions are rare and the applied methodology for stimulation is inconsistent.[25] Hence, conclusive recommendations are not possible. In our experience, areas of pain in CNeP conditions are usually too large to allow for significant pain relief from TENS.

REFERENCES

1. Treede RD, Jensen TS, Campbell JN, et al. Neuropathic pain: redefinition and a grading system for clinical and research purposes. *Neurology.* 2008;70(18):1630–1635.
2. Boivie J, Leijon G, Johansson I. Central poststroke pain—a study of the mechanisms through analyses of the sensory abnormalities. *Pain.* 1989;37(2):173–185.
3. Österberg A, Boivie J. Central pain in multiple sclerosis—sensory abnormalities. *Eur J Pain.* 2010;14(1):104–110.

4. Beiske AG, Loge JH, Ronningen A, Svensson E. Pain in Parkinson's disease: prevalence and characteristics. *Pain*. 2009;141(1–2):173–177.

5. Svendsen KB, Jensen TS, Overvad K, Hansen HJ, Koch-Henriksen N, Bach FW. Pain in patients with multiple sclerosis: a population-based study. *Arch Neurol*. 2003;60(8):1089–1094.

6. Attal N, Cruccu G, Haanpaa M, et al. EFNS guidelines on pharmacological treatment of neuropathic pain. *Eur J Neurol*. 2006;13(11): 1153–1169.

7. Vierck CJ Jr., Siddall P, Yezierski RP. Pain following spinal cord injury: animal models and mechanistic studies. *Pain*. 2000;89(1):1–5.

8. Hansson P. Difficulties in stratifying neuropathic pain by mechanisms. *Eur J Pain*. 2003;7(4): 353–357.

9. Jensen TS, Lenz FA. Central post-stroke pain: a challenge for the scientist and the clinician. *Pain*. 1995;61(2):161–164.

10. Dejerine J, Roussy G. La syndrome thalamique. *Rev Neurol*. 1906(14):521–532.

11. Bowsher D. Central post-stroke ("thalamic syndrome") and other central pains. *Am J Hosp Palliat Care*. 1999;16(4):593–597.

12. Leijon G, Boivie J, Johansson I. Central post-stroke pain—neurological symptoms and pain characteristics. *Pain*. 1989;36(1):13–25.

13. Andersen G, Vestergaard K, Ingeman-Nielsen M, Jensen TS. Incidence of central post-stroke pain. *Pain*. 1995;61(2):187–193.

14. MacGowan DJ, Janal MN, Clark WC, et al. Central poststroke pain and Wallenberg's lateral medullary infarction: frequency, character, and determinants in 63 patients. *Neurology*. 1997;49(1):120–125.

15. Hansson P. Neuropathic pain: clinical characteristics and diagnostic workup. *Eur J Pain*. 2002;6(suppl A):47–50.

16. Hansson P, Haanpaa M. Diagnostic work-up of neuropathic pain: computing, using questionnaires or examining the patient? *Eur J Pain*. 2007;11(4):367–369.

17. Marchettini P, Marangoni C, Lacerenza M, Formaglio F. The Lindblom roller. *Eur J Pain*. 2003;7(4):359–364.

18. Leijon G, Boivie J. Central post-stroke pain—a controlled trial of amitriptyline and carbamazepine. *Pain*. 1989;36(1):27–36.

19. Vestergaard K, Andersen G, Gottrup H, Kristensen BT, Jensen TS. Lamotrigine for central poststroke pain: a randomized controlled trial. *Neurology*. 2001;56(2):184–190.

20. Vranken JH, Dijkgraaf MG, Kruis MR, van der Vegt MH, Hollmann MW, Heesen M. Pregabalin

in patients with central neuropathic pain: a randomized, double-blind, placebo-controlled trial of a flexible-dose regimen. *Pain*. 2008;136 (1–2):150–157.

21. Attal N, Gaude V, Brasseur L, et al. Intravenous lidocaine in central pain: a double-blind, placebo-controlled, psychophysical study. *Neurology*. 2000;54(3):564–574.

22. Tsubokawa T, Katayama Y, Yamamoto T, Hirayama T, Koyama S. Chronic motor cortex stimulation for the treatment of central pain. *Acta Neurochir Suppl (Wien)*. 1991;52:137–139.

23. Katayama Y, Fukaya C, Yamamoto T. Poststroke pain control by chronic motor cortex stimulation: neurological characteristics predicting a favorable response. *J Neurosurg*. 1998;89(4):585–591.

24. Nguyen JP, Lefaucheur JP, Decq P, et al. Chronic motor cortex stimulation in the treatment of central and neuropathic pain. Correlations between clinical, electrophysiological and anatomical data. *Pain*. 1999;82(3):245–251.

25. Cruccu G, Aziz TZ, Garcia-Larrea L, et al. EFNS guidelines on neurostimulation therapy for neuropathic pain. *Eur J Neurol*. 2007;14(9): 952–970.

26. Ehde DM, Gibbons LE, Chwastiak L, Bombardier CH, Sullivan MD, Kraft GH. Chronic pain in a large community sample of persons with multiple sclerosis. *Mult Scler*. 2003;9(6):605–611.

27. Österberg A, Boivie J, Thuomas KA. Central pain in multiple sclerosis—prevalence and clinical characteristics. *Eur J Pain*. 2005;9(5):531–542.

28. Moulin DE. Pain in multiple sclerosis. *Neurol Clin*. 1989;7(2):321–331.

29. Vermote R, Ketelaer P, Carton H. Pain in multiple sclerosis patients. A prospective study using the McGill Pain Questionnaire. *Clin Neurol Neurosurg*. 1986;88(2):87–93.

30. Clifford DB, Trotter JL. Pain in multiple sclerosis. *Arch Neurol*. 1984;41(12):1270–1272.

31. Stenager E, Knudsen L, Jensen K. Acute and chronic pain syndromes in multiple sclerosis. A 5-year follow-up study. *Ital J Neurol Sci*. 1995;16(9):629–632.

32. Kassirer MR, Osterberg DH. Pain in multiple sclerosis. *Am J Nurs*. 1987;87(7):968–969.

33. Rog DJ, Nurmikko TJ, Friede T, Young CA. Randomized, controlled trial of cannabis-based medicine in central pain in multiple sclerosis. *Neurology*. 2005;65(6):812–819.

34. Svendsen KB, Jensen TS, Bach FW. Does the cannabinoid dronabinol reduce central pain in multiple sclerosis? Randomised double blind placebo controlled crossover trial. *BMJ*. 2004;329(7460):253–260.

35. Rog DJ, Nurmikko TJ, Young CA. Oromucosal delta9-tetrahydrocannabinol/cannabidiol for neuropathic pain associated with multiple sclerosis: an uncontrolled, open-label, 2-year extension trial. *Clin Ther.* 2007;29(9):2068–2079.

36. Cruccu G, Gronseth G, Alksne J, et al. AAN-EFNS guidelines on trigeminal neuralgia management. *Eur J Neurol.* 2008;15(10):1013–1028.

37. Siddall PJ, Taylor DA, McClelland JM, Rutkowski SB, Cousins MJ. Pain report and the relationship of pain to physical factors in the first 6 months following spinal cord injury. *Pain.* 1999;81(1–2): 187–197.

38. Siddall PJ, McClelland JM, Rutkowski SB, Cousins MJ. A longitudinal study of the prevalence and characteristics of pain in the first 5 years following spinal cord injury. *Pain.* 2003;103(3):249–257.

39. Nepomuceno C, Fine PR, Richards JS, et al. Pain in patients with spinal cord injury. *Arch Phys Med Rehabil.* 1979;60(12):605–609.

40. Finnerup NB, Johannesen IL, Fuglsang-Frederiksen A, Bach FW, Jensen TS. Sensory function in spinal cord injury patients with and without central pain. *Brain.* 2003;126 (pt 1):57–70.

41. Frisbie JH, Aguilera EJ. Chronic pain after spinal cord injury: an expedient diagnostic approach. *Paraplegia.* 1990;28(7):460–465.

42. Siddall P, Yezierski RP, Loeser JD. Taxonomy and epidemiology of spinal cord injury pain. In: Yezierski RP, Burchiel K, eds. *Spinal Cord Injury Pain: Assessment, Mechanisms, Management.* Vol. 23. Seattle: IASP Press; 2002:9–24.

43. Levendoglu F, Ogun CO, Ozerbil O, Ogun TC, Ugurlu H. Gabapentin is a first line drug for the treatment of neuropathic pain in spinal cord injury. *Spine (Phila, Pa 1976).* 2004;29(7):743–751.

44. Siddall PJ, Cousins MJ, Otte A, Griesing T, Chambers R, Murphy TK. Pregabalin in central neuropathic pain associated with spinal cord injury: a placebo-controlled trial. *Neurology.* 2006;67(10):1792–1800.

45. Norrbrink C, Lundeberg T. Tramadol in neuropathic pain after spinal cord injury: a randomized, double-blind, placebo-controlled trial. *Clin J Pain.* 2009;25(3):177–184.

46. Eide PK, Stubhaug A, Stenehjem AE. Central dysesthesia pain after traumatic spinal cord injury is dependent on *N*-methyl-D-aspartate receptor activation. *Neurosurgery.* 1995;37(6): 1080–1087.

47. Kvarnstrom A, Karlsten R, Quiding H, Gordh T. The analgesic effect of intravenous ketamine and lidocaine on pain after spinal cord injury. *Acta Anaesthesiol Scand.* 2004;48(4):498–506.

48. Herman RM, D'Luzansky SC, Ippolito R. Intrathecal baclofen suppresses central pain in patients with spinal lesions. A pilot study. *Clin J Pain.* 1992;8(4):338–345.

49. Siddall PJ, Molloy AR, Walker S, Mather LE, Rutkowski SB, Cousins MJ. The efficacy of intrathecal morphine and clonidine in the treatment of pain after spinal cord injury. *Anesth Analg.* 2000;91(6):1493–1498.

50. Denkers MR, Biagi HL, Ann O'Brien M, Jadad AR, Gauld ME. Dorsal root entry zone lesioning used to treat central neuropathic pain in patients with traumatic spinal cord injury: a systematic review. *Spine (Phila, Pa 1976).* 2002;27(7): E177–E184.

51. Hansson PT, Dickenson AH. Pharmacological treatment of peripheral neuropathic pain conditions based on shared commonalities despite multiple etiologies. *Pain.* 2005;113(3): 251–254.

52. Dib-Hajj SD, Black JA, Waxman SG. Voltage-gated sodium channels: therapeutic targets for pain. *Pain Med.* 2009;10(7):1260–1269.

53. Hains BC, Waxman SG. Sodium channel expression and the molecular pathophysiology of pain after SCI. *Prog Brain Res.* 2007;161:195–203.

54. Flor H, Elbert T, Knecht S, et al. Phantom-limb pain as a perceptual correlate of cortical reorganization following arm amputation. *Nature.* 1995;375(6531):482–484.

55. Wrigley PJ, Press SR, Gustin SM, et al. Neuropathic pain and primary somatosensory cortex reorganization following spinal cord injury. *Pain.* 2009;141(1–2):52–59.

21

Spinal Root Disease

Radiculopathy and Arachnoiditis

JOHN D. MARKMAN AND HALEH VAN VLIET

INTRODUCTION

RADICULAR LOW BACK pain is widely considered to be the most common neuropathic syndrome.[1] Despite their minute anatomical extent and seemingly secure location within the spinal canal, the anterior (ventral) and posterior (dorsal) nerve roots are subject to mechanical, inflammatory, infectious, and even vascular insults. Injury to the posterior roots arising from degenerative conditions of spinal structures such as the lumbar discs is by far the most prevalent cause of painful radicular syndromes.[1,2] The degree to which chronic low back pain syndromes involve the nerve roots and may therefore be characterized as neuropathic, or "a direct consequence of a lesion or disease affecting the somatosensory system," remains a matter of vigorous debate. Estimates range widely from a high of 4.5% of all adults over age 30 in one sample to fewer than 5% of patients experiencing low back pain.[3,4] There is

no definitive clinical tool to localize neuropathic pain to the nerve root level; however, there is an enduring, broad consensus that radicular syndromes constitute a major health and socioeconomic problem worldwide.

The archetypal clinical presentation of radicular pain, commonly referred to as *sciatica* in lay terms, is distinctive and the pain may localize to either the dorsal root or its ganglion. Animal models have linked radicular pain to ectopic discharge and neuronal hyperexcitability in the dorsal root or its ganglion.[5] Introduction of the proinflammatory nucleus propulsus into the epidural space, even in the absence of nerve root compression, is a well-established cause of this pain pattern.[6] In contrast, radiculopathy is defined by conduction block in the distribution of a spinal nerve or its roots.[7] Radiculopathy may result in weakness when motor fibers are blocked or numbness when sensory fibers are involved. The resulting myotomal or dermatomal patterns of deficit on clinical exam are not necessarily associated with the symptom of pain.

Arachnoiditis is a more narrowly defined clinical entity in which fibrosis, adhesions, and scarring transform neural tissue. This pathology was named for the arachnoid membrane because (1) the small vasculature of this meningeal layer permits the immune reaction necessary for late proliferative phase changes and (2) it is more predisposed to undergo inflammatory and edematous responses to injury as well as to induce fibroblast proliferation.[8] The prevalence of these syndromes has surged in tandem with the rates of surgical treatment of painful radicular syndromes.[9]

The challenge confronted by clinicians and researchers alike is that lateralized lancinating pain radiating from the low back to the distal leg has numerous putative causes, anatomical correlates, and neurobiological mechanisms. This diversity of cause and mechanism is invoked to account for the significant variation in both the chronicity and intensity of radiating low back pain symptoms in the clinical context. Chronic pain intensity often fluctuates in individual patients without a demonstrable change in the root lesion as characterized by neurological exam. Conversely, many patients with persistent sensory and motor deficits localizing to a nerve root territory are pain free for extended periods of time.[10] Further complicating the study of chronic low back pain in an era of readily accessible axial imaging is that radicular pain is frequently endorsed without a radiographic correlate.[11] Neurophysiological and pathological studies lack sufficient sensitivity and specificity to rule in or exclude the experience of radicular pain in a definitive fashion. It is widely recognized that painful symptoms with an inflammatory mechanism often localize to nonneural tissue, thereby earning the description *pseudoradicular*.[12] This heterogeneity of symptoms and signs is frequently used to explain the lack of analgesic benefit repeatedly found in clinical trials of chronic low back pain treatments.[13,14]

Despite the variability of the clinical presentation, the claim that a significant proportion of chronic low back pain cases should be considered *neuropathic* is supported by the observation that the core positive signs (e.g., numbness) and symptoms (e.g., burning quality, spontaneous pain) often resemble those of other neuropathic pain syndromes, such as mononeuropathy and polyneuropathy. Regardless of the cause, the vast majority of acute radicular pain syndromes resolve with specific treatment of the underlying etiology, whether attributed to a disc protrusion, Lyme disease, varicella-zoster virus infection, or acute inflammatory demyelinating polyneuropathy (i.e., Guillain-Barré syndrome). The responsiveness of acute radicular syndromes to specific treatments offers compelling evidence of distinct pain mechanisms. The colossal public health burden in terms of poorly controlled pain, health care utilization, and disability results from the sizable population in all of these various syndromes that continues to experience chronic symptoms even after the inciting cause has resolved. For this reason, this chapter focuses on painful radicular syndromes characterized as chronic.

The organization of this chapter presupposes that there are clinically relevant subgroups of chronic neuropathic low back pain syndromes with a diverse, but likely overlapping, set of corresponding underlying neuropathic mechanisms. As a consequence, a range of index painful neuropathic chronic low back pain syndromes, ranging from episodic neurogenic claudication in the context of lateral recess stenosis to nonspecific chronic low back pain are considered in each section to cover the spectrum of etiological diversity, prevalence, and clinical presentations.

EPIDEMIOLOGY

Chronic low back pain is the most prevalent type of neuropathic pain syndrome by a wide margin, even if the most conservative estimate of 1 out of every 10 cases is so classified.[4,15] Because acute low back pain has an annual incidence of up to one-third in most population samples, with more than 80% of adults experiencing at least a single episode of low back pain within their lifetime,[16–20] the number of patients endorsing symptoms with neuropathic features is high. Many recent symptom-based cross-sectional surveys have attempted to confirm this clinical impression. A large Egyptian study employing the Leeds Assessment of Neuropathic Symptoms and Signs scale found that 54.7% of patients presenting with chronic low back pain experienced a significant neuropathic pain component.[21] A series of German studies in over 21,000 patients used symptom-based screening tools to model the neuropathic component of chronic low back pain at 4% of the general adult population.[22] Survey data from the United States characterize a rapidly rising prevalence trend in chronic low back pain cases over the past two decades regardless of race, gender, or socioeconomic status.[20] The segment of the population older than 60 years comprises the largest proportion of chronic low back pain cases by adult age strata.[23,24]

Among the anatomical conditions known to induce low back pain, spinal stenosis (SpS), intervertebral disc herniation (IDH), and degenerative spondylolisthesis (DS) of the lumbar region are three of the most significant contributors to low back and leg symptoms (i.e., radicular) for which surgery is performed.[25–27] In general, epidemiological estimates derived from the vast surgical literature on radicular syndromes emphasize somatic distribution over symptom quality. Patients in these samples tend to have more advanced neurocompressive disease, as well as imaging correlates of a known structural cause, and are far more likely to have neurological deficits indicative of radiculopathy. This selection bias limits the specificity of studies for the presence of neuropathic pain since many patients with symptom-predominant clinical presentations are excluded from these samples. The epidemiology of a given subpopulation of patients with chronic, neuropathic low back pain varies widely by pathoanatomical correlate. For example, the incidence of lumbar disc herniations peaks among individuals aged 40 to 60 years,[28] whereas lateral recess stenosis giving rise to neurogenic claudication in a polyradicular distribution peaks after age 60.[29,30]

A dramatic rise in the number of surgical procedures, most notably in the United States, for the treatment of chronic low back pain has translated into a concomitant increase in the incidence of painful iatrogenic syndromes of the nerve roots. Chronic neuropathic syndrome after spine surgery, the so-called failed back surgery syndrome (FBSS), is a relatively common complication of lumbosacral spine surgery.[31] This condition, while also very heterogeneous, tends to have a disproportionately higher number of patients with severe neuropathic symptoms seeking ongoing treatment.[32] Following spinal fusion procedures, as many as 30% to 40% of patients report recurrent or chronic low back pain.[33] Using 2007 estimates of life expectancy, about one-third of laminectomy patients initially endorsing relief of symptoms related to stenosis may expect to experience recurrent neurogenic claudication for up to a decade postoperatively.[30]

NATURAL HISTORY

The vast majority of patients experiencing an episode of acute low back pain recover quickly, without long-term loss of function; however, if low back and leg pain continue for more than 12 weeks, recovery is slow and uncertain. The challenge of determining the relevance and likelihood of resolution of a structural cause of severe acute or subacute low back pain continues to bedevil clinicians in spite of steady progress in imaging technology.[34] In other words, there is no reliable way to predict which pars fracture will fuse spontaneously with bracing alone or which disc extrusion will resorb without local intervention. In many cases of chronic neuropathic low back pain, these structural causes decisively inform the natural history. To the extent that acute nerve root compression resulting from grade II spondylolisthesis or a disc fragment gives rise to a "direct consequence of a lesion or disease of the somatosensory system," the trajectory of neuropathic symptoms in specific chronic low back pain syndromes is driven by nonneural causes.

Recent cross-sectional surveys of the neuropathic symptom component in chronic low back pain population samples are a novelty compared with decades of research in the surgical literature comparing surgical treatments to reasonable alternatives. These point prevalence surveys reveal little about the natural history of neuropathic low back pain. The currently available information about neuropathic chronic low back pain lends itself to a discussion of a natural history anchored in the inciting etiology, be it neural or otherwise. For the chronic low back pain cases with axial- or radicular-predominant symptom patterns in which there is no clear neurocompressive correlate (i.e., nonspecific low back pain), the etiological lesion or disease is less important from a clinical standpoint.

The Spine Outcomes Research Trial (SPORT) investigators conducted a large multicenter comprehensive study of patients with low back and leg pain and the three most common structural causes: SpS, IDH, and DS. In their evaluation of baseline patient characteristics, they found that most patients experienced symptoms for 3 to 6 months, thereby meeting most of the criteria for chronic pain. In this cohort (n = 1441), a significantly larger percentage of those with SpS and DS had symptom durations exceeding 1 year (33%) relative to those with IDH (9%).[26] Older clinical studies have found a similarly distinctive pattern of spontaneous amelioration in IDH, with 90% of patients reporting substantial alleviation of their pain over 5–6 weeks[23] with nonoperative treatment.[35,36] Within the SPORT IDH group, 35% of patients had symptoms that resolved within 3 months. At onset, IDH patients typically had higher levels of pain intensity and were significantly more likely to have sought care in a hospital emergency department (21%), to have employed opioid medications (49%), and to have used antidepressants and muscle relaxants (29%) relative to DS and SpS patients.

To evaluate this spectrum of natural histories, one study (n = 69) measured herniation reduction as a percentage of intraspinal volume using magnetic resonance imaging (MRI), and more than two-thirds of these patients endorsed radicular pain.[37] Reductions as large as 70% were found in 63% of patients, while no change (29%) or an increase in herniated material (8%) was observed in the remaining study participants. Studies from this era lack data about neuropathic symptom characteristics. Radicular pain from IDH is often recurrent.[38] In his analysis of 280 patients with herniated lumbar discs, Weber found that 90% of them (ages 25 to 55) reported a prior attack of low back pain; an average of 10 years had passed before the onset of radicular symptoms.[38] This investigator did not identify prognostic factors that could distinguish between a temporary case of low back pain and one that was the harbinger of sciatica.[38] The course of the majority of these IDH patients from acute through chronic symptoms was summarized as a transition from "annoying pain to a more endurable back insufficiency in which pain only was provoked through certain movements."[38]

In contrast to the rapid onset of radicular neuropathic symptoms attributed to acute IDH, lumbar SpS is characterized by insidious onset and gradual progression.[39,40] The cardinal neuropathic symptom of SpS is neurogenic claudication, a distinctive symptom pattern of low back and leg pain that is induced with standing and walking and remits when the person is seated. As such, neurogenic claudication is an episodic symptom pattern; its impact on mobility tends to wax and wane over extended periods ranging from months to years. Inexorable progression is not the norm. In fact, multiple clinical studies have shown that deferring decompressive surgery does not result in an irreversible neurological deficit.[41,42] In several series, those patients who elected not to undergo surgery tended to demonstrate modest improvement,[43] although one analysis of 19 untreated patients found that 60% had unchanged symptom severity over a mean period of 4 years.[44] With the most prevalent, form, DS, peak onset occurs in patients over age 60 and is the leading motive for spine surgery in seniors.[45] Those individuals with congenitally narrow canals, thickened laminae, and stunted pedicles are more susceptible to acquired forms of stenosis and will likely experience neurogenic claudication at a younger age.[30]

Arachnoiditis with prominent neuropathic symptoms is most commonly associated with lumbar surgery in the modern era. It is the most persistent neuropathic symptom and, like other common neuropathic syndromes, is notable for the severity of the associated spontaneous pain.[23] Lumbosacral adhesive arachnoiditis may be secondary to numerous different medical conditions or insults, including structural abnormalities of the vertebral column, physical trauma to the spine such as that incurred during surgery, or introduction of noxious substances into the epidural space.[46,47] Two phases describe the disease process: acute inflammatory and chronic proliferative.[8,48] The latter phase may be defined as the end-stage repair process of the former.[49,50] Epidural scarring can also accompany inflammation and fibrosis of the arachnoid, particularly after spinal surgery, resulting in the condition called *epiduro-arachnoiditis*.[50] One retrospective study evaluated the histories of 38 patients with diagnosed epiduro-arachnoiditis.[50] All had undergone at least one laminectomy for disc herniation, and persistent or recurrent sciatica among all 38 ultimately led to repeat operation. Fourteen of the patients had experienced no symptom-free intervals prior to this repeat intervention; the remaining patients had experienced anywhere from 2 months to 10 years of temporary relief.[50]

SOCIETAL IMPACT

Chronic low back pain is the second most common cause of disability among adults in the United States and a leading cause of lost work days.[51-53] In fact, cost estimates of total lost work days in the United States per year due to LBP approach $150 million.[54] In some samples, up to 80% of workers reported lost time from their occupations due to LBP.[55] Although most cases involve only a brief clinical course, the subpopulation of patients with chronic low back pain represents a disproportionately high percentage of medical consultations and is responsible for the colossal burden that has been imposed on health care systems.[56-60] Like other chronic neuropathic pain syndromes, chronic low back pain has significant adverse effects on health-related quality of life and mental health.[61] Psychological factors are also fundamental modifiers of the experience of chronic low back pain that have been identified as barriers to pain resolution and promoters of progression to chronicity.[62,63] In patients with specific syndromes such as lumbar SpS, rates of depression exceed those of age-matched controls and have been linked to increased pain severity, poorer functional status, and poorer surgical outcomes.[64] In a comparison of surgically and conservatively treated IDH patients, individuals with various forms of psychopathology (e.g., major depressive disorder) had inferior results regardless of treatment type.[38]

Nearly $40 billion is spent annually on spinal pain in the United States.[9] Despite an upward cost trend for the care of these patients, there does not appear to be a corresponding improvement in self-reported health status.[65,66] When reduced productivity and wages are taken into consideration, the estimated total annual cost of this condition approximately triples to between $100 and $200 billion.[67] The neuropathic component of spinal pain syndromes has been identified as a key driver of cost based on an analysis of a representative U.S. health insurance database.[2] Cost calculations from a recent survey modeling the neuropathic component of low back pain valued its contribution to the total cost of care as greater than 10%.[22]

Given that senior citizens represent a large proportion of those affected by certain spinal pain syndromes, such as lumbar SpS, expenditures for this condition are expected to grow fourfold by the year 2050.[68] Likewise, it is anticipated that the extended life expectancy will increase not only the neuropathic symptoms related to degenerative causes but also the number of office visits for recurrent postoperative symptoms following interventions such as laminectomy.[69]

CLINICAL AND DIAGNOSTIC FEATURES

Lateralized pain radiating from the low back into the distal lower extremity is the classic clinical presentation equated with segmental localization to the level of the nerve root or dorsal root ganglion. Because of the distinctive anatomical distribution (e.g., dermatomal), the quality of the corresponding pain symptoms, and the frequent association with motor deficits and diminished deep tendon reflexes, the clinical diagnosis of pain radiculopathy is considered a direct consequence of a lesion or disease affecting the somatosensory system. As such, the predominant mechanism of the pain is considered neuropathic. As demonstrated in evoked perioperative studies in patients undergoing discectomy, the clinical hallmarks of radicular pain include lateralization, radiation from the low back to the distal extremity along a narrow band, and a lancinating quality.[70] It is important to recognize that radiculopathy is defined by conduction block and often results in sensory disturbance, motor deficit, or diminished reflexes but not necessarily radicular pain. Radicular pain is most commonly a defining feature of the syndrome when there is local inflammation in the region of the nerve root or direct compression of the dorsal root ganglion in the absence of inflammation.

One clinical challenge is to distinguish this pattern from nociceptive pain referred from spinal structures such as the sacroiliac or facet joints and nonspinal joint spaces such as the hip. Additionally, there is a need to discriminate between peripheral mononeuropathies (e.g., sciatic nerve compression) and lumbosacral plexopathies (e.g., diabetic amotrophy). Neurophysiological studies are helpful in differentiating radiculoneuropathies from peripheral neuropathies through evaluation of features such as sensory action potentials. Because it only assesses the function of heavily myelinated peripheral nerve fibers, and not the $\alpha\delta$ and c fibers that likely play an important role in subserving the experience of radicular pain, electromyography has limited value as a confirmatory test for the diagnosis of radicular pain. Other ancillary studies, such as skin biopsy and quantitative sensory testing, may be useful for ruling out other localizations, but they are not conclusive for the diagnosis or exclusion of radicular pain.[71]

There is growing recognition that neuropathic low back pain cannot simply be equated with radiculopathy. Several lines of clinical evidence bolster this claim.

- Nociceptive pain referred from nonneural spinal structures (e.g., a facet joint) often radiates into the distal lower extremities.[10]
- Subclinical sensory loss is often detectable in these "pseudoradicular" presentations.[12]
- Neuropathic pain qualities are often endorsed in chronic axial low back pain syndromes in the absence of associated neurological deficits.[72]
- Multiple published and unpublished clinical trials of drugs with demonstrated efficacy in other neuropathic pain syndromes (e.g., postherpetic neuralgia and diabetic peripheral neuropathy) lack analgesic benefit for strictly defined radicular neuropathic pain syndromes.[73]

In fact, some experts have argued that underestimation of the high prevalence of nociceptive low back pain referred from somatic structures has led clinicians and clinical trial experts alike to overdiagnose radicular neuropathic pain when "it should be regarded as the exception rather than somatic referred pain being relegated to some irregularity of radicular pain."[10]

Several research groups have recently developed novel clinical tools to define the clinical and diagnostic features of neuropathic low back pain.[13,74] These tools rely on clusters of symptoms and signs with the aim of teasing apart neuropathic from nociceptive pain independent of etiology. Together these tools represent an effort to reframe neuropathic low back symptoms in terms of underlying molecular pain mechanisms rather than macroscopic, pathoanatomical treatment targets (e.g., disc extrusions, spondylolisthesis) that have understandably been the historical focus of the vast surgical literature. These instruments combine qualitative symptom reports and physical tests and generally marry older diagnostic maneuvers such as radicular pain evoked with the straight-leg-raising test and sensory responses (e.g., to vibration and pinprick) with approaches borrowed from standard assessment of other neuropathic pain conditions such as an abnormal response to brush movement (e.g., decrease or allodynia). As bedside tests, these screening tools do not include quantification of sensory fiber loss using skin biopsy, electrophysiological tests of nociceptive pathways, or functional brain imaging used by other investigators attempting to unite pain signs and symptoms with underlying biological mechanisms. The Standardized Evaluation of Pain (StEP) tool identifies a positive straight-leg-raising test and abnormal responses to cold stimulation and pinprick as key indicators of radicular low back pain. A burning pain quality and dynamic tactile allodynia were not found to be characteristic features of radicular neuropathic low back pain using their validation model. Overall, StEP found physical examination measures to be more valuable in discriminating neuropathic from nonneuropathic pain and from subtypes of neuropathic pain. Spontaneous burning pain in a radicular distribution has proved to be more important using other diagnostic methods, such as the DN4 and painDETECT tools.[75] The painDETECT questionnaire evaluates the intensity of low back pain using the numerical rating scale, the presence of radiating symptoms, and physical function. Further validation of these important screening and assessment tools is still needed, and important issues such as test-retest reproducibility of the findings and inter- and intrarater reliability have yet to be evaluated.

Imaging is an essential tool for differentiating among chronic neuropathic syndromes associated with specific spinal pathology and nonspecific low back pain (see Figures 21.1–21.5). In patients with marked or progressive neurological deficits, or with suspected concomitant medical illnesses such as cancer and infection (e.g., vertebral body osteomyelitis), early imaging with MRI or computed tomography (CT) is

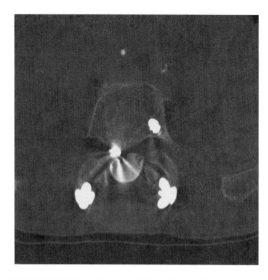

FIGURE 21.2   Chronic L5 lumbar radicular pain following spine surgery attributed to nerve root trauma in the lateral recess caused by pedicle screw placement.

required.[76,77] In cases with high pain intensity persisting for more than 4 weeks, such imaging is routine. In the absence of macroscopic direct nerve root impingement by severe lateral recess stenosis, direct compression by disc protrusion, segmental instability in the setting of

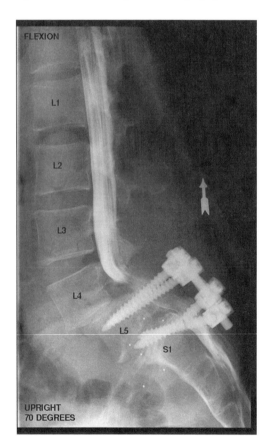

FIGURE 21.1   Chronic bilateral L4 radicular pain after lumbar fusion due to hardware failure resulting in recurrent spondylolisthesis.

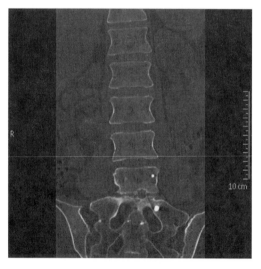

FIGURE 21.3   Persistent axial low back pain worsened with loading after spinal fusion due to failure of bony fusion.

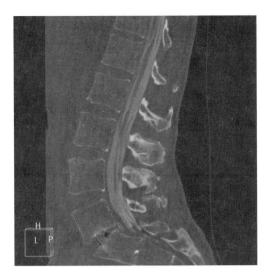

FIGURE 21.4 Persistent axial low back pain worsened with loading after spinal fusion due to failure of bony fusion.

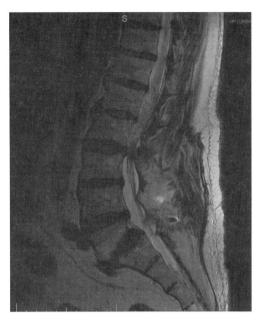

FIGURE 21.5 Recurrent neurogenic claudication attributed to L2/3 segment lumbar stenosis 2 years following L3–5 decompressive laminectomy.

spondylolisthesis, or a space-occupying lesion (e.g., tumor or abscess), imaging has minimal value in distinguishing radicular from non-radicular pain and a predominantly nociceptive underlying mechanism from a neuropathic one. The extent of disc herniation or mechanical deformation of the dorsal root ganglion does not appear to correlate with pain severity[19]; some patients with only minimal disruption to the external morphology of the annulus present with severe radicular pain and signs of dural irritation.[19] With regard to biomarkers in the cerebrospinal fluid of IDH patients, none of definitive diagnostic value have been identified, although interesting evidence has been brought forth on neurofilament and S-100 protein[78] as well as interleukin-8 (IL-8)[79] as indicators of the local inflammatory disease process. As the discussion of neuropathic low back pain screening tools above affirms, patient-reported dysesthesia, paroxysmal symptoms, altered sensory function on physical exam, and historical factors such as prior spinal surgery are among the most common indicators that pain is neuropathic in origin.[15,21] Pain associated with inflamed nerve roots has long been evoked with clinical maneuvers that further narrow neuroforamina or generate a reaction on the nerve roots and thus elicit or augment pain.[80] Evoked symptoms associated with increased intra-abdominal pressure, such as occur with coughing, sneezing, and straining during bowel movements, and the lifting of heavy items are common in patients with radicular pain.

The clinical and diagnostic features of lumbar SpS are distinct from those of other chronic neuropathic low back pain syndromes. Neurogenic claudication is the predominant symptom pattern of lumbar SpS.[40,45] This unique pain pattern typically involving the low back and legs in a nondermatomal distribution is evoked with an upright posture when the patient is standing and walking, thereby causing greater pain-related interference with activity as the syndrome progresses. The pain quality is most often described as dull or aching and carries an impression of heaviness. Multiple clinical studies have shown that neurogenic claudication, with its distinctive clinical phenomenology, is highly specific for the diagnosis of lumbar SpS.[81] In contrast to a prototypical neuropathic radicular pain syndrome, neurogenic claudication is most commonly associated with advanced age and improves when the patient is in a seated or recumbent position.[40] Similar to a radicular syndrome, severe low back and leg pain is the prevailing anatomical distribution. When the lateral recess alone is stenotic, the unpleasant symptoms are typically lateralized as seen with classic radicular pain in the setting of inflammation. The differential diagnosis is also distinctive: vascular claudication due to peripheral vascular disease (e.g., aortoiliac ischemia) must be considered in these patients.

Advanced imaging techniques offers exhaustive anatomical information, but this rich detail tends to be nonspecific for the experience of pain, especially in older patients with extensive degenerative pathology including facet hypertrophy, ligamentous infolding, and extensive osteophyte formation.[82] Because of the postural consequences for intraspinal canal volume, pressure, and resultant symptoms, axial images may underrate narrowing when taken in a supine position as opposed to an upright, load-bearing position.[83] Frequently, radiographic diagnoses of lumbar SpS with minimal clinical relevance are made after imaging an acute nonspecific LBP episode.[84] It is well known that the mild to moderate narrowing often evident on imaging does not correlate with symptom severity. When MRI does reveal a narrowing canal and surgery becomes probable, CT combined with myelography (CTM) offers the best resolution of anatomical posture-dependent targets.[30] Myelography has the drawback of being an invasive procedure with a slight increase in risk. This liability is largely offset by the nuanced characterization of bony and soft tissue advancement against the dural sac with the patient is in the symptomatic posture. Such information may be a valuable adjunct to surgical decision making if decompressive surgery is performed.[85]

Many older patients with imaging evidence of lumbar SpS have no symptoms associated with narrowing, so the clinician's history taking is critical to understanding the experience of pain. Alleviation of chronic low back and leg pain with forward flexion that increases the dimensions of the canal is often a critical detail. Investigators have validated the use of functional tests of walking tolerance as a way to evaluate neurogenic claudication as a screen prior to surgery and as measure of the treatment response after laminectomy.[86-88] Formal treadmill testing has several advantages in addition to minimizing recall bias: it induces the symptoms for which patients seek medical attention, provides a well-studied, quantifiable assessment of functional status, possesses an excellent safety record, and is easy to administer.[89] Treadmill testing has the distinct advantage of being a highly clinically relevant measure since it reproduces the neuropathic claudicatory symptom pattern for which patients seek medical treatment.[90]

The chronic neuropathic low back pain syndrome associated with arachnoiditis is most commonly linked to a prior history of lumbar surgery in the modern era. During the second half of the twentieth century, it was more frequently linked to certain contrast media used for myelography. Arachnoiditis may be a feature of the heterogeneous group of diagnoses encompassed by the term *failed back surgery syndrome* or *postlaminectomy pain syndrome* (See Table 21-1). Arachnoiditis was commonly associated with tuberculosis or syphilis infections up to the early 1900s.[8] Postinfectious inflammatory syndromes following tuberculosis and syphilis were the leading causes before imaging and surgery of the lumbar spine for pain indications became routine. Despite the absence of a consistent clinical picture of arachnoiditis,[91] many practitioners have looked to certain symptoms and signs as clues to this disease process, which is widely considered to have a neuropathic mechanism because of the quality of the spontaneous dysesthetic symptoms. Intense burning pain (particularly in the sacral area or inner aspects of the knees), throbbing, stabbing, or clawing sensations at the calves and ankles, and dysesthesias have all been attributed to arachnoiditis.[46,92,93] These symptoms commonly continue during rest and into the night.[46] Neurogenic claudication has also been reported among patients with arachnoiditis.[94] Involvement of the sympathetic nervous system can occur as well in the form of asymmetric perineal numbness, incontinence of urine or excrement, and/or sexual dysfunction.[8,46] Other common symptoms include back pain, leg pain that may or may not be radicular, and motor and sensory loss.[91,94]

In contrast to other disorders affecting the lumbosacral spinal roots, arachnoiditis is a radiologically and pathologically defined entity that lacks a consistent clinical presentation.[23,91,95]

Table 21-1. Unique Differential Diagnosis of Persistent Neuropathic Pain Following Lumbar Surgery

LACK OF REDUCTION IN PAIN INTENSITY	RECURRENCE OF PAIN
Wrong patient	Recurrence of disc herniation
Wrong lumbar segment	New disc herniation
Insufficient removal of herniated disc	Epidural fibrosis
Inadequate decompression	Arachnoiditis
Unrecognized second disc herniation/pathology	Symptomatic osteoarthritis/adjacent level disease
Nerve root trauma	Secondary spinal stenosis
	Microinstability
	Macroinstability

Imaging with CTM and MRI offers good discrimination of soft tissue densities and thus the possibility of identifying the chronic dural changes associated with arachnoiditis[8,95]; failure of the myelographic medium to fill the subarachnoid space immediately after injection or only filiform passage of the medium can be suggestive of arachnoiditis.[94,96] Even in the domain of radiology, however, this condition has considerable variability.[97–99] Pathologically, differing degrees of severity can present, "from mild thickening of the pia and arachnoid membrane to severe adhesions binding the roots to each other and to the dura, causing obliteration of the subarachnoid space."[94] Only when a fibrinous exudate causes the subarachnoid membrane to adhere to encapsulated nerve roots or causes the roots to adhere to one another will the pathological changes of arachnoiditis be radiologically observable.[95] Alternatively, fibrosis and scarring must distort the spinal neural anatomy enough for the abnormalities to be visible on imaging.[95] Thus, the spectrum of radiological arachnoiditis varies from a condition of no observable alteration to one of dramatic change.[95] The first radiological abnormalities to be observable include arachnoid adhesion within the nerve root sleeves, adhesion of neighboring roots of the cauda equina or of roots and the arachnoid within the theca, or a mixture of such adhesions.[95] The ensuing stage presents as disfigurement of the lumbosacral cul de sac, signifying some concentric fibrotic tightening of the theca.[95] While Delamarter et al. established three categories to delineate the various MRI appearances, ranging from mild to severe, of arachnoiditis, these groupings are not associated with clinical histories.[95,98] Several studies have highlighted this lack of correlation between radiological findings and symptomatic presentation.[100,101] Canine models have also highlighted a lack of correlation between clinical presentation and postmortem pathological changes.[102]

PATHOGENESIS

The relationship between chronic low back symptoms in patients and underlying mechanisms of neuropathic pain is poorly understood. It is widely presumed that most chronic low back pain syndromes have multiple underlying mechanisms, that is, a mixture of inflammatory and neuropathic processes, giving rise to chronic symptoms.[16] Attribution of a *mixed* mechanism does not suffice to reconcile the diverging lines of evidence with regard to the neuropathic component of chronic low back pain. The debate turns on the precise localization of the lesion or disease affecting the somatosensory system that gives rise to chronic low back pain. The *lesion-based* line of research emphasizes specific spinal pathologies and their direct consequences for neural structures in the periphery. By contrast, the *disease* or *dysfunction* school focuses on on the preponderance of nonspecific chronic low back pain cases and posits a disorder of altered nociceptive processing at the level of the central nervous system.

Animal models of radiculopathy highlight the importance of ectopic discharges at the level of the dorsal spinal root and its ganglion in αβ, αδ, and C fibers as a cause of neuropathic low back pain.[103] Various canine and porcine animal models using autologous nucleus pulposus injected into the epidural space induce features of radiculopathy such as nerve fiber degeneration and reduced conduction velocity.[104,105] Nerve roots exposed to nucleus pulposus but not mechanically compressed have been shown to induce lesions consistent with neuropathic pain, including axonal degeneration, myelin edema, intravascular coagulation, increased endoneurial pressure, reduced intraneural blood flow, and diminished nerve conduction velocity.[106] Inflammatory mediators such as prostaglandin E2 produce ectopic impulses in canine models, and other lines of evidence support the role of IL-6 and IL-8.[107]

Inflammation of the symptomatic nerve roots in humans appears to figure prominently in the pathophysiology of highly prevalent radicular pain syndromes associated with both compressive and noncompressive disc lesions.[6] This insight is of critical importance because it offers an explanation for nerve root pain that would not be disclosed with advanced imaging techniques. Ongoing inflammation within and outside neural structures may have important implications for the neurobiological transformation that occurs in nociceptive pathways during the transition from acute to chronic low back pain. Both animal models and studies of radicular pain in humans suggest that inflammation around the nerve root may induce a lowering of the pain threshold, thereby rendering subsequent mechanical compression more painful.[6,108] The Guanosine triphosphate (GTP) cyclohydrase gene has already been identified as a possible modifier of chronicity in patients with low back pain.[109] Inflammatory pain is mediated by GTP cyclohydrolase, and the end product of the synthesis cascade that it initiates, tetrahydrobiopterin (BH4), is a cofactor essential for the production of nitric oxide, catecholamine, and serotonin as well as for metabolism of phenylalanine.[109,110]

Over the past decade, studies of the pathogenesis of neuropathic chronic low back pain have increasingly concentrated on altered nociceptive processing at the spinal and supraspinal levels rather than on nociceptive foci in the spine, the so-called *end-organ dysfunction models*. This shift in emphasis from the study of local injury implicating structures such as the nerve root, ganglion, and intervertebral disc to neuroplasticity at the level of the dorsal horn and cortical processing has been propelled largely by the lack of a clear relationship between macroscopic pathology, as disclosed by imaging, and pain intensity. Other key drivers for this redirection of research focus include the pivotal role of psychological vulnerabilities as a risk factor for chronic low back pain and a predictor of the treatment outcome; the elevated rates of co-occurring pain syndromes (e.g., headache, Temporomandibular joint disorder); emerging genetic evidence for the heritability of heightened pain sensitivity; and lack of a biological explanation for the persistence of symptoms in patients with nonspecific low back pain.[111-114] Functional MRI studies of patients with low back pain highlight the importance of the medial prefrontal cortex in modulating the intensity of spontaneous pain and its duration; however, the claim for a causative role of these alterations in regional brain metabolism and other morphometric observations in the dorsolateral prefrontal cortex in low back pain is purely speculative.[115,116] Countering this trend toward classification of nonspecific chronic low back pain as neuropathic at the level of the cortex is the argument that these cases are most aptly classified as nociceptive axial syndromes referred from paraspinal musculature, ligaments, and joint surfaces or somatic referred pain reflecting the convergence of afferent input at the level of the second-order neurons in the spinal cord.[10] Research on the neuropathic mechanism of neurogenic claudication associated with SpS has resolved the tension between lesion and dysfunction altogether differently by focusing on the peripheral neurovascular changes that correlate with that distinctive syndrome's evoked symptoms.

For much of the twentieth century, the pathogenesis of neurogenic claudication was attributed to direct mechanical compression of the cauda equina and nerve roots in a narrowed lumbar bony canal. This explanation provided the rationale for decompressive laminectomy in the 1950s. The bony and soft tissue overgrowth associated with a variety of disease processes, such as Paget's disease, are known to cause stenosis and may be the targets of surgical decompression. These nonneural changes alone are not widely considered to be a source of pain. The simplistic direct neurocompressive explanation for claudicating pain further unraveled in the ensuing decades because several clinical features of the pain were not consistent with a neural entrapment syndrome. These included the rapid symptom relief with change of posture, absence of fixed sensory and motor deficits in many patients with significant narrowing, and lack of analgesic or functional benefit in up to a third of patients with neurogenic claudication undergoing extensive surgical decompression. Although direct mechanical compression of neural structures may cause symptoms in a subpopulation of patients with the most severely narrowed canals, it fails to account for the episodic pain experienced by the vast majority of patients with symptoms that rapidly remit with postural adjustment. Earlier theories of mechanical compression have given way to more refined studies relating the effects of increased intraspinal pressure on local neural conduction, homeostasis, and inflammation.

The underlying pain mechanism of the neuropathic symptom pattern known as *neurogenic claudication* remains a matter of controversy, but the animal and human evidence for a neurovascular mechanism continues to build. The direct relationship between increased intraspinal pressure and extensor postures is the best-understood aspect of the syndrome's pathophysiology; it has been quantified with manometry and directly observed with myeloscopy in symptomatic and asymptomatic patients.[117,118] The reproducible correspondence of symptom onset and resolution with pressure changes (e.g., postural adjustment) underscores the clinical significance of this association. Cadaveric studies describe the specific nerve lesions, such as hypertrophy of the pia-arachnoid, as well as characteristic venous changes indicative of chronic congestion that would constitute the basis for a neuropathic pain syndrome.[119] The clinical significance of the adhesive pia-arachnoiditis is thought to impede normal cerebrospinal fluid (CSF) flow and compound the metabolic derangement associated with episodic neuroischemia. Reduced permeability coupled with compromised CSF flow may provoke a localized hypometabolic state in the nerve root(s) at symptomatic levels. The cumulative effects of inflammation may explain why progression of neuropathic symptoms in lumbar SpS is gradual compared with other radicular syndromes. Gradual decomposition of the blood-nerve barrier has been demonstrated in a canine model of chronic constriction and results in intraradicular edema.[120] This edema is mediated by macrophage invasion of the nerve root and has been linked to heightened vascular permeability; it seems to instigate a transient inflammatory neuritis.[121]

Olmarker et al. revealed that mechanical pressure in a porcine could cause disturbances in the blood supply and in the nutrition of the nerve roots; they characterized the direct relationship between increased pressure and impairment of nerve conduction.[105] These pathophysiological findings have been replicated in nerve conduction studies of patients with neurogenic claudication (e.g., transient loss of f waves), thereby providing a basis for this pain syndrome's somatosensory dysfunction.[122] Ikawa et al. linked venous stasis to ectopic nerve root activity in a rat model of two-level chronic lumbar spinal canal stenosis by demonstrating antidromically propagated sural nerve impulses following clamping of the inferior vena cava.[123] This model aimed to replicate the venous congestion observed in ambulating patients with stenosis and claudication.[18-20] Sekiguchi and colleagues have shown that a neuropathic pain syndrome localizing to the cauda equina does not have the characteristic apoptosis of dorsal root ganglion cells important for the generation and maintenance of mechanical allodynia or hyperalgesia.[124] The lack of mechanical allodynia in these models is consistent with the clinical presentation of neurogenic claudication in the human, in which these neuropathic signs are also absent.

In contrast to the evoked pain pattern of neurogenic claudication, the neuropathic pain syndromes following lumbar spine surgery are marked by ongoing spontaneous pain. The list of hypothesized causes for this diverse group of syndromes is extensive and includes a range of specific structural spinal pathologies in addition to nonspecific syndromes defined primarily by symptom quality and duration. Residual lateral spinal stenosis,[32,125–127] spondylolisthesis as a late sequela of laminectomy or pseudoarthrosis in the context of fusion,128 recurrent/residual disc herniation,[127] epidural scar formation,[31] and arachnoiditis are the most common structural and macroscopically visible etiological factors following spine surgery (i.e., FBSS).[46,127] As the name reveals, inflammation and impaired CSF flow are thought to figure prominently in the pain of arachnoiditis. This radiologically defined condition has been attributed to a multitude of etiological agents including surgery of the spine,[49,50,97,129,130] contrast media used in imaging,[91,95,131–133] spinal anesthesia,[8,49,131] infections,[49,134,135] intrathecal hemorrhage,[94] and intervertebral disc herniation.[132,136,137] Ultimately, "the introduction of virtually any foreign material into the subarachnoid space is likely to result in some degree of arachnoiditis."[95]

While the pathology of lumbosacral arachnoiditis has been meticulously described,[46] the relationship of physiological, cellular, and/or molecular factors to neuropathic pain remains elusive. Fibrinous bands and cauda equina adhesions that develop in this condition alter both CSF and blood flow.[47] Postlaminectomy rat models demonstrate dilated nutrient vessels, augmented vascular permeability, and eosinophilic exudation in the cauda equina soon after surgery.[138,139] Ultrastructural examination of the rat cauda equina following laminectomy has revealed opening of tight junctions and heightened vesicular transport within endothelial cells of nutrient vessels, which could point to a compromised blood-nerve barrier.[138,139] Such evidence has led some investigators to believe that extradural inflammation as part of the process of wound healing may induce cauda equina adhesion.[140] Anti-inflammatory drugs delivered both pre- and postoperatively in the laminectomy rat model inhibited protein leakage through nutrient vessels as well as cauda equina adhesion.[140] Such findings lend support to the proposal that increasing permeability in the cauda equina arises from epidural inflammation and leads to cauda equina adhesion.[140] Nerve degeneration has also been associated with prolonged lumbar adhesive arachnoiditis,[139] while human patients have demonstrated neurological involvement including hyporeflexia and weakness.[141] With the goal of identifying the mechanism underpinning nerve degeneration, Miaki and colleagues examined the glucose supply to the adhered cauda equina in rats.[47] Interestingly, the glucose supply from blood was elevated by 153%, while that from CSF was dramatically diminished to 28% (of the supply to the healthy cauda equina). Such conditions may be responsible for the pathological and functional alterations observed in lumbar adhesive arachnoiditis.[47]

MANAGEMENT, TREATMENT, AND PREVENTION

The evidence base for the management of radicular pain and radiculopathy may be broadly divided into two groups: (1) medication therapy and (2) surgical, interventional, and multidisciplinary rehabilitation approaches. Treatments in the latter group include a range of surgical techniques, spinal injections, and neuromodulating therapies, as well as non-pharmacological interventions mostly targeting specific spinal structures, radicular pain, and neuropathic symptoms. The accuracy of these varied approaches for addressing specific spinal causes of radicular pain and radiculopathy, as well as the evidence for their efficacy, raise controversial questions.[142] Approaches for nonspecific low back pain, such as interdisciplinary rehabilitation for which the level of evidence has been favorably rated, are beyond the scope of this chapter. Of note, there are multiple analgesic studies of opioids, tramadol, and, more recently, duloxetine demonstrating drug efficacy for nonspecific chronic low back pain syndromes.[143–146] To the extent that these therapies reduce pain intensity and improve function in chronic nonspecific low back pain, it may be reasonable to infer that there are specific treatment effects for syndromes with *mixed* mechanisms.

Most therapies in widespread use, such as nonsteroidal anti-inflammatory drugs (NSAIDs) and muscle relaxants, have not been specifically tested in populations enriched for the neuropathic symptom profiles or signs discussed above. In many cases, their benefit for chronic pain has been extrapolated from *acute* treatment trials. The external validity of these results for a population of patients with chronic low back pain cannot be assumed since the clinical features and underlying neurobiological mechanisms are largely distinct. This claim is supported by the fact that currently there are no published double-blind, repeated-dose trials of pharmacotherapy specifically for radicular pain demonstrating the superiority of active drug to placebo. For example, the authors of a recent evidence-based review of medications for chronic low back pain could not draw a definite conclusion about therapy for radiculopathy or radicular pain due to the paucity of studies designed for this indication.[76] A recent systematic review of analgesic studies in low back pain highlighted other problems with the evidence base, including lack of clinically relevant back-related functional endpoints, such as walking tolerance in patients with neurogenic claudication associated with lumbar SpS.[147]

There are multiple international consensus guidelines for the evidence-based treatment of neuropathic pain, but insofar as their recommendations pertain to spinal conditions, they are derived from syndromes such as postherpetic neuralgia and diabetic peripheral neuropathy.[148] There are multiple negative trials for drugs with demonstrated efficacy in other neuropathic pain syndromes including recent well-designed trials of pregabalin for radiculopathy.[73] The screening tools discussed earlier, such as DN4 and StEP, were designed and validated for epidemiological studies and patient screening. In clinical practice, the results of these screens may support further clinical investigation and consultation with a specialist, but they should not serve as the basis for prescribing neuropathic pain medications. This lack of analgesic efficacy may reflect an absence of pain-relieving benefit for these drugs in spinal syndromes with neuropathic mechanisms or possibly methodological flaws in these studies. Many of these published studies and other, unpublished negative clinical trials have rigorously defined the neuropathic low back pain study population in accordance with the symptoms and signs

of painful radiculopathy. Such a grouping of patients with pain may still be too diverse from a mechanistic standpoint for these methods to detect benefit. Of note, three trials of corticosteroids for acute radiculopathy (i.e., oral steroid taper or single infusion) did not have a clinically significant analgesic benefit compared with placebo.[150,151] A small double-blind, single-dose trial of acute lidocaine infusion was shown to significantly reduce pain intensity in patients with a diagnosis of sciatica,[152] but a comprehensive review of the literature found that bed rest, NSAIDs, intramuscular steroids, tizandine, and traction are not superior to placebo.[153]

In patients with persistent radicular pain in the context of disc herniation, consensus guidelines recommend a trial of epidural steroid injections on the basis of moderate evidence of short-term benefit.[142] The evidence is less robust for the role of this modality in neurogenic claudication. A retrospective review of 140 patients found that approximately 33% reported relief for over 2 months, and 50% exhibited improved walking tolerance.[154] A prospective, randomized study found that the injections provided improvement in approximately 50% of lumbar IDH patients who had a previous 6-week trial of noninvasive care.[155] No differences in regression or herniation size were found between patients who improved and those who did not.[155] The therapy remained effective for as long as 3 years. Further research has confirmed the benefits of epidural steroid injections in relieving the radicular pain of IDH,[156–158] with one study even reporting a higher success rate.[156]

There is high-quality evidence favoring decompressive surgery for the treatment of persistent radicular pain in the setting disc herniation with standard open discectomy or microdiscectomy at 3 months compared with nonsurgical approaches.[159,160] Although surgery is associated with better short-term results, over time the beneficial effects wane and may be less advantageous than those offered by other approaches.[161,162] Other investigators have found more prolonged benefit, with the caveat that the patient with a radicular syndrome has not had previous lumbar surgery.[69] There is strong evidence for up to at least 2 years of increased benefit relative to conservative treatment with decompressive laminectomy for the treatment of disabling neurogenic claudication in the context of lumbar SpS with or without spondylolisthesis.[163,164] The trade-off of benefit and risk appears to be far less favorable for instrumented fusion for lumbar SpS and axial low back pain syndromes.[9,165]

There is evidence for the role of spinal cord stimulation (SCS) in patients with prominent radicular neuropathic symptoms following laminectomy. Two randomized, prospective studies of SCS in FBSS have shown significant reductions in pain intensity and have demonstrated SCS to be superior to reoperation in alleviating target symptoms. A recent study examined 100 FBSS patients with leg pain of neuropathic radicular orgin and self-rated pain greater than 50 mm by visual analog scale of at least 6 months' duration.[166] Patients were randomized to receive SCS plus conventional medical management (CMM) or CMM alone.

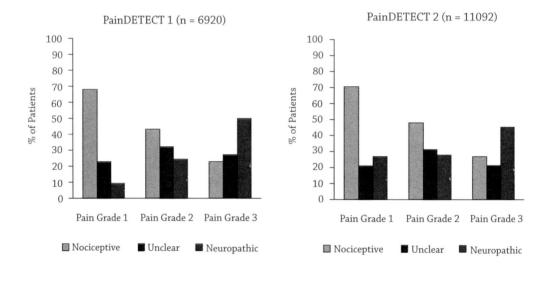

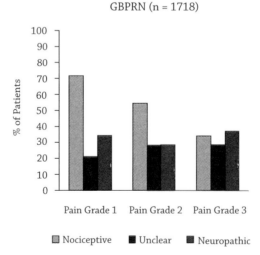

FIGURE 21.6 These data from three German Back Pain Research Network surveys demonstrate the consistent relationship between higher pain grade and phenotypic features of a neuropathic mechanism using the Pain Dectect instrument.

Source: Reprinted from Schmidt CO et al. Modelling the prevalence and cost of back pain with neuropathic components in the general population. *Eur J Pain*. 2009;13(10):1030–10355, with permission from Elsevier.

The primary outcome of at least 50% pain reduction in the legs was achieved in 48% of SCS patients compared to only 9% of CMM patients using an intention to treat analysis ($P < .001$). Patients in the SCS arm of the trial also experienced a significantly improved health-related quality of life and superior outcomes on the Oswestry low back pain disability measure. An earlier study of 50 enrolled FBSS patients who had been selected for reoperation by standard criteria and randomized them to receive either reoperation or SCS.[167] Patients randomized to SCS were significantly less likely to cross over to surgery compared to reoperation patients who crossed over to SCS (5 of 24 patients vs. 14 of 26 patients, $P = .02$), and the proportion of patients experiencing 50% pain relief was greater in the SCS group. In addition, the patients randomized to SCS also required less opioid analgesia than those undergoing reoperation. The benefit of SCS must be weighed against the technical complications such as lead migration and the need for repeat interventions (e.g., battery replacement). Uncertainty about the subgroup of patients most likely to benefit from this treatment and the lack of blinding of patients in a controlled fashion must be taken into account when interpreting these study results.

FUTURE DIRECTIONS

There are many barriers to improving the care of patients with neuropathic LBP that will only be addressed by further research. Firstly, the process of defining the relationship between clinical pain phenotypes and underlying pain mechanisms begun in the past decade with the development of screening tools must continue. Refining this understanding will not only improve the ability of clinical trials to detect meaningful effects of novel therapies but also enhance treatment matching in clinical practice. Most chronic neuropathic low back pain syndromes originate in acute nociceptive pain syndromes localizing to specific spinal structures. Future research efforts must reconcile the large treatment effect sizes of local approaches targeting neurocompressive causes of neuropathic pain with the growing body of evidence that nonspecific chronic low back pain, often with neuropathic features, may result from dysfunctional nociceptive processing at the cortical, subcortical, and spinal levels within the central nervous system. The neurobiology of the transition from acute to chronic pain is the least well understood aspect of the neuropathic chronic low back pain enigma. Since neuropathic low back pain is both expensive and disabling, it is imperative that trials of currently available and new therapies incorporate comprehensive outcome measures including back-specific functional endpoints. These trials must be reported in such a way as to facilitate estimates of effect size and other comparisons of clinical relevance (see Figure 21.6).

REFERENCES

1. Khoromi S et al. Topiramate in chronic lumbar radicular pain. *J Pain*. 2005;6(12):829–836.
2. Berger A, Dukes EM, Oster G. Clinical characteristics and economic costs of patients with painful neuropathic disorders. *J Pain*. 2004;5(3):143–149.
3. Deyo RA. Drug therapy for back pain. Which drugs help which patients? *Spine (Phila Pa 1976)*. 1996;21(24):2840–2849; discussion 2849–2850.
4. Heliovaara M et al. Lumbar disc syndrome in Finland. *J Epidemiol Community Health*. 1987;41(3):251–258.
5. Xie WR et al. Robust increase of cutaneous sensitivity, cytokine production and sympathetic sprouting in rats with localized inflammatory irritation of the spinal ganglia. *Neuroscience*. 2006;142(3):809–822.
6. Peng B et al. Chemical radiculitis. *Pain*. 2007;127(1–2):11–16.
7. Merskey H, Bogduk N, and International Association for the Study of Pain, Task Force on Taxonomy. *Classification of Chronic Pain: Descriptions of Chronic Pain Syndromes and Definitions of Pain Terms*. 2nd ed. Seattle: IASP Press; 1994:xvi.
8. Aldrete JA. Neurologic deficits and arachnoiditis following neuroaxial anesthesia. *Acta Anaesthesiol Scand*. 2003;47(1):3–12.
9. Deyo RA et al. Trends, major medical complications, and charges associated with surgery for lumbar spinal stenosis in older adults. *JAMA*. 2010;303(13):1259–1265.
10. Bogduk N. On the definitions and physiology of back pain, referred pain, and radicular pain. *Pain*. 2009;147(1–3):17–19.

11. Jensen MC et al. Magnetic resonance imaging of the lumbar spine in people without back pain. *N Engl J Med*. 1994;331(2):69–73.

12. Freynhagen R et al. Pseudoradicular and radicular low-back pain—a disease continuum rather than different entities? Answers from quantitative sensory testing. *Pain*. 2008;135(1–2): 65–74.

13. Scholz J et al. A novel tool for the assessment of pain: validation in low back pain. *PLoS Med*. 2009;6(4):e1000047.

14. Butler SH. Back pain is complicated. *Pain*. 2010; 150(3):380–381.

15. Bennett GJ. Neuropathic pain: new insights, new interventions. *Hosp Pract (Minneap)*. 1998;33(10):95–8, 101–104, 107–110 passim.

16. Deyo RA, Weinstein JN. Low back pain. *N Engl J Med*. 2001;344(5):363–370.

17. Rubin DI, Epidemiology and risk factors for spine pain. *Neurol Clin*. 2007;25(2):353–371.

18. van Tulder M, Koes B, Bombardier C. Low back pain. *Best Pract Res Clin Rheumatol*. 2002;16(5):761–775.

19. Zhang JM, Munir M. Radicular low back pain: what have we learned from recent animal research? *Anesthesiology*. 2008;108(1):5–6.

20. Freburger JK et al. The rising prevalence of chronic low back pain. *Arch Intern Med*. 2009;169(3):251–258.

21. Kaki AM, El-Yaski AZ, Youseif E. Identifying neuropathic pain among patients with chronic low-back pain: use of the Leeds Assessment of Neuropathic Symptoms and Signs pain scale. *Reg Anesth Pain Med*. 2005;30(5):422–428.

22. Schmidt CO et al. Modelling the prevalence and cost of back pain with neuropathic components in the general population. *Eur J Pain*. 2009;13(10):1030–1035.

23. Shipton EA. Low back pain and the postlaminectomy pain syndrome. *S Afr Med J*. 1989;76(1):20–23.

24. Kauffman C, Garfin SR., Spinal stenosis: pathophysiology and symptom complex update 1999. Semin Spine Surg. 1999;11:209–214.

25. Cherkin DC et al. An international comparison of back surgery rates. *Spine (Phila Pa 1976)*. 1994;19(11):1201–1206.

26. Cummins J et al. Descriptive epidemiology and prior healthcare utilization of patients in the Spine Patient Outcomes Research Trial's (SPORT) three observational cohorts: disc herniation, spinal stenosis, and degenerative spondylolisthesis. *Spine (Phila Pa 1976)*. 2006;31(7):806–814.

27. Epter RS et al. Systematic review of percutaneous adhesiolysis and management of chronic low back pain in postlumbar surgery syndrome. *Pain Physician*. 2009;12(2):361–378.

28. Frymoyer JW. Back pain and sciatica. *N Engl J Med*. 1988;318(5):291–300.

29. Hart LG, Deyo RA, Cherkin DC. Physician office visits for low back pain. Frequency, clinical evaluation, and treatment patterns from a U.S. national survey. *Spine (Phila Pa 1976)*. 1995;20(1):11–19.

30. Markman JD, Gaud KG. Lumbar spinal stenosis in older adults: current understanding and future directions. *Clin Geriatr Med*. 2008;24(2):369–388, viii.

31. Fiume D et al. Treatment of the failed back surgery syndrome due to lumbo-sacral epidural fibrosis. *Acta Neurochir Suppl*. 1995;64:116–118.

32. Djukic S et al. The postoperative spine. Magnetic resonance imaging. *Orthop Clin North Am*. 1990;21(3):603–624.

33. Frymoyer JW et al. Failed lumbar disc surgery requiring second operation. A long-term follow-up study. *Spine (Phila Pa 1976)*. 1978;3(1):7–11.

34. Chou R et al. Imaging strategies for low-back pain: systematic review and meta-analysis. *Lancet*. 2009;373(9662):463–472.

35. Saal JA, Saal JS. Nonoperative treatment of herniated lumbar intervertebral disc with radiculopathy. An outcome study. *Spine (Phila Pa 1976)*. 1989;14(4):431–437.

36. Fager CA. Observations on spontaneous recovery from intervertebral disc herniation. *Surg Neurol*. 1994;42(4):282–286.

37. Bozzao A et al. Lumbar disk herniation: MR imaging assessment of natural history in patients treated without surgery. *Radiology*. 1992;185(1):135–141.

38. Weber H. Lumbar disc herniation. A controlled, prospective study with ten years of observation. *Spine (Phila Pa 1976)*. 1983;8(2):131–140.

39. Atlas SJ et al. Surgical and nonsurgical management of lumbar spinal stenosis: four-year outcomes from the Maine lumbar spine study. *Spine (Phila Pa 1976)*. 2000;25(5):556–562.

40. Katz JN et al. Degenerative lumbar spinal stenosis. Diagnostic value of the history and physical examination. *Arthritis Rheum*. 1995;38(9):1236–1241.

41. Simotas AC et al. Nonoperative treatment for lumbar spinal stenosis. Clinical and outcome results and a 3-year survivorship analysis. *Spine (Phila Pa 1976)*. 2000;25(2):197–203; discussions 203–204.

42. Amundsen T et al. Lumbar spinal stenosis: conservative or surgical management? A prospective

10-year study. *Spine (Phila Pa 1976)*. 2000;25(11): 1424–1435; discussion 1435–1436.

43. Haig AJ et al. The sensitivity and specificity of electrodiagnostic testing for the clinical syndrome of lumbar spinal stenosis. *Spine (Phila Pa 1976)*. 2005;30(23):2667–2676.

44. Johnsson KE, Uden A, Rosen I. The effect of decompression on the natural course of spinal stenosis. A comparison of surgically treated and untreated patients. *Spine (Phila Pa 1976)*. 1991;16(6):615–619.

45. Siebert E et al. Lumbar spinal stenosis: syndrome, diagnostics and treatment. *Nat Rev Neurol*. 2009;5(7):392–403.

46. Bourne IH. Lumbo-sacral adhesive arachnoiditis: a review. *J R Soc Med*. 1990;83(4):262–265.

47. Miaki K et al. Nutritional supply to the cauda equina in lumbar adhesive arachnoiditis in rats. Eur Spine J. 1999;8(4):310–316.

48. Horax G. Generalised cisternal arachnoiditis simulating cerebellar tumour: its surgical treatment and end results. *Arch Surg*. 1924;9:95–112.

49. Quiles M, Marchisello PJ, Tsairis P. Lumbar adhesive arachnoiditis. Etiologic and pathologic aspects. *Spine (Phila Pa 1976)*. 1978;3(1):45–50.

50. Benoist M et al. Postoperative lumbar epiduro-arachnoiditis. Diagnostic and therapeutic aspects. *Spine (Phila Pa 1976)*. 1980;5(5):432–436.

51. Ricci JA et al. Back pain exacerbations and lost productive time costs in United States workers. *Spine (Phila Pa 1976)*. 2006;31(26):3052–3060.

52. Rowe ML. Low back pain in industry. A position paper. *J Occup Med*. 1969;11(4):161–169.

53. Stewart WF et al. Lost productive time and cost due to common pain conditions in the U.S. workforce. *JAMA*. 2003;290(18):2443–2454.

54. Guo HR et al. Back pain prevalence in U.S. industry and estimates of lost workdays. *Am J Public Health*. 1999;89(7):1029–1035.

55. Bigos SJ, United States Agency for Health Care Policy and Research. *Acute Low Back Problems in Adults*. Clinical Practice Guideline No. 14. Rockville, MD: U.S. Department of Health and Human Services, Public Health Service, Agency for Health Care Policy and Research; 1994:viii.

56. Andersson GB. Epidemiological features of chronic low-back pain. *Lancet*. 1999;354(9178): 581–585.

57. Croft PR et al. Outcome of low back pain in general practice: a prospective study. *BMJ*. 1998;316(7141):1356–1359.

58. Tang PC et al. Comparison of methodologies for calculating quality measures based on administrative data versus clinical data from an elec-

tronic health record system: implications for performance measures. *J Am Med Inform Assoc*. 2007;14(1):10–15.

59. Ehrlich GE. Low back pain. *Bull World Health Org*. 2003;81(9):671–676.

60. Woolf AD, Pfleger B. Burden of major musculoskeletal conditions. *Bull World Health Org*. 2003;81(9):646–656.

61. Jensen MP, Chodroff MJ, Dworkin RH. The impact of neuropathic pain on health-related quality of life: review and implications. *Neurology*. 2007;68(15):1178–1182.

62. Pincus T et al. A systematic review of psychological factors as predictors of chronicity/disability in prospective cohorts of low back pain. *Spine (Phila Pa 1976)*. 2002;27(5):E109–E120.

63. Linton SJ. A review of psychological risk factors in back and neck pain. *Spine (Phila Pa 1976)*. 2000;25(9):1148–1156.

64. Herron LD et al. The differential utility of the Minnesota Multiphasic Personality Inventory. A predictor of outcome in lumbar laminectomy for disc herniation versus spinal stenosis. *Spine (Phila Pa 1976)*. 1986;11(8):847–850.

65. Brook RH. Health policy and public trust. *JAMA*. 2008;300(2):211–213.

66. Frymoyer J, Durett C. The economics of spinal disorders. Philadelphia , PA: Lippincott-Raven. 1997.

67. Katz JN. Lumbar disc disorders and low-back pain: socioeconomic factors and consequences. *J Bone Joint Surg Am*. 2006;88(suppl 2):21–24.

68. Kinsella K, Velkoff V. *An Aging World*. In: Bureau USC (ed), Washington, DC. 2001.

69. Atlas SJ et al. Long-term outcomes of surgical and nonsurgical management of lumbar spinal stenosis: 8 to 10 year results from the Maine lumbar spine study. *Spine (Phila Pa 1976)*. 2005;30(8):936–943.

70. Smyth MJ, Wright V. Sciatica and the intervertebral disc; an experimental study. *J Bone Joint Surg Am*. 1958;40-A(6):1401–1418.

71. Cruccu G et al. EFNS guidelines on neuropathic pain assessment. *Eur J Neurol*. 2004;11(3): 153–162.

72. Markman J et al. Characterization of neuropathic pain in post laminectomy pain syndromes. Presented at the 13th World Congress on Pain. Montreal, Ontario, Canada; 2010.

73. Baron R et al. The efficacy and safety of pregabalin in the treatment of neuropathic pain associated with chronic lumbosacral radiculopathy. *Pain*. 2010;150(3):420–427.

74. Bouhassira D et al. Comparison of pain syndromes associated with nervous or somatic

lesions and development of a new neuropathic pain diagnostic questionnaire (DN4). *Pain*. 2005;114(1–2):29–36.

75. Freynhagen R et al. painDETECT: a new screening questionnaire to identify neuropathic components in patients with back pain. *Curr Med Res Opin*. 2006;22(10):1911–1920.

76. Chou R et al. Medications for acute and chronic low back pain: a review of the evidence for an American Pain Society/American College of Physicians clinical practice guideline. *Ann Intern Med*. 2007;147(7):505–514.

77. Chou R et al. Diagnosis and treatment of low back pain: a joint clinical practice guideline from the American College of Physicians and the American Pain Society. *Ann Intern Med*. 2007;147(7):478–491.

78. Brisby H et al. Markers of nerve tissue injury in the cerebrospinal fluid in patients with lumbar disc herniation and sciatica. *Spine (Phila Pa 1976)*. 1999;24(8):742–746.

79. Brisby H et al. Proinflammatory cytokines in cerebrospinal fluid and serum in patients with disc herniation and sciatica. *Eur Spine J*. 2002;11(1):62–66.

80. Brown JR. Radicular pain including the Guillain-Barré syndrome. *Lancet*. 1955;75(7):315–319.

81. Turner JA et al. Surgery for lumbar spinal stenosis. Attempted meta-analysis of the literature. *Spine*. 1992;17(1):1–8.

82. Boden SD et al. Abnormal magnetic-resonance scans of the cervical spine in asymptomatic subjects. A prospective investigation. *J Bone Joint Surg Am*. 1990;72(8):1178–1184.

83. Saint-Louis LA. Lumbar spinal stenosis assessment with computed tomography, magnetic resonance imaging, and myelography. *Clin Orthop Relat Res*. 2001;(384):122–136.

84. Jinkins JR. MR evaluation of stenosis involving the neural foramina, lateral recesses, and central canal of the lumbosacral spine. *Magn Reson Imaging Clin North Am*. 1999;7(3):493–511, viii.

85. Willen J et al. Dynamic effects on the lumbar spinal canal: axially loaded CT-myelography and MRI in patients with sciatica and/or neurogenic claudication. *Spine (Phila Pa 1976)*. 1997;22(24):2968–2976.

86. Dong G, Porter RW. Walking and cycling tests in neurogenic and intermittent claudication. *Spine (Phila Pa)*. 1989;14(9):965–969.

87. Dyck P, Doyle JB Jr. "Bicycle test" of van Gelderen in diagnosis of intermittent cauda equina compression syndrome. Case report. *J Neurosurg*. 1977;46(5):667–670.

88. Fritz JM et al. Preliminary results of the use of a two-stage treadmill test as a clinical diagnostic tool in the differential diagnosis of lumbar spinal stenosis. *J Spinal Disord*. 1997;10(5):410–416.

89. Deen HG et al. Use of the exercise treadmill to measure baseline functional status and surgical outcome in patients with severe lumbar spinal stenosis. *Spine (Phila Pa 1976)*. 1998;23(2):244–248.

90. Deen HG Jr et al. Test-retest reproducibility of the exercise treadmill examination in lumbar spinal stenosis. *Mayo Clin Proc*. 2000;75(10):1002–1007.

91. Long DM. Chronic adhesive spinal arachnoiditis: pathogenesis, prognosis, and treatment. *Neurosurg Q*. 1992;2:296–319.

92. Malmberg AB, Yaksh TL. Hyperalgesia mediated by spinal glutamate or substance P receptor blocked by spinal cyclooxygenase inhibition. *Science*. 1992;257(5074):1276–1279.

93. Lin Q et al. Involvement of cGMP in nociceptive processing by and sensitization of spinothalamic neurons in primates. *J Neurosci*. 1997;17(9):3293–3302.

94. Roca J et al. The results of surgical treatment of lumbar arachnoiditis. *Int Orthop*. 1993;17(2):77–81.

95. Petty PG, Hudgson P, Hare WS. Symptomatic lumbar spinal arachnoiditis: fact or fallacy? *J Clin Neurosci*. 2000;7(5):395–399.

96. Shikata J et al. Surgical treatment for symptomatic spinal adhesive arachnoiditis. *Spine (Phila Pa 1976)*. 1989;14(8):870–875.

97. Benner B, Ehni G. Spinal arachnoiditis. The postoperative variety in particular. *Spine (Phila Pa 1976)*. 1978;3(1):40–44.

98. Delamarter RB et al. Diagnosis of lumbar arachnoiditis by magnetic resonance imaging. *Spine (Phila Pa 1976)*. 1990;15(4):304–310.

99. Jorgensen J et al. A clinical and radiological study of chronic lower spinal arachnoiditis. *Neuroradiology*. 1975;9(3):139–144.

100. Dullerud R, Morland TJ. Adhesive arachnoiditis after lumbar radiculography with Dimer-X and Depo-Medrol. *Radiology*. 1976;119(1):153–155.

101. Mooij JJ. Spinal arachnoiditis: disease or coincidence? *Acta Neurochir (Wien)*. 1980;53(3–4):151–160.

102. Hoffman RM, Wheeler KJ, Deyo RA. Surgery for herniated lumbar discs: a literature synthesis. *J Gen Intern Med*. 1993; 8(9):487–496.

103. Howe JF, Loeser JD, Calvin WH. Mechanosensitivity of dorsal root ganglia and chronically

injured axons: a physiological basis for the radicular pain of nerve root compression. *Pain*. 1977;3(1):25–41.

104. McCarron RF et al., The inflammatory effect of nucleus pulposus. A possible element in the pathogenesis of low-back pain. *Spine (Phila Pa 1976)*. 1987;12(8):760–764.

105. Olmarker K, Rydevik B, Nordborg C. Autologous nucleus pulposus induces neurophysiologic and histologic changes in porcine cauda equina nerve roots. *Spine (Phila Pa 1976)*. 1993;18(11):1425–1432.

106. Kayama S et al. Incision of the anulus fibrosus induces nerve root morphologic, vascular, and functional changes. An experimental study. *Spine (Phila Pa 1976)*. 1996;21(22):2539–2543.

107. Burke JG et al. Intervertebral discs which cause low back pain secrete high levels of proinflammatory mediators. *J Bone Joint Surg Br*. 2002;84(2):196–201.

108. Takahashi N et al. Pathomechanisms of nerve root injury caused by disc herniation: an experimental study of mechanical compression and chemical irritation. *Spine (Phila Pa 1976)*. 2003;28(5):435–441.

109. Tegeder I et al. GTP cyclohydrolase and tetrahydrobiopterin regulate pain sensitivity and persistence. *Nat Med*. 2006;12(11):1269–1277.

110. Thony B, Auerbach G, Blau N. Tetrahydrobiopterin biosynthesis, regeneration and functions. *Biochem J*. 2000;347(pt 1):1–16.

111. Sambrook PN, MacGregor AJ, Spector TD. Genetic influences on cervical and lumbar disc degeneration: a magnetic resonance imaging study in twins. *Arthritis Rheum*. 1999;42(2):366–372.

112. Mustard CA et al. Childhood and early adult predictors of risk of incident back pain: Ontario Child Health Study 2001 follow-up. *Am J Epidemiol*. 2005;162(8):779–786.

113. Wiesinger B et al. Back pain in relation to musculoskeletal disorders in the jaw-face: a matched case-control study. *Pain*. 2007;131(3):311–319.

114. Von Korff M et al. Chronic spinal pain and physical-mental comorbidity in the United States: results from the national comorbidity survey replication. *Pain*. 2005;113(3):331–339.

115. Baliki MN et al. Chronic pain and the emotional brain: specific brain activity associated with spontaneous fluctuations of intensity of chronic back pain. *J Neurosci*. 2006;26(47):12165–12173.

116. Apkarian AV et al. Chronic back pain is associated with decreased prefrontal and thalamic gray matter density. *J Neurosci*. 2004;24(46): 10410–10415.

117. Takahashi K et al. Changes in epidural pressure during walking in patients with lumbar spinal stenosis. *Spine (Phila Pa 1976)*. 1995;20(24):2746–2749.

118. Ooi Y, Mita F, Satoh Y. Myeloscopic study on lumbar spinal canal stenosis with special reference to intermittent claudication. *Spine (Phila Pa 1976)*. 1990;15(6): 544–549.

119. Watanabe R, Parke WW. Vascular and neural pathology of lumbosacral spinal stenosis. *J Neurosurg*. 1986;64(1):64–70.

120. Kobayashi S et al. Imaging of cauda equina edema in lumbar canal stenosis by using gadolinium-enhanced MR imaging: experimental constriction injury. *AJNR Am J Neuroradiol*. 2006;27(2):346–353.

121. Kobayashi S et al. Localization and changes of intraneural inflammatory cytokines and inducible-nitric oxide induced by mechanical compression. J *Orthop Res*. 2005;23(4): 771–778.

122. London SF, England JD. Dynamic F waves in neurogenic claudication. *Muscle Nerve*. 1991;14(5):457–461.

123. Ikawa M, Atsuta Y, Tsunekawa H. Ectopic firing due to artificial venous stasis in rat lumbar spinal canal stenosis model: a possible pathogenesis of neurogenic intermittent claudication. *Spine (Phila Pa 1976)*. 2005;30(21):2393–2397.

124. Sekiguchi M, Kikuchi S, Myers RR. Experimental spinal stenosis: relationship between degree of cauda equina compression, neuropathology, and pain. *Spine (Phila Pa 1976)*. 2004;29(10):1105–1111.

125. Burton CV et al. Causes of failure of surgery on the lumbar spine. *Clin Orthop Relat Res*. 1981:(157):191–199.

126. Pheasant HC, Dyck P. Failed lumbar disc surgery: cause, assessment, treatment. *Clin Orthop Relat Res*. 1982:(164):93–109.

127. Burton CV Lumbosacral arachnoiditis. *Spine (Phila Pa 1976)*. 1978;3(1):24–30.

128. Bundschuh CV et al. Epidural fibrosis and recurrent disk herniation in the lumbar spine: MR imaging assessment. *AJR Am J Roentgenol*. 1988;150(4):923–932.

129. Seaman WB, Marder SN, Rosenbaum HE. The myelographic appearance of adhesive spinal arachnoiditis. *J Neurosurg*. 1953;10(2):145–153.

130. Smolik EA, Nash FP. Lumbar spinal arachnoiditis: a complication of the intervertebral disc operation. *Ann Surg*. 1951;133(4):490–495.

131. Bergeron RT et al. Experimental pantopaque arachnoiditis in the monkey. *Radiology*. 1971;99(1):95–101.

132. Fisher RL. An experimental evaluation of pantopaque and other recently developed myelographic contrast media. *Radiology*. 1965;85(3):537–545.

133. Howland WJ, Curry JL, Richey D. Experimental studies of pantopaque arachnoiditis. 3. Clinical studies in progress. *Radiology*. 1966;87(2):258–261.

134. Cosan TE et al. Spinal toxoplasmic arachnoiditis associated with osteoid formation: a rare presentation of toxoplasmosis. *Spine (Phila Pa 1976)*. 2001;26(15):1726–1728.

135. Elkington JS. [Traumatic lesions of peripheral nerves; prognosis and treatment.]. *Ann Med Psychol (Paris)*. 1951;109(1:2):233–234.

136. Ransford AO, Harries BJ. Localised arachnoiditis complicating lumbar disc lesions. *J Bone Joint Surg Br*. 1972;54(4):656–665.

137. French J. Clinical manifestations of lumbar spinal arachnoiditis. Surgery. 1946;:718–729.

138. Nakano M et al. Postlaminectomy adhesion of the cauda equina. Changes of postoperative vascular permeability of the equina in rats. *Spine (Phila Pa 1976)*. 1997;22(10):1105–1114.

139. Yamagami T et al. Effects of laminectomy and retained extradural foreign body on cauda equina adhesion. *Spine (Phila Pa 1976)*. 1993;18(13):1774–1781.

140. Nakano M et al. Postlaminectomy adhesion of the cauda equina. Inhibitory effects of anti-inflammatory drugs on cauda equina adhesion in rats. *Spine (Phila Pa 1976)*. 1998;23(3):298–304.

141. Jayson MI. Vascular damage, fibrosis, and chronic inflammation in mechanical back pain problems. *Semin Arthritis Rheum*. 1989;18(4 suppl 2):73–76.

142. Chou R et al. Nonsurgical interventional therapies for low back pain: a review of the evidence for an American Pain Society clinical practice guideline. *Spine (Phila Pa 1976)*. 2009;34(10):1078–1093.

143. Dellemijn PL, van Duijn H, Vanneste JA. Prolonged treatment with transdermal fentanyl in neuropathic pain. *J Pain Symptom Manage*. 1998;16(4):220–229.

144. Skljarevski V et al. Efficacy and safety of duloxetine in patients with chronic low back pain. *Spine (Phila Pa 1976)*. 2010;35(13):E578–E585.

145. Hale M et al. Once-daily OROS hydromorphone ER compared with placebo in opioid-tolerant patients with chronic low back pain. *Curr Med Res Opin*. 2010;26(6):1505–1518.

146. Moore RA et al. Chronic low back pain analgesic studies—a methodological minefield. *Pain*. 2010;149(3):431–434.

147. Machado LA et al. Analgesic effects of treatments for non-specific low back pain: a meta-analysis of placebo-controlled randomized trials. *Rheumatology (Oxford)*. 2009;48(5):520–527.

148. O'Connor AB, Dworkin RH. Treatment of neuropathic pain: an overview of recent guidelines. *Am J Med*, 2009;122(10 suppl):S22–S32.

149. Podichetty VK et al. Effectiveness of salmon calcitonin nasal spray in the treatment of lumbar canal stenosis: a double-blind, randomized, placebo-controlled, parallel group trial. *Spine (Phila Pa 1976)*. 2004;29(21):2343–2349.

150. Haimovic IC, Beresford HR. Dexamethasone is not superior to placebo for treating lumbosacral radicular pain. *Neurology*. 1986;36(12):1593–1594.

151. Finckh A et al. Short-term efficacy of intravenous pulse glucocorticoids in acute discogenic sciatica. A randomized controlled trial. *Spine (Phila Pa 1976)*. 2006;31(4):377–381.

152. Medrik-Goldberg T et al. Intravenous lidocaine, amantadine, and placebo in the treatment of sciatica: a double-blind, randomized, controlled study. *Reg Anesth Pain Med*. 1999;24(6):534–540.

153. Vroomen PC et al. Conservative treatment of sciatica: a systematic review. *J Spinal Disord*. 2000;13(6):463–469.

154. Delport EG et al. Treatment of lumbar spinal stenosis with epidural steroid injections: a retrospective outcome study. *Arch Phys Med Rehabil*. 2004;85(3):479–484.

155. Buttermann GR. Treatment of lumbar disc herniation: epidural steroid injection compared with discectomy. A prospective, randomized study. *J Bone Joint Surg Am*. 2004;86-A(4):670–679.

156. Wang JC et al. Epidural injections for the treatment of symptomatic lumbar herniated discs. *J Spinal Disord Tech*. 2002;15(4):269–272.

157. Autio RA et al. Effect of periradicular methylprednisolone on spontaneous resorption of intervertebral disc herniations. *Spine (Phila Pa 1976)*. 2004;29(15):1601–1607.

158. Bush K et al. The natural history of sciatica associated with disc pathology. A prospective study with clinical and independent radiologic follow-up. *Spine (Phila Pa 1976)*. 1992;17(10):1205–1212.

159. Weinstein JN et al. Surgical vs. nonoperative treatment for lumbar disk herniation: the Spine Patient Outcomes Research Trial (SPORT) observational cohort. *JAMA*. 2006;296(20): 2451–2459.

160. Osterman H et al. Effectiveness of microdiscectomy for lumbar disc herniation: a randomized controlled trial with 2 years of follow-up. *Spine (Phila Pa 1976)*. 2006;31(21):2409–2414.

161. Weinstein JN et al. Surgical versus nonsurgical treatment for lumbar degenerative spondylolisthesis. *N Engl J Med*. 2007;356(22): 2257–2270.

162. Postacchini F. Surgical management of lumbar spinal stenosis. *Spine (Phila Pa 1976)*. 1999;24(10):1043–1047.

163. Weinstein JN et al. Surgical versus nonsurgical therapy for lumbar spinal stenosis. N Engl J Med. 2008;358(8):794–810.

164. Malmivaara A et al. Surgical or nonoperative treatment for lumbar spinal stenosis? A randomized controlled trial. *Spine (Phila Pa 1976)*. 2007;32(1):1–8.

165. Martin BI et al. Reoperation rates following lumbar spine surgery and the influence of spinal fusion procedures. *Spine (Phila Pa 1976)*. 2007;32(3):382–387.

166. Kumar K et al. Spinal cord stimulation versus conventional medical management for neuropathic pain: a multicentre randomised controlled trial in patients with failed back surgery syndrome. *Pain*. 2007;132(1–2): 179–188.

167. North RB et al. Spinal cord stimulation versus repeated lumbosacral spine surgery for chronic pain: a randomized, controlled trial. *Neurosurgery*. 2005;56(1):98–106; discussion 106–107.

22

The Complex Regional Pain Syndrome

STEVEN H. HOROWITZ AND ANNE LOUISE OAKLANDER

COMPLEX REGIONAL PAIN syndrome (CRPS) is a dramatic chronic pain syndrome rich in history and in unexplicated clinical features, with great variability in clinical presentation. Mildly affected patients often recover without care, severely affected patients are disabled, and the worst have disfigurements and severe chronic pain. The cause of most symptoms remains uncertain, and much treatment is palliative. Sympathetic blockade had been the standard treatment for decades despite unclear utility, but new research findings offer hope of efficacious disease-modifying therapies.

The term *complex regional pain syndrome* was created by a consensus panel of the International Association for the Study of Pain (IASP) in 1993 to incorporate two distinct pain conditions, causalgia (now CRPS Type II) and reflex sympathetic dystrophy (RSD; now CRPS Type I), under one umbrella with specific descriptive criteria.[1] However, the medical perception of CRPS as a legitimate clinical entity was compromised by the vagueness of these criteria. Fortunately, the pathophysiology is emerging from multiple sources—epidemiological study of digital records, advanced brain imaging, pathology, and animal models—further diagnostic revisions seem probable. A brief historical background is followed by the clinical presentation and current treatment options, and this review concludes with an overview of this active and diverse research field.

HISTORY

Following earlier fragmentary reports, S. Weir Mitchell and his colleagues Morehouse and Keen provided the first detailed characterization of this syndrome in American Civil War soldiers with bullet or shrapnel injuries to their peripheral nervous system (PNS). Between 1864 and 1872 they described cases of severe or persistent regional pain in injured limbs that had a unique burning quality (Fig 22.1).[2–6]

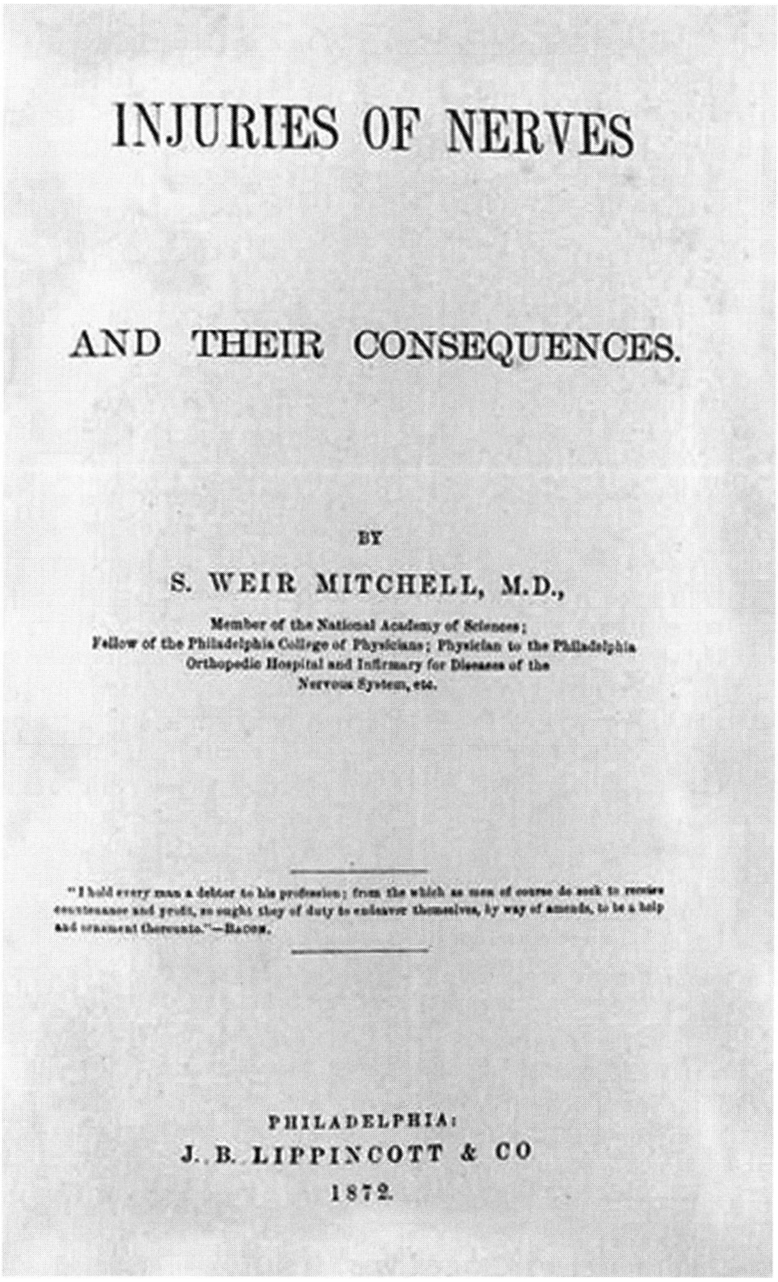
INJURIES OF NERVES

AND THEIR CONSEQUENCES.

BY

S. WEIR MITCHELL, M.D.,

Member of the National Academy of Sciences;
Fellow of the Philadelphia College of Physicians; Physician to the Philadelphia
Orthopedic Hospital and Infirmary for Diseases of the
Nervous System, etc.

"I hold every man a debtor to his profession; from the which as men of course do seek to receive countenance and profit, so ought they of duty to endeavor themselves, by way of amends, to be a help and ornament thereunto."—BACON.

PHILADELPHIA:
J. B. LIPPINCOTT & CO
1872.

FIGURE 22.1. The frontispiece of the original edition of Weir Mitchell's most important publication on causalgia, currently known as CRPS-II.

Medical lexicographer Robley Dunglison helped Mitchell combine the Greek terms for burning (*kausos*) and pain (*algos*) into *causalgia*, Mitchell's name for this symptom complex.[5,6] His meticulous depictions of the clinical, anatomical, and psychosocial effects of this syndrome remain unsurpassed today.

In our early experience with nerve wounds, we met a small number of men who were suffering from a pain, which they described as "burning" or as "mustard red-hot" or as "red-hot file rasping the skin." In all of these patients, and in many later cases, this pain was an associate of the glossy skin....The burning comes first, the visible skin-change afterwards....Its intensity varies from the most trivial burning to a state of torture...which reacts on the whole economy, until the general health is seriously affected. The part itself is not alone subject to an intense burning sensation, but becomes exquisitely hyperaesthetic, so that a touch or a tap of the finger increases the pain....As the pain increases, the general sympathy becomes more marked. The temper changes and grows irritable, the face becomes anxious....The sleep is restless....Motion of the part was unendurable in some of the very worst cases.[4]

The cardinal and inviolate symptom described by S. Weir Mitchell and coworkers was burning pain. They noted that this usually resolved over weeks or months, but 25 years later his son, John Mitchell, described pain persistence in some of the original patients.[7] S. W. Mitchell and his coworkers[2-4] described additional features that distinguished this syndrome from standard posttraumatic neuralgia, including abnormalities in vascular regulation and in sweating. Progress on causalgia resumed after the First World War, as new cases emerged, when it was formally defined by the Nerve Injuries Committee of the British Medical Research Council.[8]

The next World War renewed awareness and in 1946, James Evans described causalgia-like symptoms in civilians with far lesser injuries, including some that are not considered injuries today, such as flat feet.[9] He built on evidence from Leriche, Livingston, and others to conclude in two seminal papers that the sympathetic nervous system is reflexively involved in posttraumatic limb disorders.[9,10] For this reason, he coined the term *reflex sympathetic dystrophy* to describe "a most disabling, often extremely painful, malady following minor sprains, ordinary fractures, or, in military or civil life, trauma to blood vessels or nerves. Pain may be moderate, mild, or absent. The true diagnostic features are those disorders initiated by perversions of reflex sympathetic stimulation, namely increased rubor or pallor, sweating, edema, atrophy of skin, and spotty

or even cystic atrophy of bone."[9] Another Evans contribution, adding response to sympathetic blockade to the diagnostic criteria, is currently viewed as a misstep that led to misdiagnosis and unnecessary procedures: "Either cervical or paralumbar sympathetic procaine block comprises a diagnostic therapeutic test. The relief of pain may be almost miraculous, but need not be so dramatic as to establish the diagnosis, provided relief of other phenomena is also noted."[9,10] Evans' term *reflex sympathetic dystrophy* quickly caught on and is far more commonly diagnosed than causalgia today in civilian practice. Nerve injury was not requisite, but reflexive sympathetic overactivity from "prolonged bombardment of pain impulses" was.[10]

Homans' 1940 and 1941 papers also emphasized civilian cases, usually caused by fractures, minor traumas, immobilization, and surgery.[11,12] Also termed *minor* or *mimocausalgia, algodystrophy, Sudeck's atrophy, posttraumatic spreading neuralgia,* and *posttraumatic neurovascular pain syndrome,* these conditions were not deemed serious, nor were they attributable to nerve injury.[11-17] In the 1980s, reports of civilian patients with symptoms as severe as those of wartime patients appeared,[18,19] after which the distinction between "major" and "minor" causalgias was abandoned.

MODERN DIAGNOSTIC CRITERIA

Despite these multiple attempts to define this syndrome, the absence of codified diagnostic criteria inhibited accurate diagnosis and research, particularly for trials of potential therapies. The term *reflex sympathetic dystrophy* was problematic in that the "reflex" component was unspecified and hypothetical, the "sympathetic" component was not always present and not clinically helpful, and the "dystrophy" was uncommon. In response, the IASP convened a consensus workshop in 1993 that developed criteria intended to be inclusive and sensitive and to standardize the diagnosis[1,20] (Table 22.1). Descriptive symptom-based consensus criteria were adopted, mostly because of the contemporary rudimentary understanding of the pathophysiology, but also because of similar recent efforts in the fields of headache and psychiatry, such as the *Diagnostic and*

Table 22-1. The current (1994) diagnostic criteria of the International Association for the Study of Pain for CRPS-I and CRPS-II.[1]

IASP DIAGNOSTIC CRITERIA FOR CRPS-I (REFLEX SYMPATHETIC DYSTROPHY)

1. The presence of an initiating noxious event, or a cause of immobilization.
2. Continuing pain, allodynia, or hyperalgesia with which the pain is disproportionate to any inciting event.
3. Evidence at some time of edema, changes in skin blood flow, or abnormal sudomotor activity in the region of pain.
4. This diagnosis is excluded by the existence of conditions that would otherwise account for the degree of pain and dysfunction. Note: Criteria 2–4 must be satisfied.[2]

IASP DIAGNOSTIC CRITERIA FOR CRPS-II (CAUSALGIA)

1. The presence of continuing pain, allodynia, or hyperalgesia after a nerve injury, not necessarily limited to the distribution of the injured nerve.
2. Evidence at some time of edema, changes in skin blood flow, or abnormal sudomotor activity in the region of pain.
3. This diagnosis is excluded by the existence of conditions that would otherwise account for the degree of pain and dysfunction. Note: All three criteria must be satisfied.[2]

Sources:

1. Merskey H, Bogduk N. Classification of chronic pain: descriptions of chronic pain syndromes and definitions of pain terms. In Merskey H, Bogduk N (eds): Task Force on Taxonomy of the International Association for the Study of Pain. Seattle: IASP Press, 1994, pp.40–43.

2. Bruehl S, Harden NR, Galer BS, Saltz S, Bertram M, Backonja M, Gayles R, Rudin N, Bhugra MK, Stanton-Hicks M. External validation of IASP diagnostic criteria for complex regional pain syndrome and proposed research diagnostic criteria. Pain 1999;81:147–154.

3. Harden NR, Bruehl S, Stanton-Hicks, Wilson PR. Proposed new diagnostic criteria for complex regional pain syndrome. Pain Med 2007;8:326–331.

Statistical Manual of Mental Disorders (DSM).[21,22] The essential unity of causalgia and RSD was acknowledged by defining a new condition: *complex regional pain syndrome* (CRPS). Reflex sympathetic dystrophy was repackaged as CRPS-I and causalgia as CRPS-II. Patients with known nerve injuries were classified as having CRPS-II and those without them as having CRPS-I, although the criteria for making this distinction remained unspecified, making this dichotomy impractical for clinical use as very few patients ever received the neurological examinations or electrodiagnostic study necessary to determine if nerve injuries were present or not. *Complex regional pain syndrome* entered the medical lexicon (although atavistic use of *reflex sympathetic dystrophy* and, to a lesser degree, *causalgia* continues).

Despite validation in subsequent studies,[21,22] criticisms of the 1994 diagnostic criteria soon arose, mostly concerning vagueness and reliance upon patient self-reporting. The reciprocal of the criteria's very high sensitivity (0.98) was low specificity (0.36), and the criteria for dysautonomia were vague.[21–23] The absence of pathophysiological understanding and lack of objective diagnostic tests devalued these descriptive criteria. Perez et al. compared three different sets of diagnostic criteria in 372 patients suspected of having CRPS-I and found poor agreement among them. They proposed a broad diagnostic approach with explicit reference to diagnostic criteria and clinical features.[24]

Accordingly, separate criteria were then proposed for research, where it is critical to obtain a homogeneous group for study, versus clinical use, where sensitivity is more essential. Adding criteria concerning motor and trophic changes and separating vasomotor and sudomotor signs and symptoms improved validity[21,23] (Table 22.2). At a 2003 Budapest consensus workshop, it was proposed to retain the CRPS I and II subtypes and add a third subtype, CRPS-not otherwise specified (CRPS-NOS) for patients previously

Table 22-2. The proposed (Budapest, 2003) new diagnostic criteria. Current distinctions between CRPS-I and CRPS-II are retained and a third subtype, CRPS-NOS (not otherwise specified) was recommended.

PROPOSED CLINICAL DIAGNOSTIC CRITERIA FOR CRPS

General Definition

CRPS describes an array of painful conditions characterized by continuing (spontaneous and/or evoked) regional pain seemingly disproportionate in time or degree to the usual course of any known trauma or other lesion. The pain is regional (not in a specific nerve territory or dermatome) and usually has a distal predominance of abnormal sensory, motor, sudomotor, vasomotor, and/or trophic findings. The syndrome shows variable progression over time.

To make the *clinical* diagnosis the following criteria must be met:

1. Continuing pain, which is disproportionate to any inciting event

2. Must report at least one symptom in *three of the four* following categories:
   Sensory: Reports of hyperesthesia and/or allodynia
   Vasomotor: Reports of temperature asymmetry and/or skin color changes and/or skin color asymmetry
   Sudomotor/Edema: Reports of edema and/or sweating changes and/or sweating asymmetry
   Motor/Trophic: Reports of decreased range of motion and/or motor dysfunction (weakness, tremor, dystonia) and/or trophic changes (hair, nail, skin)

3. Must display at least one sign **at time of evaluation** in *two or more* of the following categories:
   Sensory: Evidence of hyperalgesia (to pinprick) and/or allodynia (to light touch and/or temperature sensation and/or deep somatic pressure and/or joint movement)
   Vasomotor: Evidence of temperature asymmetry (>1°C) and/or skin color changes and/or asymmetry
   Sudomotor/Edema: Evidence of edema and/or sweating changes and/or sweating asymmetry
   Motor/Trophic: Evidence of decreased range of motion and/or motor dysfunction (weakness, tremor, dystonia) and/or trophic changes (hair, nail, skin)

4. There is no other diagnosis that better explains the signs and symptoms

   For research purposes: Must report at least one symptom ***in all four*** symptom categories and at least one sign (observed at evaluation) ***in two or more*** sign categories.

Modified from:

1. Harden R, Bruehl S. Diagnostic criteria: the statistical derivation of the four criterion factors. In: Wilson PR, Stanton-Hicks M, Harden RN, eds. CRPS: Current Diagnosis and Therapy. Seattle, WA: IASP Press; 2005:45–58.

2. Harden NR, Bruehl S, Stanton-Hicks, Wilson PR. Proposed new diagnostic criteria for complex regional pain syndrome. Pain Med 2007;8:326–331.

diagnosed with CRPS who now "did not fully meet the new clinical criteria, but whose symptoms could not better be explained by another diagnosis" (~15%).[25,26] This paralleled the methods of the DSM and appeased concern about disenfranchising some patients, but the value of CRPS-NOS was unclear and this term did not achieve widespread use. A recurring concern was that these criteria continue to make CRPS a diagnosis of exclusion when no better diagnosis can be established. This waste basket approach perverts the utility of identifying patients' causative lesions because as soon as a cause is identified, the patient no longer has CRPS! Furthermore, the new CRPS-NOS subtype is tautological; nobody presenting with regional chronic pain can be definitively excluded from having CRPS. As with other diseases, phenotype-based diagnoses will gradually yield to objective pathophysiologically based diagnostic criteria. However, it remains uncertain which medical specialty's organization is best qualified to issue those criteria.

Recent validation efforts are no more successful. Regarding the 2003 Budapest criteria, Harden et al.[26a] compared CRPS I patients to patients with non-CRPS neuropathic pain, most of whom had specific nerve injuries or radiculopathies secondary to surgical or crush injuries. While the manuscript does not describe the non-CRPS patients in detail, it is noted in a table that many had hyperesthesias, temperature asymmetry, edema and motor changes, suggesting that some of them had CRPS II; if such was the case it compromises the sensitivity and specificity calculations on which the validation estimates are based. Additionally, Sumitani et al.[26b] studied the validity of the 1993 IASP/CRPS criteria in Japanese patients and did not find the criteria to be valid. They created new Japan-specific criteria, raising the daunting possibility of regionally specific criteria.

EPIDEMIOLOGY

The primary epidemiological characteristic of CRPS is that it is a very rare outcome of a very common situation: injury. No kind of injury is exempt, although fracture, particularly of the long bones of the limbs, is disproportionately common. In a retrospective analysis of 134 patients meeting the 1994 IASP CRPS criteria, 70% were female. The most common inciting injuries were sprains/strains (29%), surgical procedures (24%), and fractures (16%), with physician-imposed physical immobilization occurring in 47%.[27] Mean age at onset was 37.7 (range, 14–64) years, 56% of causative injuries occurred on the job, and 17% involved lawsuits.[27]

Other demographic analyses confirm these sex and age predilections. Females consistently comprise 75%–80% of patients, reflecting more than just reporting bias. The disease is rare in young children and the elderly; the median age of onset is near 40 in most studies. The incidence and prevalence are only estimates because of diagnostic imprecision,

nomenclature, and the variable presentation of patients across multiple specialties. Sandroni et al. generated the first community-based data.[28] In one county in the midwestern United States, the incidence of CRPS was 5.46 per 100,000 person-years and the prevalence was 20.57 per 100,000, with median age of onset of 46 years.[28] De Mos and colleagues published the second epidemiological study using electronic records from primary care physicians in the Netherlands. They found an incidence of 26.2 per 100,000 person-years, which was greatest in the 61- to 70-year-old group, with a mean age of onset of 52.7 years.[29] The explanation of the fivefold disparity in incidence and the substantially older age of onset is unclear. Both studies concurred that females comprise 75%–80% of patients and that fractures are the most common precipitant. Mild CRPS-I has been reported to follow 30%–40% of fractures of the radial head,[30,31] although severe and long-lasting CRPS-I probably occurs after only 1%–2% of fractures.[30–32] It is not clear if bone fracture is an epiphenomenon or mere marker for severe trauma that also damages nerves or other soft tissues, or whether transection of interosseous axons by the fracture contributes directly. The Sandroni study additionally reported that the CRPS-II diagnosis (CRPS associated with major nerve injury) is much less common, with an estimated incidence of 0.82 per 100,000 person-years at risk and a prevalence of 4.2 per 100,000 without a sex effect.[28] It reportedly occurs in approximately 2%–5% of peripheral nerve injuries.[33] Sumitani et al.[26b] raised the possibility of cultural, regional or sampling differences to account for widely divergent incidence.

Limited data suggest that CRPS is a complex disorder with both genetic and environmental contributions. Because environmental influences are so strong—with trauma being required to trigger it—genetic contributions are obscured. In the Netherlands, human leukocyte antigen (HLA)-DQ1 is more prevalent amongst CRPS patients than in the general population,[34] and an association between CRPS-I and Ehlers-Danlos syndrome, an inherited disorder of collagen, has been proposed but not quantified.[35] Rare family clusters have been reported; familial CRPS may be more severe, with earlier onset, more affected extremities, and more dystonia.[36]

CLINICAL PRESENTATION

Chronic Pain, Hyperalgesia, and Allodynia

As expected given its name, the cardinal feature of CRPS is pain—pain disproportionate to the intensity of the inciting event.[1,25,26] Early descriptions characterized this pain as "burning"[37,38]; other adjectives more recently applied are "shooting," "lancinating," "electrical," "tearing," "stinging," "squeezing," "pulsating," and "aching," often deep in the limb.[39–41] As with other neuropathic pain conditions, there is a spectrum of pain symptoms. In analyzing 145 patients meeting the 1994 IASP CRPS criteria, Birklein et al. found that the most frequent pain descriptor used by CRPS-I patients was "tearing" (25.4%), followed by "stinging" (17.2%), "burning" (16.4%), and others.[42] Among CRPS-II patients, the percentages were 30.4%, 21.7%, and 26.1%, respectively.[42] Spontaneous (stimulation-independent) pain occurred in 74.6% of CRPS-I patients and 91.3% of CRPS-II patients.[42] The pain of CRPS usually begins immediately after injury or shortly thereafter, and its characteristics change over time, usually gradually improving then resolving. Some patients report that "burning" and "electrical" qualities gradually metamorphose into "dull," "boring," "aching," or "tingling," with the severe constant pain becoming intermittent, usually after mechanical stimulation.[39] The pain is often exacerbated by external stimuli, movement of the affected limb, and temperature changes.[33,37,39,42] As is characteristic of neuropathic pain, many patients report worsening during cold weather and improvement in warm seasons. Medication needs may vary accordingly. Modern studies document the frequency of hyperalgesia in CRPS: 93.4% in CRPS-I and 95.7% (Birklein et al.[42]), 75% (Veldman et al.[33]), and 65.1% (Harden et al.[23]) in CRPS-II. The wide variations among these studies, each of which (except Veldman et al.[33]) enrolled subjects meeting the 1994 IASP/CRPS criteria, attest to the fluidity of the diagnosis.

Further, patients recruited at university hospitals are, on average, more severely affected than patients identified in community-based studies.

Not all patients have all forms of pain. Sieweke et al.[43] found marked mechanical hyperalgesia without static mechanical hyperalgesia or hyperalgesia to heat and thought this implicated central mechanisms. It is significant that sensory deficits (numbness or hypoesthesia) often colocalize with the pain, frequently in a pattern that extends outside of individual nerve territories. Some patients who otherwise meet CRPS criteria lack pain: this was reported variously as 6.6% of CRPS-I patients and 4.3% of CRPS-II patient,[42] and as 7% of CRPS I patients.[33] These patients represent a conundrum. Although some may have a *forme fruste*, others may have partly recovered from a full CRPS syndrome. The vasomotor changes often improve before the pain to leave garden-variety neuralgia, testifying to the overlap between CRPS and posttraumatic neuralgia.

Other CRPS symptoms also fluctuate, sometimes from hour to hour. This led earlier scholars to propose three sequential stages: acute, dystrophic, then an atrophic stage,[44,45] a concept not supported by later studies.[46] Eberle et al. proposed warm and cold subgroups according to skin temperature differences in the affected area. Complex regional pain syndrome that begins cold usually remains cold, whereas warm CRPS often turns cold over time.[47] Modern science places these transient phenotypes in the context of microcirculatory abnormalities. Paradoxically, CRPS-affected skin that is warm, red, and seemingly hyperperfused can conceal tissues below left hypoxic by pathological diversion of blood through arteriovenous shunts that bypass the capillary exchange beds.[48]

Vasomotor Changes (Edema, Color, and Temperature Changes)

Vasomotor or sudomotor phenomena are requisite at some point for the diagnosis of CRPS. Typical vasomotor changes comprise regional edema, color changes including erythema, pallor, blueness, or fluctuating combinations thereof (Figure 22.2). Veldman et al. found discolored skin in 91%, altered skin temperature

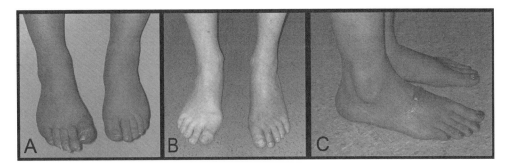

FIGURE 22.2.   Reflex sympathetic dystrophy/CRPS-I is a complex of symptoms of varying severity and location, most commonly affecting the distal limbs. Few patients have all symptoms, and these usually gradually abate so that many patients pass from a CRPS diagnosis to one of simple neuralgia en route to recovery—evidence unifying these conditions. (A) A laborer in his 30s 4 years after right-foot crush by a steel beam. His premorbid neurological history showed remote ileostomy for childhood megacolon. Severe ongoing and touch-induced pain in his great toe spread to his entire foot, which he guarded from contact even with bath water. Poor hygiene and mild edema, color change, and toe dystonia are visible. His history and a persistent Tinel's sign at his right fibular head suggested peroneal nerve injury, but he declined electromyography/nerve conduction studies. (B) A researcher in her 30s with chronic pain, edema, and vasodysregulation in her left foot and lower leg following bunionectomy several years ago. She also developed benign ectopic bone growth of her proximal left tibia. Her history is notable for migraines and asthma, linked through epidemiological study to CRPS.[9] (C) An otherwise healthy woman in her 40s several years after a well-healed second-degree burn from a hot coffee spill on her right foot. Ever since, any prolonged contact triggers severe pain and blister formation (shown), and the resulting ulcer takes weeks to heal. Inability to wear a shoe precludes employment.

in 92%, and edema in 69% of their CRPS I patients.[33] Birklein et al. found side-to-side temperature differences in 90% of their subjects, and when skin color or edema was included, 98% of subjects had vasomotor abnormalities.[42] However, these were not constant and varied with disease duration; edema prevalence was 92% within the first 5 weeks but only 55% in patients with durations between 25 and 468 weeks. Warmer limbs and erythema were more common in acute CRPS, with a colder and bluer appearance more common in chronic cases. Veldman et al.[33] found that the longer the interval between the beginning of CRPS and the first examination, the greater the likelihood of limb coldness. However, these findings are relative and cannot be used to stage the disease. They are also strongly influenced by environmental conditions and clearly, disuse and prolonged limb dependency will worsen symptoms. Skin temperature has been studied by infrared thermography, and interlimb temperature differences of 1.5–2.2°C[49–51] between affected and unaffected homonymous areas are considered

indicative of CRPS, but this is a nonspecific finding associated with other conditions (*vide infra*). Controlled thermoregulation (body warming or cooling with a thermal suit) may increase the temperature asymmetries in research studies.[50,51]

Sweating (Sudomotor) Abnormalities

A minority of patients notice sweating changes in their affected limb. This finding supports a CRPS diagnosis and because it is caused by small-fiber axonopathy, may help localize the involved nerve(s).[52] Localization and characterization of CRPS-related sweating abnormalities has provided insights into the mechanisms, although the situation is complex and there is no one single pattern, debunking the common view that hyperhydrosis (excessive sweating) is characteristic.[53] Patients are far more likely to notice and be disabled by hyperhydrosis than hypohydrosis (reduced or absent sweating). Focal hypohydrosis triggered by nerve injury can generate compensatory hyperhydrosis in surrounding normal skin, and it is often this that the patient notices and reports. Botulinum toxin injections are increasingly being used to treat disabling focal areas of neuropathic hyperhydrosis,[54,55] and there is intriguing early evidence of their independent efficacy against neuropathic pain.[56] Other caveats in interpreting this literature are that there are different types of sweating regulated by different mechanisms and mediators; CRPS (and other lesions) can affect one type of sweating but not another; and hyperhydrosis may be present in one situation, whereas hypohydrosis develops in other circumstances. The complexity occurs because sweating is under both CNS and PNS control for varied purposes, and varied mechanisms are involved. There are several ways to measure sweating. These include measuring resting sweat output; thermoregulatory sweat testing, which evaluates combined central and peripheral sweat control; and quantitative sudomotor axon reflex testing, which measures focal output after cholinergic stimulation. The results of these tests can vary, making composite scores valuable.

Effects on Movement

Movement abnormalities in CRPS are of increasing interest. Their presence was not required in the 1994 IASP diagnostic criteria whereas they are given equal weight to other criteria in the proposed 2003 revisions. Earlier disregard reflected the widespread misperception that motor signs and symptoms were psychogenic or merely protective withdrawal reflexes.[57] Accreted descriptions of weakness, bradykinesia, dystonia, myoclonus, tremor, and motor neglect, along with new imaging evidence of brain dysfunction, adaptation, and reorganization in CRPS, finally demonstrated that movement abnormalities are intrinsic to CRPS, though present only in a minority of patients. Schwartzman and Kerrigan described 43 of 200 CRPS patients with major motor symptoms: weakness, spasms, tremor, inability to initiate movements, and painful dystonic posturing.[58] Veldman et al.[33] found weakness in 95%, tremor in 49%, muscular incoordination in 54%, and severe muscle spasms in 25% of affected limbs. They labeled the paresis and incoordination

that progressed to inability to move at all *pseudoparalysis*, "because during careful examination, discrete muscle contractions could regularly be felt and because we found no changes on electromyography."[33] Birklein et al.[42] found motor dysfunction in 97% of affected limbs (CRPS-I and -II): 79% had weakness, 87% had limited range of motion, 46% had exaggerated tendon reflexes, 48% had enhanced tremor, 30% had myoclonic jerks and dystonic contractions, and 45% had difficulty initiating movement. Myoclonic jerks and dystonia were almost twice as common in CRPS-II as in CRPS-I.[42] Van Rijn et al.[59] found movement abnormalities in 121 of 185 (65.4%) CRPS-I patients, with dystonia comprising 90.9%. Other series corroborate these findings,[23] although prevalences would be much less in community-based surveys.

Dystonia, or sustained involuntary cocontracture of agonist and antagonist muscles to produce abnormal painful positions, is the most common major CRPS movement disorder. It differs significantly from the dystonias familiar to movement disorder specialists, which are usually of central origin, axial, and not fixed (constant). It more closely resembles the focal dystonias of distal limb musculature, some of which are triggered by trauma. Few of these are fixed though.[60]

Complex regional pain syndrome/dystonia usually remains in the affected limb, but can spread to axial muscles in severe cases.[61] We find dystonia to be present in less than 10% of CRPS patients, but some specialized clinics report higher prevalences. Dutch physicians have described spread to other limbs not always linked to trauma; this may represent a distinct phenotype.[59] Compared to CRPS patients without dystonia, those with dystonia are younger, with longer disease duration. Nonmotor symptoms of CRPS can improve as dystonia develops.[62] Dystonia is an independent source of chronic pain that may require treatment using specific algorithms for dystonia rather than neuralgia. Verdugo and Ochoa[63] described 58 patients with movement abnormalities (out of a total of 686 CRPS patients) without structurally based CNS or PNS abnormalities, each exhibiting at least one "pseudoneurologic sign," and interpreted this as evidence of psychogenic origin. Interestingly, all of these patients had CRPS-I rather than CRPS-II, in contrast to Birklein et al.'s[42] finding that movement abnormalities were very common in both. Schrag et al. studied 103 patients with fixed dystonia, 20% of whom met criteria for CRPS, and found subjects with and without evidence of psychogenic causality.[64] Van der Laan et al.[65] did not find increased psychopathology in CRPS/dystonia secondary to fracture, and reduced central inhibition has been found in CRPS/dystonia patients,[57] in keeping with current concepts of dystonia as a central circuit disorder.[60,66] Impaired reciprocal inhibition and markedly reduced stretch reflexes were seen on electromyography, as was vibratory inhibition of the H-reflex, in CRPS/dystonic patients, each finding suggesting impairment of interneuronal circuits that mediate presynaptic inhibition.[67] Munts et al.[67a] used computer modeling to simulate the fixed dystonia seen in 85 CRPS I patients, concluding that aberrant force feedback regulation from Golgi tendon organs involving an inhibitory interneuron may be present. Cortical reorganization, involving primary motor (both ipsilateral and contralateral), supplemental motor, and posterior parietal cortices, has been found on functional magnetic resonance imaging in CRPS/dystonia patients. This correlates with kinematic evaluations of motor impairment.[68] However, Hawley and Weiner[68a] find such pathophysiologic evidence weak, note a marked "overlap between fixed painful dystonia and psychogenic movement disorders," and conclude that CRPS dystonia is psychogenic. Finally, Galer and colleagues described motor or cognitive neglect in 84% of 224 CRPS patients (a finding often associated with parietal cortical disorders) and linked this to difficulty initiating movements and bradykinesia.[69,70]

Effects on Bones and Joints

Bone and joint abnormalities were recognized early, and are consistent with the hypothesis that small-fiber nerve injuries are central in CRPS as bones and joints are densely innervated, predominantly by small fibers.[71,72] Animal data implicate substance P secretion in the development of these abnormalities.[73] The severe pain of bone fracture testifies to the density of osseous innervation. Bone is exquisitely sensitive to loss of small-fiber innervation.[74,75] The dependence of bone integrity on its innervation is evident in the development of Charcot joints, where distal bones and joints collapse in advanced sensory neuropathies and in the malunion of bone fractures if innervation of the fracture site is lost.[76]

The characteristic bone abnormalities in CRPS that contribute to deep pain include endosteal and intracortical excavations, as well as demineralization and resorption of subperiosteal and trabecular bone.[77] These processes reflect excess osteoclast activity that causes resorption. Rare patients develop focal bone overgrowth if remodeling is prolonged. Bone is resorbed by lowering the local pH to 4; this affects demineralization, and this low pH stimulates nearby cheminociceptors to trigger bone pain. Other neurogenic changes, including bone hyperperfusion and bone marrow edema, are sometimes radiologically detectable. These often localize to the sclerotome innervated by an injured nerve, and they are more prominent when the damaged nerve has a large sclerotome. Bisphosphonates and calcitonin, inhibitors of bone resorption, have been found to be effective for treating CRPS pain in preliminary studies. More extensive studies of bone should be performed in patients with severe deep CRPS pain.[78]

PEDIATRIC CRPS

Complex regional pain syndrome is well described in school-age children and teenagers and differs little from adult CRPS in presentation. The major difference is that the prognosis for rapid and complete recovery is much better in children.[79,80] Case series demonstrate consistent features:[79–83] 70%–95% of patients are female; onset is usually in the 8–16 age group; the lower extremities are more commonly affected, especially the foot (57%–100%); and movement disorders such as dystonia, tremors, and myoclonus, while rare, can occur alone or together.[84] Most quantitative sensory text studies document abnormal sensory patterns similar to those of adult patients, although heat and cold allodynia may be less common.[83] The rapid recovery of most children has facilitated detection of changes in brain function during recovery.[85]

Treatment algorithms differ for children, with more physical therapy and behavioral support and less medication and surgery. This reflects not only the increased caution of pediatric medicine, but also the far better spontaneous recovery rate in children. Even medication therapy may be targeted to enable participation in physical therapy.[81] Full or partial recovery occurs in the vast majority of patients (~80%–90%), but recurrence has been documented (20%–50%).[81,82,86,87] Seven pediatric patients had good outcomes with spinal cord stimulation.[88]

DIFFERENTIAL DIAGNOSIS

The diagnosis of CRPS is currently so ill defined that it is often applied generically by physicians and patients alike to any unexplained chronic pain syndrome, particularly one with swelling or color changes. In our experience, the majority of patients labeled with this diagnosis do not actually meet the IASP criteria. In evaluating such patients, we formulate a differential diagnosis and conduct appropriate testing. Correcting a misdiagnosis can suggest entirely different treatments. Arthritis (which can be posttraumatic) and other late sequelae of joint, bone, or muscle injury should always be considered. Particularly problematic are the many patients who attribute widespread CRPS-like symptoms to earlier focal trauma. This is called *spreading* or *total-body CRPS*, but there are currently no known mechanisms that can explain it. Far more likely alternatives include spinal-cord injury or small-fiber polyneuropathy. If autoimmunity is confirmed in CRPS, it should be investigated whether focal injuries that breach the blood-nerve barrier might trigger widespread autoimmune polyneuropathy. A precedent might be the relationship between shoulder-region injuries and brachial plexitis (Parsonage-Turner syndrome[89]).

Small-fiber-predominant polyneuropathies produce "pain plus" signs and symptoms identical to those of CRPS but more widely distributed, usually symmetrically and bilaterally in contrast to CRPS.[90] These tend to begin distally, and affect upper extremities later and not as severely. If large ($A\alpha\beta$) nerve fibers are also affected, there is loss of reflexes, weakness, and vibratory and proprioceptive deficits. There is no history of trauma, and most peripheral neuropathies develop and worsen gradually, in contrast to CRPS, which has a sudden onset and then tends to improve. However, in a study of the specificity of the 1994 IASP CRPS criteria, Galer et al. found that up to 37% of patients with painful diabetic neuropathy also met diagnostic criteria for CRPS.[22] Polyneuropathy increases the risk of focal or entrapment neuropathies such as carpal tunnel, cubital tunnel, or thoracic outlet syndromes which might be misdiagnosed as CRPS, despite the absence of inciting trauma. Systemic autoimmune diseases must always be considered, as these are increasingly treatable with new immunomodulatory treatments. Chronic subclinical problems can suddenly become symptomatic after a seemingly minor trauma, such as whiplash. Focal conditions including gout, pseudogout, and tenosynovitis must also be excluded.

Vascular abnormalities such as deep vein thrombosis or thrombophlebitis can present similarly to CRPS and can be precipitated by trauma. Unilateral arterial insufficiency can cause painful, blue, cold limbs. Vascular problems must be rapidly diagnosed and definitively treated because of the possibility of tissue loss, pulmonary embolism, and other serious complications. Ultrasound vascular studies should be immediately performed if these diagnoses are at all likely. In contrast, lymphedema after surgery, radiation therapy, or infection develops insidiously, and the pain is usually aching and without neuropathic qualities. It can be diagnosed with lymphoscintigraphy.

DIAGNOSTIC TESTS

Currently, there are no objective diagnostic tests for CRPS and the diagnosis remains clinical. However, the following tests can help support the clinical impression, eliminate the alternatives discussed above, and identify specific CRPS features that influence treatment decisions.

Neurophysiological Studies

Nerve conduction studies and electromyography are often used to document peripheral nerve damage. However, standard (surface) electrodes only detect action potentials from large (rapidly conducting) myelinated Aαβ fibers within mixed peripheral nerves, *not* the small Aδ and C fibers primarily affected in CRPS. If nerve conduction studies are abnormal, revealing large nerve fiber damage, coincident small-fiber dysfunction can be inferred, but normal nerve conduction studies do not rule out small-fiber damage and thus do not differentiate between CRPS-I and -II, despite their common use for this purpose.[21,23,25,91,92] The same points also apply to electromyography, in which "neurogenic" patterns of muscle electrophysiology only identify axonal injuries to large myelinated motor axons. The role of these studies in CRPS diagnosis needs to be clarified, as the current CRPS-I/CRPS-II dichotomy does not differentiate between patients with normal electromyographic/nerve conduction studies and the majority who have never undergone electrophysiological testing, leaving their nerve injury status unexplored.

Sympathetic Nerve Blocks

Sympathetic nerve blocks are a controversial subject whose complicated history has been addressed *vide supra*. For an affected upper limb, the stellate ganglion is blocked with local anesthetic with or without corticosteroids, and for a lower limb the lumbar sympathetic chain is blocked. Following Evans' enthusiasm, for decades not only were these blocks used for treatment, but a positive response was required for the diagnosis of RSD.[9,10] Few if any early studies of sympathetic nerve blocks are considered adequate today; they were unblinded and generally uncontrolled. The importance of the placebo response, which is particularly strong for therapeutic interventions, was unknown at the time. Later, patients with temporary post-block pain reduction were described as having sympathetically maintained pain; those not responding had sympathetically independent pain. As the technical and interpretational limitations of this method became known, and it became apparent that somatic axons coinnervated most structures traditionally thought to be only autonomically innervated, use of sympatholytic procedures waned.

Radiological Studies

Useful studies include bone scintigraphy and, to a lesser extent, x-ray and bone densitometry, as these can reveal the focal subchondral or subperiosteal osteoporosis discussed above. These are underutilized for identifying patients whose bone remodeling is a source of pain that can be treated with nasal calcitonin or bisphosphonates.[93–97] Computed tomography and magnetic resonance imaging are less often useful, but they can identify neurogenic edema of affected bones, joints, and deep tissues. Magnetic resonance neurography and ultrasound are emerging techniques for visualizing nerves.[98] They can help identify potentially surgical causes of persistent CRPS such as entrapment neuropathies.[99,100]

Quantitative Sensory Testing

Quantitative sensory testing (QST) is a more formal and sensitive method of characterizing sensory thresholds (most commonly thermal, mechanical, and vibratory) than the clinical examination. However, the technique is entirely subjective and dependent upon the patient's motivation and alertness.[101] While some authors think no characteristic pattern has emerged, and QST has only research utility at present,[92] more recently Maier et al.[101a] found thermal and mechanical hyperalgesias were most frequent in CRPS.

Punch Skin Biopsy

This increasingly popular method involves removing a small piece of skin under local anesthesia. This is sectioned and immunolabeled with a pan-axonal marker that permits evaluation and quantitation of the unmyelinated sensory axons, the type of axon most implicated in CRPS.[102] Neurodiagnostic skin biopsy, currently the best diagnostic test for small-fiber polyneuropathy,[102] has provided critical research evidence of small-fiber nerve injury in CRPS-I, obviating its distinction from CRPS-II.[103] But because normative densities differ at different body locations, and because of high interindividual variability, skin biopsy is not a useful clinical diagnostic test except for rare situations in which comparison of biopsy specimens from patients' CRPS-affected and matching unaffected areas confirms focal small-fiber losses.

PATHOPHYSIOLOGY OF CRPS

Recent research is illuminating many aspects of the pathophysiology of CRPS, but a final common pathway remains elusive (reviewed in refs. 104–106) As discussed above, the long-prevalent theory that CRPS was caused by excess sympathetic activity thought to be due to increased sympathetic outflow or α-adrenoreceptor hypersensitivity is not sustainable in the face of newer data, and in fact, sympathetic vasoconstrictor activity is often reduced rather than increased in acute CRPS (reviewed in ref. 107). Other proposed mechanisms now have experimental support, and these may all contribute to varying degrees in individual patients and perhaps at different times during the course of illness.

Multiple lines of evidence suggest that some CRPS features reflect neurogenic inflammation. Small-fiber axons are intimately coupled to the immune system, with feed-forward loops that potentiate pain, swelling, and vasodysregulation. Active primary nociceptive fibers release neuropeptides including substance P (SP) and calcitonin gene-related peptide (CGRP), along with cytokines and reactive oxygen scavengers.[108] These can trigger or maintain inflammation locally, which then augments nociceptor firing.

Neurogenic inflammation has been identified in the affected limb and, to a lesser degree, in the nonaffected limbs of CRPS patients[109–111] where it produces axon reflex vasodilatation and plasma extravasation that cause limb edema. Neuropeptide release in the dorsal horn may mediate central sensitization, resulting in pain and hyperalgesia in chronic CRPS. Neurogenic inflammation may, in turn, be triggered by hypoxia/ischemia and associated with ischemia-reperfusion.[104,112,113] A rat model of CRPS-I based on bone fracture and casting has highlighted the importance (and complexity) of neuropeptide changes.[114] Ischemia-reperfusion in animal models leads to free radical formation, endothelial cell damage, and arterial norepinephrine hypersensitivity. There is also clinical evidence for oxidative stress in CRPS-I patients.[115] Additionally, some peripheral nerve injuries activate Schwann cells with upregulation of cell-surface antigens (e.g., glial fibrillary acidic protein) and release multiple inflammatory mediators.[113a]

What might cause primary afferents to fire ectopically and release these proinflammatory messengers? Mounting evidence implicates structural neuronal abnormalities—nerve damage—particularly affecting the primary afferent small fibers as the link between causative traumas and this molecular mayhem, at least in susceptible people. Pathological study of amputated legs from eight patients with advanced CRPS revealed partial injuries, particularly to small-fiber axons, neurogenic changes in muscle, and marked thickening of capillaries, as seen in diabetic small-fiber polyneuropathy.[116] Skin samples from two additional amputated limbs of CRPS-I patients revealed partial loss of epidermal, sweat gland, and vascular small fibers, as well as altered patterns of neuropeptide expression in remaining fibers[117] (Figure 22.2). A larger study of skin biopsy specimens from the affected limbs of 19 more representative CRPS-I patients revealed average losses of 29% of intraepidermal nerve fibers compared to unaffected control sites[103] (Figure 22.3). These studies suggest that in CRPS, patients' limb traumas have initiated chronic focal axonal degeneration, predominantly affecting small fibers, and that CRPS-I, like CRPS-II, is associated with nerve injury.

Damage to some small fibers appears to trigger ectopic activity in surviving fibers and in central postsynaptic targets in the dorsal horn and higher centers via early long-term potentiation, chronic facilitation, and disinhibition. The final result is spontaneous pain, allodynia, hyperalgesia, and spread of symptoms to nearby areas.[118] This ectopia is unlikely to arise from sympathetic involvement; a very recent microneurographic study of single nerve fibers did not find evidence for C nociceptor activation by sympathetic efferent fibers in either CRPS-I or CRPS-II patients.[119] An autopsy study of the spinal cord of a patient with long-standing CRPS

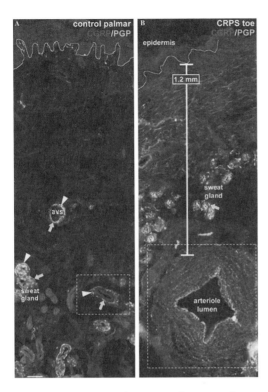

FIGURE 22.3. Complex regional pain syndrome and PGP9.5 immunolabeling of cutaneous innervation. (A) Control palmar skin demonstrating normal abundant innervation of sweat glands, arteries (box), and arteriovenous shunts (avs) located within 2 mm of the epidermis (basement membrane delineated by the white line). All contain abundant PGP⁺ innervation (arrows), and some coexpress CGRP (arrowheads). (B) In contrast, CRPS-affected skin contains sweat glands with reduced PGP⁺ innervation (arrow), no coexpression of CGRP, and denervated arteries (box) that are extremely hypertrophied. Scale bar = 100 lM.

Source: From Albrecht PJ, Hines S, Eisenberg E, et al. Pathologic alterations of cutaneous innervation and vasculature in affected limbs from patients with complex regional pain syndrome. *Pain.* 2006;120:244–266. This figure has been reproduced with permission of the International Association for the Study of Pain (IASP®). The figure may not be reproduced for any other purpose without permission.

demonstrated significant microglial and astrocyte activation, plus neuronal loss in the posterior horn, with decreased posterior horn size, most prominent at the level of original injury (L4-S2) but extending throughout the spinal cord.[120]

The most exciting new development in this field is the increasing evidence that implicates the host immune response to injury in determining who will be left with CRPS.[121] Several human leukocyte antigen alleles have been associated with CRPS,[34,122] and the recent epidemiological evidence supporting a role for inflammation was reviewed earlier. One laboratory has found antineuronal antibodies in serum from CRPS patients, although this awaits independent confirmation.[123] These surface-binding autoantibodies appear to target autonomic neurons.[123] Evidence of efficacy from a small trial of IVIG (*vide infra*) further supports this hypothesis.[124]

Functional brain imaging in CRPS has found evidence of reorganization of the primary sensorimotor cortex similar to that seen in other neuropathic and chronic pain syndromes. Use of prescription opioids may be responsible in some patients.[124a] Magnetoencephalographic studies of CRPS patients have shown increased responses of the primary sensory cortex to tactile stimulation of the affected side, increased cortical inhibition, and shrinkage of cortical hand representation,[125] which correlated with pain intensity.[126] In a group of 10 patients, these cortical changes reverted toward normal as CRPS resolved.[127] Moseley and colleagues have demonstrated that CRPS patients have disorders of higher cortical function more commonly associated with strokes and other brain injuries.[128-131] At this time, it is not yet clear whether these cortical abnormalities are triggered primarily by peripheral injuries that affect the PNS or by secondary factors such as disuse, muscle atrophy, depression, or medication use, but they are likely to contribute to the spread of pain and sensory abnormalities outside the distributions of individual peripheral nerves, and they provide a new target for therapy and rehabilitation.[127]

Postvenipuncture CRPS: A Human Model of CRPS

Rare patients undergoing phlebotomy for blood sampling, blood donation, insertion of intravenous lines, or intravenous administration of medication develop CRPS as the consequence of needlestick nerve injuries (axotomies) during the procedure. The superficial veins at the usual phlebotomy sites—antecubital fossa, radial surface of the wrist, and dorsum of the hand—are near cutaneous nerves containing sensory and autonomic axons. These can be punctured, causing unintentional axotomy, even with good technique.[132,133] The consequences of this vary broadly. Most patients probably never come to medical attention. One of us experienced several months of intermittent deep forearm pain and pinpointed the cause—uncomplicated phlebotomy at the antecubital fossa—only because of our extensive experience. No medical care was sought and this gradually resolved spontaneously. Patients who seek medical care most often report "burning," "lancinating," "shooting," "electrical" pain during their procedure,[39,134] followed by gradual resolution over weeks to months.[134,135] Rare patients develop full-blown CRPS with sensory, vasomotor, sudomotor, and motor/trophic symptoms and signs that can last for years.[39,132,134] The incidence of self-reported needlestick nerve injury is estimated by the American Red Cross as 1 in 6300 blood donations, most of which are mild and recover spontaneously.[135] The most severe cases have a self-reported incidence of 1 in 1.5 million procedures.[136] Because of its highly stereotyped wound, postvenipuncture CRPS can be viewed as a model for other cases of CRPS caused by penetrating nerve injury, of which many are iatrogenic. It also provided the rationale for a rodent model of CRPS-I based on needlestick nerve injury.[137]

THERAPY

Functional Restoration/Physiotherapy

Pharmacotherapy for CRPS has its limitations and should be used as an adjunct to functional restoration. This may be all that is needed for early, mild, or pediatric cases. Therapies including desensitization, physical therapy to increase range of motion and limb strength, postural and balance normalization, general aerobic conditioning, and occupational therapy share the primary goal of increasing function, as well as secondary goals including minimizing effects of disuse such as contractures, osteoporosis, weight gain, skin and muscle atrophy, depression, and disability. If pain limits patient participation, better pain management may improve participation.[138–140] A recent literature review suggests that the physiotherapy guidelines should be interpreted cautiously, as there is little evidence of efficacy.[141] Only graded motor imagery had good-quality (Level II) evidence in CRPS, and none had Level I evidence.[141,142] Graded motor imagery consists of limb-laterality recognition, imagined movement, and mirror movement phases over 6 weeks.[142] The mechanisms of effectiveness are unknown but are thought to be cortical and are possibly related to the neglect discussed earlier.[69,70] A preliminary study reports utility of mirror therapy in reducing CRPS-I pain in the paretic arm of stroke patients,[143] but recent reviews have questioned its efficacy.[143a,143b]

Evidence-Based Pharmacotherapy for CRPS

The uncertainties about CRPS pathogenesis, definition, and diagnosis have made it difficult to conduct clinical trials. Complex regional pain syndrome, a rare condition, is not attractive for pharmaceutical development, so the few trials performed have been investigator-initiated, small, and often without placebo controls or double blinding. The United States has no drugs approved by the Food and Drug Administration for a CRPS indication. Although some patients improve without treatment, particularly pediatric patients and those with acute conditions, most patients with chronic severe symptoms should consider pharmacotherapy. A 1997 analysis of controlled clinical trials for peripheral neuropathic pain and CRPS concluded that studies conducted for other forms of peripheral neuropathic pain had far better methodology.[144] Nonetheless, the CRPS trials do support the use of the same medications found effective for peripheral neuropathic pain.

Treatment Options for Acute CRPS

Some randomized clinical trials (RCTs) have been conducted for acute CRPS. A few small trials have evaluated agents that reduce bone resorption, calcitonin, and several bisphosphonates. These studies generally focused on improving movement rather than providing pain relief. It is unclear to what extent the actions of these agents in CRPS involve reducing bone resorption. Calcitonin, for instance, is a neuroactive peptide with centrally mediated analgesic effects independent of bone activity.[145,146] Systematic meta-analyses of several placebo-controlled trials for intranasal calcitonin 100–400 IU support its use in early CRPS.[147] Other small studies and case series support the use of intravenous bisphosphonates in early CRPS.[78,148] Pamidronate, 30 mg daily for 3 days, was reportedly helpful in a case series of chronic as well as acute patients.[149] A meta-analysis of the use of bisphosphonates in CRPS concluded that the very limited data available was promising but not sufficient to recommend usage in practice.[149a] Long-term bisphosphonates, usually for osteoporosis, rarely may increase fracture risk[149b] and intravenous use has been associated with jaw necrosis.[149c]

Two small unblinded trials provide preliminary evidence for efficacy of oral corticosteroids.[150,151] Several groups have studied antioxidants and free radical scavengers such as topical dimethylsulfoxide,[152] and one large randomized trial found that vitamin C reduced the incidence of CRPS after wrist fracture.[153] There are weak or uncertain results of trials of several α-adrenergic antagonists and vasodilators, including phenoxybenzamine and nifedipine.[154,155]

Treatment Options for Pain in Chronic CRPS

The lack of strong therapeutic trials in chronic CRPS forces physicians to be guided by the results of high-quality RCTs for other neuralgias, such as postherpetic neuralgia (PHN) after shingles and painful diabetic neuropathy. The PHN trials may be most relevant since PHN is also a focal (or regional) neuralgia that follows a monophasic insult, and most patients are otherwise healthy. Systematic meta-analyses of PHN trials enable physicians to compare the efficacy and safety of different treatments, something that individual trials do not usually permit. Currently, the best meta-analysis is that of Hempenstall et al.[156] (free download

from medicine.plosjournals.org). Many CRPS patients will require polypharmacy, but it is best to start with the single medication most likely to be effective and safe and to increase it to the full recommended or maximal tolerated dose. If it is not clearly effective, it should be discontinued before a second medication is tried. In general, if several drugs are used, they should be from different classes or treat different symptoms. Rarely, a second medication is needed to counteract the adverse effects of an otherwise useful medication.

There are currently four classes of medications with documented efficacy against neuralgia in multiple RCTs: the tricyclics and serotonin-noradrenaline reuptake inhibitors, the opioids, the gabapentinoids, and topical or systemic local anesthetics. Although sympathetic nerve blocks have long been a common CRPS treatment, meta-analysis shows no long-term benefit.[157] In contrast, systemic local anesthetics may be underutilized for patients with severe refractory pain including CRPS. Lidocaine cannot be given orally, but it can be delivered by continuous subcutaneous injection using external metered pumps of the kind used for insulin.[158] Topical local anesthetics, available as viscous lidocaine gels, creams, and sprays, may be helpful. The strongest evidence is for the 5% lidocaine patch, whose use is supported by large studies in PHN, a study of 40 patients with peripheral neuropathic pain including CRPS,[159]and as an uncontrolled open-label add-on study that included six patients with CRPS.[160]

Treatment Options for Other Symptoms in Chronic CRPS

Treatment of dystonia is complicated because prolonged tonic postures can lead to fixed contractures that require additional orthopedic therapy, such as serial casting or tendon release. Although trihexylphenidate can be considered, baclofen is the oral treatment of choice. Because it is sedating, many patients cannot tolerate the high doses often needed to lessen dystonia. Administration by intrathecal pump is an effective option that is underutilized, although pharmacological and mechanical complications are common.[161,162] There is no evidence of efficacy with long-term use of muscle relaxants such as benzodiazepines or cyclobenzaprine. Botulinum toxin injections can be very useful for focal dystonias limited to small areas, but they are impractical and too expensive for widespread dystonias. Amantadine can be considered for tremor. Rare CRPS patients have edema severe enough to distort their tissues and prevent adequate tissue oxygenation and nutrition. This can lead to skin ulceration and infection; treatment usually involves limb elevation, compressive garments, or exercise as tolerated. Trials of nitric oxide synthase inhibitors are underway.

Promising Pharmacological Therapies

The N-methyl-D-aspartate antagonist ketamine has achieved widespread attention and use for refractory CRPS. While subanesthetic doses did not help four CRPS patients,[163] higher doses (up to 100 mg for 4 hours x 10 days) in a randomized double-blind, placebo-controlled study[164] produced significant pain reduction. Administering anesthetic doses over a 5-day period was also beneficial in an open-label phase II study of 20 patients. Complete remission occurred at 1 month in all patients, at 3 months in 17 patients, and at 6 months in 16 patients, although complications ensued.[165] At present, there is tempered enthusiasm,[165a] tempered concern,[165b] and a lack of meta-analytic evidence for efficacy of ketamine in neuropathic pain states and CRPS.[165c] Recent reports of hepatotoxicity and transaminitis developing in 3/6 CRPS-I patients treated with 2 continuous intravenous 100-hour S(+)-ketamine infusions (infusion rate 10–20 mg/h) separated by 16 days suggest caution with prolonged infusions or those repeated at short intervals. At a minimum, liver function monitoring is indicated.[165d]

A small but intriguing crossover study has reported modest benefit (pain relief) from treatment of long-standing CRPS with intravenous immunoglobulin (IVIg), and provides additional evidence consistent with a role for autoimmunity in CRPS.[124] The high cost of IVIg will preclude routine use, but with confirmation, this might develop into an added tool for patients who are refractory to other treatments or for those with strong evidence of autoimmunity. It should also prompt reconsideration of other modes of immunosuppression. Implication of cytokines in CRPS has prompted consideration of new classes of therapies. Infliximab, a tumor necrosis factor-α (TNF-α) inhibitor, reduced cytokine levels and pain in two patients with CRPS.[166] Unexpected improvement in a CRPS patient being treated for multiple myeloma with thalidomide (which inhibits proinflammatory cytokines such as TNF-α),[167] plus two promising open-label thalidomide trials in patients refractory to other therapies[168,169] prompted a trial of its more potent analog, lenalidomide, in CRPS. The trial was completed but never published, so lack of efficacy is inferred.

Botulinum toxin type A (Botox) has been used for years to weaken focal muscles in conditions including movement disorders and spasticity by blocking acetylcholine exocytosis at cholinergic synapses. However, it also inhibits noncholinergic neurotransmitter (e.g., glutamate) and neuropeptide (e.g., SP and CGRP) release from sensory nerve terminals by blocking transient receptor potential vanilloid 1 exocytosis,[170,171] prompting recent evaluation for neuropathic pain. Regional intradermal injections of Botox improved spontaneous pain, as well as brush allodynia and cold pain thresholds at the painful site of 25 patients with focal painful neuropathies[56] and, when used in conjunction with sympathetic blockade with bupivicaine, extended the duration of analgesia in a subset of CRPS patients.[172] These findings await confirmation.

Neurosurgical Treatments

Rare patients with ongoing nerve injury from compression or a lesion within or near a nerve (e.g., tumor, vascular malformation) may benefit from surgical exploration, but such lesions need to be definitively localized first. The only role for ablative neurosurgery (cutting the nerves or roots innervating a painful area) is in patients with short life expectancies, because pain relief tends to be transient after this procedure, whereas the functional loss is permanent, and anesthesia dolorosa can develop in denervated body parts. Similarly, results of limb amputation are disappointing, with stump pain persisting in 28 of 34 limb amputations performed for CRPS.[173]

Much better results have been obtained with implanted neural stimulators, which augment the function of surviving neurons; spinal cord stimulation has been used for almost half a century to treat CRPS pain. This is a minimally invasive technique that involves inserting a stimulator close to the spinal cord, most frequently in the lumbar or thoracic areas, usually through an epidural needle. It is usually considered only when the disease persists despite maximal medical and rehabilitation therapy. Several recent reviews and meta-analyses demonstrate long-term reductions in pain intensity, increased function of affected extremities, and improvements in the quality of life.[174–177] However, RCTs are few, and complications such as infections and mechanical problems with the lead position often cause difficulties including need for reoperation .

Peripheral nerve stimulation is another reasonable option, especially in patients who qualify for dorsal column stimulation but are not able to achieve persistent coverage.[178] Because there are currently no commercially available leads for stimulating nerves in the limbs, some jury-rigging is needed, and the leads not infrequently shift position.[179] Chronic motor cortex stimulation by implanted electrode or repetitive transcranial magnetic stimulation has shown beneficial effects in neuralgia,[180–183] but has not been sufficiently evaluated for CRPS. One meta-analysis found that invasive brain stimulation produces greater pain reduction than noninvasive brain stimulation, but the advantage was small.[182]

CONCLUSIONS

Complex regional pain syndrome is an uncommon chronic pain syndrome with an illustrious history. Because its pathophysiology is only beginning to emerge, its present definition and diagnostic criteria are phenotypically based and therefore imprecise. Recent experimental and clinical findings, particularly regarding small-fiber dysfunction and neurogenic inflammation, have advanced the field by disproving earlier hypotheses that CRPS is primarily

psychosomatic or sympathetically mediated. The discovery of a small-fiber-predominant axonopathy in CRPS-I by three independent groups so far[103,116,117] should prompt elimination of the CRPS-I versus CRPS-II dichotomy in future definitions. Both types can now be firmly defined as peripheral neuropathic pain syndromes. It is not clear if we should persist in distinguishing between CRPS and posttraumatic neuralgia. The fact that CRPS and posttraumatic neuralgia are caused by the same injuries and respond to the same medical and surgical treatments argues for their fundamental unity. They may be endophenotypes of a spectrum disorder in which patients have different combinations of neuralgia, microvascular instability, and motor dysfunction. Individual patients' positions on that spectrum may change over time as some signs and symptoms resolve before others. Patients should be treated with whatever medications are most effective for their particular blend of symptoms. Given that CRPS is a rare consequence of common injuries, it appears likely that endogenous factors governing the internal response to injury determine susceptibility, as in other areas of medicine such as asthma and allergy. Development of treatments directed at suppressing neuroinflammation, central sensitization, and brain plasticity have potential to be more effective than current palliative therapies. We are beginning to see the light at the end of the tunnel.

ACKNOWLEDGMENTS

Supported in part by the Public Health Service R01NS052754 (A.L.O.) and K24NS059892 (A.L.O.).

REFERENCES

1. Merskey H, Bogduk N. Classification of chronic pain: descriptions of chronic pain syndromes and definitions of pain terms. In: Merskey H, Bogduk N, eds. *Task Force on Taxonomy of the International Association for the Study of Pain*. Seattle: IASP Press; 1994:40–43.
2. Mitchell SW, Morehouse GR, Keen WW. *Gunshot Wounds and Other Injuries of Nerves*. Philadelphia: Lippincott; 1864.

3. Mitchell SW. On the diseases of nerves resulting from injuries. In: Flint A, ed. *Contributions Relating to the Causation and Prevention of Disease, and to Camp Diseases*. New York: U.S. Sanitary Commission Memoirs; 1867.

4. Mitchell SW. *Injuries of Nerves and Their Consequences*. Philadelphia: Lippincott; 1872 (Dover Publication edition 1965):197–198.

5. Richards RL. Causalgia: a centennial review. *Arch Neurol*. 1967;16:339–350.

6. Wilkins RH, Brody IA. Causalgia. *Arch Neurol*. 1970;22:89–94.

7. Mitchell JK. *Remote Consequences of Injuries of Nerves and Their Treatment*. Philadelphia: Lea Brothers, 1895.

8. Medical Research Council. The diagnosis and treatment of peripheral nerve injuries. *Med Res Counc Spec Rep*. 1920;54:1–59.

9. Evans J. Reflex sympathetic dystrophy. *Surg Gynecol Obstet*. 1946;82:36–44.

10. Evans J. Reflex sympathetic dystrophy; report on 57 cases. *Ann Intern Med*. 1947;26:417–426.

11. Homans J. Minor causalgia: a hyperesthetic neurovascular syndrome. *N Engl J Med*. 1940;222:870–874.

12. Homans J. Minor causalgia following injuries and wounds. *Ann Surg*. 1941;113:932–941.

13. Echlin F, Owens FM Jr, Wells WL. Observations on "major" and "minor" causalgia. *Arch Neurol Psychiatry*. 1949;62:183–203.

14. Hardy WG, Posch JL, Webster JE, Gurdjian ES. The problem of minor and major causalgias. *Am J Surg*. 1958;95:545–551.

15. Wirth FP Jr, Rutherford RB. A civilian experience with causalgia. *Arch Surg*. 1970;100:633–638.

16. Patman RD, Thompson JE, Persson AV. Management of posttraumatic pain syndromes: report of 113 cases. *Ann Surg*. 1973;177;780–787.

17. Thompson JE, Patman RD, Persson AV. Management of posttraumatic pain syndromes (causalgia). *Am Surg*. 1975;41:599–602.

18. Tahmoush AJ. Causalgia: redefinition as a clinical pain syndrome. *Pain*. 1981;10:187–197.

19. Horowitz SH. Iatrogenic causalgia: classification, clinical findings, and legal ramifications. *Arch Neurol*. 1984;41:821–824.

20. Stanton-Hicks M, Janig W, Hassenbusch S, Haddox JD, Boas R, Wilson P. Reflex sympathetic dystrophy: changing concepts and taxonomy. *Pain*. 1995;63:127–133.

21. Bruehl S, Harden NR, Galer BS, Saltz S, Bertram M, Backonja M, Gayles R, Rudin N, Bhugra MK, Stanton-Hicks M. External validation of IASP diagnostic criteria for complex regional pain syndrome and proposed research diagnostic criteria. *Pain*. 1999;81:147–154.

22. Galer BS, Bruehl S, Harden RN. IASP diagnostic criteria for complex regional pain syndrome: a preliminary empirical validation study. *Clin J Pain*. 1998;14:48–54.

23. Harden RN, Bruehl S, Galer BS, Saltz S, Bertram M, Backonja M, Gayles R, Rudin N, Bhugra MK, Stanton-Hicks M. Complex regional pain syndrome: are the IASP diagnostic criteria valid and sufficiently comprehensive? *Pain*. 1999;83:211–219.

24. Perez RSGM, Collins S, Marinus J, Zuurmond WWA, de Lange JJ. Diagnostic criteria for CRPS I: differences between patient profiles using three different diagnostic sets. *Eur J Pain*. 2007;11:895–902.

25. Harden R, Bruehl S. Diagnostic criteria: the statistical derivation of the four criterion factors. In: Wilson PR, Stanton-Hicks M, Harden RN, eds. *CRPS: Current Diagnosis and Therapy*. Seattle: IASP Press; 2005:45–58.

26. Harden NR, Bruehl S, Stanton-Hicks, Wilson PR. Proposed new diagnostic criteria for complex regional pain syndrome. *Pain Med*. 2007;8:326–331.

26a. Harden RN, Bruehl S, Perez RSGM, Birklein F, Marinus J, Maihofner C, Lubenow T, Buvanendran A, Mackey S, Graciosa J, Mogilevski M, Ramsden C, Chont M, Vatine JJ. Validation of proposed diagnostic criteria (the "Budapest Criteria") for complex regional pain syndrome. *Pain*. 2010;150:268–274.

26b. Sumitani M, Shibata M, Sakaue G, Mashimo T. Development of comprehensive criteria for complex regional pain syndrome in the Japanes population. *Pain*. 2010;150:243–249.

27. Allen G, Galer BS, Schwartz L. Epidemiology of complex regional pain syndrome: a retrospective chart review of 134 patients. *Pain*. 1999; 80:539–544.

28. Sandroni P, Benrud-Larson LM, McClelland RL, Low PA. Complex regional pain syndrome type I: incidence and prevalence in Olmstead County, a population-based study. *Pain*. 2003; 103:199–207.

29. de Mos M, de Bruijn AG, Huygen FJ, et al. The incidence of complex regional pain syndrome: a population-based study. *Pain*. 2007;129:12–20.

30. Atkins RM, Duckworth T, Kanis JA. Features of algodystrophy after Colles fracture. *J Bone Joint Surg Br*. 1990;72:105–110.

31. Bickerstaff DR, Kanis JA. Algodystrophy: an under-recognized complication of minor trauma. *Br J Rheumatol*. 1994;33:240–248.

32. Atkins RM. Complex regional pain syndrome. *J Bone Joint Surg Br.* 2003;85:1100–1106.

33. Veldman PH, Reynen HM, Arntz IE, Goris RJ. Signs and symptoms of reflex sympathetic dystrophy: prospective study of 829 patients. *Lancet.* 1993;342:1012–1016.

34. van de Beek WJ, van Hilten JJ, Roep BO. HLA-DQ1 associated with reflex sympathetic dystrophy. *Neurology.* 2000;55:457–458.

35. Stoler JM, Oaklander AL. Patients with Ehlers Danlos syndrome and CRPS: a possible association? *Pain.* 2006;123:204–209.

36. de Rooij AM, de Mos M, Sturkenboom MCJM, Marinus J, van den Maagdenberg AMJM, van Hilten JJ. Familial occurrence of complex regional pain syndrome. *Eur J Pain.* 2009;13: 171–177.

37. Wasner G, Schattschneider J, Binder A, Baron R. Complex regional pain syndrome—diagnostic, mechanisms, CNS involvement and therapy. *Spinal Cord.* 2003;41:61–75.

38. Schott GD. Complex? Regional? Pain? Syndrome? *Pract Neurol.* 2007;7:145–157.

39. Horowitz SH. Venipuncture-induced neuropathic pain: the clinical syndrome, with comparisons to experimental nerve injury models. *Pain.* 2001;94:225–229.

40. Birklein F, Handwerker, HO. Complex regional pain syndrome: how to resolve the complexity? *Pain.* 2001;94:1–6.

41. Albazaz R, Wong YT, Homer-Vanniasinkam S. Complex regional pain syndrome: a review. *Ann Vasc Surg.* 2008;22:297–306.

42. Birklein F, Riedl N, Sieweke N, Weber M, Neundorfer B. Neurological findings in complex regional pain syndromes—analysis of 145 cases. *Acta Neurol Scand.* 2000;101:262–269.

43. Sieweke N, Birklein F, Riedl B, Neundorfer B, Handwerker HO. Patterns of hyperalgesia in complex regional pain syndrome. *Pain.* 1999;80:171–177.

44. Bonica JJ. Causalgia and other reflex sympathetic dystrophies. In: Bonica JJ, ed. *Advances in Pain Research and Therapy.* Vol. 3. New York: Raven Press; 1979: 141–166.

45. Schwartzman RJ, McLellan TL. Reflex sympathetic dystrophy. *Arch Neurol.* 1987;44:555–561.

46. Bruehl S, Harden RN, Galer BS, Saltz S, Backonja M, Stanton-Hicks M. Complex regional pain syndrome: are there distinct subtypes and sequential stages of the syndrome? *Pain.* 2002;95:119–124.

47. Eberle T, Doganci B, Kramer HH, Geber C, Fechir M, Magerl W, Birklein F. Warm and cold complex regional pain syndromes: differences beyond skin temperature? *Neurology.* 2009;72:505–512.

48. Heerschap A, den Hollander JA, Reynen H, Goris RJ. Metabolic changes in reflex sympathetic dystrophy: a ^{31}P NMR spectroscopy study. *Muscle Nerve.* 1993;16(4):367–373.

49. Rommel O, Habler H-J, Schurmann M. Laboratory tests for complex regional pain syndrome. In: Wilson PR, Stanton-Hicks M, Harden RN, eds. *CRPS: Current Diagnosis and Therapy.* Seattle: IASP Press; 2005:139–159.

50. Wasner G, Schattschneider J, Heckmann K, Maier C, Baron R. Vascular abnormalities in reflex sympathetic dystrophy (CRPS I): mechanisms and diagnostic value. *Brain.* 2001; 124:587–599.

51. Wasner G, Schattschneider J, Baron R. Skin temperature side differences: a diagnostic tool for CRPS? *Pain.* 2002;98:19–26.

52. Low VA, Sandroni P, Fealey RD, Low PA. Detection of small-fiber neuropathy by sudomotor testing. *Muscle Nerve.* 2006;34(1):57–61.

53. Birklein F, Sittl R, Spitzer A, Claus D, Neundorfer B, Handwerker HO. Sudomotor function in sympathetic reflex dystrophy. *Pain.* 1997;68 (1–2):49–54.

54. Bergmann I, Dauphin M, Naumann M, Flachenecker P, Mullges W, Koltzenburg M, Sommer C. Selective degeneration of sudomotor fibers in Ross syndrome and successful treatment of compensatory hyperhidrosis with botulinum toxin. *Muscle Nerve.* 1998;21: 1790–1793.

55. Restivo DA, Lanza S, Patti F, Giuffrida S, Marchese-Ragona R, Bramanti P, Palmeri A. Improvement of diabetic autonomic gustatory sweating by botulinum toxin type A. *Neurology.* 2002;59:1971–1973.

56. Ranoux D, Attal N, Morain F, Bouhassira D. Botulinum type A induces direct analgesic effects in chronic neuropathic pain. *Ann Neurol.* 2008;64:274–283.

57. van Hilten JJ, Blumberg H, Robert Schwartzman RJ. Factor IV: movement disorders and dystrophy—pathophysiology and measurement. In: Wilson PR, Stanton-Hicks M, Harden RN, eds. *CRPS: Current Diagnosis and Therapy.* Seattle: IASP Press; 2005:119–137.

58. Schwartzman RJ, Kerrigan J. The movement disorder of reflex sympathetic dystrophy. *Neurology.* 1990;40:57–61.

59. van Rijn MA, Marinus J, Putter H, van Hilten JJ. Onset and progression of dystonia in complex regional pain syndrome. *Pain.* 2007;130: 287–293.

60. Tarsy D, Simon DK. Current concepts: dystonia. *N Engl J Med*. 2006;355:818–829.

61. Schott GD. Peripherally-triggered CRPS and dystonia. *Pain*. 2007;130:203–207.

62. Bhatia KP, Bhatt MH, Marsden CD. The causalgia-dystonia syndrome. *Brain*. 1993;116:843–851.

63. Verdugo RJ, Ochoa JL. Abnormal movements in complex regional pain syndrome: assessment of their nature. *Muscle Nerve*. 2000;23:198–205.

64. Schrag A, Trimble M, Quinn N, Bhatia K. The syndrome of fixed dystonia: an evaluation of 103 patients. *Brain*. 2004;127:2360–2372.

65. van der Laan L, van Spaendonck K, Horstinnk MW, Goris RJ. The Symptom Checklist-90 Revised questionnaire: no psychological profiles in complex regional pain syndrome-dystonia. *J Pain Symptom Manage*. 1999;17:357–362.

66. Mink JW. Abnormal circuit function in dystonia. *Neurology*. 2006;66:959.

67. van de Beek WJT, Vein A, Hilgevoord AAJ, van Dijk, van Hilten JJ. Neurophysiological aspects of patients with generalized or multifocal dystonia in reflex sympathetic dystrophy. *J Clin Neurophysiol*. 2002;19:77–83.

67a. Munts AG, Mugge W, Meurs TS, et al. Fixed dystonia in complex regional pain syndrome: a descriptive and computational modeling approach. *BMC Neurol*. 2011;11:53.

68. Maihofner C, Baron R, DeCol R, Binder A, Birklein F, Deuschl G, Handwerker HO, Schattschneider J. The motor system shows adaptive changes in complex regional pain syndrome. *Brain*. 2007;130:2671–2687.

68a. Hawley JS, Weiner WJ. Psychogenic dystonia and peripheral trauma. *Neurology*. 2011;77:496–502.

69. Galer BS, Butler S, Jensen M. Case reports and hypothesis: a neglect-like syndrome may be responsible for the motor disturbance in reflex sympathetic dystrophy (complex regional pain syndrome-I). *J Pain Symptom Manage*. 1995;10:385–391.

70. Galer BS, Jensen M. Neglect-like symptoms in complex regional pain syndrome: results of a self-administered survey. *J Pain Symptom Manage*. 1999;18:213–217.

71. Kuntz A, Richens CA. Innervation of the bone marrow. *J Comp Neurol*. 1945;83:213–222.

72. Serre CM, Farlay D, Delmas PD, Chenu C. Evidence for a dense and intimate innervation of the bone tissue, including glutamate-containing fibers. *Bone*. 1999;25:623–629.

73. Kingery WS, Offley SC, Guo TZ, Davies MF, Clark JD, Jacobs CR. A substance P receptor (NK1) antagonist enhances the widespread osteoporotic effects of sciatic nerve section. *Bone*. 2003;33:927–936.

74. Hukkanen M, Konttinen YT, Santavirta S, Paavolainen P, Gu XH, Terenghi G, Polak JM. Rapid proliferation of calcitonin gene-related peptide-immunoreactive nerves during healing of rat tibial fracture suggests neural involvement in bone growth and remodelling. *Neuroscience*. 1993;54:969–979.

75. Offley SC, Guo TZ, Wei T, Clark JD, Vogel H, Lindsey DP, Jacobs CR, Yao W, Lane NE, Kingery WS. Capsaicin-sensitive sensory neurons contribute to the maintenance of trabecular bone integrity. *J Bone Miner Res*. 2005;20:257–267.

76. Santavirta S, Konttinen YT, Nordstrom D, Makela A, Sorsa T, Hukkanen M, Rokkanen P. Immunologic studies of nonunited fractures. *Acta Orthop Scand*. 1992;63:579–586.

77. Kozin F, Genant HK, Bekerman C, McCarty DJ. The reflex sympathetic dystrophy syndrome. II. Roentgenographic and scintigraphic evidence of bilaterality and of periarticular accentuation. *Am J Med*. 1976;60:332–338.

78. Adami S, Fossaluzza V, Gatti D, Fracassi E, Braga V. Bisphosphonate therapy of reflex sympathetic dystrophy syndrome. *Ann Rheum Dis*. 1997;56:201–204.

79. Wilder RT, Olsson G. Management of pediatric patients with CRPS. In: Wilson PR, Stanton-Hicks M, Harden RN, eds. *CRPS: Current Diagnosis and Therapy*. Seattle: IASP Press; 2005:275–289.

80. Wilder RT. Management of pediatric patients with complex regional pain syndrome. *Clin J Pain*. 2006;22:413–418.

81. Low AK, Ward K, Wines AP. Pediatric complex regional pain syndrome. *J Pediatr Orthop*. 2007:27:567–572.

82. Kachko L, Efrat R, Ben Ami S, Mukamel M, Katz J. Complex regional pain syndrome in children and adolescents. *Pediatr Int*. 2008;50:523–527.

83. Sethna NF, Meier PM, Zurakowski D, Berde CB. Cutaneous sensory abnormalities in children and adolescents with complex regional pain syndromes. *Pain*. 2007;131:153–161.

84. Agrawal SK, Rittey CD, Harrower NA, Goddard JM, Mordekar SR. Movement disorders associated with complex regional pain syndrome in children. *Dev Med Child Neurol*. 2009;51: 557–562.

85. Lebel A, Becerra L, Wallin D, Moulton EA, Morris S, Pendse G, Jasciewicz J, Stein M, Aiello-Lammens M, Grant E, Berde C, Barsook D. fMRI reveals distinct CNS processing during symptomatic and recovered complex

regional pain syndrome in children. *Brain*. 2008;131:1854–1879.

86. Sherry DD, Wallace CA, Kelley C, Kidder M, Sapp L. Short- and long-term outcomes of children with complex regional pain syndrome type 1 treated with exercise therapy. *Clin J Pain*. 1999;15:218–233.

87. Lee BH, Scharff L, Sethna NF, McCarthy CF, Scott-Sutherland J, Shea AM, Sullivan P, Meier P, Zurakowski D, Masek BJ, Berde CB. Physical therapy and cognitive-behavioral treatment for complex regional pain syndrome. *J Pediatr*. 2002;141:135–140.

88. Olsson GL, Meyerson BA, Linderoth B. Spinal cord stimulation in adolescents with complex regional pain syndrome type I (CRPS-I). *Eur J Pain*. 2008;12:53–59.

89. Beghi E, Kurland LT, Mulder DW, Nicolosi A. Brachial plexus neuropathy in the population of Rochester, Minnesota, 1970–1981. *Ann Neurol*. 1985;18:320–323.

90. Mendell JR, Sahenk Z. Clinical practice. Painful sensory neuropathy. *N Engl J Med*. 2003;348(13):1243–1255.

91. Bruehl S, Harden RN, Galer BS, Saltz S, Backonja M, Stanton-Hicks M. Complex regional pain syndrome: are there distinct subtypes and sequential stages of the syndrome? *Pain*. 2002;95:119–124.

92. Rommel O, Habler H-J, Schurmann M. Laboratory tests for complex regional pain syndrome. In: Wilson PR, Stanton-Hicks M, Harden RN, eds. *CRPS: Current Diagnosis and Therapy*. Seattle: IASP Press; 2005: 139–159.

93. Hamamci N, Dursun E, Ural C, Cakci A. Calcitonin treatment in reflex sympathetic dystrophy: a preliminary study. *Br J Clin Pract*. 1996;50(7):373–375.

94. Gobelet C, Waldburger M, Meier JL. The effect of adding calcitonin to physical treatment on reflex sympathetic dystrophy. *Pain*. 1992;48(2):171–175.

95. Bickerstaff DR, Kanis JA. The use of nasal calcitonin in the treatment of post-traumatic algodystrophy. *Br J Rheumatol*. 1991;30(4): 291–294.

96. Maillefert JF, Cortet B, Aho S. Pooled results from 2 trials evaluating bisphosphonates in reflex sympathetic dystrophy. *J Rheumatol*. 1999;26(8):1856–1857.

97. Cortet B, Flipo RM, Coquerelle P, Duquesnoy B, Delcambre B. Treatment of severe, recalcitrant reflex sympathetic dystrophy: assessment of efficacy and safety of the second gen-

eration bisphosphonate pamidronate. *Clin Rheumatol*. 1997;16(1):51–56.

98. Aagaard BD, Maravilla KR, Kliot M. MR neurography. MR imaging of peripheral nerves. *Magn Reson Imaging Clin North Am*. 1998;6(1):179–194.

99. Thimineur MA, Saberski L. Complex regional pain syndrome type I (RSD) or peripheral mononeuropathy: a discussion of three cases. *Clin J Pain*. 1996;12:145–150.

100. Grant GA, Goodkin R, Maravilla KR, Kliot M. MR neurography: diagnostic utility in the surgical treatment of peripheral nerve disorders. *Neuroimaging Clin North Am*. 2004;14(1):115–133.

101. Freeman R, Chase KP, Risk MR. Quantitative sensory testing cannot differentiate simulated sensory loss from sensory neuropathy. *Neurology*. 2003;60:465–470.

101a. Maier C, Baron R, Tolle TR, et al. Quantitative sensory testing in the German Research Network on Neuropathic Pain (DFNS): somatosensory abnormalities in 1236 patients with different neuropathic pain syndromes. *Pain*. 2010;150:439–450.

102. England JD, Gronseth GS, Franklin G, et al. Practice parameter: evaluation of distal symmetric polyneuropathy: role of autonomic testing, nerve biopsy, and skin biopsy (an evidence-based review). Report of the American Academy of Neurology, American Association of Neuromuscular and Electrodiagnostic Medicine, and American Academy of Physical Medicine and Rehabilitation. *Neurology*. 2009;72(2):177–184.

103. Oaklander AL, Rissmiller JG, Gelman LB, Zheng L, Chang Y, Gott R. Evidence of focal small-fiber axonal degeneration in complex regional pain syndrome-I (reflex sympathetic dystrophy). *Pain*. 2006;120(3):235–243.

104. de Mos M, Sturkenboom MCJM, Huygen FJPM. Current understandings on complex regional pain syndrome. *Pain Pract*. 2009;9:86–99.

105. Oaklander AL, Fields HL. Is reflex sympathetic dystrophy/complex regional pain syndrome type I a small fiber neuropathy? *Ann Neurol*. 2009;65:629–638.

106. Smith HS, Albrecht PJ, Rice FL. Complex regional pain syndrome: pathophysiology. In Smith HS, ed. *Current Therapy in Pain*. Philadelphia: Saunders Elsevier; 2009:295–309.

107. Wasner G, Baron R. Factor II: vasomotor changes—pathophysiology and measurement. In: Wilson PR, Stanton-Hicks M,

Harden RN, eds. *CRPS: Current Diagnosis and Therapy*. Seattle: IASP Press; 2005:81–106.

108. Price TJ, Flores CM. Critical evaluation of the colocalization between calcitonin gene-related peptide, substance P, transient receptor potential vanilloid subfamily type I immunoreactivities, and isolectin B4 binding in primary afferent neurons of the rat and mouse. *J Pain*. 2007;8(3):263–272.

109. Weber M, Birklein F, Neundorfer B, Schmelz M. Facilitated neurogenic inflammation in complex regional pain syndrome *Pain*. 2001;91:251–257.

110. Leis S, Weber M, Schmelz M, Birklein F. Facilitated neurogenic inflammation in unaffected limbs of patients with complex reginal pain syndrome. *Neurosci Lett*. 2004;359:163–166.

111. Heijmans-Antonissen C, Wesseldijk F, Munnikes RJ, Huygen FJ, van der Meijden P, Hop WC, Hooijkaas H, Zijistra FJ. Multiplex bead array assay for detection of 25 soluble cytokines in blister fluid of patients with complex regional pain syndrome type I. *Mediators Inflamm*. 2006;2006(1):28398.

112. Coderre TJ, Xantlhos DN, Francis L, Bennett GJ. Chronic post-ischemia pain (CPIP): a novel animal model of complex regional pain syndrome-type I (CRPS-I; reflex sympathetic dystrophy) produced by prolonged hind paw ischemia and reperfusion in the rat. *Pain*. 2004;112:94–105.

113. Coderre TJ, Bennett GJ. Objectifying CRPS-I. *Pain*. 2008;138:3–4.

113a. Saab CY, Hains BC. Remote neuroimmune signaling: a long-range mechanism of nociceptive network plasticity. *Trends Neurosci*. 2009;32(2):110–117.

114. Wei T, Li WW, Guo TZ, Zhao R, Wang L, Clark DJ, Oaklander AL, Schmelz M, Kingery WS. Post-junctional facilitation of Substance P signaling in a tibia fracture rat model of complex regional pain syndrome type I. *Pain*. 2009;144(3):278–286.

115. Eisenberg E, Shtahl S, Geller R, Reznick AZ, Sharf O, Rabinovich M, Ehrenreich A, Nagler RM. Serum and salivary oxidative analysis in complex regional pain syndrome. *Pain*. 2008;138:226–232.

116. van der Laan L, ter Laak HJ, Gabreels-Festen A, Gabreels F, Goris RJA. Complex regional pain syndrome type I (RSD): pathology of skeletal muscle and peripheral nerve. *Neurology*. 1998;51(1):20–25.

117. Albrecht PJ, Hines S, Eisenberg E, Pud D, Finlay DR, Connolly MK, Pare M, Davar G, Rice FL. Pathologic alterations of cutaneous innervation and vasculature in affected limbs from patients with complex regional pain syndrome. *Pain*. 2006;120:244–266.

118. Woolf CJ. Pain: moving from symptom control toward mechanism-specific pharmacologic management. *Ann Intern Med*. 2004;140:441–451.

119. Campero M, Bostock H, Baumann TK, Ochoa JL. A search for activation of C nociceptors by sympathetic fibers in complex regional pain syndrome. *Clin Neurophysiol*. 2010;121(7):1072–1079.

120. Del Valle L, Schwartzman RJ, Alexander G. Spinal cord histopathological alterations in a patient with longstanding complex regional pain syndrome. *Brain Behav Immun*. 2009;23:85–91.

121. Blaes F, Tschernatsch M, Braeu ME, Matz O, Schmitz K, Nascimento D, Kaps M, Birklein F. Autoimmunity in complex regional pain syndrome. *Ann NY Acad Sci*. 2007;1107:168–173.

122. Kemler MA, van de Vusse AC, van den Berg-Loonen EM, Barendse GA, van Kleef M, Weber WE. HLA-DQ1 associated with reflex sympathetic dystrophy. *Neurology*. 1999;53(6):1350–1351.

123. Kohr D, Tschernatsch M, Schmitz K, et al. Autoantibodies in complex regional pain syndrome bind to a differentiation-dependent neuronal surface autoantigen. *Pain*. 2009;143(3):246–251.

124. Goebel A, Baranowski A, Maurer K, Ghiai A, McCabe C, Ambler G. Intravenous immunoglobulin treatment of the complex regional pain syndrome: a randomized trial. *Ann Intern Med*. 2010;152:152–158.

124a. Younger JW, Chu LF, D'Arcy NT, Trott KE, Jastrzeb LE, Mackey SC. Prescription opioids analgesics rapidly change the human brain. *Pain*. 2011;152(8):1803–1810.

125. Juottonen K, Gockel M, Silen T, Hurri H, Hari R, Forss N. Altered central sensorimotor processing in patients with complex regional pain syndrome. Pain 2002;98:315–323.

126. Maihofner C, Handwerker HO, Neundorfer B, Birklein F. Patterns of cortical reorganization in complex regional pain syndrome. *Neurology*. 2003;61:1707–1715.

127. Maihofner C, Handwerker HO, Neundorfer B, Birklein F. Cortical reorganization during recovery from complex regional pain syndrome. *Neurology*. 2004;63:693–701.

128. Acerra NE, Moseley GL. Dysynchiria: watching the mirror image of the unaffected limb

elicits pain on the affected side. *Neurology.* 21005;65:751–753.

129. Moseley GL. Distorted body image in complex regional pain syndrome. *Neuroogy.* 2005;65:773.

130. Moseley GL Olthof N, Venema A, Don S, Wijers M, Gallace A, Spence C. Psychologically induced cooling of a specific body part caused by the illusory ownership of an artificial counterpart. *Proc Natl Acad Sci USA.* 2008;105:13169–13173.

131. Moseley GL, Gallace A, Spence C. Space-based, but not arm-based, shift in tactile processing in complex regional pain syndrome and its relationship to cooling of the affected limb. *Brain.* 2009;132:3142–3151.

132. Horowitz SH. Venipuncture-induced causalgia: anatomic relations of upper extremity superficial veins and nerves, and clinical considerations. *Transfusion.* 2000;40:1036–1040.

133. Yamada K, Yamada K, Katsuda I, Hida T. Cubital fossa venipuncture sites based on anatomical variations and relationships of cutaneous veins and nerves. *Clin Anat.* 2008;21:307–313.

134. Horowitz SH. Venipuncture-induced nerve injury: a review. *J Neuropathol Pain Symptom Manage.* 2005;1(1):109–114.

135. Newman BH, Waxman DA. Blood donation-related neurologic needle injury: evaluation of 2 years' worth of data from a large blood center. *Transfusion.* 1996;36:213–215.

136. Newman B. Venipuncture nerve injuries after whole-blood donation. *Transfusion.* 2001;41:571.

137. Siegel SM, Lee JW, Oaklander AL. Needlestick distal nerve injury in rats models: symptoms of complex regional pain suyndrome. *Anesth Analg.* 2007;105(6):1820–1829.

138. Harden RN. Pharmacotherapy of complex regional pain syncrome. *Am J Phys Med Rehabil.* 2005;84:S17–S28.

139. Harden RN. The rationale for integrated functional restoration. In: Wilson PR, Stanton-Hicks M, Harden RN, eds. *CRPS: Current Diagnosis and Therapy.* Seattle: IASP Press; 2005:163–171.

140. Geertzen JHB, Harden RN. Physical and occupational therapies. In: Wilson PR, Stanton-Hicks M, Harden RN, eds. *CRPS: Current Diagnosis and Therapy.* Seattle: IASP Press; 2005:173–179.

141. Daly AE, Bialocerkowski AE. Does evidence support physiotherapy management of adult complex regional pain syndrome type one?

A systematic review. *Eur J Pain.* 2009;13: 339–353.

142. Moseley GL. Graded motor imagery for pathologic pain: a randomized controlled trial. *Neurology.* 2006;67:2129–2134.

143. Cacchio A, De Blasis E, Necozione S, di Orio F, Santilli V. Mirror therapy for chronic complex regional pain syndrome type 1 and stroke. *N Engl J Med.* 2009;361:634–636.

143a. Moseley GL, Gallace A, Spence C. Is mirror therapy all it is cracked up to be? Current evidence and future directions. *Pain.* 2008;138:7–10.

143b. Rothgangel AS, Braun SM, Beurskens AJ, Seitz RJ, Wade DT. The clinical aspects of mirror therapy in rehabilitation: a systematic review of the literature. *Int J Rehabil Res.* 2011;34:1–13.

144. Kingery WS. A critical review of controlled trials for peripheral neuropathic pain and complex regional pain syndromes. *Pain.* 1997;73(2):123–139.

145. Fraioli F, Fabbri A, Gnessi L, Moretti C, Santoro C, Felici M. Subarachnoid injection of salmon calcitonin induces analgesia in man. *Eur J Pharmacol.* 1982;78(3):381–382.

146. Clemento G, Amico Roxas M, Rasiparda E. The analgesic activity of calcitonin and the central serotonergic system. *Eur J Pharmacol.* 1985;108:71–75.

147. Perez RS, Kwakkel G, Zuurmond WW, de Lange JJ. Treatment of reflex sympathetic dystrophy (CRPS type 1): a research synthesis of 21 randomized clinical trials. *J Pain Symptom Manage.* 2001;21(6):511–526.

148. Varenna M, Zucchi F, Ghiringhelli D, Binelli L, Bevilacqua M, Bettica P, Sinigaglia L. Intravenous clodronate in the treatment of reflex sympathetic dystrophy syndrome. A randomized, double blind, placebo controlled study. *J Rheumatol.* 2000;27(6):1477–1483.

149. Kubalek I, Fain O, Paries J, Kettaneh A, Thomas M. Treatment of reflex sympathetic dystrophy with pamidronate: 29 cases. *Rheumatology (Oxford).* 2001;40(12):1394–1397.

149a. Brunner F, Schmid A, Kissling R, Held U, Bachmann LM. Bisphosphonates for the therapy of complex regional pain syndrome I—systematic review. *Eur J Pain* 2009;13(1):17–21.

149b. Sellmeyer DE. Atypical fractures as a potential complication of long-term bisphosphonates therapy. *JAMA.* 2010; 304(13):1480–1484.

149c. Baqain ZH, Sawair FA, Tamimi Z, et al. Osteonecrosis of jaws related to intravenous bisphosphonates: the experience of a Jordanian teaching hospital. *Ann R Coll Surg Engl.* 2010;92(6):489–494.

150. Christensen K, Jensen EM, Noer I. The reflex dystrophy syndrome response to treatment with systemic corticosteroids. *Acta Chir Scand.* 1982;148(8):653–655.

151. Braus DF, Krauss JK, Strobel J. The shoulder-hand syndrome after stroke: a prospective clinical trial. *Ann Neurol.* 1994;36(5):728–733.

152. Zuurmond WW, Langendijk PN, Bezemer PD, Brink HE, de Lange JJ, van Loenen AC. Treatment of acute reflex sympathetic dystrophy with DMSO 50% in a fatty cream. *Acta Anaesth Scand.* 1996;40(3):364–367.

153. Zollinger PE, Tuinebreijer WE, Kreis RW, Breederveld RS. Effect of vitamin C on frequency of reflex sympathetic dystrophy in wrist fractures: a randomized trial. *Lancet.* 1999;354(9195):2025–2028.

154. Muizelaar JP, Kleyer M, Hertogs IA, deLange DC. Complex regional pain syndrome (reflex sympathetic dystrophy and causalgia): management with the calcium channel blocker nifedipine and/or the alpha-sympathetic blocker phenoxybenzamine in 59 patients. *Clin Neurol Neurosurg.* 1997;99(1):26–30.

155. Prough DS, McLeskey CH, Poehling GG, Korman LA, Weeks DB, Whitworth T, Semble EL. Efficacy of oral nifedipine in the treatment of reflex sympathetic dystrophy. *Anesthesiology.* 1985;62(6):796–799.

156. Hempenstall K, Nurmikko TJ, Johnson RW, A'Hern RP, Rice AS. Analgesic therapy in postherpetic neuralgia: a quantitative systematic review. *PloS Med.* 2005;2(7):e164.

157. Cepeda MS, Lau J, Carr DB. Defining the therapeutic role of local anesthetic sympathetic blockade in complex regional pain syndrome: a narrative and systematic review. *Clin J Pain.* 2002;18(4):216–233.

158. Challapalli V, Tremont-Lukats IW, McNicol ED, Lau J, Carr DB. Systemic administration of local anesthetic agents to relieve neuropathic pain. *Cochrane Database Syst Rev.* 2005;(4):CD003345.

159. Meier T, Wasner G, Faust M, Kuntzer T, Ochsner F, Hueppe M, Bogousslavsky J, Baron R. Efficacy of lidocaine patch 5% in the treatment of focal peripheral neuropathic pain syndromes: a randomized, double-blind, placebo-controlled study. *Pain.* 2003;106:151–158.

160. Devers A, Galer BS. Topical lidocaine patch relieves a variety of neuropathic pain

conditions: an open-label study. *Clin J Pain.* 2000;16:205–208.

161. van Rijn MA, Munts AG, Marinus J, Voormolen JHC, de Boer KS, Teepe-Twiss IM, van Dasselaar NT, Delhaas EM, van Hilgten JJ. Intrathecal baclofen for dystonia of complex regional pain syndrome. *Pain.* 2009;143:41–47.

162. Raja SN. Motor dysfunction in CRPS and its treatment. *Pain.* 2009;143:3–4.

163. Kiefer RT, Rohr P, Ploppa A, Nohe B, Dieterich HJ, Grothusen J, Altemeyer KH, Unertl K, Schwartzman RJ. A pilot open-label study of the efficacy of subanesthetic isomeric S (+)-ketamine in refractory CRPS patients. *Pain Med.* 2008;9:44–54.

164. Schwartzman RJ, Alexander GM, Grothusen JR, Paylor T, Reichenberger E, Perreault M. Outpatient intravenous ketamine for the treatment of complex regional pain syndrome: a double-blind placebo controlled study. *Pain.* 2009;147:107–115.

165. Kiefer RT, Rohr P, Ploppa A, Dieterich HJ, Grothusen J, Koffler S, Altemeyer KH, Unertl K, Schwartzman RJ. Efficacy of ketamine in anesthetic dosage for the treatment of refractory complex regional pain syndrome: an open-label phase II study. *Pain Med.* 2008;9:1173–1201.

165a. Schwartzman RJ, Alexander GM, Grothusen JR. The use of ketamine in CRPS: possible mechanisms. *Expert Rev Neurother.* 2011;11:719–734.

165b. Bell RF, Moore RA. Intravenous ketamine for CRPS: making too much of too little. *Pain.* 2010;150:10–11.

165c. Collins S, Sigtermans MJ, Dahan A, Zuurmond WW, Perez RS. NMDA receptor antagonists for the treatment of neuropathic pain. *Pain Med.* 2010;11:1726–1742.

165d. Noppers IM, Niesters M, Aarts LPHJ, Bauer MCR, Drewes AM, Dahan A, Sarton EY. Drug-induced liver injury following a preated course of ketamine treatment for chronic pain in CRPS type I patients. A report of 3 cases. *Pain.* 2011;152(9): 2173–2178.

166. Huygen FJ, Niehof S, Zijlstra FJ, van Hagen PM, van Daele PL. Successful treatment of CRPS 1 with anti-TNF. *J Pain Symptom Manage.* 2004;27:101–103.

167. Rajkumar SV, Fonseca R, Witzig TE. Complete resolution of reflex sympathetic dystrophy with thalidomide treatment. *Arch Intern Med.* 2001;161:2502–2503.

168. Schwartzman RJ, Chevlen E, Bengtson K. Thalidomide has activity in treating complex regional pain syndrome. *Arch Intern Med.* 2003;163:1487–1488.

169. Prager J, Fleischman J, Lingua G. Open label trial of thalidomide in the treatment of complex regional pain. *J Pain.* 2003;4 (suppl 1):76.

170. Aoki KR. Review of a proposed mechanism for the antinociceptive action of botulinum toxin type A. *Neurotoxicology.* 2005;26:785–793.

171. Tugnoli V, Capone JG, Eleopra R, Quatrale R, Sensi M, Gastaldo E, Tola MR, Geppetti P. Botulinum toxin type A reduces capsaicin-evoked pain and neurogenic vasodilatation in human skin. *Pain.* 2007;130:76–83.

172. Carroll I, Clark JD, Mackey S. Sympathetic block with botulinum toxin to treat complex regional pain syndrome. *Ann Neurol.* 2009;65:348–351.

173. Dielssen PW, Claassen AT, Veldman PH, Goris RJ. Amputation for reflex sympathetic dystrophy. *J Bone Joint Surg Br.* 1995; 77-B(2):270–273.

174. Forouzanfar T, Kemler MA, Weber WE, Kessels AG, van Kleef M. Spinal cord stimulation in complex regional pain syndrome: cervical and lumbar devices are comparably effective. *Br J Anaesth.* 2004;92:348–353.

175. Turner JA, Loeser JD, Deyo RA, Sanders SB. Spinal cord stimulation for patients with failed back surgery syndrome or complex regional pain syndrome: a systematic review of effectiveness and complications. *Pain.* 2004;108:137–147.

176. Taylor RS, Van Buyten JP, Buchser E. Spinal cord stimulation for complex regional pain syndrome: a systematic review of the clinical cost-effectiveness literature and assessment of prognostic factors. *Eur J Pain.* 2006;10: 91–101.

177. Stanton-Hicks M. Complex regional pain syndrome: manifestations and the role of neurostimulation in its management. *J Pain Symptom Manage.* 2006;31(4 suppl): S20–S24.

178. Hassenbusch SJ, Schoppa D, Walsh JG, Covington EC. Long-term results of peripheral nerve stimulation for reflex sympathetic dystrophy. *J Neurosurg.* 1996;84(3):415–423.

179. Ishizuka K, Oaklander AL, Chiocca EA. A retrospective analysis of reasons for reoperation following initially successful peripheral nerve stimulation. *J Neurosurg.* 2007;106(3): 388–390.

180. Brown JA, Pilitsis JG. Motor cortex stimulation. *Pain Med.* 2006;7:S140–S145.

181. Lefaucheur JP, Hatem S, Nineb A, Menard-Lefaucheur I, Wending S, Keravel Y, Nguyen JP. Somatotopic organization of the analgesic effects of motor cortex rTMS in neuropathic pain. *Neurology.* 2006;67: 1998–2004.

182. Lima MC, Fregni F. Motor cortex stimulation for chronic pain: systematic review and meta-analysis of the literature. *Neurology.* 2008;70:2329–2337.

183. Andre-Obadia N, Mertens P, Gueguen A, Peyron R, Garcia-Larrea L. Pain relief by rTMS. *Neurology.* 2008;71:833–840.

23

Trigeminal Neuralgia and Atypical Facial Pain

TRANG NGUYEN, PABLO F. RECINOS, AND MICHAEL LIM

INTRODUCTION

THE EARLIEST DOCUMENTED cases of trigeminal neuralgia (TN) can be inferred from the writings of Galen, Hippocrates, and Aretaeus describing unilateral headaches.[1] Trigeminal neuralgia was first commonly known as *tic douloureux*, a term coined by Nicolous Andre in 1756 that means "painful spasms" in French.[2,3] In 1773, John Fothergill gave the first detailed clinical description of this painful disease in a paper to the Medical Society of London.[2,4] Decades later, his great-nephew, Samuel Fothergill, would localize *tic douloureux* to the trigeminal nerve.[1] Trigeminal neuralgia has a characteristic presentation, and successful treatment depends on an accurate clinical diagnosis.[5] Pain syndromes that do not localize to the trigeminal nerve or other cranial nerve sensory distributions are labeled *atypical facial pain* or, more appropriately, *persistent idiopathic facial pain*, since these syndromes still conform to a pattern.[6]

Epidemiology (Incidence and Prevalence)

There have only been a few epidemiological studies on this relatively rare disease.[7] In a 40-year examination of the population of Rochester, Minnesota, the annual age and gender-adjusted incidence of TN was 4.3 per 100,000.[8] A prospective study in London reported the incidence as 6 per 100,000.[9] More females are affected than males, with a ratio of 1.7–2.2:1.[8,9] The incidence of TN increases with age and peaks at around 70 years.[7] The prevalence of TN may be increasing, as more recent studies have shown an incidence rate of 27–28.9, although it is unclear whether these are adjusted rates.[10,11] Fewer than 1% of TN cases are familial.[12]

There is an association between multiple sclerosis (MS) and TN. Multiple sclerosis patients have a relative risk of 20 of developing TN.[11] From 2% to 4% of TN patients have MS; conversely, 1%–5% of MS patients have TN.[7,8,13] In practice, a young person presenting with TN should mandate a search for MS. Other, less common associations with TN include arterial hypertension, Charcot-Marie-Tooth disorder, and bony skull base abnormalities.[7]

Other facial pain syndromes, excluding temporomandibular disease, have a prevalence of 1.4%.[14]

NATURAL HISTORY

Patients with TN do not have a decreased survival rate.[11] Historically, before the advent of adequate pharmacological and surgical management, TN was called the "suicide disease" by the press. While there are occasional tragic anecdotes, there is little evidence to suggest a dramatic increase in the rate of depression or suicide in TN patients. The pain is episodic, and the frequency of attacks is variable.[15] The episodes may last for seconds to minutes and range from a few to hundreds of times a day. Some patients may go into remission for months or years.[11] The natural history of the disorder has yet to be analyzed, but reports suggest that over time the pain increases in severity and becomes less responsive to treatment.[16] Many patients may exhaust medical management and require an interventional procedure.

SOCIETAL IMPACT

Trigeminal neuralgia imposes a great burden on the patient that can interfere with daily functioning and general health status. Eighty-two TN patients from six European countries were questioned to determine the impact of their disease on their lives. Thirty-four percent of these patients responded that their pain affected their employment through decreased work time, disability, unemployment, or early retirement. For those who were employed, an average of 3.9 days were missed from work in the past month due to pain. The disease also had a great impact on health care resources. More than three-quarters of the patients surveyed said that they had visited their physician at least once in the past month. Forty-five percent had two or more physician visits and a quarter had made at least four visits.[17]

CLINICAL AND DIAGNOSTIC FEATURES

The pain elicited by TN is very distinctive. The International Association for the Study of Pain (IASP) defines TN as "sudden, usually unilateral, severe, brief, stabbing, recurrent pains in the distribution of one or more branches of the fifth cranial nerve."[18] The International Headache Society (IHS) categorizes TN as classical or symptomatic.[6] *Classical TN* is idiopathic or due to vascular compression of the trigeminal nerve. The IHS criteria for *classical TN* are:

1. Paroxysmal pain attacks lasting for up to 2 minutes
2. Distribution along at least one branch of the trigeminal nerve
3. Pain characterized by one of the following:

   a. Intense, sharp, superficial, or stabbing quality
   b. Elicited by stimuli to trigger areas
   c. Precipitated by trigger factors

4. Attacks are stereotyped for each patient
5. Not attributable to a clinically evident neurological deficit or other disorder.

The majority of patients, 70%–95%, will use the term "sharp," "cutting," or "shooting" to describe their pain.[19] The presence of provoking factors and trigger areas helps to distinguish TN from other pain syndromes since 96% of TN patients have trigger factors and half have trigger areas.[19,20] The most common TN triggers are chewing and talking, but other common provocations include washing, shaving, smoking, and brushing teeth. Most patients, 73%, are asymptomatic between episodes, although some patients with long-standing disease may have dull, persistent background pain.[6,19] The pain may also progress to having a more aching, throbbing, or burning quality than seen at initial presentation.[21] The asymptomatic period can last for as long as a few years, and more than 50% of TN patients will have at least a 6-month remission period.[15,21] The pain is usually unilateral and in only 1%–2% of instances bilateral. In these rare cases, a central cause such as MS should be considered.[6] Trigeminal neuralgia should not be diagnosed in cases of bilateral continuous pain.[19]

Pain on the right side is more common than on the left.[15,22] Pain can occur along any branch or combination of branches of the fifth cranial nerve (see the accompanying chart). The second and third branches of the trigeminal nerve are most commonly affected, correlating with pain along the cheek and jaw, respectively.[6,15] Less than 5% of TN patients have pain along the ophthalmic division.[6]

Pain Distribution in TN[15]

V1	4%
V2	17%
V3	15%
V1 + V2	14%
V2 + V3	15%
V1 + V2 + V3	17%

In up to 15% of patients, there may be a secondary cause.[19] Trigeminal neuralgia that is due to a known structural lesion other than vascular compression is termed *symptomatic TN*.[6] Causes include benign and malignant tumors of the middle and posterior fossa and MS. Unlike *classical TN*, there may be no refractory period after a paroxysm.[19] Electrophysiological trigeminal reflex testing is highly diagnostic for identifying patients who have *symptomatic TN* versus *classical TN*.[23] Young age, bilateral involvement, and trigeminal sensory deficits are more common in *symptomatic TN* but are not sufficiently specific indicators to rule out *classical TN*.[24]

Eller et al. have proposed a classification scheme for TN that further delineates idiopathic TN and the various causes of secondary TN.[21] Idiopathic TN type 1 encompasses what was previously known as *classical* or *typical TN*. Trigeminal neuralgia type 2 is consistent with more longstanding TN with its more constant and burning pain. Trigeminal neuralgia due to secondary causes is divided into neuropathic pain due to unintentional nerve injury, deafferentation pain due to iatrogenic injury, symptomatic TN associated with MS, postherpetic TN, and atypical TN due to a somatoform pain disorder.

The differential diagnosis is very broad and includes dental causes, glossopharyngeal neuralgia, headache syndromes, migraines, and temporomandibular disorders.[19] Thalamic pain syndromes should also be considered if there is any limb involvement.

Idiopathic or Atypical Facial Pain

Atypical facial pain is poorly defined and is considered a diagnosis of exclusion.[25] Atypical facial pain was renamed *persistent idiopathic facial pain* (PIFP) by IHS in 2004.[6] The diagnostic criteria are:

1. Daily facial pain, which persists for most of the day
2. Unilateral pain confined to one area that is deep and poorly localized
3. Not associated with sensory loss or other physical signs
4. Investigations, including x-rays, do not demonstrate any relevant abnormality.

The pain most often begins in a nasolabial fold or a side of the chin. Although the pain may start after surgery or injury, it continues without any identifiable cause.

PATHOGENESIS

The cause of TN remains unclear.[15] However, the proposal that it is due to the proximity of a vessel near the trigeminal nerve dates as far back as the eleventh century to an Arab physician, Jujani.[13] The prevailing theory is that chronic focal demyelination of the trigeminal nerve from vascular compression near the dorsal root entry zone may lead to the increased firing of trigeminal primary afferents and decreased inhibition at the trigeminal brainstem complex.[13,15] The dorsal root entry zone is a vulnerable area due to the transition from oligodendrocyte-produced central myelin to Schwann cell-produced peripheral myelin.[22] This theory is supported by the success of microvascular decompression and by evidence from specialized magnetic resonance imaging (MRI) sequences or from intraoperative visualization of an offending vessel in TN cases.[13,26–28] The vascular compression seen during surgery

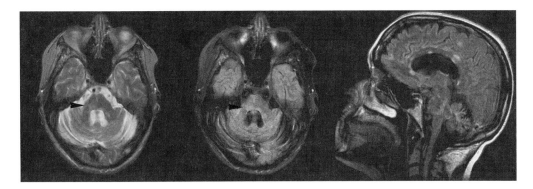

FIGURE 23.1   Axial T2 (left), axial fluid attenuated inversion recovery (FLAIR; middle), and sagittal FLAIR (right) MRI sequences of a patient with right-sided TN and MS. Characteristic demyelinating plaques are seen diffusely throughout. Specifically, a demyelinating plaque is present in the right pons near the root entry zone of the trigeminal nerve (arrowhead), which is a specific finding in patients with TN and MS.

is in most cases by the superior cerebellar artery or vein. Other offending vessels include the anterior inferior cerebellar artery, basilar artery, veretebral artery, and petrosal artery.[29–31] However, vascular compression is a common finding in MRI and autopsy studies of asymptomatic individuals, and a more proximal location and a severe degree of compression may determine TN development.[32–34]

Demyelinating plaques at the root entry zone is a specific finding in MS patients with TN[35–37] (Figure 23.1). Plaques found in other areas of the central nervous system are not associated with TN.[13] While neurovascular compression is still a common finding in this subset of patients as well, microvascular decompression is not as effective as in patients without MS.[38] In TN secondary to a tumor, invasion of the peripheral branches or the gasserian ganglion usually causes additional sensory deficits and continual pain consistent with neuropathy, whereas a more typical TN presentation occurs if there is only tumor abutment.[13,39]

Elevated vasoactive intestinal peptide levels and sodium channel mutations have also been implicated in TN occurrence.[40,41]

MANAGEMENT, TREATMENT, AND PREVENTION

Successful treatment of TN relies on an accurate diagnosis. The diagnosis is primarily based on clinical judgment. Although the neurological

examination is usually normal, a thorough assessment of the cranial nerves should be performed.[42] Particular attention should to be paid to corneal reflex testing and a sensory examination of all three branches of the trigeminal nerve.[5] A routine MRI scan is necessary to exclude a nonvascular structural cause, such as MS plaques or a tumor.[24,43] A high-resolution MRI scan that can identify neurovascular compression may be useful, but the sensitivity and specificity achieved in correlating this finding with TN are highly variable. The use of high-resolution MRI is suggested only for patients who are being considered for surgery.[43] Neurovascular compression can be demonstrated in a significantly higher number of patients with TN than in those with PIFP.[44]

Pharmacological Therapy

Once a diagnosis of TN has been established, treatment begins with pharmacological therapy, usually consisting of pain-modifying anticonvulsants.[45] Carbamazepine is considered the first-line therapy since it has been shown to achieve good pain control in placebo-controlled trials.[11,24,46] A dose of 200–800 mg/day in two to three divided doses is usually given, but doses can range from 100–2400 mg/day.[47] Carbamazepine, a voltage-sensitive sodium channel blocker, is thought to work by decreasing the responsiveness of trigeminal mechanoreceptive neurons to peripheral stimulation.

Relief can occur in as little as several hours.[15,46] Carbamazepine decreases the frequency and severity of pain attacks and is effective for both spontaneous and triggered paroxysms.[48] However, it becomes less effective after 5 years, and additional or alternative therapy may be necessary.[11] This is most likely due to the drug's pharmacokinetic properties. Carbamazepine not only causes its own induction, but also has a decreased half-life with chronic usage. A therapeutic level is therefore difficult to maintain at a constant dosage. Eventually, patients may become intolerant or require doses that exceed safe levels. The most common side effect is drowsiness, which usually improves after several days.[15] Other side effects include impaired mental and motor function, nausea, vomiting, dizziness, nystagmus, ataxia, diplopia, rashes, and abnormal liver function tests.[11,15] Hematological dysfunction, including aplastic anemia and self-resolving leukopenia, may occur.[15,46]

While oxcarbazepine has not been studied in a placebo-controlled trial, it has been found to have efficacy similar to that of carbamazepine in randomized, controlled trials.[43,49] Pain relief occurs in 24–72 hours.[50] Oxcarbazepine (900–1800 mg/day), a keto derivative of carbamazepine, may be preferred due to its better side effect profile, greater tolerability, and decreased drug interactions.[15,24,43] It has also been found to reduce pain in patients who switched from or were refractory to carbamazepine.[51,52] It is considered a first-line drug in Scandinavian countries and a second-line drug in North America.[11] Like carbamazepine, oxcarbazepine also becomes less effective over the long term.

If carbamazepine or oxcarbazepine is ineffective in controlling TN pain, surgical consultation is reasonable. Other drugs may be prescribed alone or used in combination therapy if the patient is not a surgical candidate.[43] Phenytoin (200–500 mg/day) was the first widely used effective drug for TN. It can be used in parenteral form for acute abortive treatment in the emergency department, but it has little beneficial role otherwise.[53] Baclofen (50–80 mg/day) can be prescribed alone or in combination with phenytoin or carbamazepine. It may be particularly useful in patients who have MS and develop TN, since these patients may already be taking baclofen.[11] Side effects include transient sedation, loss of muscle tone, drowsiness, dizziness, and gastrointestinal discomfort.[11,15] Rapid withdrawal may cause hallucinations, anxiety, and seizures.[15,25] Lamotrigine (200–400 mg/day) is also used as alternative or combination therapy. Its advantages are that it has a better side effect profile than carbamazepine and phenytoin, and its dosing can remain stable over time since it has no autoinduction and does not interfere with the metabolism of other drugs.[15] It has also been studied as combination therapy with carbamazepine or phenytoin in patients with refractory TN. While pain control was improved, the study followed patients for only 2 weeks.[54] Lamotrigine doses should be tapered up very slowly due to the risk of Stevens-Johnson syndrome and should be discontinued if a rash develops.[11,15]

Pimozide was found to be more effective than carbamazepine in a double-blind crossover trial. However, 83% of patients experienced adverse effects.[55] Pimazone has severe side effects, including mental retardation, hand tremor, memory impairment, and parkinsonism, and is no longer in use.[15,43] Tocainide may be effective, but it has been removed from the market due to severe hematological side effects.[56,57] Tizanidine has been shown to be better than placebo, but the pain relief was limited to 1 to 3 months.[58] Small studies have shown that levetiracetam, pregabalin, and sumatriptan may be effective for controlling pain in TN.[24,59–62] In a study of seven patients, misoprostol was able to relieve pain in six patients with refractory TN related to MS.[63] There is little evidence that clonazepam, gabapentin, sodium valproate, or topical capsaicin is useful for TN.[24] Topical ophthalmic anesthesia is also not useful for TN.[64]

Procedural Therapy

Once medical therapy becomes ineffective or no longer tolerated, invasive treatment is reasonable. Eventually, surgical therapy will be indicated in about 75% of patients.[16] Many options exist, ranging from minimally invasive therapy to an open neurosurgical procedure. There are five procedures in current use: percutaneous radiofrequency (RF) treatment, percutaneous glycerol rhizolysis, percutaneous balloon microcompression, stereotactic radiotherapy, and surgical microvascular decompression.[42] The percutaneous procedures all are ablative, and the sensory function of the trigeminal nerve is intentionally destroyed at the level of the gasserian ganglion.[65] While it has the highest morbidity and mortality, microvascular decompression narrowly is the best therapeutic option, with the highest long-term efficacy and improvement in quality of life, followed by balloon compression, glycerol rhizolysis, and RF thermocoagulation.[42,65]

Nicolous Andre is credited not only with coining the term *tic douloureux* but also with being one of the first to use ablative therapy. He used caustic substances to destroy the infraorbital nerve at the infraorbital foramen, based on the theory of Marechal, Louis XIV's surgeon, that cutting this nerve would relieve the tics.[1,66] In the nineteenth century, neurectomy of the peripheral branches of the trigeminal nerve was the preferred treatment for TN, even though there was little long-term success.[3] John Carnochan is credited with the first successful surgery in 1856 for TN by excising the entire maxillary division of the trigeminal nerve through the maxillary sinus.[67] Walter Dandy would refine the technique of partial resection of the trigeminal nerve through a posterior fossa approach that allowed adequate visualization of the nerve.[3,66] While Dandy would note the impingement of vascular loops at the root entry zone of the trigeminal nerve in many of his patients, it was not until 1967 that decompression of nerve was developed by Peter Jannetta.[66,68] Since the 1960s, percutaneous ablative procedures and microvascular decompression have become acceptable treatments for TN.[66] Around the turn of the twenty-first century, the use of stereotactic radiotherapy became effective as the treatment target moved from the ganglion to the preganglionic root adjacent to the brainstem, similar to where decompression is performed.[66]

RF Thermocoagulation

Radiofrequency thermocoagulation is the most common surgical treatment for TN and has the highest rate of complete pain relief among the minimally invasive treatment options.[69,70] It is preferable to microvascular decompression for elderly patients.[42] The advantages of this procedure are that the patient may go home the same day and that the relief is immediate. The objective of RF thermocoagulation is to use electric current to locally heat a portion of the trigeminal root in or near the gasserian root. The thermocoagulation destroys some but not all nerve fibers. This results in near-total to complete pinprick analgesia and partial light touch hypesthesia in the sensory distribution of the trigeminal root. The amount of analgesia correlates with the success of pain relief in the affected area. Total anesthesia is unnecessary for pain relief, but some degree of hypesthesia is required for successful treatment.[69,71] The procedure involves local anesthesia and short-acting intravenous sedation. A needle is fluoroscopically guided from the buccal mucosa through the foramen ovale to reach the gasserian ganglion.[72] Thermocoagulation is then delivered in stepwise increments until hypesthesia is produced.[69] Theoretically, RF thermocoagulation destroys the pain-producing smaller Aδ and C fibers while preserving the larger Aβ fibers that are responsible for light touch and the corneal reflex.[72] Other image guidance systems have also been used, including computed tomography (CT) and virtual reality assisted imaging.[73,74] With preoperative CT guidance, RF thermocoagulation has also been performed to isolated branches of the trigeminal nerve with great success.[75,76]

In a study of 2138 RF thermocoagulation procedures in 1600 patients over a 25-year period, 97.6% of patients had acute pain relief, but this decreased to 57.7% at 5-year follow-up and to 52.3% at 10-year follow-up for patients who had only a single procedure.[77] The procedure can be repeated in cases of recurrence, with the same success as for the first treatment.[69,71] Complications include diminished corneal reflex, masseter weakness, and paralysis. Rare but severe (<1%) complications include dysesthesia, anesthesia dolorosa, keratitis, intracranial hemorrhage, meningitis, and transient paralysis of the third and sixth cranial nerves.[78,79] Reactivation of H. simplex virus can also occur and may require antiviral therapy. The risk of anesthesia dolorosa is higher than that of other procedures.[25] There is a low mortality with this procedure, and it often results from intracranial hemorrhage.[69] Pulsed RF therapy, with an average lower temperature delivery, has been studied in an effort to reduce complications from conventional RF thermocoagulation. However, it has been shown not to be effective in the treatment of TN.[80]

Glycerol Rhizolysis

The use of glycerol to ablate the trigeminal nerve was discovered accidentally. When the Leksell Gamma Knife was first studied for the stereotactic radiotherapy of TN, glycerol was used as a vehicle for the radiopaque metal dust and it was noted that the injection of this mixture alone could produce pain relief. The neurolytic effect of glycerol is thought to be due to its hypertonicity. As with the other percutaneous techniques, a needle is initially used for localization of the retro-ganglionic fibers in the trigeminal cistern. Glycerol (0.18–0.30 cc) is injected with the patient in the sitting position to limit spillover outside of the cistern. Selective rhizolysis of individual branches may be attempted by varying the volume of glycerol injected, injecting contrast medium to fill the bottom of the cistern to protect the third branch, changing the needle tip position, or altering the degree of the patient's head flexion.[81]

Glycerol rhizolysis has been reported to have mixed results, possibly dependent on the surgeon's experience. Acute pain relief is achieved in more than 80% of patients, and long-term relief is varied. One-year recurrence rates range from 10% to 53% and 5-year rates range from 34% to 83%.[69,79] Half of the patients have pain relief within 24 hours, but others may not have relief for 7–10 days.[15] The most common complication is facial sensation deficit.[79] Other complications are similar to those of RF thermocoagulation, although with a lower risk of facial sensory loss.[81,82] Glycerol rhizolysis is the preferred surgical treatment for MS-related TN.[83,84]

Balloon Microcompression

For balloon microcompression, a Fogarty catheter is inflated into Meckel's cave under anesthesia and fluoroscopic guidance. Compression is applied for 1–7 minutes.[69] It differs from the other percutaneous approaches in that the guide needle is not advanced beyond the foramen ovale and the procedure is considered to be technically easier.[13,69,85] There is immediate pain relief in almost all patients accompanied by mild, usually self-resolving, sensory loss.[13,86–88] Even without sensory change, there may be complete relief.[85] Since the compression likely preserves Aδ and C fibers, the corneal reflex is not affected, making this procedure particularly useful for TN of the first branch.[85,89] Recurrence rates have varied in different studies, with a 6%–14% 1-year recurrence. Mean time to recurrence ranges from 7.3 months for those with recurrent TN to 4.3 years for all treated patients.[87,90] Studies with long-term follow-up demonstrate a 20% recurrence rate at 5 years.[86–88] Masseter weakness is common but resolves within a year.[13,91] Other reported complications include minor dysesthesia, hearing difficulties, corneal anesthesia, anesthesia dolorosa, and subarachnoid hemmorhage.[87,88,90] Balloon compression pressure monitoring can reduce the rates of complications.[91]

Stereotactic Radiosurgery

Ionizing radiation for the treatment of TN dates back to within a few years of the time when x-rays were discovered but eventually grew out of favor.[92] When stereotactic radiosurgery was invented, the use of radiation for TN was revisited. Results were initially unsatisfactory until the target was moved from the gasserian ganglion to the proximal trigeminal root near the pons.[13] Use of stereotactic radiosurgery, usually with the Gamma Knife machine, became widely acceptable in 1996 after a multi-institutional study demonstrated favorable results.[93]

Gamma Knife radiation involves the placement of a stereotactic frame under local anesthesia, followed by an MRI scan to identify the trigeminal nerve.[94] The target is a single 4-mm isocenter positioned at the trigeminal nerve root entry zone, 2–4 mm from the junction of the nerve and the pons[93–95] (Figure 23.2). Doses of radiation range from 70–90 Gy since patients treated with doses below 70 Gy have significantly lower pain control.[92] However, there is a higher risk of facial numbness and dysesthesias as doses

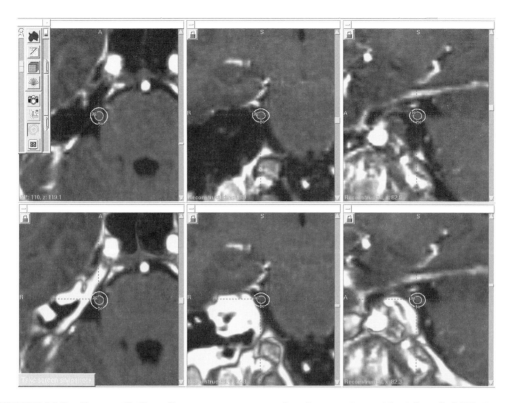

FIGURE 23.2 Gamma Knife radiosurgery treatment plan for a patient with right-sided TN. Image panes demonstrate T1 contrast-enhanced MRI (top panes) and MRI/CT fusion (bottom panes) in the axial (left), coronal (middle), and sagittal (right) planes. A 4 mm isocenter along the trigeminal nerve is targeted 2–4 mm from the root entry zone to minimize the radiation to the brainstem. The 90% isodose line (green) and the 50% isodose line (yellow) are seen centered on the trigeminal nerve and in reference to the brainstem.

approach 90 Gy and the target is more proximally located.[96] Baboon studies have shown that radiosurgery at the root entry zone works by causing focal axonal degeneration and necrosis of the trigeminal nerve without affecting the gasserian ganglion.[97]

While stereotactic radiosurgery is noninvasive, pain relief is not immediate and may take months.[94] Initially, 75% of patients may be free of pain, but that decreases to less than 50% at 5 years.[98] Most patients studied had undergone prior procedures.[13] Those who had no prior invasive treatment had a significantly longer duration without pain.[99] Repeat radiosurgery at a reduced dose for those who have pain recurrence provides pain relief rates similar to those of the first procedure, but with an increased risk of sensory symptoms.[100,101] For TN that is refractory after microvascular

decompression, salvage Gamma Knife therapy can provide pain relief for 50% of patients and complete resolution for 20% at 5 years.[102] The most common side effect is facial paresthesia in 6%–13%.[93,98] There have been no reported complications outside of the trigeminal nerve, and 88% of patients were satisfied with their treatment.[15,103] Overall, stereotactic radiosurgery appears to be the safest technique for treating TN, particularly in elderly patients.[92]

CyberKnife radiosurgery, a frameless delivery system developed in 1994, has also been used for TN treatment.[104–106] Time to pain relief is arguably faster than with Gamma Knife therapy.[106] As a first interventional treatment, CyberKnife radiosurgery at doses of 55–75 Gy demonstrated pain relief in 94% of patients at a median time of 30 days (range, 1–180 days), with recurrence in 33% of patients at a mean time of 9 months (range, 1–43 months).[104] The early results of a multicenter trial reported pain relief in 67% of TN patients at a median time of 14 days. Of these patients, 47% had numbness after therapy, and treatment with higher doses or of longer segments correlated with both better pain alleviation and a greater risk of hypesthesia. Half of the patients still experienced pain relief at a mean follow-up time of 2 years.[105] As with other interventions, the effectiveness of treating atypical TN with CyberKnife radiosurgery is not as great as for typical TN. In a series of seven patients with atypical TN, four had complete pain relief at a mean follow-up time of 28 months.[107]

Microvascular Decompression

Microvascular decompression (MVD) is the only treatment for TN that directly addresses the neurovascular compression of the trigeminal nerve, the prevailing theory of the underlying cause of TN. It is the most aggressive therapy available and has the best success rates at relieving pain due to TN.[65,108-111] With the use of a microscope, Janetta is credited with standardizing the procedure of relieving the compression of offending vessels on the trigeminal nerve at the root entry zone.[68] Since MVD is an open neurosurgical operation, it has the greatest perioperative morbidity and mortality of all the TN treatments, but it is a nondestructive procedure compared to the percutaneous therapies.[112]

Patients selected for MVD should be surgical candidates, ideally younger than 70 years old, who have *classical TN*. High-resolution MRI is useful in determining if there is an offending vessel before surgery. Due to the risk of hearing impairment, other recommended preoperative measures include baseline audiometry and brainstem auditory evoked potential measurement (BAEP).[112] The procedure involves a suboccipital retromastoid craniotomy under general endotracheal anesthesia with BAEP monitoring. More than 90% of patients are found to have vessel compression during surgery.[113] The vessel is displaced from the trigeminal nerve using synthetic material, usually Teflon felt. It is debatable if the trigeminal nerve should be intentionally injured if no vascular compression is found.[13,112] Exploration alone can sometimes relieve pain, albeit with a high recurrence rate, for patients in whom no neurovascular compression is found.[114]

Significant pain relief immediately after surgery is high, ranging from 88.6% to 98.9% in various studies.[112] After 10 years, 70% of patients are still pain-free without medication and an additional 4% have occasional pain.[31] Most recurrences occur within 2 years of surgery and are very unlikely to develop afterward.[29,31] The annual rate of recurrence 10 years after surgery is less than 1%.[31] Factors that are associated with an improved prognosis after MVD include a preoperative finding of an offending vessel, arterial compression instead of compression by a vein, symptom duration of less than 8 years prior to surgery, presence of trigger points, symptoms consistent with *classical TN*, male sex, and immediate postoperative resolution of pain.[29,31,115-117] Patients with type 1 TN are more likely to have arterial compression, better pain relief, and less recurrence than those with type 2 TN.[118,119] The presence of constant pain should not prevent patients from receiving MVD since 77% of these patients will have complete pain relief.[120] In two studies of MVD performed on elderly patients, the rate of success in alleviating pain and the risk of morbidity and mortality were similar to those in younger patients, but this treatment is still debatable for patients older than 70 years.[121-123]

Microvascular decompression is not as effective for patients who do not exhibit *classical TN* findings. For patients who have atypical TN, MVD may provide immediate postoperative pain relief in up to 90%, but only 35% will have favorable long-term outcomes and half will have poorly controlled recurrent pain.[115] For patients with MS-related TN, rhizotomy appears to have greater success in alleviating pain than MVD, although some argue that MVD treatment is still acceptable.[38,84,124]

The use of intraoperative BAEP monitoring has greatly decreased complication rates.[31,112] Mortality rates range from 0% to 1.43%.[112] One of the most common operative complications is a cerebrospinal fluid (CSF) leak, which occurs in 0.9%–12% of patients.[29] A CSF leak can lead to reexploration and meningitis.[22,29] Other frequent complications occurring in approximately 1% of patients include cerebellar injury, facial numbness, transient extraocular muscle palsy, and hearing loss.[29,112] Rare complications include facial nerve palsy, cerebellar and supratentorial hematomas, hydrocephalus, and pseudomeningocele.[29]

Peripheral Therapies

Previously, extracranial peripheral denervation was the most common procedure for treating TN before the advent of the percutaneous procedures and MVD.[15] The peripheral nerve treatments involve using acupuncture, cryotherapy, laser surgery, or nerve blocks.[11] The location of TN pain or trigger zones determines which nerve is targeted. Denervation is done at the supraorbital notch for ophthalmic pain, the infraorbital notch for maxillary pain, and the mental foramen for mandibular pain. Temporary measures include using lidocaine and bupivocaine, while permanent nerve damage is induced with neurectomy, cryotherapy, or alcohol block. While pain relief is immediate and the success rate is 50%–100%, pain relief is almost always brief, ranging from hours with lidocaine to 30 months with neurectomy.[15] While the morbidity with peripheral techniques is low, pain recurs in at least 50% of patients at 1 year, and the only two randomized, controlled trials demonstrated that there was no long-term effect on pain using streptomycin and lidocaine.[24] Currently, peripheral denervation is recommended only for patients who cannot undergo percutaneous procedures, stereotactic radiosurgery, or MVD due to serious medical problems or for patients who need emergency treatment.[11,15,69]

Persistent Idiopathic Facial Pain

The diagnosis of PIFP, formerly known as *atypical facial pain*, is based on a thorough history and examination. It is a diagnosis of exclusion. Imaging should be done to rule out cranial or pulmonary lesions.[125] In rare cases, atypical facial pain, especially around the ear or temple, may be due to referred pain from lung cancer invasion of the vagus nerve.[6]

The treatment of PIFP is often less successful than that for TN. Tricyclic antidepressants are moderately effective.[126,127] Amitriptyline is often used as first-line treatment at doses (10–100 mg/day) lower than those needed for antidepressant effects with analgesia, taking effect within 4 weeks.[128,129] Other antidepressants that have been studied and found to have some effect include dothiepine, venlafaxine, gabapentin, iprazochrome, and fluoxetine.[126] In a case report, topiramate was demonstrated to be effective for relieving PIFP.[130] Other antiepileptics, including lamotrigine, gabapentin, clonazepam, phenytoin, and valproic acid, may also offer some pain relief, but they have not been well studied.[131,132]

Transcutaneous electrical stimulation and intranasal cocaine may also be effective.[126] Calcitonin and sumatripan have been found not to be efficacious in treating PIFP.[133–135] Nonsteroid anti-inflammatory can be used for short periods.[132]

Hypnotic treatment, especially in patients who are susceptible to hypnosis, can significantly reduce pain and decrease the use of analgesics compared to simple relaxation techniques.[136] Surgical treatments, including MVD, are generally avoided since they are less effective for PIFP compared to TN, even if neurovascular compression is found.[44,129,137,138] Microvascular decompression may be used in select cases where there are mixed symptoms of paroxysmal and constant pain and MRI evidence of neurovascular compression.[138] Percutaneous techniques, such as RF treatment or balloon microcompression, and stereotactic radiosurgery should be avoided since the risk of causing neuropathic pain that is more severe than the initial pain is very high.[138]

FUTURE DIRECTIONS IN RESEARCH AND TREATMENT

Although there are many treatment options for patients with TN, there is still a need for randomized, controlled trials to evaluate the efficacy of newer pharmacological and interventional treatments. Experimental therapies that appear to have some promise include an implantable gasserian ganglion electrical stimulator, botulinum toxin injections at trigger areas, motor cortex stimulation, and intravenous immunoglobin.[139–143] More evidence is also needed on determining when patients should be referred for surgical treatment or whether patients who no longer tolerate first-line medical therapy should be given alternative drugs or surgery. Treatment options for atypical TN and for patients who are not surgical candidates can also be improved.

RESOURCES FOR PATIENTS AND FAMILIES

The Facial Pain Association (formerly The Trigeminal Neuralgia Association) serves as an advocate and a resource for patients living with neuropathic facial pain, including TN, by providing information, encouraging research, and offering support. (http://www.fpa-support.org/)

REFERENCES

1. Eboli P, Stone JL, Aydin S, Slavin KV. Historical characterization of trigeminal neuralgia. *Neurosurgery.* 2009;64(6):1183–1186; discussion 1186–1187.
2. Pearce JM. Trigeminal neuralgia (Fothergill's disease) in the 17th and 18th centuries. *J Neurol Neurosurg Psychiatry.* 2003;74(12):1688.
3. Dandy WE. An operation for the cure of tic douloureux. *Arch Surg.* 1920;18(2):687–734.
4. Chad CD, Liu JK, Apfelbaum RI. Historical perspectives on the diagnosis and treatment of trigeminal neuralgia. Neurosurg Focus. 2005;18(5):E4.
5. Casey KF. Role of patient history and physical examination in the diagnosis of trigeminal neuralgia. *Neurosurg Focus.* 2005;18(5):E1.
6. The International Classification of Headache Disorders: 2nd edition. *Cephalalgia.* 2004;24(suppl 1): 9–160.
7. Sadosky A, McDermott AM, Brandenburg NA, Strauss M. A review of the epidemiology of painful diabetic peripheral neuropathy, postherpetic neuralgia, and less commonly studied neuropathic pain conditions. *Pain Pract.* 2008;8(1):45–56.
8. Katusic S, Beard CM, Bergstralh E, Kurland LT. Incidence and clinical features of trigeminal neuralgia, Rochester, Minnesota, 1945–1984. *Ann Neurol.* 1990;27(1):89–95.
9. MacDonald BK, Cockerell OC, Sander JW, Shorvon SD. The incidence and lifetime prevalence of neurological disorders in a prospective community-based study in the UK. *Brain.* 2000;123(pt 4):665–676.
10. Hall GC, Carroll D, McQuay HJ. Primary care incidence and treatment of four neuropathic pain conditions: a descriptive study, 2002–2005. *BMC Fam Pract.* 2008;9:26.
11. Zakrzewska JM, Linskey ME. Trigeminal neuralgia. *Clin Evid (Online).* 2009. pii:1207. http://www.clinicalevidence.bmj.com/ceweb/pmc/2009/03/1207. Accessed July 17, 2009.
12. Ebner FH, Tatagiba M, Roser F. Familial trigeminal neuralgia—microsurgical experience and psychological observations. *Acta Neurochir.* 2010;152(2):381–382.
13. Nurmikko TJ, Eldridge PR. Trigeminal neuralgia—pathophysiology, diagnosis and current treatment. *Br J Anaesth.* 2001;87(1):117–132.
14. Lipton JA, Ship JA, Larach-Robinson D. Estimated prevalence and distribution of reported orofacial pain in the United States. *J Am Dent Assoc.* 1993;124(10):115–121.
15. Rozen TD. Trigeminal neuralgia and glossopharyngeal neuralgia. *Neurol Clin.* 2004;22(1): 185–206.
16. Zakrzewska JM, Patsalos PN. Long-term cohort study comparing medical (oxcarbazepine) and surgical management of intractable trigeminal neuralgia. *Pain.* 2002;95(3):259–266.
17. Tölle T, Dukes E, Sadosky A. Patient burden of trigeminal neuralgia: results from a cross-sectional survey of health state impairment and treatment patterns in six European countries. *Pain Pract.* 2006;6(3):153–160.
18. Merskey H, Bogduk N. *Classification of Chronic Pain: Descriptions of Chronic Pain Syndromes and Definitions of Pain Terms.* 2nd ed. Seattle: IASP Press; 1994.
19. Zakrzewska JM. Diagnosis and differential diagnosis of trigeminal neuralgia. *Clin J Pain.* 2002;18(1):14–21.
20. Rasmussen P. Facial pain. IV. A prospective study of 1052 patients with a view of: precipitating factors, associated symptoms, objective psychiatric and neurological symptoms. *Acta Neurochir (Wien).* 1991;108(3–4):100–109.
21. Eller JL, Raslan AM, Burchiel KJ. Trigeminal neuralgia: definition and classification. *Neurosurg Focus.* 2005;18(5):E3.
22. Tomasello F, Alafaci C, Angileri FF, Calisto A, Salpietro FM. Clinical presentation of trigeminal neuralgia and the rationale of microvascular decompression. *Neurol Sci.* 2008;29(suppl 1): S191–S195.
23. Cruccu G, Biasiotta A, Galeotti F, Iannetti GD, Truini A, Gronseth G. Diagnostic accuracy of trigeminal reflex testing in trigeminal neuralgia. *Neurology.* 2006;66(1):139–141.

24. Gronseth G, Cruccu G, Alksne J, et al. Practice parameter: the diagnostic evaluation and treatment of trigeminal neuralgia (an evidence-based review): report of the Quality Standards Subcommittee of the American Academy of Neurology and the European Federation of Neurological Societies. *Neurology.* 2008;71(15):1183–1190.

25. Zakrzewska JM. Facial pain: neurological and non-neurological. *J Neurol Neurosurg Psychiatry.* 2002;72(suppl 2):ii27–ii32.

26. Boecher-Schwarz HG, Bruehl K, Kessel G, Guenthner M, Perneczky A, Stoeter P. Sensitivity and specificity of MRA in the diagnosis of neurovascular compression in patients with trigeminal neuralgia. A correlation of MRA and surgical findings. *Neuroradiology.* 1998;40(2):88–95.

27. Meaney JF, Eldridge PR, Dunn LT, Nixon TE, Whitehouse GH, Miles JB. Demonstration of neurovascular compression in trigeminal neuralgia with magnetic resonance imaging. Comparison with surgical findings in 52 consecutive operative cases. *J Neurosurg.* 1995;83(5): 799–805.

28. Chun-Cheng Q, Qing-Shi Z, Ji-Qing Z, Zhi-Gang W. A single-blinded pilot study assessing neurovascular contact by using high-resolution MR imaging in patients with trigeminal neuralgia. *Eur J Radiol.* 2009;69(3):459–463.

29. Kabatas S, Karasu A, Civelek E, Sabanci AP, Hepgul KT, Teng YD. Microvascular decompression as a surgical management for trigeminal neuralgia: long-term follow-up and review of the literature. *Neurosurg Rev.* 2009;32(1):87–93; discussion 93–84.

30. Barker FG, Jannetta PJ, Babu RP, Pomonis S, Bissonette DJ, Jho HD. Long-term outcome after operation for trigeminal neuralgia in patients with posterior fossa tumors. *J Neurosurg.* 1996;84(5):818–825.

31. Barker FG, Jannetta PJ, Bissonette DJ, Larkins MV, Jho HD. The long-term outcome of microvascular decompression for trigeminal neuralgia. *N Engl J Med.* 1996;334(17):1077–1083.

32. Ramesh VG, Premkumar G. An anatomical study of the neurovascular relationships at the trigeminal root entry zone. *J Clin Neurosci.* 2009;16(7):934–936.

33. Peker S, Dinçer A, Necmettin Pamir M. Vascular compression of the trigeminal nerve is a frequent finding in asymptomatic individuals: 3-T MR imaging of 200 trigeminal nerves using 3D CISS sequences. *Acta Neurochir.* 2009;151(9): 1081–1088.

34. Miller JP, Acar F, Hamilton BE, Burchiel KJ. Radiographic evaluation of trigeminal neurovascular compression in patients with and without trigeminal neuralgia. *J Neurosurg.* 2009;110(4): 627–632.

35. Gass A, Kitchen N, MacManus DG, Moseley IF, Hennerici MG, Miller DH. Trigeminal neuralgia in patients with multiple sclerosis: lesion localization with magnetic resonance imaging. *Neurology.* 1997;49(4):1142–1144.

36. Cruccu G, Biasiotta A, Di Rezze S, et al. Trigeminal neuralgia and pain related to multiple sclerosis. *Pain.* 2009;143(3):186–191.

37. Nurmikko TJ. Pathophysiology of MS-related trigeminal neuralgia. *Pain.* 2009;143(3):165–166.

38. Broggi G, Ferroli P, Franzini A, Pluderi M, La Mantia L, Milanese C. Role of microvascular decompression in trigeminal neuralgia and multiple sclerosis. *Lancet.* 1999;354(9193): 1878–1879.

39. Cheng TM, Cascino TL, Onofrio BM. Comprehensive study of diagnosis and treatment of trigeminal neuralgia secondary to tumors. *Neurology.* 1993;43(11):2298–2302.

40. Siqueira SR, Alves B, Malpartida HM, Teixeira MJ, Siqueira JT. Abnormal expression of voltage-gated sodium channels Nav1.7, Nav1.3 and Nav1.8 in trigeminal neuralgia. *Neuroscience.* 2009;164(2):573–577.

41. Zhao Y, Jiang X, Liu Y. [Observation of vasoactive intestinal polypeptide in patients with trigeminal neuralgia: a 16-cases report]. *Hua Xi Kou Qiang Yi Xue Za Zhi.* 2002;20(1):33–34, 38.

42. van Kleef M, van Genderen WE, Narouze S, et al. 1. Trigeminal neuralgia. *Pain Pract.* 2009;9(4):252–259.

43. Cruccu G, Gronseth G, Alksne J, et al. AAN-EFNS guidelines on trigeminal neuralgia management. *Eur J Neurol.* 2008;15(10):1013–1028.

44. Kuncz A, Vörös E, Barzó P, et al. Comparison of clinical symptoms and magnetic resonance angiographic (MRA) results in patients with trigeminal neuralgia and persistent idiopathic facial pain. Medium-term outcome after microvascular decompression of cases with positive MRA findings. *Cephalalgia.* 2006;26(3):266–276.

45. Zakrzewska JM. Trigeminal neuralgia and facial pain. *Semin Pain Med.* 2004;2(2):76–84.

46. Wiffen PJ, McQuay HJ, Moore RA. Carbamazepine for acute and chronic pain. *Cochrane Database Syst Rev.* 2005(3):CD005451.

47. Krafft RM. Trigeminal neuralgia. *Am Fam Physician.* 2008;77(9):1291–1296.

48. Campbell FG, Graham JG, Zilkha KJ. Clinical trial of carbazepine (Tegretol) in trigeminal neuralgia. *J Neurol Neurosurg Psychiatry.* 1966;29(3):265–267.

49. Beydoun A. Safety and efficacy of oxcarbazepine: results of randomized, double-blind trials. *Pharmacotherapy.* 2000;20(8 pt 2):152S–158S.

50. Farago F. Trigeminal neuralgia: its treatment with two new carbamazepine analogues. *Eur Neurol.* 1987;26(2):73–83.

51. Gomez-Arguelles JM, Dorado R, Sepulveda JM, et al. Oxcarbazepine monotherapy in carbamazepine-unresponsive trigeminal neuralgia. *J Clin Neurosci.* 2008;15(5):516–519.

52. Zakrzewska JM, Patsalos PN. Oxcarbazepine: a new drug in the management of intractable trigeminal neuralgia. *J Neurol Neurosurg Psychiatry.* 1989;52(4):472–476.

53. Sindrup SH, Jensen TS. Pharmacotherapy of trigeminal neuralgia. *Clin J Pain.* 2002;18(1): 22–27.

54. Zakrzewska JM, Chaudhry Z, Nurmikko TJ, Patton DW, Mullens EL. Lamotrigine (Lamictal) in refractory trigeminal neuralgia: results from a double-blind placebo controlled crossover trial. *Pain.* 1997;73(2):223–230.

55. Lechin F, van der Dijs B, Lechin ME, et al. Pimozide therapy for trigeminal neuralgia. *Arch Neurol.* 1989;46(9):960–963.

56. Lindstrom P, Lindblom U. The analgesic effect of tocainide in trigeminal neuralgia. *Pain.* 1987;28(1):45–50.

57. Pascual J, Berciano J. Failure of mexiletine to control trigeminal neuralgia. *Headache.* 1989;29(8):517–518.

58. Fromm GH, Aumentado D, Terrence CF. A clinical and experimental investigation of the effects of tizanidine in trigeminal neuralgia. *Pain.* 1993;53(3):265–271.

59. Jorns TP, Johnston A, Zakrzewska JM. Pilot study to evaluate the efficacy and tolerability of levetiracetam (Keppra) in treatment of patients with trigeminal neuralgia. *Eur J Neurol.* 2009;16(6):740–744.

60. Pérez C, Navarro A, Saldaña MT, Martínez S, Rejas J. Patient-reported outcomes in subjects with painful trigeminal neuralgia receiving pregabalin: evidence from medical practice in primary care settings. *Cephalalgia.* 2009;29(7): 781–790.

61. Kanai A, Saito M, Hoka S. Subcutaneous sumatriptan for refractory trigeminal neuralgia. *Headache.* 2006;46(4):577–582; discussion 583–574.

62. Kanai A, Suzuki A, Osawa S, Hoka S. Sumatriptan alleviates pain in patients with trigeminal neuralgia. *Clin J Pain.* 2006;22(8):677–680.

63. Reder AT, Arnason BG. Trigeminal neuralgia in multiple sclerosis relieved by a prostaglandin E analogue. *Neurology.* 1995;45(6):1097–1100.

64. Kondziolka D, Lemley T, Kestle JR, Lunsford LD, Fromm GH, Jannetta PJ. The effect of single-application topical ophthalmic anesthesia in patients with trigeminal neuralgia. A randomized double-blind placebo-controlled trial. *J Neurosurg.* 1994;80(6):993–997.

65. Spatz AL, Zakrzewska JM, Kay EJ. Decision analysis of medical and surgical treatments for trigeminal neuralgia: how patient evaluations of benefits and risks affect the utility of treatment decisions. *Pain.* 2007;131(3):302–310.

66. Cole CD, Liu JK, Apfelbaum RI. Historical perspectives on the diagnosis and treatment of trigeminal neuralgia. *Neurosurg Focus.* 2005;18(5):E4.

67. Tubbs RS, Loukas M, Shoja MM, Cohen-Gadol AA. John Murray Carnochan (1817–1887): the first description of successful surgery for trigeminal neuralgia. *J Neurosurg.* 2010;112(1): 199–201.

68. Jannetta PJ. Arterial compression of the trigeminal nerve at the pons in patients with trigeminal neuralgia. *J Neurosurg.* 1967;26(1 suppl): 159–162.

69. Peters G, Nurmikko TJ. Peripheral and gasserian ganglion-level procedures for the treatment of trigeminal neuralgia. *Clin J Pain.* 2002;18(1):28–34.

70. Lopez BC, Hamlyn PJ, Zakrzewska JM. Systematic review of ablative neurosurgical techniques for the treatment of trigeminal neuralgia. *Neurosurgery.* 2004;54(4):973–982; discussion 982–973.

71. Taub E. Radiofrequency rhizotomy for trigeminal neuralgia. In: Lozano AM GP, Tasker RR, eds. *Textbook of Stereotactic and Functional Neurosurgery.* Berlin, Heidelberg: Springer Berlin Heidelberg; 2009:2421–2428.

72. Sweet WH, Wepsic JG. Controlled thermocoagulation of trigeminal ganglion and rootlets for differential destruction of pain fibers. 1. Trigeminal neuralgia. *J Neurosurg.* 1974;40(2):143–156.

73. Meng FG, Wu CY, Liu YG, Liu L. Virtual reality imaging technique in percutaneous radiofrequency rhizotomy for intractable trigeminal neuralgia. *J Clin Neurosci.* 2009;16(3):449–451.

74. Koizuka S, Saito S, Sekimoto K, Tobe M, Obata H, Koyama Y. Percutaneous radio-frequency thermocoagulation of the Gasserian ganglion guided by high-speed real-time CT fluoroscopy. *Neuroradiology.* 2009;51(9):563–566.

75. Fraioli MF, Cristino B, Moschettoni L, Cacciotti G, Fraioli C. Validity of percutaneous controlled radiofrequency thermocoagulation in the treatment of isolated third division trigeminal neuralgia. *Surg Neurol.* 2009;71(2):180–183.

76. Huibin Q, Jianxing L, Guangyu H, Dianen F. The treatment of first division idiopathic trigeminal neuralgia with radiofrequency thermocoagulation of the peripheral branches compared to conventional radiofrequency. *J Clin Neurosci.* 2009;16(11):1425–1429.

77. Kanpolat Y, Savas A, Bekar A, Berk C. Percutaneous controlled radiofrequency trigeminal rhizotomy for the treatment of idiopathic trigeminal neuralgia: 25-year experience with 1,600 patients. *Neurosurgery.* 2001;48(3): 524–532; discussion 532–524.

78. van Boxem K, van Eerd M, Brinkhuize T, Patijn J, van Kleef M, van Zundert J. Radiofrequency and pulsed radiofrequency treatment of chronic pain syndromes: the available evidence. *Pain Pract.* 2008;8(5):385–393.

79. Tatli M, Satici O, Kanpolat Y, Sindou M. Various surgical modalities for trigeminal neuralgia: literature study of respective long-term outcomes. *Acta Neurochir* (Wien). 2008;150(3):243–255.

80. Erdine S, Ozyalcin NS, Cimen A, Celik M, Talu GK, Disci R. Comparison of pulsed radiofrequency with conventional radiofrequency in the treatment of idiopathic trigeminal neuralgia. *Eur J Pain.* 2007;11(3):309–313.

81. Linderoth BL, Lind G. Retrogasserian glycerol injection for trigeminal neuralgia. In: Lozano AM, Gildenberg PL, Tasker RR, eds. *Textbook of Stereotactic and Functional Neurosurgery.* Berlin, Heidelberg: Springer Berlin Heidelberg; 2009:2429–2456.

82. Kondziolka D, Lunsford LD. Percutaneous retrogasserian glycerol rhizotomy for trigeminal neuralgia: technique and expectations. *Neurosurg Focus.* 2005;18(5):E7.

83. Kondziolka D, Lunsford LD, Bissonette DJ. Long-term results after glycerol rhizotomy for multiple sclerosis-related trigeminal neuralgia. *Can J Neurol Sci.* 1994;21(2):137–140.

84. Antic B, Peric P. Posterior fossa exploration in treatment of trigeminal neuralgia associated with multiple sclerosis. *Surg Neurol.* 2009;71(4):419–423; discussion 423.

85. Brown J, Pilitsis J. Balloon compression for trigeminal neuralgia. In: Lozano AM, Gildenberg PL, Tasker RR, eds. *Textbook of Stereotactic and Functional Neurosurgery.* Berlin, Heidelberg: Springer Berlin Heidelberg; 2009:2457–2464.

86. Skirving DJ, Dan NG. A 20-year review of percutaneous balloon compression of the trigeminal ganglion. *J Neurosurg.* 2001;94(6):913–917.

87. Abdennebi B, Mahfouf L, Nedjahi T. Long-term results of percutaneous compression of the gasserian ganglion in trigeminal neuralgia (series of 200 patients). *Stereotact Funct Neurosurg.* 1997;68(1–4 pt 1):190–195.

88. Lichtor T, Mullan JF. A 10-year follow-up review of percutaneous microcompression of the trigeminal ganglion. *J Neurosurg.* 1990;72(1):49–54.

89. Cruccu G, Inghilleri M, Fraioli B, Guidetti B, Manfredi M. Neurophysiologic assessment of trigeminal function after surgery for trigeminal neuralgia. *Neurology.* 1987;37(4):631–638.

90. Omeis I, Smith D, Kim S, Murali R. Percutaneous balloon compression for the treatment of recurrent trigeminal neuralgia: long-term outcome in 29 patients. *Stereotact Funct Neurosurg.* 2008;86(4):259–265.

91. Brown JA, Pilitsis JG. Percutaneous balloon compression for the treatment of trigeminal neuralgia: results in 56 patients based on balloon compression pressure monitoring. *Neurosurg Focus.* 2005;18(5):E10.

92. de Lotbiniere A. Gamma knife surgery for trigeminal neuralgia and facial pain. In: Lozano AM, Gildenberg PL, Tasker RR, eds. *Textbook of Stereotactic and Functional Neurosurgery.* Berlin, Heidelberg: Springer Berlin Heidelberg; 2009:2475–2481.

93. Kondziolka D, Lunsford LD, Flickinger JC, et al. Stereotactic radiosurgery for trigeminal neuralgia: a multi-institutional study using the gamma unit. *J Neurosurg.* 1996;84(6):940–945.

94. Kondziolka D, Perez B, Flickinger JC, Habeck M, Lunsford LD. Gamma knife radiosurgery for trigeminal neuralgia: results and expectations. *Arch Neurol.* 1998;55(12):1524–1529.

95. Kondziolka D, Flickinger JC, Lunsford LD, Habeck M. Trigeminal neuralgia radiosurgery: the University of Pittsburgh experience. *Stereotact Funct Neurosurg.* 1996;66(suppl 1):343–348.

96. Pollock BE, Phuong LK, Foote RL, Stafford SL, Gorman DA. High-dose trigeminal neuralgia radiosurgery associated with increased risk of trigeminal nerve dysfunction. *Neurosurgery.* 2001;49(1):58–62; discussion 62–54.

97. Kondziolka D, Lacomis D, Niranjan A, et al. Histological effects of trigeminal nerve radiosurgery in a primate model: implications for trigeminal neuralgia radiosurgery. *Neurosurgery.* 2000;46(4):971–976; discussion 976–977.

98. Han JH, Kim DG, Chung HT, et al. Long-term outcome of gamma knife radiosurgery for treatment of typical trigeminal neuralgia. *Int J Radiat Oncol Biol Phys.* 2009;75(3):822–827.

99. Dhople AA, Adams JR, Maggio WW, Naqvi SA, Regine WF, Kwok Y. Long-term outcomes of Gamma Knife radiosurgery for classic trigeminal neuralgia: implications of treatment and critical

review of the literature. Clinical article. *J Neurosurg.* 2009;111(2):351–358.

100. Hasegawa T, Kondziolka D, Spiro R, Flickinger JC, Lunsford LD. Repeat radiosurgery for refractory trigeminal neuralgia. *Neurosurgery.* 2002;50(3):494–500; discussion 500–492.

101. Dvorak T, Finn A, Price LL, et al. Retreatment of trigeminal neuralgia with Gamma Knife radiosurgery: is there an appropriate cumulative dose? Clinical article. *J Neurosurg.* 2009;111(2):359–364.

102. Little AS, Shetter AG, Shetter ME, Kakarla UK, Rogers CL. Salvage gamma knife stereotactic radiosurgery for surgically refractory trigeminal neuralgia. *Int J Radiat Oncol Biol Phys.* 2009;74(2):522–527.

103. Regis J, Metellus P, Hayashi M, Roussel P, Donnet A, Bille-Turc F. Prospective controlled trial of gamma knife surgery for essential trigeminal neuralgia. *J Neurosurg.* 2006;104(6):913–924.

104. Fariselli L, Marras C, De Santis M, Marchetti M, Milanesi I, Broggi G. CyberKnife radiosurgery as a first treatment for idiopathic trigeminal neuralgia. *Neurosurgery.* 2009;64 (2 suppl):A96–A101.

105. Villavicencio AT, Lim M, Burneikiene S, et al. Cyberknife radiosurgery for trigeminal neuralgia treatment: a preliminary multicenter experience. *Neurosurgery.* 2008;62(3):647–655; discussion 647–655.

106. Romanelli P, Heit G, Chang SD, Martin D, Pham C, Adler J. Cyberknife radiosurgery for trigeminal neuralgia. *Stereotact Funct Neurosurg.* 2003;81(1–4):105–109.

107. Patil CG, Veeravagu A, Bower RS, et al. CyberKnife radiosurgical rhizotomy for the treatment of atypical trigeminal nerve pain. *Neurosurg Focus.* 2007;23(6):E9.

108. Linskey ME, Ratanatharathorn V, Peñagaricano J. A prospective cohort study of microvascular decompression and Gamma Knife surgery in patients with trigeminal neuralgia. *J Neurosurg.* 2008;109(suppl):160–172.

109. Jellish WS, Benedict W, Owen K, Anderson D, Fluder E, Shea JF. Perioperative and long-term operative outcomes after surgery for trigeminal neuralgia: microvascular decompression vs. percutaneous balloon ablation. *Head Face Med.* 2008;4:11.

110. Meglio M, Cioni B, Moles A, Visocchi M. Microvascular decompression versus percutaneous procedures for typical trigeminal neuralgia: personal experience. *Stereotact Funct Neurosurg.* 1990;54–55:76–79.

111. Tronnier VM, Rasche D, Hamer J, Kienle AL, Kunze S. Treatment of idiopathic trigeminal neuralgia: comparison of long-term outcome after radiofrequency rhizotomy and microvascular decompression. *Neurosurgery.* 2001;48(6):1261–1267; discussion 1267–1268.

112. Chung SS. Microvascular decompression for trigeminal neuralgia. In: Lozano AM, Gildenberg PL, Tasker RR, eds. *Textbook of Stereotactic and Functional Neurosurgery.* Berlin, Heidelberg: Springer Berlin Heidelberg; 2009:2465–2474.

113. Hamlyn PJ, King TT. Neurovascular compression in trigeminal neuralgia: a clinical and anatomical study. *J Neurosurg.* 1992;76(6):948–954.

114. Baechli H, Gratzl O. Microvascular decompression in trigeminal neuralgia with no vascular compression. *Eur Surg Res.* 2007;39(1):51–57.

115. Tyler-Kabara EC, Kassam AB, Horowitz MH, et al. Predictors of outcome in surgically managed patients with typical and atypical trigeminal neuralgia: comparison of results following microvascular decompression. *J Neurosurg.* 2002;96(3):527–531.

116. Bederson JB, Wilson CB. Evaluation of microvascular decompression and partial sensory rhizotomy in 252 cases of trigeminal neuralgia. *J Neurosurg.* 1989;71(3):359–367.

117. Han-Bing S, Wei-Guo Z, Jun Z, Ning L, Jian-Kang S, Yu C. Predicting the outcome of microvascular decompression for trigeminal neuralgia using magnetic resonance tomographic angiography. *J Neuroimag.* 2010;20(4):345–349.

118. Miller JP, Acar F, Burchiel KJ. Classification of trigeminal neuralgia: clinical, therapeutic, and prognostic implications in a series of 144 patients undergoing microvascular decompression. *J Neurosurg.* 2009;111(6):1231–1234.

119. Miller JP, Magill ST, Acar F, Burchiel KJ. Predictors of long-term success after microvascular decompression for trigeminal neuralgia. *J Neurosurg.* 2009;110(4):620–626.

120. Sandell T, Eide PK. Effect of microvascular decompression in trigeminal neuralgia patients with or without constant pain. *Neurosurgery.* 2008;63(1):93–99; discussion 99–100.

121. Gunther T, Gerganov VM, Stieglitz L, Ludemann W, Samii A, Samii M. Microvascular decompression for trigeminal neuralgia in the elderly: long-term treatment outcome and comparison with younger patients. *Neurosurgery.* 2009;65(3):477–482; discussion 482.

122. Sekula RF, Marchan EM, Fletcher LH, Casey KF, Jannetta PJ. Microvascular decompression for trigeminal neuralgia in elderly patients. *J Neurosurg.* 2008;108(4):689–691.

123. Burchiel KJ. Microvascular decompression for trigeminal neuralgia. *J Neurosurg.* 2008;108(4):687–688; discussion 688.

124. Athanasiou TC, Patel NK, Renowden SA, Coakham HB. Some patients with multiple sclerosis have neurovascular compression causing their trigeminal neuralgia and can be treated effectively with MVD: report of five cases. *Br J Neurosurg.* 2005;19(6):463–468.

125. Agostoni E, Frigerio R, Santoro P. Atypical facial pain: clinical considerations and differential diagnosis. *Neurol Sci.* 2005;26(suppl 2): s71–s74.

126. Sardella A, Demarosi F, Barbieri C, Lodi G. An up-to-date view on persistent idiopathic facial pain. *Minerva Stomatol.* 2009;58(6):289–299.

127. Pettengill CA, Reisner-Keller L. The use of tricyclic antidepressants for the control of chronic orofacial pain. *Cranio.* 1997;15(1):53–56.

128. Sharav Y, Singer E, Schmidt E, Dionne RA, Dubner R. The analgesic effect of amitriptyline on chronic facial pain. *Pain.* 1987;31(2): 199–209.

129. Evans RW, Agostoni E. Persistent idiopathic facial pain. *Headache.* 2006;46(8):1298–1300.

130. Volcy M, Rapoport AM, Tepper SJ, Sheftell FD, Bigal ME. Persistent idiopathic facial pain responsive to topiramate. *Cephalalgia.* 2006;26(4):489–491.

131. Delvaux V, Schoenen J. New generation antiepileptics for facial pain and headache. *Acta Neurol Belg.* 2001;101(1):42–46.

132. Frediani F. Pharmacological therapy of atypical facial pain: actuality and perspective. *Neurol Sci.* 2005;26(Suppl 2):s92–94.

133. Schwartz G, Galonski M, Gordon A, Shandling M, Mock D, Tenenbaum HC. Effects of salmon calcitonin on patients with atypical (idiopathic) facial pain: a randomized controlled trial. *J Orofac Pain.* 1996;10(4):306–315.

134. al Balawi S, Tariq M, Feinmann C. A double-blind, placebo-controlled, crossover, study to evaluate the efficacy of subcutaneous sumatriptan in the treatment of atypical facial pain. *Int J Neurosci.* 1996;86(3–4):301–309.

135. Harrison SD, Balawi SA, Feinmann C, Harris M. Atypical facial pain: a double-blind placebo-controlled crossover pilot study of subcutaneous sumatriptan. *Eur Neuropsychopharmacol.* 1997;7(2):83–88.

136. Abrahamsen R, Baad-Hansen L, Svensson P. Hypnosis in the management of persistent idiopathic orofacial pain—clinical and psychosocial findings. *Pain.* 2008;136(1–2):44–52.

137. Lang E, Naraghi R, Tanrikulu L, et al. Neurovascular relationship at the trigeminal root entry zone in persistent idiopathic facial pain: findings from MRI 3D visualisation. *J Neurol Neurosurg Psychiatry.* 2005;76(11): 1506–1509.

138. Broggi G, Ferroli P, Franzini A, Galosi L. The role of surgery in the treatment of typical and atypical facial pain. *Neurol Sci.* 2005;26(Suppl 2): s95–100.

139. Ebel H, Rust D, Tronnier V, Boker D, Kunze S. Chronic precentral stimulation in trigeminal neuropathic pain. *Acta Neurochir* (Wien). 1996;138(11):1300–1306.

140. Lefaucheur JP, Drouot X, Cunin P, et al. Motor cortex stimulation for the treatment of refractory peripheral neuropathic pain. *Brain.* 2009;132(pt 6):1463–1471.

141. Goebel A, Moore A, Weatherall R, Roewer N, Schedel R, Sprotte G. Intravenous immunoglobulin in the treatment of primary trigeminal neuralgia refractory to carbamazepine: a study protocol [ISRCTN33042138]. *BMC Neurol.* 2003;3(1):1.

142. Piovesan EJ, Teive HG, Kowacs PA, Della Coletta MV, Werneck LC, Silberstein SD. An open study of botulinum-A toxin treatment of trigeminal neuralgia. *Neurology.* 2005;65(8):1306–1308.

143. Holsheimer J. Electrical stimulation of the trigeminal tract in chronic, intractable facial neuralgia. *Arch Physiol Biochem.* 2001;109(4):304–308.

24

Metabolic, Endocrine, and Other Toxic Neuropathies

AMANDA PELTIER AND JUSTIN C. MCARTHUR

INTRODUCTION

THIS CHAPTER WILL review the more common causes of peripheral nerve toxicity, specifically their clinical features, differential diagnosis, and management. Diabetes mellitus and nerve toxicity from chemotherapy agents or human immune deficiency virus (HIV) medications will be covered, respectively, in Chapters 11 and 12.

First, we will review the general principles of toxic nerve injury, and then the unique signs and symptoms of individual toxic agents. There have been substantial social and regulatory actions in developed countries that have altered the frequency of environmental and workplace toxic exposures. Unfortunately, in many parts of the world, the regulation of potentially toxic chemicals is either rudimentary or nonexistent, and workers or consumers may still be exposed to dangerous levels of nerve-injuring chemicals (as reported, for example, in the *New York Times* article "Cheap Lead Paint Common on Chinese Goods").[1]

EPIDEMIOLOGY

The incidence and prevalence of toxic neuropathy in the United States are difficult to quantify due to the lack of a central agency and a uniform reporting method. In 2001 there were 1293 cases of reported peripheral nervous system illnesses, excluding carpal tunnel syndrome; 121 cases were identified as "inflammatory and toxic neuropathy, toxic polyneuropathy," while the rest were described as "not specified" (Bureau of Labor Statistics). In Olmstead County, MN., fewer than 10 cases of lead neuropathy were identified between 1949 and 1989.[2] This does not include cases of iatrogenic polyneuropathy, which can be more difficult to estimate given that literally hundreds of drugs have been associated with toxic peripheral neuropathy. Frequently, medication-induced polyneuropathy is often not apparent until the medication receives U.S. Food and Drug Administration approval and is in widespread use, such as with the 3-hydroxy-3-methyl-glutaryl-CoA reductase (HMG CoA) inhibitors (statin drugs).

CLINICAL AND DIAGNOSTIC FEATURES

Principles of Nerve Toxicity

The principles of peripheral nerve damage from toxic chemicals or metabolic/endocrine causes guide our approach to understanding the pathophysiology. Theoretically, any toxic exposure may damage the peripheral nerves, but *dose, duration,* and *comorbid conditions* modulate the expression of that toxicity. Comorbidities may include underlying conditions such as diabetes mellitus, HIV infection, inherited neuropathy, or even a genetic susceptibility to metabolize drugs in a particular manner. Schaumburg and Albers have described different patterns of "pseudointoxication," including the coincidental co-occurrence of a naturally occurring neurological disorder or psychiatric/psychological disorders associated with chemical exposure.[3]

The relationship of exposure dose and duration is illustrated in Figure 24.1; a single large exposure may rapidly produce irreversible nerve damage. In contrast, smaller, frequent exposures over many months may produce only mild, and potentially reversible, damage (Figure 24.1). One important principle is the phenomenon of *coasting,* defined as the continued development of nerve damage despite withdrawal of the offending agent. This represents the lag in nerve damage after exposure. A second principle is *fiber selectivity,*[4,5] in which there is a differential effect on either sensory or motor fibers and on large- versus small-caliber nerve fibers. A third principle is *reversibility,* since many toxic neuropathies are associated with significant recovery of function and reduction in symptoms after withdrawal of the offending agent.

In general, the association between a potentially toxic agent and the development of neuropathy must satisfy the traditional causality criteria: the strength of the association, the temporal sequence, and the evidence for a dose-response relationship.[6]

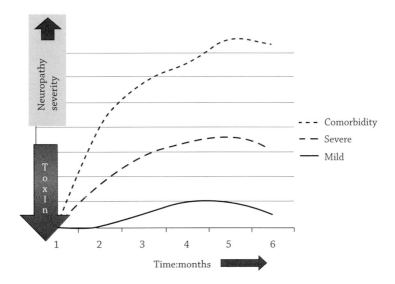

FIGURE 24.1   Different theoretical trajectories for toxic neuropathies: (1) mild: mild neuropathy develops after low-dose exposure with partial reversal; (2) severe: severe neuropathy develops after repeated high-dose exposure; there is minimal reversal; (3) comorbidity: very severe neuropathy in a setting of, for example, diabetic neuropathy; reversal is negligible.

PATHOPHYSIOLOGY

Jortner has reviewed the different patterns of toxic neuropathies.[7] The most common pattern is a distal *dying-back* axonopathy. Typically, these neuropathies progress toward the Wallerian-like degeneration of affected fibers. The pathological changes are usually more severe in the distal regions of the neurite, and they affect both peripheral and central fibers. Examples of such distal axonopathies are organophosphorous ester-induced delayed neuropathy, hexacarbon neuropathy, and *p*-bromophenylacetylurea intoxication. In neuronopathies, the primary nerve injury is in the neuronal cell bodies. This is exemplified by pyridoxine neurotoxicity, in which there is sublethal or lethal damage to larger neurons in the sensory ganglia. Demyelinating neuropathies are uncommon. An example of this is tellurium intoxication, in which demyelination is caused by toxin-induced interference with cholesterol synthesis by Schwann cells.

Different agents produce damage to the nervous system in different, and sometimes unique, patterns. For example, acrylamide appears to affect retrograde transport of proteins, including neurotrophic factors such as nerve growth factor. Certain antiretrovirals used to suppress HIV replication produce nerve injury by inhibiting gamma DNA polymerase and producing mitochondrial injury. Table 24.1 lists some of the mechanisms that have been well defined.

CLINICAL FEATURES OF TOXIC NEUROPATHIES

Toxic neuropathies typically affect sensory fibers more than motor function; however, this is dependent upon the agent in question. For example, lead and botulism classically affect motor fibers predominantly. Tables 24.2 and 24.3 describe some of the general features of toxic neuropathies (see also Chapter 14).

SPECIFIC NERVE TOXINS

This section is not designed to review every potential neurotoxin, but rather to provide illustrative examples, either where the clinical features are distinctive, the pathophysiology is unique, or there are specific management strategies that hasten recovery. For details of antiretroviral agents see Chapter 12, and for chemotherapy agents see Chapter 14.

TOXIC MEDICATIONS

Antibiotics

Nitrofurantoin is an antibiotic that is still very widely used for treating urinary tract infections caused by several types of bacteria. Despite the ubiquity of its usage, relatively little attention has been given to the toxicity that can occur, especially because this drug is widely used for long periods of time for urinary

Table 24-1. Examples of Specific Mechanisms of Nerve Damage from Toxins or Metabolic Derangements

AGENT	MECHANISM
Acrylamide[8]	Inhibition of axonal retrograde transport
Nucleoside reverse transcriptase inhibitors[9]	Inhibition of gamma DNA polymerase leads to mitochondrial dysfunction
Lead[10,11]	Disruption of calcium processes, especially protein kinase C
Agent Orange[12]	Possible effect of dioxin acting via an intracellular protein (the Ah receptor) on transcription levels
Hypothyroidism[13]	Accumulation of mucinous material deposited in the endoneurium
Uremia[14]	Inhibition of axolemma-bound Na$^+$/K$^+$-ATPase
Linezolid[15]	Mitochondrial inhibition of protein synthesis

Table 24-2 Clinical Features of Fiber-Specific Neuropathies

AUTONOMIC FIBERS	SMALL-FIBER SENSORY	LARGE-FIBER SENSORY
Orthostatic hypotension	Spontaneous burning pain	Loss of vibratory and proprioceptive function
Poorly responsive pupils or Horner's syndrome*	Evoked pain with allodynia	Reduced or absent stretch reflexes
Heart rate variability	Spontaneous/evoked paresthesias	Sensory ataxia with pseudoathetosis
Lack of R-R variability on electrocardiogram	Lancinating pains	Weakness
Disturbed sweating	Hypesthesia with diminished pain and temperature sensibility	Slowed nerve conduction velocities on nerve conduction velocity studies
Erectile dysfunction	Loss of protective sensation with foot ulceration	Demyelination or axonal abnormalities on sural nerve biopsy
Abnormal ejaculation	Visceral pain loss	
Constipation or gastroparesis	Epidermal denervation on skin biopsies	

*Bremner FD, Smith SE . Pupil abnormalities in selected autonomic neuropathies. *J Neuro-Ophthalmol.* 2006;26(3):209–219.

Source: Modified from Rutchik JS. Toxic neuropathy treatment and Management. 2009. Medscape from WebMD. http://emedicine.medscape.com/article/1175276-treatment. Accessed November 26, 2011.

prophylaxis.[16,17] The typical presentation is with features of a painful sensory neuropathy with prominent dysesthesias. Neuropathy appears to be more common and more severe with renal impairment. Skin biopsies can show prominent changes in epidermal nerves (Figure 24.2). Discontinuation of the medication usually allows recovery over a few weeks.

Linezolid is the first of a new class of antimicrobial agents, the oxazalinodones, which bind to the 50s subunit of the prokaryotic ribosome, blocking protein synthesis.[18] Linezolid was introduced in 2000 to treat resistant gram-positive cocci and was also found to be effective in treating drug-resistant *Mycobacterium tuberbulosis*.[19] Nineteen cases have been reported of a predominantly sensory, sometimes irreversible polyneuropathy.[20–23] Multiple cases of optic neuropathy have also been reported with linezolid.[20,24] The risk of development of polyneuropathy is significantly increased with long-term treatment. Patients in the initial phase II and III clinical trials limited to 28-day exposure had no reported polyneuropathy.[25] The optic neuropathy and polyneuropathy are most likely related to

mitochondrial inhibition of protein synthesis, as chloramphenicol has similar toxicities and a similar mechanism.[15]

Other drugs for tuberculosis treatment, such as isoniazid and ethambutol, have a well-documented risk of polyneuropathy.[26,27] However, there may be an increased risk of development of neuropathy when other medications associated with neuropathy, such as stavudine, are introduced.[28] Patients who are "slow inactivators" due to acetyltransferase variants are also at higher risk of developing polyneuropathy.[29]

HMG-CoA Reductase Inhibitors (Statins)

The first statin, lovastatin, was introduced in 1987, followed by multiple other statins including pravastatin, simvastatin, fluvastatin, atorvastatin, rosuvastatin, and cervastatin. Multiple case reports and series have been published suggesting statins as a class to be a risk factor for peripheral neuropathy[30–32] despite the lack of polyneuropathy reported in multiple clinical trials of statins.[33–37] Gaist et al. reported United Kingdom data and Danish data suggesting an

Table 24-3 Potential Causes of Toxic Neuropathies and Fiber Selectivity

	AXONAL PATHOLOGY		DEMYELINATING PATHOLOGY	MIXED PATHOLOGY
SENSORY	SENSORIMOTOR	MOTOR		
Almitrine	Acrylamide	β-Bungarotoxin	Buckthorn	**Amiodarone**
Bortezomib	Allyl chloride	Botulism	**Chloroquine**	Diethylene
Chloramphenicol	Arsenic Cadmium	Dimethylamine	Diphtheria	glycol Ethylene
Dioxin	Carbon disulfide	Borane	Hexachlorophene	glycol 1,1'-
Doxorubicin	Chlorphenoxy	Gangliosides	Muzolimine	Ethylidinebis
Ethambutol	Ciguatoxin	Latrotoxin (black	Perhexiline	(L-tryptophan
Ethionamide	**Colchicine**	widow spider)	Procainamide	contaminant)
Etoposide	Cyanide Dapsone	**Lead**	**Tacrolimus**	Gold
(VP-16)	Dimethylamino-	Mercury	Tellurium	Hexacarbons
Gemcitabine	propionitrile	Misoprostol	Zimeldine	n-Hexane
Glutethimide	Dichloroacetate	Tetanus Tick		Na+ cyanate
Hydralazine	Disulfiram	paralysis		Suramin
Ifosfamide	**Ethanol** Ethylene			
Interferon-α	oxide Heroin			
Isoniazid	(Lead) Lithium			
Leflunomide	Methyl bromide			
Metronidazole	**Nitrofurantoin**			
Misonidazole	**Organophosphates**			
Nitrous oxide	Podophyllin			
Nucleosides	PCBs Saxitoxin			
HIV ddC, ddI,	Spanish toxic oil			
d4T Phenytoin	**Taxol** Tetrodotoxin			
Platinum analogs	Thallium Trichlo-			
Propafenone	roethylene			
Pyridoxine	TOCP Vacor (PNU)			
Statins	**Vinca alkaloids**			
Thalidomide				

Note: Common toxins are highlighted.

Dideoxycytidine (ddc); didanosine (ddI); stavudine (d4T); PCBs, polychlorinated biphenyls; tri-ortho-cresyl-phosphate (TOCP); N-3-pyridylmethyl N'-p-nitrophenyl urea (PNU).

Source: Modified from the Washington University Web site. http://neuromuscular.wustl.edu/ Accessed November 26, 2011.

increased risk of peripheral neuropathy in statin users up to 12 times that of the population in some groups.[38,39]

The most common type of polyneuropathy reported with statin use is a sensorimotor axonal polyneuropathy, although small-fiber neuropathies have also been reported. Most patients experienced improvement of symptoms when the statin was discontinued; however, some had permanent neuropathy. A recent case exemplifies the typical findings in statin-associated neuropathies. A 60-year-old nondiabetic male presented with symptoms of neuropathy after simvastatin was initiated. Electromyography testing was normal. Blood testing revealed no other cause of neuropathy. Quantitative sudomotor axon reflex testing (QSART) showed a length-dependent loss of sweat volume. Simvastatin was stopped, and the symptoms improved. An intervening QSART test showed normal sweat volumes. One month later, rosuvastatin was initiated and peripheral neuropathy symptoms returned. Once again, QSART demonstrated significant loss of sweat

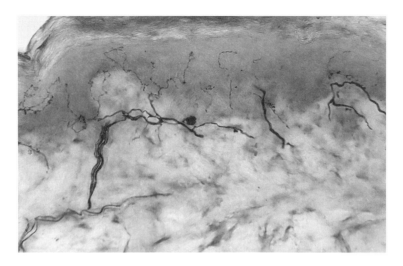

FIGURE 24.2   Photomicrograph of epidermal nerve fibers and swellings.

volume distally (Boger MS, Hulgan T, Donofrio P. **Peltier AC**. QSART for diagnosis of statin-associated polyneuropathy. Muscle Nerve. 2011 Feb;43(2):295-6.) (see Figures 24.3a and b).

Recently, the Fremantle Diabetes Study suggested that lipid-lowering agents were protective for peripheral neuropathy, with a hazard ratio of 0.30, 95% CI (0.10–0.86) for fibrates and 0.70, 95% CI (0.49–0.997) for statins. Age, body mass index, and ethnicity (aboriginal ancestry) were the largest risk factors for development of peripheral neuropathy in the study.[40] This suggests that the overall the risk of development of peripheral neuropathy with the statin class is low and should not be an impediment to treating hyperlipidemia unless there is a time-linked association with statins. It is unclear from the literature if there are specific genetic risk factors for statin neuropathy.

ENVIRONMENTAL TOXINS

Acrylamide Neuropathy

The neurotoxic effects of acrylamide have been well documented for almost 50 years, and although most industrialized nations now restrict the use of this agent, it still serves as an important model for toxic neuropathies. Most acrylamide is used to synthesize nontoxic polyacrylamides, which find many uses as water-soluble thickeners in wastewater treatment, gel electrophoresis, papermaking, and ore processing. Acrylamide also occurs in many cooked starchy foods, and some years ago was discovered in certain fried foods. The monomer is the toxic form, whereas the polymer is innocuous. Acrylamide is readily absorbed by inhalation, ingestion, or dermal contact, often preceded by a contact dermatitis. The clinical features include distal numbness and widespread hyporeflexia. Large-fiber sensory dysfunction with loss of vibration and proprioception is common, whereas dysesthesias and paresthesias are rare.[41] High-level exposure often results in encephalopathy and autonomic dysfunction. In chronic exposures, autonomic dysfunction is milder and usually produces disturbance of sweating on the hands and feet.

Acrylamide neuropathy has been used as a reproducible experimental animal model for studying axonal transport[42,43] and dying-back neuropathy.[41,44] Acrylamide-induced defects in retrograde transport could augment axonal injury, because growth factors are normally transported back to neuronal perikaryon through the retrograde transport system.

Herbicides: Agent Orange

Agent Orange is the code name for an herbicide and defoliant used by the U.S. military in its herbicidal program during the Vietnam War from 1962 to 1971. It was by far the most widely used of the so-called "Rainbow Herbicides." Dioxins

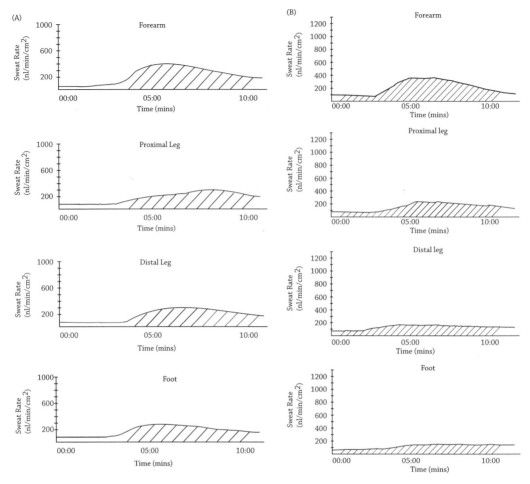

FIGURE 24.3   Sweat volumes determined by QSART before (A) and after statin use (B). Note the marked reduction in sweat production.

were a contaminant of the production process of Agent Orange (as well as Agents Purple, Pink, and Green), and according to the postwar Vietnamese government, 4.8 million Vietnamese people were exposed to Agent Orange, resulting in 400,000 deaths and disabilities and 500,000 children born with birth defects.[45]

In their initial 1993 report *Veterans and Agent Orange*, the National Academy of Sciences did not find convincing evidence for an association between peripheral neuropathy and herbicide exposure. However, in an updated 1996 report, they concluded in *Agent Orange— Health Effects of Herbicides Used in Vietnam* that "there is some evidence to suggest that neuropathy of acute or subacute onset may be associated with herbicide exposure." A further

update was released in 2009 (*Veterans and Agent Orange: Update 2008*). Today, veterans may be eligible for disability compensation and health care benefits for neuropathy, ischemic heart disease, Parkinson's disease, and other diseases that the Veterans Administration now recognizes as being associated with exposure to Agent Orange and other herbicides. The clinical features of the neuropathy are similar to those of other types of toxic neuropathy.

Dioxins are produced through a variety of industrial processes including chlorine bleaching processes at pulp and paper mills, wastewater and drinking water treatment, chemical manufacturing, and the uncontrolled combustion of household wastes. The half-life of dioxins is more than 8 years, and there are clear-cut associations with lung and other cancers, chloracne, and liver enzyme and reproductive hormone abnormalities. Dioxins act via an intracellular protein (the Ah receptor), which is a ligand-dependent transcription factor that functions with a second protein (known as Arnt). The adverse effects of Agent Orange, and of related herbicides, appear to reflect sustained alterations in gene expression. The mechanisms by which dioxins might induce neuropathy are uncertain and remain controversial.

Organophosphate Pesticides

Organophosphate pesticides have largely replaced organochlorines in the past two decades and are widely used in domestic, agricultural, and structural applications. Occupational use yields the highest exposures, but the public can also be exposed during structural applications, domestic use, or by drift from aerial spraying. The acute toxic effects of organophosphates are based on inhibition of acetylcholinesterase, leading to dysfunction of the autonomous nervous system (abdominal cramps, nausea, diarrhea, salivation, miosis) and the central nervous system (dizziness, tremor, anxiety, confusion). Some organophosphates (such as methamidophos, leptophos, fenthion, and merphos) inhibit a second enzyme, neuropathy target esterase. Significant inhibition of this enzyme may be accompanied by a peripheral neuropathy 10–14 days after exposure. An infamous human epidemic of neuropathy induced by organophosphate occurred in the United States in 1930 after ingestion of a popular headache remedy ("Ginger Jake") contaminated with triortho-cresyl phosphate. Almost 5000 cases of delayed neuropathy were reported, often with significant residua.[46] Chronic lower-level exposures may also lead to neuropathy, although the results of epidemiological studies are less consistent than those of the studies of poisoned subjects. In fact, it is controversial whether chronic neuropathy can occur with a preceding acute intoxication.[47]

Stokes et al. studied 68 long-term (mean, 20 years) pesticide applicators and 68 matched controls, tested during the off season. The principal organophosphates used were guthion, chlorpyrifos, and diazinon. The applicators showed a significant decrease in vibratory sensitivity.[48]

Lead and Heavy Metals

Lead poisoning (also known as *plumbism* or *painter's colic*) is caused by excessive levels of the heavy metal in the body. Lead is toxic to many organs and tissues including the heart, bones, intestines, kidneys, and reproductive and nervous systems. While classically lead intoxication produces a motor neuropathy, there may be sensory involvement with neuropathic pain. In the developing nervous system, it interferes with appropriate central nervous system development and is therefore particularly toxic to children, causing encephalopathy with acute high-dose exposure and, with chronic lower-dose exposure, permanent learning and behavior disorders. Other symptoms include abdominal pain, headache, anemia, and, in severe cases, encephalopathy, seizures, coma, and death. Exposure has typically been either occupational, such as in painters chronically exposed to lead-containing paints, or in children who ingest flakes of lead-containing paint in their homes. Lead has been banned from paint and gasoline in many developed countries since the 1960s, and lead abatement programs have successfully screened millions of children in the United States. Nonetheless, in some countries with less rigorous chemical safety regulations, lead-containing paint is still available for industrial purposes or children are not adequately protected from exposure to industrial uses. For example, in 2007, toys made in China were found to have been painted with lead-containing industrial paint.[49] The diagnosis of lead exposure is based on the blood lead level. The U.S. Centers for Disease Control and Prevention and the World Health Organization state that a blood lead level of 10 µg/dL or above is potentially harmful. However, lead may impair development and have harmful health effects even at lower levels, and there is no known safe exposure level.

In acute lead poisoning, typical neurological features are pain, muscle weakness, paresthesias, and encephalopathy. Abdominal pain, nausea, vomiting, diarrhea, and constipation can occur. Lead can also cause a distinctive metallic taste. Chronic lead poisoning usually presents with symptoms affecting multiple systems, typically gastrointestinal and neurological. The neuropathy associated with lead typically involves heavily used muscles; thus, in painters, the forearm muscles are particularly affected, with resulting wrist drop.[2] One study in which exposed individuals had an unusually long duration of exposure to inorganic lead suggested that the presentation was different from that traditionally attributed to lead toxicity. In this series, patients had a mild sensory and autonomic polyneuropathy rather than the pure motor neuropathy.[50] Other signs of chronic lead exposure include memory loss, reduced concentration, depression, nausea, abdominal pain, and loss of coordination. Fatigue, sleep disturbance, refractory headaches, sluggish behavior, slurred speech, and anemia are also found. Children with chronic lead poisoning may have behavioral changes including aggressive behavior.

The chelating agents used for the treatment of acute lead poisoning are edetate disodium calcium, injected dimercaprol, and the oral agents succimer and D-penicillamine. Chelation therapy is typically considered in cases of acute lead poisoning, severe poisoning, and encephalopathy, and also when blood lead levels are above 25 μg/dL. Chelation therapy appears to be of very limited value for chronic exposure to low levels of lead or in treating neuropathy.

Arsenic and Thallium Neuropathy

Neuropathy linked to exposure to these heavy metals is similar, so they will be discussed together in this section. Thallium was used in many pesticides and in rat poison, and exposures still occur either accidentally in children or from purposeful poisoning. Arsenic was widely used as a lumber preservative and in pesticides, and there have also been documented toxic exposures from contaminated wells, traditional Chinese herbal balls, Korean herbal preparations, and kelp supplements. Both thallium and arsenic induce prominent gastrointestinal symptoms when ingested. Both also produce a distal symmetric axonopathy that selectively damages large-caliber nerve fibers. Sensory symptoms predominate over motor symptoms, and pain is a particularly prominent feature.

Ingestion of a large dose of thallium will induce severe gastrointestinal distress, diarrhea, and vomiting, followed within 2–5 days by length-dependent neuropathic symptoms.[51,52] Thallium is also classically associated with alopecia developing 2–4 weeks after ingestion. A delayed autonomic neuropathy may develop after acute thallium intoxication.[53] Inorganic arsenic produces skin hyperpigmentation or an eczematous dermatitis.

The treatment of poisoning includes hydration, supportive care, and the use of chelating agents including succimer (Chemet®), penicillamine, and dimercaprol. The safe selection and use of these agents requires supervision by a toxicologist.

METABOLIC AND ENDOCRINE DISORDERS PRODUCING NEUROPATHIES

Uremic Polyneuropathy

After diabetes mellitus, uremia is one of the most common causes of peripheral neuropathy, with prevalence figures ranging from 10% to 80%. Comorbidities are common, obviously, including exposures to toxic agents. There has been a significant reduction in incidence and prevalence with the use of newer dialysis membranes.[54] Typically, uremic polyneuropathy presents as a distal symmetrical process with greater lower-limb than upper-limb involvement. The condition develops slowly over many months. Neuropathy generally develops only at glomerular filtration rates of less than 12 mL/min. Large-fiber involvement predominates, with paresthesias, reduced stretch reflexes, impaired vibration sense, wasting, and weakness. Nerve conduction studies demonstrate axonal injury. Some patients may also develop autonomic dysfunction and deficits in pain/temperature perception. For many years, the prevailing theory underlying uremic polyneuropathy was the *middle molecule hypothesis*, based on observations that neuropathy was less frequent in individuals undergoing peritoneal dialysis rather than hemodialysis. This suggested that the hemodialysis membranes might not be removing the neurotoxic substance. Substances with a molecular weight of 300–12,000 Da were considered the putative toxic agents, and parathyroid hormone has been suspected but toxicity was never convincingly proven.[55,56] Mechanisms of uremic polyneuropathy include nerve dysfunction from the inhibition of axolemma-bound Na^+/K^+-ATPase by uremic toxins, leading to intracellular sodium accumulation and altered resting membrane potentials. The current concept is that uremic neuropathy is a dying-back neuropathy, with metabolic failure of the neuron causing distal axonal degeneration.[57] The use of thinner dialysis membranes and longer dialysis times to attempt to better clear middle molecular weight has led to significant reductions in the rate of severe neuropathy.[58] Transplantation can reverse uremic polyneuropathy,[59] and the tremendous increase in successful renal transplantations may have impacted the overall prevalence of neuropathy.

Thyroid Neuropathy

While frank, severe myxedema is rarely encountered today, patients with very mild thyroid dysfunction are relatively common. The worldwide prevalence of subclinical hypothyroidism has been estimated at up to 10%.[60] These subclinically hypothyroid patients may have normal serum levels of thyroxine and triiodothyronine and only mildly elevated serum thyrotropin levels. However, despite the term *subclinical,* typically these patients do have systemic complaints. Neuropathy can occur in these patients and may reverse with thyroid replacement.[61] The clinical features of thyroid neuropathy include an insidious or sometimes subacute onset of sensory symptoms. Sensory complaints include painful acral dysesthesias and radiating lancinating pain, sometimes mimicking the pain of nerve root compression. Examination findings include a distal "glove-and-stocking" sensory loss, delayed or absent stretch reflexes (classically the ankle reflex), and occasionally ataxia. Weakness is usually from an accompanying myopathy. Superimposed entrapment neuropathy of the median nerve is also a very common

neuropathy associated with hypothyroidism (see Chapter 11), and dysfunction of the eighth nerve can also occur.

Microvascular and endoneurial ischemic involvement like that seen in diabetes can also develop. In animals with experimental hypothyroidism, the earliest abnormalities appear to be the deposit of mucopolysaccharide-protein complexes within the endoneurium and perineurium. Reduced densities of myelinated fibers, mostly large diameter, and Renaut bodies have also been noted, and other studies have shown axonal degeneration.

CRITICAL ILLNESS NEUROPATHY

Critical illness polyneuropathy (CIP) occurs in 30 to 50% of patients in the intensive care unit (ICU).[62–64] It commonly coexists with critical illness myopathy (CIM), and the two conditions may be difficult to differentiate.[65] Critical illness polyneuropathy may be associated with a poorer prognosis than CIM, as 6 of 15 patients had significant weakness or disability 1 year after hospitalization,[63] although the Lacomis study demonstrated a similar outcome of CIM and CIP posthospitalization.[64]

The cause of CIP is not well understood. Sepsis and the systemic inflammatory response syndrome (SIRS) have been put forth as significant risk factors.[66] The manifestations of SIRS include (1) a body temperature above 38°C or below 36°C; (2) a heart rate above 90 beats per minute; (3) a respiratory rate greater than 20 or a carbon dioxide partial pressure of less than 32; and (4) an abnormal white blood cell count: either more than 12,000 cells/mm^3 or less than 4000 cells/mm^3. Critical illness polyneuropathy is associated with a lengthy stay in the ICU, multiple organ failure, elevated serum glucose levels, decreased serum albumin, and a high Acute Physiology, Age, Chronic Health Evaluation III score.[67]

Nerve biopsies of patients with CIP typically show relatively intact myelin with reduced numbers of axons distally.[68] Nerve conduction values are often difficult to obtain in the ICU but, when present, are typically low in amplitude. Electromyography often shows evidence of predominantly myopathic units due to the common coexistence of CIM with

CIP.[64] Neuromuscular blocking agents such as vecuronium have been associated with motor neuropathies[69] and are linked with an increased risk of development of CIM, especially in conjunction with corticosteroid use.[70] There is no specific therapy for CIP other than to avoid muscle relaxants, neuromuscular blocking agents, and corticosteroids.

ACROMEGALY AND HUMAN GROWTH HORMONE REPLACEMENT

There is a high incidence (up to 50%) of carpal tunnel syndrome in those with acromegaly, or adults treated with human growth hormone (hGH) replacement therapy.[71,72] Older studies in acromegaly have documented peripheral neuropathy with demyelinating lesions and hypertrophic formations affecting Schwann cells associated with small-caliber fibers, with marked onion bulb formation.[73] More frequent today than frank acromegaly is the common use of hGH, a polypeptide hormone used clinically for growth failure in children who have inadequate endogenous hGH secretion. There have been occasional case reports of median nerve entrapment in children receiving hGH.[74] This agent is also used illicitly by athletes because it is thought that hGH can provide the muscle-building benefits of anabolic steroids without their serious adverse effects. The risk of neuropathy in this setting is uncertain, but there are emerging case reports of entrapment neuropathies.[75]

HEPATITIS C AND CHRONIC LIVER DISEASE

Nonalcoholic chronic liver disease may be associated with an asymptomatic or mild sensorimotor demyelinating polyneuropathy in approximately 45%–50% of patients. Guillain-Barré syndrome has also been reported, although the causal link remains unclear. Peripheral neuropathy can occur with primary biliary cirrhosis and following acute viral hepatitis. Hepatitis C is associated with sensory neuropathy, especially when cryoglobulinemia is present. Despite the frequency of coinfection with hepatitis C and HIV, there does not appear to be an additive or synergistic effect of both viruses.[76]

VITAMIN DEFICIENCIES AND EXCESS

Vitamin B_{12} Deficiency

Vitamin B_{12} is a water-soluble vitamin with a key role in the normal functioning of the brain and nervous system and in blood formation. It is found in meats (especially lamb's liver and shellfish), milk, and eggs. Normally, it is critical for the metabolism of every cell of the body, especially affecting DNA synthesis and regulation but also fatty acid synthesis and energy production. Cyanocobalamin is one component of the vitamin B_{12} complex, and it is metabolized in the body to an active coenzyme form. Vitamin B_{12} functions as a methyl donor and works with folic acid in the synthesis of DNA and red blood cells; it is also vitally important in maintaining the health of the myelin sheath. The classic vitamin B_{12} deficiency disease is pernicious anemia, characterized by macrocytic anemia. It is now clear, however, that a vitamin B_{12} deficiency can have serious consequences long before anemia is evident. The body stores up to 3–5 years' worth of vitamin B_{12} and several months' supply of folate in the liver; thus, deficiencies and their associated symptoms can take months to years to manifest in adults. Diagnosis is made, of course, by measurement of blood levels of vitamin B_{12}, and folate. Vitamin B_{12} levels below 200 pg/mL are considered abnormal, but a deficiency can also occur at levels within a normal range, especially if folate is deficient. Blood markers of intracellular deficiency include elevated levels of methylmalonic acid and homocysteine. The Schilling test for absorption is no longer generally available. Other informative tests include the intrinsic factor binding antibody, which is present in pernicious anemia. The intrinsic factor binding antibody is present in more than 50% of patients with pernicious anemia and parietal cell antibody. Dietary deficiency in vegans is much more common today than pernicious anemia or tapeworm infestation, but other causes of deficiency or malabsorption should be searched for, including the inadequate utilization of folate and vitamin B_{12}

Table 24-4 Evaluation of Toxic Neuropathy

Algorithm for clinical assessment of neurotoxic disease

- Begin the evaluation by noting the chief complaint or complaints. Consider when they began and how they relate to an exposure.
- Take a thorough medical history that includes an occupational and environmental history to consider all sources of exposure to all possible agents. List details of all jobs and job tasks within the jobs and what symptoms and medical problems began when.
- Consider a review of systems and how eating, bowel movements, sexual activity, sleep, and emotional status varied during exposure incidents.
- List medical complaints on a timeline and relate each to exposure dates, duration, and intensity. Consider other occupational, environmental, and drug exposures. Include vitamin supplements, hobbies, and traditional practices.
- Include the birth history, pregnancy, and extensive family history to uncover any genetic or congenital diseases.
- Consider how symptoms change as they relate to exposures. How often do flare-ups occur? Are the symptoms persistent or do they improve?
- Do colleagues or coworkers have similar complaints?
- List all potential sources of exposure: from where, what form, and how they are used.
- Obtain MSDSs and scientific data on each chemical agent.
- Perform a neurological examination. A general medical examination including an assessment of the autonomic system, hair, teeth, nails, skin color, and lymph system is important. Are any objective neurological signs or other systemic findings noted?
- Arrange for confirmatory neurophysiological, neuropsychological, and imaging tests.
- Arrange for serum and biological monitoring when appropriate.
- Review regulatory information for this chemical. What have the Occupational Health and Safety Administration (OSHA), the Environmental Protection Agency (EPA), the National Institute of Occupational Safety and Health (NIOSH), the American Conference of Governmental Industrial Hygienists (ACGIH), and other international organizations published as a safe level?
- Consider contacting an industrial hygienist for air and water sampling.
- Consider removal from exposure.
- Consider whether the exposure and the medical problem may be consistent chronologically. First, did the exposure precede the complaint or dysfunction?
- Exclude all other common causes of the diagnosis. Are the findings consistent with a primary neurological or other medical condition? Are the findings explained by other historical or familial factors? Other exposures, illnesses, or stressors?
- Search the literature for epidemiological and case studies and series that describe an association between the exposure and the dysfunction.
- Are the dose and duration of exposure consistent with the described dysfunction? Focus on details of the literature.
- What is the proposed mechanism for this exposure-induced dysfunction?
- Estimate the patient's functional status and the medical treatment options and whether a consultation is necessary for support.
- Reevaluate by examination and neurological and neuropsychological tests. Do the results remain consistent?

Source: Adapted from Toxic Neuropathy: Follow-up. Jonathan S Rutchik, MD, MPH, Assistant Professor, Department of Occupational and Environmental Medicine, University of California at San Francisco. February 24, 2009.

with the use of antimetabolites for cancer such as pemetrexed (Alimta®), a recently developed chemotherapy drug indicated for pleural mesothelioma and non-small cell lung cancer. Bowel surgery, including gastric bypass and resection surgery, can lead to small bowel overgrowth and interference with vitamin B_{12} absorption in the ileum.

Clinical features of vitamin B_{12} deficiency include optic neuropathy, behavioral and neurocognitive dysfunction, subacute combined degeneration of the spinal cord, and sensory neuropathy. A retrospective cohort study was done of 581 patients presenting with polyneuropathy over a 2-year period; 4% had definite vitamin B_{12} deficiency, and 32% had possible deficiency (elevated methylmalonic acid levels) as the sole or contributing cause for their polyneuropathy. For the patients treated with supplemental vitamin B_{12}, subjective improvement was seen in 87% of those with definite vitamin B_{12} deficiency and in 43% of those with possible deficiency.[77]

Most multivitamin pills contain 100–200 µg of the cyanocobalamin form of vitamin B_{12}. This must be converted to methylcobalamin or adenosylcobalamin before it can be used by the body. The actual absorption of vitamin B_{12} is also restricted, and even taking 500 µg of cyanocobalamin may permit absorption of as little as 1.8 µg. Thus, most multivitamins do not provide an adequate daily intake of vitamin B_{12}. The deficiency is treated with intramuscular cyanocobalamin 1000 µg weekly for 1 month, then twice monthly. Alternatively, intranasal cyanocobalamin (Nasacobal®) 500 µg weekly can be used.

Vitamin B_6 Excess

Vitamin B_6 is a water-soluble vitamin and is part of the vitamin B complex group. Vitamin B_6 is found in a wide variety of foods including fortified cereals, beans, meat, poultry, fish, and some fruits and vegetables. The daily requirement for adults is 2.0 µg. Pyridoxal phosphate, the active form, is involved in many aspects of macronutrient metabolism, protein synthesis, and specifically neurotransmitter synthesis (serotonin, epinephrine, norepinephrine and gamma-aminobutyric acid). Pyridoxal phosphate serves as a coenzyme for many reactions including decarboxylation, deamination, and transamination. Pyridoxine is used to prevent neuropathy in patients receiving isoniazid for tuberculosis, and it can be taken in excess if multiple doses of vitamin supplements are used (megavitamin therapy). Excessive amounts of pyridoxine can cause a sensory neuropathy.[78]

Symptoms include pain, paresthesias, and numbness of the limbs. In severe forms, sensory ataxia may occur without weakness. Sensory neuropathy typically develops at doses of pyridoxine in excess of 50 mg/day. The Food and Nutrition Board of the Institute of Medicine set the tolerable upper intake level for pyridoxine at 100 mg/day for adults

In conclusion, a very large number of medications, environmental chemicals, and nutritional agents have been associated with painful neuropathies and other neuromuscular complications. Careful history taking is key if the offending agent is to be identified and further exposure prevented. A systematic screening questionnaire can be useful when exposure is suspected. Table 24.4 illustrates an algorithm for the evaluation of a potential toxic neuropathy.

Resources for Patients

The Neuropathy Association: peripheral neuropathies including toxic neuropathy and idiopathic neuropathy. 212-692-0662 or info@neuropathy.org or http://www.neuropathy.org/.

The Foundation for Peripheral Neuropathy: http://www.foundationforpn.org/.

Poison control centers: for a poison emergency in the United States, call 1-800-222-1222.

The American Association of Poison Control Centers call 1-800-222-1222 or http://www.aapcc.org/dnn/NewsandEvents/GuidelinesforUseof18002221222Number.aspx

REFERENCES

1. Barboza D. Cheap lead paint common on Chinese goods. *New York Times*. Monday, September 10, 2007:B1.
2. Dyck PJ, Thomas PK. Neuronal atrophy and degeneration predominantly affecting peripheral

sensory and autonomic neurons. In: PJ Dyck, PK Thomas, eds. *Peripheral Neuropathy*. Philadelphia: WB Saunders; 1993:1065–1093.

3. Schaumburg HH, Albers JW. Pseudoneurotoxic disease. *Neurology*. 2005;65(1):22–26.

4. Berger AR et al. Dose response, coasting, and differential fiber vulnerability in human toxic neuropathy: a prospective study of pyridoxine neurotoxicity. *Neurology*. 1992;42(7):1367–1370.

5. Windebank AJ et al. Pyridoxine neuropathy in rats: specific degeneration of sensory axons. *Neurology*. 1985;35(11):1617–1622.

6. Hill AB. *A Short Textbook of Medical Statistics*. 11th ed. 1985, London: Hodder Arnold; 1985.

7. Jortner BS. Mechanisms of toxic injury in the peripheral nervous system: neuropathologic considerations. *Toxicol Pathol*. 2000;28(1):54–69.

8. Miller MS, Spencer PS. The mechanisms of acrylamide axonopathy. *Annu Rev Pharmacol Toxicol*. 1985;25:643–666.

9. Kohler JJ, Lewis W. A brief overview of mechanisms of mitochondrial toxicity from NRTIs. *Environ Mol Mutagen*. 2007;48(3–4):166–172.

10. Silbergeld EK. Mechanisms of lead neurotoxicity, or looking beyond the lamppost. *FASEB J*. 1992;6(13):3201–3206.

11. Bressler J et al. Molecular mechanisms of lead neurotoxicity. *Neurochem Res*. 1999;24(4):595–600.

12. Landers JP, Bunce NJ. The Ah receptor and the mechanism of dioxin toxicity. *Biochem J*. 1991;276(pt 2):273–287.

13. Cavaletti G et al. Blood-nerve barrier of endoneural vessels in experimentally-induced hypothyroidism in rats. *Int J Tissue React*. 1989;11(3):137–142.

14. Bolton CF, Young GB. *Neurological Complications of Renal Disease*. Stoneham, MA: Butterworth-Heinemann; 1990.

15. Godel V, Nemet P, Lazar M. Chloramphenicol optic neuropathy. *Arch Ophthalmol*. 1980;98(8):1417–1421.

16. Jacknowitz A. Nitrofurantoin and peripheral neuropathy. *Ann Intern Med*. 1985;102(1):138 139.

17. Spring PJ, Sharpe DM, Hayes MW. Nitrofurantoin and peripheral neuropathy: a forgotten problem? *Med J Aust*. 2001;174(3):153–154.

18. Livermore DM. Linezolid in vitro: mechanism and antibacterial spectrum. *J Antimicrob Chemother*. 2003;51(suppl 2):ii9–ii16.

19. Dietze R et al. Early and extended early bactericidal activity of linezolid in pulmonary tuberculosis. *Am J Respir Crit Care Med*. 2008;178(11):1180–1185.

20. Rucker JC et al. Linezolid-associated toxic optic neuropathy. *Neurology*. 2006; 66(4):595–598.

21. Ferry T, et al. Possibly linezolid-induced peripheral and central neurotoxicity: report of four cases. *Infection*. 2005;33(3):151–154.

22. Fortun J et al. Linezolid for the treatment of multidrug-resistant tuberculosis. *J Antimicrob Chemother*. 2005;56(1):180–185.

23. Lee E et al. Linezolid-associated toxic optic neuropathy: a report of 2 cases. *Clin Infect Dis*. 2003;37(10):1389–1391.

24. Kulkarni K, Del Priore LV. Linezolid induced toxic optic neuropathy. *Br J Ophthalmol*. 2005;89:1664–1665.

25. French G. Safety and tolerability of linezolid. *J Antimicrob Chemother*. 2003;51(Suppl 2):ii45–ii53.

26. Dixon GJ, Roberts GB, Tyrrell WF. The relationship of neuropathy to the treatment of tuberculosis with isoniazid. *Scott Med J*. 1956;1(11):350–354.

27. Tugwell P, James SL. Peripheral neuropathy with ethambutol. *Postgrad Med J*. 1972;48(565):667–670.

28. Breen RA, Lipman MC, Johnson MA. Increased incidence of peripheral neuropathy with co-administration of stavudine and isoniazid in HIV-infected individuals. *AIDS*. 2000;14(5):615.

29. Goel UC et al. Isoniazid induced neuropathy in slow versus rapid acetylators: an electrophysiological study. *J Assoc Physicians India*. 1992;40(10):671–672.

30. Jacobs MB. HMG-CoA reductase inhibitor therapy and peripheral neuropathy. *Ann Intern Med*. 1994;120(11):970.

31. Ahmad S. Lovastatin and peripheral neuropathy. *Am Heart J*. 1995;130(6):1321.

32. Phan T et al. Peripheral neuropathy associated with simvastatin. *J Neurol Neurosurg Psychiatry*. 1995;58(5):625–628.

33. Lovastatin 5-year safety and efficacy study. Lovastatin Study Groups I through IV. *Arch Intern Med*. 1993;153(9):1079–1087.

34. Randomised trial of cholesterol lowering in 4444 patients with coronary heart disease: the Scandinavian Simvastatin Survival Study (4S). *Lancet*. 1994; 344(8934):1383–1389.

35. Shepherd J et al. Prevention of coronary heart disease with pravastatin in men with hypercholesterolemia. West of Scotland Coronary Prevention Study Group. *N Engl J Med*. 1995;333(20):1301–1307.

36. Sacks FM et al. The effect of pravastatin on coronary events after myocardial infarction in patients with average cholesterol levels. Cholesterol and

Recurrent Events Trial investigators. *N Engl J Med*. 1996;335(14):1001–1009.

37. MRC/BHF Heart Protection Study of cholesterol lowering with simvastatin in 20,536 high-risk individuals: a randomised placebo-controlled trial. *Lancet*. 2002;360(9326):7–22.

38. Gaist D et al. Are users of lipid-lowering drugs at increased risk of peripheral neuropathy? *Eur J Clin Pharmacol*. 2001;56(12):931–933.

39. Gaist D et al. Statins and risk of polyneuropathy: a case-control study. *Neurology*. 2002;58(9):1333–1337.

40. Davis TM et al. Lipid-lowering therapy and peripheral sensory neuropathy in type 2 diabetes: the Fremantle Diabetes Study. *Diabetologia*. 2008;51(4):562–566.

41. Schaumburg HH, Wisniewski HM, Spencer PS. Ultrastructural studies of the dying-back process. I. Peripheral nerve terminal and axon degeneration in systemic acrylamide intoxication. *J Neuropathol Exp Neurol*. 1974;33(2):260–284.

42. Miller MS, Spencer PS. Single doses of acrylamide reduce retrograde transport velocity. *J Neurochem*. 1984;43(5):1401–1408.

43. Gold BG, Griffin JW, Price DL. Slow axonal transport in acrylamide neuropathy: different abnormalities produced by single-dose and continuous administration. *J Neurosci*. 1985;5(7):1755–1768.

44. Ko MH, Chen WP, Hsieh ST. Neuropathology of skin denervation in acrylamide-induced neuropathy. *Neurobiol Dis*. 2002;11(1):155–165.

45. Last ghost of the Vietnam War. *The Globe and Mail*. July 12, 2008:1.

46. Cherniack MG. Toxicological screening for organophosphorus-induced delayed neurotoxicity: complications in toxicity testing. *Neurotoxicology*. 1988;9(2):249–271.

47. Moretto A, Lotti M. Poisoning by organophosphorus insecticides and sensory neuropathy. *J Neurol Neurosurg Psychiatry*. 1998;64(4):463–468.

48. Stokes L et al. Neurotoxicity among pesticide applicators exposed to organophosphates. *Occup Environ Med*. 1995;52(10):648–653.

49. Mattel CEO: "Rigorous standards" after massive toy recall. 2007. http://articles.cnn.com/2007-08-14/us/recall_1_polly-pocket-mattel-ceo-toys?_s=PM:US. Accessed November 26, 2011.

50. Rubens O et al. Peripheral neuropathy in chronic occupational inorganic lead exposure: a clinical and electrophysiological study. *J Neurol Neurosurg Psychiatry*. 2001;71(2):200–204.

51. Zhao G et al. Clinical manifestations and management of acute thallium poisoning. *Eur Neurol*. 2008;60(6):292–297.

52. Kuo HC et al. Acute painful neuropathy in thallium poisoning. *Neurology*. 2005;65(2):302–304.

53. Nordentoft T, Andersen EB, Mogensen PH. Initial sensorimotor and delayed autonomic neuropathy in acute thallium poisoning. *Neurotoxicology*. 1998;19(3):421–426.

54. Krishnan AV, Kiernan MC. Uremic neuropathy: clinical features and new pathophysiological insights. *Muscle Nerve*. 2007;35(3):273–290.

55. Di Giulio S et al. Parathormone as a nerve poison in uremia. *N Engl J Med*. 1978; 299(20):1134–1135.

56. Vanholder R et al. Uremic toxicity: the middle molecule hypothesis revisited. *Semin Nephrol*. 1994;14(3):205–218.

57. Dyck PJ et al. Segmental demyelination secondary to axonal degeneration in uremic neuropathy. *Mayo Clin Proc*. 1971;46(6):400–431.

58. Ginn HE et al. Clinical experience with small surface area dialyzers (SSAD). *Proc Clin Dial Transplant Forum*. 1971;1:53–60.

59. Oh SJ et al. Rapid improvement in nerve conduction velocity following renal transplantation. *Ann Neurol*. 1978;4(4):369–373.

60. Cooper DS. Clinical practice. Subclinical hypothyroidism. *N Engl J Med*. 2001;345(4):260–265.

61. Misiunas A et al. Peripheral neuropathy in subclinical hypothyroidism. *Thyroid*. 1995;5(4):283–286.

62. Bolton CF, Young GB, Zochodne DW. The neurological complications of sepsis. *Ann Neurol*. 1993;33(1):94–100.

63. Guarneri B, Bertolini G, Latronico N. Long-term outcome in patients with critical illness myopathy or neuropathy: the Italian multicentre CRIMYNE study. *J Neurol Neurosurg Psychiatry*. 2008;79(7):838–841.

64. Lacomis D, Petrella JT, Giuliani MJ. Causes of neuromuscular weakness in the intensive care unit: a study of ninety-two patients. *Muscle Nerve*. 1998;21(5):610–617.

65. Bolton CF. Neuromuscular manifestations of critical illness. *Muscle Nerve*. 2005;32(2):140–163.

66. Bolton CF. Neuromuscular complications of sepsis. *Intensive Care Med*. 1993;19(suppl 2):S58–S63.

67. de Letter MA et al. Risk factors for the development of polyneuropathy and myopathy in critically ill patients. *Crit Care Med*. 2001;29(12):2281–2286.

68. Zochodne DW, Bolton CF, Wells GA, Gilbert JJ, Hahn AF, Brown JD, Sibbald WA. Polyneuropathy in critical illness: pathological features. *Ann Neurol*. 1985;18(1):160.

69. Geller TJ et al. Vecuronium-associated axonal motor neuropathy: a variant of critical illness polyneuropathy? *Neuromuscul Disord.* 2001; 11(6–7):579–582.

70. Danon MJ, Carpenter S. Myopathy with thick filament (myosin) loss following prolonged paralysis with vecuronium during steroid treatment. *Muscle Nerve.* 1991;14(11): 1131–1139.

71. Cohn L et al. Carpal tunnel syndrome and gynaecomastia during growth hormone treatment of elderly men with low circulating IGF-I concentrations. *Clin Endocrinol (Oxford).* 1993;39(4):417–425.

72. Jamal GA et al. Generalised peripheral nerve dysfunction in acromegaly: a study by conventional and novel neurophysiological techniques. *J Neurol Neurosurg Psychiatry.* 1987;50(7): 886–894.

73. Dinn JJ, Dinn EI. *Natural history of acromegalic peripheral* neuropathy. *Q J Med.* 1985;57(224):833–842.

74. Ong BC et al. Bilateral carpal tunnel syndrome in a child on growth hormone replacement therapy: a case report. *Bull Hosp Joint Dis.* 2001;60(2):94–95.

75. Dickerman RD, Douglas JA, East JW. Bilateral median neuropathy and growth hormone use: a case report. *Arch Phys Med Rehabil.* 2000;81(12):1594–1595.

76. Cherry CL et al. Antiretroviral use and other risks for HIV-associated neuropathies in an international cohort. *Neurology.* 2006;66(6):867–873.

77. Nardin RA, Amick AN, Raynor EM. Vitamin B_{12} and methylmalonic acid levels in patients presenting with polyneuropathy. *Muscle Nerve.* 2007;36:532–535.

78. Schaumburg H et al. Sensory neuropathy from pyridoxine abuse. A new megavitamin syndrome. *N Engl J Med.* 1983;309(8):445–448.

79. Rutchik J. Toxic neuropathy treatment and management. Medscape from WebMD. 2001. http://emedicine.medscape.com/article/1175276-treatment. Accessed November 26, 2011.

25

Complementary and Alternative Medicine for Neuropathic Pain

JOHN M. MAYER AND SCOTT HALDEMAN

INTRODUCTION

Background

COMPLEMENTARY AND ALTERNATIVE medicine (CAM) is "a group of diverse medical and health care systems, practices, and products that are not generally considered to be part of conventional medicine."[1] The CAM interventions typically fall into the following categories:[1] (1) whole medical systems (e.g., traditional Chinese medicine including acupuncture, homeopathy, and Ayurveda), (2) mind-body medicine (e.g., yoga, meditation, prayer), (3) biologically based practices (e.g., herbs, foods, vitamin supplements), (4) manipulative and body-based practices (e.g., spinal manipulation, massage), and (5) energy medicine (e.g., biofield and bioelectromagnetic-based therapies such as Reiki, magnetic therapy, and electrical field stimulation).

The use of CAM by individuals with neuropathic pain appears to be widespread. In a 2004 survey,[2] 43% of patients with peripheral neuropathy indicated that they had used CAM therapies for this disorder. The most frequent reasons cited by patients for seeking CAM therapies included the following: neuropathic pain was insufficiently controlled (32%), prescription medications did not relieve the pain (22%), more control of their medical care was sought (21%), and excessive side effects with conventional treatments were experienced (12%).[2] Of the respondents, 48% used multiple CAM therapies, 35% used vitamins, 30% used magnetic therapy, 30% used acupuncture, 22% used herbal remedies, and 21% used chiropractic manipulation. However, despite the widespread use of CAM therapies by patients with neuropathic pain, there has been relatively little research into the effectiveness of the multiple treatment approaches used by the public to manage these complaints.

Purpose

Given that patients with neuropathic pain frequently seek CAM approaches for their condition, it is important for all stakeholders, including patients, clinicians, researchers, and third-party payers, to be informed of the available evidence for CAM therapies for neuropathic pain. The purpose of this chapter is to review and assess the current scientific literature that has been published on the effectiveness of the common CAM therapies being used by the public for the treatment of neuropathic pain.

Description of Interventions

Considering the diversity of CAM therapies, it is not possible to discuss all of them in one short chapter. The interventions that were selected for this review are those that appear to be used frequently by patients with neuropathic pain, have some published controlled clinical trials evaluating their effectiveness, or have a compelling proposed mechanism of action. The following therapies fulfill these criteria and are the focus of this chapter: acupuncture, alpha-lipoic acid (ALA), B vitamins, manipulation, transcutaneous electrical nerve stimulation (TENS), and transcranial magnetic stimulation (TMS).

ACUPUNCTURE

Acupuncture involves stimulation of anatomical points through penetration of the skin with solid metallic needles that are manually or electrically manipulated.[3] Acupuncture originated in China more than 2000 years ago and has many different styles with distinct characteristics. In traditional Chinese medicine, acupuncture is based on the belief that health is maintained by a balance of vital energy (*Qi*). Needles are applied along vital energy pathways in the body (meridians) with associated acupuncture points in order to achieve balance in the flow of *Qi* within the body.[4] In Western medicine, there are several theories about acupuncture's mechanism of action regarding

pain inhibition, but the specific mechanism remains uncertain.[3]

ALPHA-LIPOIC ACID

Alpha-lipoic acid is a natural compound that is found in high concentrations in animal organs, such as heart, liver, and kidney.[5] Alpha-lipoic acid (also known as *thioctic acid*) is administered orally as a dietary supplement or by injection as a regulated drug. It is a strong antioxidant and is used for various conditions linked to oxidative stress, such as nerve degeneration, cataracts, human immune deficiency virus (HIV), and radiation injury. The proposed mechanism of action of ALA for pain relief centers on its ability to prevent oxidative damage to cell membranes, reduce deficits in blood flow and nerve conduction, and reduce lipid peroxidation.[5]

B VITAMINS

The B vitamins are a group of water-soluble vitamins including thiamine (B_1), riboflavin (B_2), nicotinic acid (B_3), pantothenic acid (B_5), pyridoxine (B_6), biotin (B_7), folic acid (B_9), cyanocobalamin (B_{12}), para-aminobenzoic acid, inositol, and choline.[6] B vitamins are administered orally as dietary supplements or by injection as regulated drugs. The B vitamins function as coenzymes in various pathways for energy metabolism and blood cell formation. The mechanism of action of B vitamins in pain management is unclear; one proposed mechanism is that nerve tissue is vulnerable to deficiencies in B vitamins due to this tissue's high energy requirements.[6]

MANIPULATION

The manual therapies, which include manipulation and mobilization applied to bony articulations, as well as soft tissue treatment approaches such as massage, have been the cornerstone of treatment for pain in most societies throughout the world before the pharmacological and interventional therapies were considered. References to manual therapies can be seen in writings from ancient China, India, and many European cultures, and references to their use can be found in the writings of Hippocrates and Galen.[7,8] Chiropractors currently administer the majority of manipulative therapies in the United States.[9] Most people seeking the care of a chiropractor do so for the management of back pain, neck pain, and headaches, while some patients seek care for symptoms of lumbar or cervical radiculopathy, and a few seek care for pain in the upper or lower extremities.[10] Manipulative therapies are also offered by a number of medical physicians, osteopathic physicians, and physical therapists who have taken advanced courses in these procedures.

There are two main subtypes of manual therapies applied to bony articulations: manipulation—which involves the application of a high-velocity, low-amplitude manual thrust to a joint slightly beyond the joint's passive range of motion—and mobilization— which involves the application of a manual force to a joint without a thrust and within a joint's passive range of motion.[11] Proposed mechanisms of action are that manipulation alters the position of anatomical structures, releases trapped structures, disrupts tissue adhesions, and impacts primary afferent neurons from paraspinal tissues to improve motor control and pain processing.[11]

TRANSCUTANEOUS ELECTRICAL NERVE STIMULATION

Transcutaneous electrical nerve stimulation is a therapeutic modality that delivers electrical current through surface electrodes placed on the skin over painful areas.[12] It is administered by various health care providers and is often prescribed for home use. Subtypes of TENS are typically classified by the frequency of current delivered; low frequency is defined as 5–10 Hz and high frequency is defined as 80–100 Hz. Low-frequency TENS produces muscle contraction and purportedly results in longer-term pain reduction, while high-frequency TENS acts as a counterirritant to temporarily block pain.[12]

TRANSCUTANEOUS MAGNETIC STIMULATION

Transcutaneous magnetic stimulation is a non-invasive modality that uses an electric coil to produce a magnetic pulse.[13] When positioned appropriately on the surface of the head, this magnetic pulse is transferred to the cortex of the brain. Typically, TMS is administered in outpatient settings via multiple 20-minute sessions of repetitive sequences of pulses. Subtypes include fast TMS, which is delivered at frequencies greater than 5 Hz, and slow TMS, which is delivered at frequencies less than 1 Hz. Possible mechanisms of action for this modality's ability to provide pain relief are that fast TMS causes cortical excitability and slow TMS induces neural inhibition.[13]

METHODS

Search Strategy

A systematic search of the literature was carried out using the search strategy and analysis procedures described in this section.

INCLUSION CRITERIA

Inclusion criteria were as follows:

• Patients: Adults with neuropathic pain originating from peripheral or central mechanisms. Conditions with unclear origins of pain or pain originating from both neuropathic and nociceptive mechanisms (e.g., complex regional pain syndrome, fibromyalgia, failed back surgery syndrome) were excluded.
• Interventions: Acupuncture, ALA, B vitamins, manipulation, TENS, TMS.
• Comparators: Any control group that did not receive the interventions listed above or that allowed for comparison of the efficacy of different types of these interventions.
• Outcomes: Patient reported outcomes including pain or pain combined with other symptoms (referred to below as *global symptoms*).
• Study design: Randomized clinical trials (RCTs) and systematic reviews.
• Published between January 1, 1990, and July 31, 2009. Randomized clinical trials with publication dates prior to 1990 found in applicable systematic reviews were deemed eligible if they met the other inclusion criteria.
• Published in English.

- Published data only.
- Independent effects of intervention can be determined from data.
- If there are mixed indications, specific data and analyses for subjects with neuropathic pain are available.
- Data are available for outcomes at least 24 hours after the first treatment (no immediate effects).
- Between-subject group comparisons of clinical outcomes are available.
- Abstracts are available for screening.

DATABASES SEARCHED

Randomized clinical trials and systematic reviews were identified through electronic searches of MEDLINE, CINAHL, and EMBASE in August 2009 through a search strategy developed by the authors (SH, JM) with assistance from medical librarians (AH, KM, JO; see the Acknowledgments). Systematic reviews were screened by one author (JM) for additional RCTs.

STUDY SELECTION

Search results were initially screened by the medical librarians (AH, KM, JO) to remove duplicates and non-English publications. One author (JM) subsequently screened the remaining articles according to the inclusion criteria. Full-text articles were retrieved for all citations deemed relevant or of uncertain relevance to confirm their eligibility.

DATA ABSTRACTION AND ANALYSIS

The data were abstracted and summarized from the eligible RCTs by one author (JM) and a research coordinator and were verified by the other author (SH). Both authors then reviewed the data together until a consensus was achieved on the validity and conclusions that could be reached from these studies.

RESULTS

Search

The initial search resulted in 1012 citations. The subsequent screening of systematic reviews uncovered three additional citations. Thirty RCTs enrolling a total of 3217 cases were found to be eligible. Details of the 30 eligible RCTs are found in Tables 25-1–25-5 (study descriptions), Tables 25-6–25-10 (clinical outcomes), and Table 25-11 (harms). Highlights of pertinent findings categorized according to peripheral, central, and mixed central and peripheral neuropathic pain are discussed in this section.

Peripheral Neuropathic Pain

Twenty-seven RCTs, which enrolled a total of 3053 cases, were uncovered for peripheral neuropathic pain, including three RCTs with 571 cases for acupuncture,[14-16] one RCT with 90 cases for acupuncture and B vitamins,[17] six RCTs with 1158 cases for ALA,[18-23] one RCT with 112 cases for ALA and B vitamins,[24] six RCTs with 433 cases for B vitamins,[25-30] five RCTs with 551 cases for manipulation,[31-35] four RCTs with 114 cases for TENS,[36-39] and in one RCT with 24 cases for TMS.[40] Details of these of these studies are discussed below.

DIABETIC NEUROPATHY (TABLES 25.1 AND 25.6)

Thirteen RCTs with 1576 cases were uncovered for neuropathic pain associated with diabetic neuropathy.[17-22,25-27,29,37-39] A 2007 systematic review on ALA for diabetic neuropathy was found,[5] which included four RCTs that met our inclusion criteria for neuropathic pain associated with diabetic neuropathy.[18,19,21,22] Our search uncovered an additional RCT.[20] Four of these studies assessed short-term outcomes. In a 3-week study that compared three doses of intravenous ALA and placebo, significant pain relief and improvements in total symptoms were noted in the 1200 mg and 600 mg dose groups of ALA, but not in the 100 mg dose group, compared with placebo.[22] In two other 3-week trials, oral administration[19] and intravenous administration[18] of 600 mg ALA were found to be superior to placebo for short-term pain relief and improvements in global symptoms and physical function. In a 5-week trial, three doses (600, 1200, and 1800 mg) of ALA were found to be superior to placebo in terms

Table 25-1. Study Descriptions: Peripheral Neuropathic Pain—Diabetic Neuropathy

REFERENCE	CONDITION NEUROPATHIC SYMPTOM DURATION POPULATION AGE	INCLUSION CRITERIA EXCLUSION CRITERIA	EXPERIMENTAL GROUP: INTERVENTION NO. OF SESSIONS (OR DOSE) TREATMENT DURATION PROVIDER SAMPLE SIZE	CONTROL GROUP 1: INTERVENTION NO. OF SESSIONS (OR DOSE) TREATMENT DURATION PROVIDER SAMPLE SIZE	CONTROL GROUP 2: INTERVENTION NO. OF SESSIONS (OR DOSE) TREATMENT DURATION PROVIDER SAMPLE SIZE
			ACUPUNCTURE AND B VITAMINS		
Jiang, 2006[17]	Diabetic neuropathy 6 months–12 years Patients from university hospitals 62.5 ± 8.6 years (46–80 years)	Inc: type 2 diabetes, peripheral neuropathy (undefined) Exc: unclear	Acupuncture-needle: wrist-ankle: bilateral upper two and lower two points and symptomatic points, 15–30 minutes 1 session/day 21 days DOM $n = 30$	Acupuncture-needle: body – local points and symptomatic points, 15–30 minutes 1 session/day 21 days DOM $n = 30$	Intramuscular injection of thiamine/B_1 & cobalamin/B_{12} 1 injection/day 21 day DOM $n = 30$
			B VITAMINS		
Abbas, 1997[25]	Diabetic neuropathy Unclear Patients from a national hospital Unclear	Inc: diabetes, peripheral neuropathy defined by various signs and symptoms Exc: history of CNS disease, pregnant	B vitamin complex (high dose) (thiamine/B_1, pyridoxine/B_6) high dose: oral Day 1-3: B_1 50 mg, B6 100 mg; days 4–28: B_1 25 mg, B_6 50 mg 28 days Unclear $n = 100$	B vitamin complex (low dose) (thiamine/B_1, pyridoxine/B_6) low dose: oral days 1-3: B_1 2 mg, B_6 2 mg; days 4–28: B_1 1 mg, B_6 1 mg 28 days Unclear $n = 100$	—

Study	Population	Intervention	Comparison	Comparison 2
Levin, 1981[26]	Diabetic neuropathy 3.1 ± 1.0 years Patients from a veterans' hospital 56.1 ± 3.4 years (43–71 years)	Inc: diabetes, clinical signs compatible with peripheral neuropathy Exc: unclear	Pyridoxine/B$_6$: oral 50 mg/3x/day (150 mg/day) 4 months Unclear $n = 9$	Placebo: oral $n = 9$	—
Winkler, 1999[27]	Diabetic peripheral neuropathy >1 year Unclear 56.7 ± 7.3 years (40–70 years)	Inc: diabetes, painful symptoms >1 year, McGill pain ≥7, vibration sensation ≤ 6 Exc: unclear	B vitamin complex (high dose) (thiamine/B$_1$, pyridoxine/B$_6$, cyano-cobalamin/B$_{12}$) high dose: oral daily dose: B$_1$ 320 mg, B$_6$ 720 mg, B$_{12}$ 2 mg 6 weeks Unclear $n = 12$	B vitamin complex (high dose) (thiamine/ B$_1$, pyridoxine/B$_6$, cyano-cobalamin/B$_{12}$) low dose: oral daily dose: B$_1$ 120 mg, B$_6$ 270 mg, B$_{12}$ 750 µg 6 weeks Unclear $n = 12$	Thiamine/B$_1$: oral 150 mg/day 6 weeks Unclear $n = 12$
Yaqub, 1992[29]	Diabetic neuropathy Unclear 53.2 years	Inc: diabetes (duration 5–20 years), peripheral neuropathy defined by various signs and symptoms Exc: other medications for neuropathy, renal failure, hereditary motor sensory polyneuropathy, lymphoma	Methylcobalamin/B$_{12}$: oral, 500 mg, 3x/day 4 months Unclear $n = 21$	Placebo: oral $n = 22$	—

(continued)

Table 25-1. (continued)

REFERENCE	CONDITION / NEUROPATHIC SYMPTOM DURATION / POPULATION / AGE	INCLUSION CRITERIA / EXCLUSION CRITERIA	EXPERIMENTAL GROUP: INTERVENTION / NO. OF SESSIONS (OR DOSE) / TREATMENT DURATION / PROVIDER / SAMPLE SIZE	CONTROL GROUP 1: INTERVENTION NO. OF SESSIONS (OR DOSE) / TREATMENT DURATION / PROVIDER / SAMPLE SIZE	CONTROL GROUP 2: INTERVENTION NO. OF SESSIONS (OR DOSE) / TREATMENT DURATION / PROVIDER / SAMPLE SIZE
			ALA		
Ametov, 2003[18]	Diabetic neuropathy 3.6 years Unclear 56.1 ± 9.2 years (18–74 years)	Inc: diabetes, TSS ≥7.5, NIS ≥2, nerve conduction or heart pulse deep breathing abnormality Exc: confounding neurological disease or neuropathy, peripheral vascular disease, complicating cardiac, pulmonary, gastrointestinal, hematological, or endocrine disease, malignancy	ALA: intravenous, 600 mg over 30 minutes 14 treatments 3 weeks MD n = 60	Placebo: intravenous n = 60	—
Ruhnau, 1999[19]	Diabetic neuropathy 4.0 ± 1.7 years Patients from a university hospital 61.3 ± 5.7 years (18–70 years)	Inc: diabetes, clinical evidence of distal polyneuropathy, moderate-severe symptoms in feet Exc: severe neuropathy, peripheral vascular disease, causes of neuropathy other than diabetes, medications and supplements likely to interfere with results, severe concomitant disease, pregnant, lactation	ALA: oral 600 mg, 3x/day (1800 mg/day) 19 days Unclear n = 12	Placebo: oral n = 12	—

Ziegler, 1995[22]	Diabetic neuropathy 3.1 ± 3.3 years Unclear 58.9 ± 7.8 years (18–70 years)	Inc: diabetes, clinical evidence of distal neuropathy, moderate-severe symptoms in feet Exc: severe neuropathy, peripheral vascular disease, causes of neuropathy other than diabetes, medications and supplements likely to interfere with results, severe concomitant disease, pregnant, lactation	ALA: 1200mg: intravenous 1200 mg/day 14 treatments 3 weeks MD $n = 65$	ALA: 600mg: intravenous 600 mg/day 14 treatments 3 weeks MD $n = 63$	Con 2: ALA: 100 mg: intravenous 100 mg/day 14 treatments 3 weeks MD $n = 66$ Con 3: placebo: intravenous $n = 66$
Ziegler, 1999[21]	Diabetic neuropathy 3.1 ± 3.0 years Patients from outpatient medical centers 56.9 ± 6.3 years (18–65 years)	Inc: diabetes, clinical evidence of symmetric distal neuropathy, TSS ≥4, NIS-LL ≥2 Exc: asymmetric neuropathy of trunk and proximal lower limb, foot ulcer, peripheral vascular disease, myopathy, causes of neuropathy other than diabetes, antioxidants or B vitamins within 1 month of study, severe concomitant disease, pregnant, lactation	ALA: intravenous+oral weeks 1–3: intravenous 600 mg/day, 14 treatments week 4–month 7: oral 600mg, 3x/day (1800 mg/day) 7 months MD $n = 167$	ALA: intravenous weeks 1–3: intravenous 600 mg/day, 14 treatments week 4–month 7: oral placebo 7 months MD $n = 174$	Placebo: intravenous+oral $n = 168$

(continued)

Table 25-1. (continued)

REFERENCE	CONDITION NEUROPATHIC SYMPTOM DURATION POPULATION AGE	INCLUSION CRITERIA EXCLUSION CRITERIA	EXPERIMENTAL GROUP: INTERVENTION NO. OF SESSIONS (OR DOSE) TREATMENT DURATION PROVIDER SAMPLE SIZE	CONTROL GROUP 1: INTERVENTION NO. OF SESSIONS (OR DOSE) TREATMENT DURATION PROVIDER SAMPLE SIZE	CONTROL GROUP 2: INTERVENTION NO. OF SESSIONS (OR DOSE) TREATMENT DURATION PROVIDER SAMPLE SIZE
Ziegler, 2006[20]	Diabetic neuropathy 4.9 ± 3.5 years Patients from outpatient medical centers 57.8 ± 11.0 years (18–74 years)	Inc: diabetes, TSS >7.5, NIS ≥2, pain sensation decreased or absent Exc: confounding neurological, neuropathy, myopathy, peripheral vascular disease, hepatic or renal disease, antioxidant or penoxyphylline therapy within 3 months, ALA or linolenic acid use within 3 months	ALA: 1800 mg: oral 1800 mg/day 5 weeks MD n = 46	ALA: 1200mg: oral 1200 mg/day 5 weeks MD n = 47	Con 2: ALA: 600 mg: oral 600 mg/day 5 weeks MD n = 45 Con 3: placebo: oral n = 43
			TENS		
Kumar, 1997[38]	Diabetic neuropathy 19 ± 6 months Unclear 56 ± 4 years (31–70 years)	Inc: diabetes, painful neuropathic symptoms in lower extremity >2 months Exc: vascular insufficiency in lower extremity, uncontrolled angina pectoris, cardiac arrhythmia, congestive heart failure, myocardial infarction within 6 months, hypertension,	TENS: leg 2–70 Hz, 25–35 V 30 minutes 1 session/day 4 weeks Unclear n = 18	Sham TENS n = 13	—

Study	Population	Inclusion/Exclusion	Intervention	Comparison
Kumar, 1998[37]	Diabetic neuropathy; 22 ± 6 months; Unclear; 59 ± 3 years (31–70 years)	Inc: diabetes, painful neuropathic symptoms in lower extremity >2 months, failed 4 weeks of amitriptiline, neurological deficit in lower extremities, pain >2; Exc: vascular insufficiency in lower extremity, uncontrolled angina pectoris, cardiac arrhythmia, congestive heart failure, myocardial infarction within 6 months, hypertension, cerebrovascular ischemia, psychiatric disease, substance abuse, renal or liver disease, current use of corticosteroids, dilantin, chemotherapy drugs	TENS+amitriptiline; TENS: leg; 2–70 Hz, ≤35 V; 30 minutes; 1 session/day; Amitripyline: 50 mg/day; 12 weeks; DPM; $n = 14$	Sham TENS+ amitriptiline; $n = 9$
Reichstein, 2005[39]	Diabetic Neuropathy; Unclear; Unclear; 61.0 ± 12.6	Inc: diabetes, HbA1c <11%, polyneuropathy; Exc: concurrent ALA, tricyclic antidepressants, anticonvulsants, ulcers, amputations caused by ischemia, malignancy	TENS; 180 Hz, ≤35 V; 30 minutes/session; 1 session/day; 3 days; Unclear; $n = 21$	Electrical muscle simulation; 4096 Hz, ≤70 V; 1 session/day; 3 days; Unclear; $n = 20$

Note: The list of abbreviations for all tables appears at the end of Table 25.12.

improvements in global symptoms but not in terms of improvements in physical function.[20]

One study assessed the longer-term efficacy of ALA for neuropathic pain associated with diabetic neuropathy. In a 7-month trial, 3 weeks of intravenous ALA (600 mg) followed by 6 months of oral ALA (600 mg) was compared with 3 weeks of intravenous ALA (600 mg) followed by 6 months of oral placebo and intravenous and oral placebo.[21] At 7 months, improvements in global symptoms and physical function were noted in all groups, and there were no differences among the groups.

A 2009 Cochrane systematic review on B vitamins for peripheral neuropathy was found,[6] which included four RCTs on neuropathic pain associated with diabetic neuropathy that met our inclusion criteria.[25-27,29] Our search uncovered an additional RCT.[17] Oral B vitamin supplementation was found to be less effective than needle acupuncture[17] and equivalent to oral placebo[26,29] on the basis of short-term improvements in global symptoms. High-dose oral B vitamin complex was found to be superior to low-dose oral B vitamin complex on the basis of short-term improvements in global symptoms in one study,[25] but no difference in short-term pain relief was found between the doses in another study.[27]

Three RCTs on TENs for neuropathic pain associated with diabetic neuropathy were uncovered that assessed short-term outcomes.[37-39] In a 4-week trial, pulsed modulating frequency TENS was shown to be more effective than sham TENS on the basis of pain relief and improvements in global symptoms.[38] In a 12-week trial, oral amitriptyline combined with pulsed modulating frequency TENS applied to the lower extremity was more effective than amitriptyline combined with sham TENS in terms of pain relief and improvements in global symptoms.[37] In a 3-day trial, electrical muscle stimulation was found to be more effective than high-frequency TENS on the basis of improvements in global symptoms.[39]

CARPAL TUNNEL SYNDROME (TABLES 25.2 AND 25.7)

Five RCTs with 338 cases were uncovered for neuropathic pain associated with carpal tunnel syndrome (CTS).[16,24,30,31,34] A 2007 systematic review[41] on conservative treatment of CTS identified two RCTs published prior to May 2006 that fit our inclusion criteria,[30,34] while our search uncovered three more recent RCTs.[16,24,31] No RCTs were found on TENS or TMS for CTS. No RCTs were found for any of the other peripheral entrapment neuropathies that met our inclusion criteria.

A recent RCT on CTS compared the efficacy of needle acupuncture applied to fixed points on the affected upper extremity with oral corticosteroids over a 4-week intervention period.[16] At 2 weeks and 4 weeks of follow-up, improvements in global symptoms were noted in both groups and there was no difference between the groups.

One RCT on B vitamins for CTS compared oral vitamin B$_6$ (pyridoxine) with oral placebo and/or no treatment for 12 weeks.[30] At follow-up, no differences in pain relief or improvements in physical function were noted between the experimental and control groups. Another RCT compared an oral B vitamin complex supplement with an oral multisupplement containing ALA, GLA, B vitamins, and other vitamins and minerals.[24] At 90 days of follow-up, improvements in global symptoms and physical function were greater in the multisupplement group compared with the B vitamin complex group.

In one RCT on manipulation for CTS, chiropractic treatment using soft tissue and bony manipulation of the neck and upper extremity was compared with ibuprofen and wrist supports.[34] Another RCT on manipulation for CTS compared two different upper extremity manipulative techniques.[31] In both of these RCTs, pain relief and improvements in physical function were noted in the experimental and control groups, but there were no significant differences in outcomes between the groups.

LUMBAR RADICULOPATHY AND/OR SCIATICA (TABLES 25.3 AND 25.8)

Five RCTs with 617 cases were uncovered for neuropathic pain associated with lumbar radiculopathy and/or sciatica.[15,23,32,33,35] The most comprehensive and recent systematic review of conservative treatments for lumbosacral radiculopathy was published in 2007.[42] This

Table 25-2. Study Descriptions: Peripheral Neuropathic Pain—CTS

REFERENCE	CONDITION NEUROPATHIC SYMPTOM DURATION POPULATION AGE	INCLUSION CRITERIA EXCLUSION CRITERIA	EXPERIMENTAL GROUP: INTERVENTION NO. OF SESSIONS (OR DOSE) TREATMENT DURATION PROVIDER SAMPLE SIZE	CONTROL GROUP 1: INTERVENTION NO. OF SESSIONS (OR DOSE) TREATMENT DURATION PROVIDER SAMPLE SIZE	CONTROL GROUP 2: INTERVENTION NO. OF SESSIONS (OR DOSE) TREATMENT DURATION PROVIDER SAMPLE SIZE
			ACUPUNCTURE		
Yang, 2009[16]	CTS 7.7 ± 3.5 months Unclear 49.6 ± 9.6 years (18–85 years)	Inc: electrodiagnostic confirmation of CTS based on median nerve sensory and motor latencies Exc: unclear	Acupuncture-needle: fixed acupuncture points on affected upper extremity, 30 minutes 8 sessions (2x/week) 4 weeks MD $n = 38$	Corticosteroid - prednisolone: oral 10–20 mg/day 4 weeks MD $n = 39$	—
			ALA AND B VITAMINS		
DiGeronimo, 2009[24]	CTS Unclear Unclear 50.2 years (18–85 years)	Inc: CTS confirmed by clinical signs and median nerve sensory and motor latencies Exc: unclear	Multisupplement: oral, ALA 300 mg, GLA 180 mg, selenium 25 mcg, Vit E 7.5 mg, B_1 1.05 mg, B_2 1.2 mg, B_5 4.5 mg, B_6 1.5 mg (total daily dose) 90 days Unclear $n = 56$	Vitamin B complex: oral, B_1 100 mg, B_6 150 mg, B_{12} 500 mcg (total daily dose) 90 days Unclear $n = 56$	—

(continued)

Table 25-2. (continued)

REFERENCE CONDITION NEUROPATHIC SYMPTOM DURATION POPULATION AGE	INCLUSION CRITERIA EXCLUSION CRITERIA	EXPERIMENTAL GROUP: INTERVENTION NO. OF SESSIONS (OR DOSE) TREATMENT DURATION PROVIDER SAMPLE SIZE	CONTROL GROUP 1: INTERVENTION NO. OF SESSIONS (OR DOSE) TREATMENT DURATION PROVIDER SAMPLE SIZE	CONTROL GROUP 2: INTERVENTION NO. OF SESSIONS (OR DOSE) TREATMENT DURATION PROVIDER SAMPLE SIZE
		B VITAMINS		
Spooner, 1993[30] CTS Unclear Patients from an outpatient university medical center 42.5 years (18–76 years)	Inc: CTS confirmed by clinical signs and median nerve sensory and motor latencies Exc: pregnant, trauma to forearm, history of alcoholism, diabetes, hypothyroidism, rheumatoid arthritis	Pyridoxine/B_6: oral, 200 mg/day 12 weeks Unclear $n = 16$	Placebo: oral $n = 16$	—

Burke, 2007[31]	CTS Unclear Patients from an outpatient medical rehabilitation center 41.6 ± 14.1 years	Inc: electrodiagnostic confirmation of CTS based on median nerve sensory and motor latencies Exc: age >50 years, surgery or injection for CTS, wrist trauma, systemic causes of symptoms, rheumatoid arthritis, litigation	Manipulation-MOB: upper extremity, home exercise, ice 1–2 sessions/week 6 weeks DC $n = 14$	Manipulation-instrument assisted: upper extremity, home exercise, ice 1–2 sessions/week 6 weeks DC $n = 12$	—
Davis, 1998[34]	CTS Unclear Patients from an outpatient medical rehabilitation center 37 ± 6 years (21–45 years)	Inc: electrodiagnostic confirmation of CTS based on median nerve sensory and motor latencies Exc: current treatment for CTS, NSAIDs, litigation, pregnant, B_6 use, systemic disorder, use of wrist brace, evidence of median nerve axonal degeneration	Manipulation-HVLA: upper extremity, cervical spine, ultrasound, massage, wrist supports 1–3 sessions/week 9 weeks DC $n = 46$	Ibuprofen, 800 mg 1–3x/day wrist supports 7 weeks MD $n = 45$	—

Note: The list of abbreviations for all tables appears at the end of Table 25.12.

Table 25-3. Study Descriptions: Peripheral Neuropathic Pain—Lumbar Radiculopathy and/or Sciatica

REFERENCE	CONDITION NEUROPATHIC SYMPTOM DURATION POPULATION AGE	INCLUSION CRITERIA EXCLUSION CRITERIA	EXPERIMENTAL GROUP: INTERVENTION NO. OF SESSIONS (OR DOSE) TREATMENT DURATION PROVIDER SAMPLE SIZE	CONTROL GROUP 1: INTERVENTION NO. OF SESSIONS (OR DOSE) TREATMENT DURATION PROVIDER SAMPLE SIZE	CONTROL GROUP 2: INTERVENTION NO. OF SESSIONS (OR DOSE) TREATMENT DURATION PROVIDER SAMPLE SIZE
ACUPUNCTURE					
Hollisaz, 2007[15]	Lumbar radiculopathy/ sciatica >6 months Patients from outpatient neurosurgery and orthopedic centers 21–50 years	Inc: LBP with confirmed sciatic origin of pain Exc: surgical indication, contraindication to acupuncture (e.g., systemic disease, prosthesis, cutaneous disorder, coagulation disorder)	Acupuncture-electro: 10–15 needles into painful and suitable points, 20 minutes 9.2 sessions Unclear MD $n = 41$	Physiotherapy: heat, ultrasound, muscle stimulation, diathermy 11.7 sessions Unclear MD $n = 38$	Sham acupuncture 8.1 sessions Unclear MD $n = 40$
ALA					
Memeo, 2008[23]	Lumbar radiculopathy/ sciatica ≤6 weeks Patients from a municipal hospital 61 years (29–85 years)	Inc: low back pain with sciatica. Sciatica confirmed with various clinical signs and symptoms, EMG, and MRI findings Exc: severe cognitive or psychological disturbances, treatment with chemotherapy, immunosuppressants, corticosteroids, NSAIDs, antiepileptics, or thioridazine drugs	ALA: oral 600 mg/day 60 days Unclear $n = 31$	Acetyl-L-carnitine: oral 1180 mg/day 60 days Unclear $n = 33$	—

		Intervention	Comparison	
Burton, 2000[32]	Lumbar radiculopathy/ sciatica 7.3 ± 8.2 months Patients from inpatient orthopaedic clinic 41.9 ± 10.6 years (18–60 years)	Inc: sciatica, slr +, imaging evidence of single-level, nonsequestered disc herniation Exc: sequestered disc herniation, multilevel, marked lumbar spine DJD, lumbar surgery, previous chemonucleolysis or SMT, active litigation	Manipulation-HVLA and MOB: lumbar spine, massage Unclear 12 weeks DO n = 20	Intradiscal injection with chymopapain 1 NA MD n = 20	—
Coxhead, 1981[33]	Lumbar radiculopathy/ sciatica 3.4 ± 3.8 months Patients from an outpatient physiotherapy center 41.9 ± 12.2 years	Inc: sciatica Exc: red flags for serious pathologies, lumbar surgery, pregnant, sacroiliac disease, vertebral fracture	*Factorial design* manipulation - undefined: lumbar spine, exercise, traction, corset Unclear 4 weeks Unclear n = 155	Exercise, traction, corset Unclear 4 weeks Unclear n = 137	—
Santilli, 2006[35]	Lumbar radiculopathy/ sciatica <10 days Patients from outpatient medical rehabilitation centers 18–65 years	Inc: LBP ≥5/10 with leg pain ≥5/10, MRI evidence of lumbar disc protrusion Exc: BMI >30, diabetic neuropathy, herniated disc, chronic LBP, leg length difference >1.5 cm, lumbar scoliosis >20°, surgical lesion, osteopenia, osteoporosis, previous SMT, spinal surgery, spondylolisthesis	manipulation-HVLA: lumbar spine up to 20 sessions 30 days DC n = 53	Sham SMT up to 20 sessions 30 days DC n = 49	—

Note: The list of abbreviations for all tables appears at the end of Table 25.12.

Table 25-4. Study Descriptions: Peripheral Neuropathic Pain—Other

REFERENCE	CONDITION / NEUROPATHIC / SYMPTOM DURATION / POPULATION / AGE / INCLUSION CRITERIA / EXCLUSION CRITERIA	EXPERIMENTAL GROUP: INTERVENTION / NO. OF SESSIONS (OR DOSE) / TREATMENT DURATION / PROVIDER / SAMPLE SIZE	CONTROL GROUP 1: INTERVENTION / NO. OF SESSIONS (OR DOSE) / TREATMENT DURATION / PROVIDER / SAMPLE SIZE	CONTROL GROUP 2: INTERVENTION / NO. OF SESSIONS (OR DOSE) / TREATMENT DURATION / PROVIDER / SAMPLE SIZE
		ACUPUNCTURE		
Shlay, 1998[14]	HIV neuropathy Unclear Patients from an outpatient medical center 40.7 ± 7.0 years Inc: HIV+, peripheral neuropathy (lower extremity) Exc: acute infection, malignancy, pregnant, current use of antidepressant medication	*Factorial design* Acupuncture-needle: various traditional points, 15–25 minutes 1–2x/week 14 weeks LAC $n = 121$	Sham acupuncture $n = 118$	Con 2: amitriptyline - oral 25–75 mg/day 14 weeks MD $n = 71$ Con 3: placebo - oral $n = 65$
		B VITAMINS		
Woelk, 1998[28]	Alcoholic peripheral neuropathy ≤ 8 years Unclear Patients from outpatient medical centers 56.6 years (30–70 years) Inc: alcoholism as defined by DSM-III-R, marked polyneuropathy defined by great toe vibratory perception threshold ≤ 2, pain ≤ 2, sensory ≤ 3 Exc: allergies to study drugs, diabetes, toxic neuropathy, Parkinson's disease, psychiatric disorder, pregnant, neurological or endocrine disorders, collagenosis, skin lesions at assessment site, vitamin replacement therapy, drug dependency	Thiamine/B_1: oral, weeks 1–4: 320 mg/day, weeks 5–8: 120 mg/day 8 weeks MD $n = 34$	B vitamin complex (thiamine/B_1, pyridoxine/ B_6, methylcobalamin/ B_{12}): oral, weeks 1–4: 320 B_1, 720 mg B_6, 2 mg B_{12}; weeks 5–8: 120 mg B_1, 270 mg B_6, 0.75 mg B_{12} 8 weeks MD $n = 35$	Placebo: oral $n = 35$

		TENS		
Cheing, 2005[36]	Peripheral neuropathy (various)	Inc: hypersensitive hands due to peripheral nerve injury	TENS: hand continuous, 100 Hz,	Sham TENS	—
	4.7 ± 0.9 weeks	Exc: causalgia, shoulder-arm	20 minutes	$n = 9$	
	Patients from a	syndrome, previous TENS,	10 sessions		
	hospital	pacemaker, sensory loss in hands	2 weeks		
	35 ± 12 years		Unclear		
			$n = 10$		

		TMS		
Khedr, 2005[40]	Trigeminal neuralgia	Inc: trigeminal neuralgia based on	TMS: 20 Hz, 80%	Sham TMS	—
	3.3 ± 2.9 years	IASP criteria, unilateral pain	resting motor threshold,	$n = 12$	
	Patients from a	Exc: intracranial metallic device,	200 pulses/minute		
	university hosp:tal	pacemaker, extensive myocardial	10 minutes/session		
	51.5 ± 10.7 years	ischemia, epilepsy	1 session/day		
			5 days		
			MD		
			$n = 12$		

Note: The list of abbreviations for all tables appears at the end of Table 25.12.

Table 25-5. Study Descriptions: Central Neuropathic Pain and Mixed Central/Peripheral Neuropathic Pain

REFERENCE	CONDITION NEUROPATHIC SYMPTOM DURATION POPULATION AGE	INCLUSION CRITERIA EXCLUSION CRITERIA	EXPERIMENTAL GROUP: INTERVENTION NO. OF SESSIONS (OR DOSE) TREATMENT DURATION PROVIDER SAMPLE SIZE	CONTROL GROUP 1: INTERVENTION NO. OF SESSIONS (OR DOSE) TREATMENT DURATION PROVIDER SAMPLE SIZE	CONTROL GROUP 2: INTERVENTION NO. OF SESSIONS (OR DOSE) TREATMENT DURATION PROVIDER SAMPLE SIZE
			CENTRAL TENS		
Noorbrink, 2009[46]	SCI neuropathy Unclear Patients from a university hospital 47.2 ± 11.2 years (29–68 years)	Inc: SCI >6 months, neuropathic pain, pain intensity ≥4/10. Exc: known cognitive impairment, previous TENS use, current acupuncture use	Crossover design TENS: high-frequency 80 Hz, 30–40 minutes 3 sessions/day 14 days Unclear n = 24	TENS: low frequency 2 Hz, 30–40 minutes 3 sessions/day 14 days Unclear n = 24	—
			TMS		
Khedr, 2005[40]	Poststroke pain 18 ± 17 months Patients from a university hospital 52.3 ± 10.3 years	Inc: history of cerebrovascular stroke diagnosed by CT scan, unilateral poststroke pain	TMS: 20 Hz, 80% resting motor threshold, 200 pulses/minute 10 minutes/session 1 session/day 5 days MD n = 12	Sham TMS n = 12	—

Andre, 2006[48]	Central and peripheral neuropathy (various) 6.9 ± 4.0 years Patients from a university hospital 53 ± 11 years (31–66 years)	Inc: chronic neuropathic pain, resistant to conventional pharmacological procedures Exc: history of seizure, pacemaker	*Crossover design* TMS: 1 Hz, 25 minutes 1 session NA Unclear *n* = 12	TMS: 20 Hz, 25 minutes 1 session NA Unclear *n* = 12	Sham TMS *n* = 12
Andre, 2008[47]	Central and peripheral neuropathy (various) 1–17 years Patients from a university hospital 31–72 years	Inc: chronic neuropathic pain, resistant to conventional pharmacological procedures Exc: history of seizure, pacemaker	*Crossover design* TMS: posterior-anterior, 20 Hz, 26 minutes 1 session NA Unclear *n* = 28	Sham TMS, 26 min 1 session NA Unclear *n* = 28	—

Note: The list of abbreviations for all tables appears at the end of Table 25.12.

Table 25-6. Study Outcomes: Peripheral Neuropathic Pain—Diabetic Neuropathy

REFERENCE	OUTCOME MEASURE RANGE	TIME POINT	INTERVENTION			P VALUE*
			EXPERIMENTAL	CONTROL 1	CONTROL 2	
ACUPUNCTURE AND B VITAMINS						
Jiang, 2006[17]	Global clinical symptoms (% of subjects "markedly relieved" from baseline)	3 weeks	56.7%	56.7%	23.3%	<.05 (exp, con 1 > con 2)
B VITAMINS						
Abbas, 1997[25]	Global symptom (NRS) 0–9 (% subjects improved from baseline)	1 month	59.1	10.1		<.001
Levin, 1981[26]	Global symptoms (NRS) -1 to +2 (improvement from baseline)	4 months	1.4	1.3	—	NS
Winkler, 1999[27]	Pain (VAS) 0–20	baseline	13.7	13.0	12.8	—
		3 weeks	9.7	9.1	10.0	NS
		6 weeks	6.5	6.8	7.2	NS
Yaqub, 1992[29]	Global symptoms (PNS) 0–140	baseline	72.2	95.5	—	—
		4 months	106.6	94.8	—	NS
ALA						
Ametov, 2003[18]	Global symptoms (TSS) 0–14.64	baseline	8.8	8.2	—	—
		3 weeks	3.1	6.4	—	<.001
	Global symptoms (NSC-severity)	baseline	18.4	20.5	—	—
		3 weeks	7.3	13.3	—	<.001
	Function (NIS) (improvement from baseline)	3 weeks	2.7	1.2	—	<.001
	Function (NIS-LL) (improvement from baseline)	3 weeks	NR	NR	—	NS

Ruhnau, 1999[19]	Pain (HPAL) 0–6	baseline	3.7	3.6	—	—
		19 days	1.5	2.5	—	NS
	Global symptoms (TSS) 0–14.64	baseline	8.0	8.2	—	—
		19 days	4.3	6.2	—	.021
	Function (NDS)	baseline	8.5	8.2	—	—
		19 days	8.2	8.4	—	.025
Ziegler, 1995[22]	Pain (HPAL) 0–6	baseline	2.0	2.1	con 2: 2.2 con 3: 2.1	—
		19 days	0.9	0.7	con 2: 1.7 con 3: 1.7	<.01 (exp, con 1 <con 3)
	Global symptoms (TSS) 0–14.64	baseline	7.6	7.8	con 2: 7.6 con 3: 6.8	—
		19 days	3.1	2.8	con 2: 4.3 con 3: 4.2	<.01 (exp, con 1 <con 3)
	Function (NDS)	baseline	6.1	6.0	con 2: 6.2 con 3: 6.2	—
		19 days	4.3	4.5	con 2: 5.3 con 3: 5.2	0.03 (exp < con 3)
Ziegler, 1999[21]	Global symptoms (TSS) 0–14.64	baseline	8.1	8.3	8.4	—
		19 days	4.4	4.6	5.4	NS
		7 months	4.1	4.3	4.4	NS
	Function (NIS-LL)	baseline	11.0	11.3	11.0	—
		19 days	7.7	8.0	8.2	NS
		7 months	6.6	7.1	7.6	NS
Ziegler, 2006[20]	Global symptoms (TSS) 0–14.64	baseline	9.0	9.4	con 2: 9.4 con 3: 9.3	—

(continued)

Table 25-6. (continued)

REFERENCE	OUTCOME MEASURE RANGE	INTERVENTION				
		TIME POINT	EXPERIMENTAL	CONTROL 1	CONTROL 2	P VALUE*
		5 weeks	4.3	4.9	con 2: 4.6 con 3: 6.4	<.05 (exp, con 1, con 2 < con 3)
	Global symptoms (NSC)	baseline	6.6	7.1	con 2: 7.0 con 3: 6.8	—
		5 weeks	3.9	4.3	con 2: 4.2 con 3: 5.1	<.05 (con 1, con 2 < con 3)
	Function (NIS-LL)	baseline	13.0	15.0	con 2: 15.4 con 3: 14.5	
		5 weeks	10.3	12.4	con 2: 11.7 con 3: 12.4	NS
TENS						
Kumar, 1997[38]	Pain (NRS) 0–5	baseline	3.2	2.9		—
		4 weeks	1.4	2.4	—	<.03
	Global symptoms (VAS) (% relief from baseline)	4 weeks	52	27		<.05

					p value
Kumar, 1998[37]	Pain (NRS) 0–5	baseline	3.2	2.8	—	—
		12 weeks	1.4	1.9	—	.03
	Global symptoms (VAS) (% relief from baseline)	12 weeks	47	24	—	<.02
	Pain (NRS - MPI-S) 0–6	baseline	3.5	3.5	—	—
		2 weeks	3.5	3.5	—	NS
Reichstein, 2005[39]	Global symptoms (TSS)	baseline	6.6	7.0	—	—
		3 days	5.4	4.6	—	<.05
	Global symptoms (VAS) 0–10 (% of subjects classified as responders, i.e., ≥3 point improvement)	3 days	33	80	—	<.05

*The *p* value reflects the comparison between groups at a specified time point.
Note: The list of abbreviations for all tables appears at the end of Table 25.12.

Table 25-7. Study Outcomes: Peripheral Neuropathic Pain—CTS

REFERENCE	OUTCOME MEASURE RANGE	TIME POINT	INTERVENTION			
			EXPERIMENTAL	CONTROL 1	CONTROL 2	P VALUE*
	ACUPUNCTURE					
Yang, 2009[16]	Global symptoms (GSS) 0–50	baseline	16.1	14.3	—	—
		2 weeks	7.5	7.0	—	NS
		4 weeks	4.4	5.0	—	NS
	ALA AND B VITAMINS					
DiGeronimo, 2009[24]	Global symptoms (BCTQ) 0–40 (improvement from baseline)	90 days	8.6	2.2	—	<.001
	Function (BTCQ) 0–20 (improvement from baseline)	90 days	2.5	-0.3	—	<.001
	B VITAMINS					
Spooner, 1993[30]	Pain-night (NRS) 0–4	baseline	2.4	2.6	—	—
		12 weeks	1.9	2.4	—	NS
	Pain-movement (NRS) 0–4	baseline	3.1	3.1	—	—
		12 weeks	1.7	2.7	—	NS
	Coordination (NRS) 0–4	baseline	1.6	1.9	—	—
		12 weeks	1.2	1.8	—	NS

MANIPULATION

Study	Measure	Time			p*
Burke, 2007[31]	Pain-Hand (VAS) 0–100	baseline	60.5	61.5	—
		6 weeks	15.4	9.8	NS
		3 months	33.7	9.2	<.05
	Function (NRS) 0–5	baseline	2.4	2.1	—
		6 weeks	1.7	1.6	NS
		3 months	1.7	1.6	NS
Davis, 1998[34]	Pain (SF-36 bodily pain) 0–100	baseline	67.7	60.8	—
		3 months	69.5	64.5	NS
	Function (CTOA-P) 0–64	baseline	12.5	14.7	—
		9 weeks	9.3	5.7	NS

*The p value reflects the comparison between groups at a specified time point.
Note: The list of abbreviations for all chapters appears at the end of Table 25.12.

Table 25-8. Study Outcomes: Peripheral Neuropathic Pain—Lumbar Radiculopathy and/or Sciatica

			INTERVENTION			
REFERENCE	OUTCOME MEASURE RANGE	TIME POINT	EXPERIMENTAL	CONTROL 1	CONTROL 2	P VALUE*
ACUPUNCTURE						
Hollisaz, 2007[15]	Pain (VAS) 0–100 (% of pain reduction from baseline)	following last treatment session	62.1	52.5	17.5	<.05 (exp > con 1, con 2; con1 > con2)
ALA						
Memeo, 2008[23]	Global symptoms (NSC-LL) (improvement from baseline)	60 days	2.2	1.4	—	<.05
	Global symptoms (TSS) (improvement from baseline)	60 days	1.9	1.2	—	<.05
	Function (NIS-LL) (improvement from baseline)	60 days	2.5	1.5	—	<.05
MANIPULATION						
Burton, 2000[32]	Pain-Leg (NRS) 0–5	baseline	4.0	3.7	—	—
		2 weeks	3.2	3.3	—	NS
		6 weeks	2.7	2.7	—	NS
		12 months	2.1	2.3	—	NS
	Pain-Low Back (NRS) 0–5	baseline	3.8	4.1	—	—
		2 weeks	3.2	4.0	—	<.05
		6 weeks	2.7	3.6	—	<.05
		12 months	2.3	2.9	—	NS
	Function (RDQ) 0–24	baseline	11.9	12.0	—	—
		2 weeks	10.2	13.9	—	<.05
		6 weeks	7.8	11.0	—	NS

Coxhead, 1981[33] Pain (VAS) –100 to +100 (improvement from baseline)	12 months	5.9	7.3	—	NS
	4 weeks	52.6	42.2	—	<.05
Function (% of subjects who returned to normal activities)	4 weeks	36	29	—	NS
Santilli, 2006[35] Pain reduction (low back) from baseline (% of subjects)	2 weeks	86	61	—	<.01
	1 month	94	85	—	NS
	6 weeks	100	92	—	NS
	3 months	98	90	—	NS
	6 months	98	94	—	NS
Pain reduction (leg) from baseline (% of subjects)	2 weeks	82	53	—	<.005
	1 month	94	77	—	<.05
	6 weeks	100	81	—	<.05
	3 months	98	77	—	<.005
	6 months	100	83	—	.01
Free of pain (low back) (% of subjects)	2 weeks	0	0	—	NS
	1 month	6	0	—	NS
	6 weeks	17	6	—	NS
	3 months	24	6	—	<.05
	6 months	28	6	—	<.005
Free of pain (leg) (% of subjects)	2 weeks	13	4	—	NS
	1 month	23	12	—	NS
	6 weeks	41	16	—	<.01
	3 months	55	12	—	<.0001
	6 months	55	20	—	<.0001

*The p value reflects the comparison between groups at a specified time point.
Note: The list of abbreviations for all tables appears at the end of Table 25.12.

Table 25-9. Study Outcomes: Peripheral Neuropathic Pain—Other

			INTERVENTION			
REFERENCE	OUTCOME MEASURE RANGE	TIME POINT	EXPERIMENTAL	CONTROL 1	CONTROL 2	P VALUE*
ACUPUNCTURE						
Shlay, 1998[14]	Pain (NRS) 0–1.75	baseline	1.1	1.1	con 2: 1.1 con 3: 1.1	—
		6 weeks	0.9	0.9	con 2: 0.9 con 3: 0.9	NS
		14 weeks	0.8	0.9	con 2: 0.8 con 3: 0.8	NS
	Function (SF36-PF) 0–100 (improvement from baseline)	6 weeks	6.0	5.6	con 2: 5.9 con 3: 5.1	NS
		14 weeks	3.4	1.3	con 2: 7.1 con 3: 0.6	NS
ACUPUNCTURE AND B VITAMINS						
Woelk, 1998[28]	Pain (NRS) 0–5 (% of subjects with no pain or mild pain)	8 weeks	77	54	54	NS
	Global symptoms (NRS) 0–16 (% of subjects ≥10)	8 weeks	93.3	76.9	67.9	NS
TENS						
Cheing, 2005[36]	Pain (VAS) 0–10	baseline	6.2	6.5	—	—
		4 days	4.3	6.1	—	.05
		7 days	3.0	5.5	—	.003
		11 days	1.7	4.6	—	.002
TMS						
Khedr, 2005[40]	Pain (VAS) 0–10	baseline	8.5	8.0	—	—
		5 days	4.5	6.8		.025
		19 days	5.0	6.8		.025
	Pain (LANSS) 0–24	baseline	21	21		—
		5 days	9	19		< .001
		19 days	12.3	18		< .001

*The p value reflects the comparison between groups at a specified time point.
Note: The list of abbreviations for all tables appears at the end of Table 25.12.

Table 25-10. Study Outcomes: Central Neuropathic Pain and Mixed Central/Peripheral Neuropathic Pain

REFERENCE	OUTCOME MEASURE RANGE	TIME POINT	INTERVENTION			P VALUE*
			EXPERIMENTAL	CONTROL 1	CONTROL 2	
CENTRAL						
Norrbrink, 2009[46]	Pain (NRS - Borg CR-10) 0–11	19 days	1.5	2.5	—	NS
		TENS				
		baseline	4	5	—	—
		2 weeks	5	4.5	—	NS
	Pain (NRS - MPI-S) 0–6	baseline	3.5	3.5	—	—
		2 weeks	3.5	3.5	—	NS
TMS						
Khedr, 2005[40]	Pain (VAS) 0–10	baseline	8.3	8.3	—	—
		5 days	4.5	7.5	—	<.001
		19 days	5.0	8.0	—	<.001
	Pain (LANSS) 0–24	baseline	20	20	—	—
		5 days	11.7	20	—	<.001
		19 days	11.7	20	—	<.001
MIXED						
		TMS				
Andre, 2006[48]	Pain (VAS) 0–10 (% improvement from baseline)	1 week	-2	11	8	0.04 (con 1, con 2 < exp)
Andre, 2008[6]	Pain (NRS) 0–10 (% improvement from baseline)	1–2 days	3	-9	—	NS
		3–4 days	5	-8	—	0.03
		4–6 days	5	-5	—	NS
	Global symptom (NRS) –3 (worse) to +3 (improved)	6 days	0.6	0		0.01

*The p value reflects the comparison between groups at a specified time point.
Note: The list of abbreviations for all tables appears at the end of Table 25.12.

Table 25-11. Harms

REFERENCE	TREATMENT-RELATED HARMS?	TREATMENT-RELATED SERIOUS AES?	INTERVENTION		
			EXPERIMENTAL	CONTROL 1	CONTROL 2
			ACUPUNCTURE		
Hollisaz, 2007[15]	NR	NR	NR	NR	NR
Shlay, 1998[14]	Harms reported; relation to treatment is unclear	Serious AEs reported; relation to treatment is unclear	Grade 4 AE - unspecified (n = 3)	Grade 4 AE - unspecified (n = 10)	Con 2: grade 4 AE - unspecified (n = 6) Con 3: grade 4 AE - unspecified (n = 2)
Yang, 2009[16]	Yes	No	Local pain, bruising, or paresthesia (n = 2)	Nausea, epigastralgia, or other unspecified (n = 7)	—
			ACUPUNCTURE AND B VITAMINS		
Jiang, 2006[17]	NR	NR	NR	NR	NR
ALA					
Ametov, 2003[18]	No	No	None	None	—
Memeo, 2008[23]	No	No	None	None	—
Ruhnau, 1999[19]	No	No	None	None	—
Ziegler, 1995[22]	Yes	Unclear	Total AEs (n = 28) Incidence > 10%: Nausea (n = 13) Vomiting (n = 8)	Total AEs (n = 14) Incidence > 10%: None	Con 2: total AEs (n = 11) Incidence > 10%: None Con 3: total AEs (n = 17) Incidence >10%: Headache (n = 8)

Study					
Ziegler, 1999[21]	Harms reported; relation to treatment is unclear	Unclear	Total AEs oral phase (n = 77) Specifics - NR	Total AEs oral phase (n = 66) Specifics - NR	Total AEs oral phase (n = 75) Specifics - NR
Ziegler, 2006[20]	Yes	Unclear	Total AEs (n = 25) Incidence > 10%: Nausea (n = 22) Vomiting (n = 12) Vertigo (n = 5)	Total AEs (n = 20) Incidence > 10%: Nausea (n = 10)	Con 2: total AEs (n = 12) Incidence >10%: Nausea (n = 6) Con 3: total AEs (n = 9) Incidence >10%: None
			ALA AND B VITAMINS		
DiGeronimo, 2009[24]	No	No	None	None	—
			B VITAMINS		
Abbas, 1997[25]	Yes: gastrointestinal irritation (n = 1);, group assignment is unclear	No	Unclear	Unclear	—
Levin, 1981[26]	NR	NR	NR	NR	—
Spooner, 1993[30]	No	No	None	None	—
Winkler, 1999[27]	No	No	None	None	None
Woelk, 1998[28]	No	No	None	None	None

(continued)

Table 25-11. (continued)

| REFERENCE | TREATMENT-RELATED HARMS? | TREATMENT-RELATED SERIOUS AES? | INTERVENTION | | |
			EXPERIMENTAL	CONTROL 1	CONTROL 2
Yaqub, 1992[29]	Yes	No	None	Gastrointestinal irritation (n = 1)	—
MANIPULATION					
Burke, 2007[31]	Yes	No	Soreness and bruising of treated forearm-wrist-hand (n = NR)	Soreness and bruising of treated forearm-wrist-hand (n = NR) Profound bruising and swelling of treated forearm-wrist-hand (n = 1)	—
Burton, 2000[32]	No	No	None	One	—
Coxhead, 1981[33]	NR	NR	NR	NR	—
Davis, 1998[34]	Yes	No	Soreness in neck (n = 1)	Intolerance to ibuprofen (e.g., gastrointestinal symptoms, headache) (n = 10)	—
Santilli, 2006[35]	No	No	None	None	—

	TENS				
Cheing, 2005[36]	NR	NR	NR	NR	—
Kumar, 1997[38]	Yes	No	None	Burning sensation at electrode site (n = 1)	—
Kumar, 1998[37]	No	No	N one	None	—
Norrbrink, 2009[46]	Yes: local discomfort (n = 3), local muscle spasms (n = 1); group assignment is unclear	No	Unclear	Unclear	
Reichstein, 2005[39]	Yes	No	None	Local muscle discomfort (n = 1)	—
TMS					
Andre, 2006[48]	No	No	None	None	None
Andre, 2008[47]	No	No	None	None	—
Khedr, 2005[40]	No	No	None	None	—

Note: The list of abbreviations for all tables appears at the end of Table 25.12.

systematic review identified two RCTs published prior to May 2004 that fit our inclusion criteria.[32,33] Our search uncovered three more recent RCTs.[15,23,35] No RCTs were found on B vitamins, TENS, or TMS for lumbar radiculopathy and/or sciatica.

No RCTs were found on cervical radiculopathy that met our inclusion criteria, in agreement with recent findings of the Bone and Joint Decade Task Force 2000–2010 on Neck Pain and Its Associated Disorders.[43–45] While there is no evidence available to confirm a benefit of acupuncture, ALA, B vitamins, manipulation, TENS, or TMS for patients with cervical radiculopathy, there also is no evidence that any other noninvasive treatment approaches are of any benefit.[44,45]

One RCT on manipulation for symptomatic lumbar disc herniation found relative benefits favoring manipulation compared with chymopapain injections in short-term pain relief in the low back and improvements in physical function.[32] No differences were found between the groups in short-term pain relief in the leg, long-term pain relief in the low back and leg, and improvements in physical function. Another RCT on manipulation for symptomatic disc herniation found that at the 6-month follow-up, manipulation was more effective than sham manipulation based on the percentage of pain-free cases for low back pain and leg pain, as well as the percentage of cases with clinically meaningful relief of leg pain. However, no difference was found between the groups in percentage of cases with clinically meaningful relief of low back pain.[35] An earlier RCT with a factorial design compared traditional physiotherapy with and without manipulation for sciatica.[33] This study reported greater pain relief at 4 weeks when manipulation was added to physiotherapy compared with physiotherapy alone, but no difference was found between the groups in terms of the percentage of patients who returned to normal activities.

An RCT assessing the efficacy of acupuncture for sciatica found that both electro-acupuncture and physiotherapy were superior to sham acupuncture for providing short-term pain relief, while there was no difference between electro-acupuncture and physiotherapy.[15] An RCT assessing the efficacy of ALA for lumbar disc herniation found that oral ALA was superior

to oral acetyl-L-carnitine in terms of improvements in global symptoms and physical function at the 2-month follow-up.[23]

ALCOHOLIC NEUROPATHY (TABLES 25.4 AND 25.9)

A 2009 Cochrane systematic review on B vitamins for peripheral neuropathy was found,[6] which included one RCT with 104 cases on B vitamins for neuropathic pain associated with alcoholic neuropathy that fit our inclusion criteria.[28] Our search did not reveal any additional studies. In an 8-week trial that compared oral vitamin B_1 (thiamine), B vitamin complex, and placebo, no differences among the groups were noted in terms of pain relief and improvements in global symptoms.[28]

HIV-RELATED NEUROPATHY (TABLES 25.4 AND 25.9)

One RCT with 375 cases was uncovered on neuropathic pain associated with HIV-related neuropathy, which compared needle acupuncture, sham acupuncture, oral amitriptyline, and oral placebo in a 14-week trial with a factorial design.[14] At the end of the trial, no differences were noted among the groups in pain relief or improvements in physical function.

TRIGEMINAL NEURALGIA (TABLES 25.4 AND 25. 9)

One RCT with 24 cases was uncovered on trigeminal neuralgia, which compared low-frequency TMS with sham TMS.[40] At the end of the 5-day trial and at the 19-day follow-up, TMS was found to provide greater pain relief than sham TMS.

VARIOUS PERIPHERAL NEUROPATHIES (TABLES 25.4 AND 25.9)

One RCT with 19 cases was uncovered for neuropathic pain associated with various peripheral neuropathies, which compared high-frequency TENS with sham TENS[36] This 2-week trial noted greater pain relief for high-frequency TENS applied to the affected hand compared with sham TENS.

Central Neuropathic Pain

Two RCTs, which enrolled a total of 72 cases, were uncovered for central neuropathic pain.[40,46] The details are discussed below.

SPINAL CORD INJURY-RELATED NEUROPATHY (TABLES 25.5 AND 25.10)

One RCT with 48 cases was uncovered on neuropathic pain associated with spinal cord injury-related neuropathy, which compared high-frequency TENS with low-frequency TENS in a 2-week crossover trial.[46] No significant pain relief was noted in either group.

POSTSTROKE PAIN SYNDROME (TABLES 25.5 AND 25.10)

One RCT with 24 cases was uncovered on neuropathic pain associated with cerebrovascular stroke,[40] which compared low-frequency TMS with sham TMS.[40] At the end of the 5-day trial and at the 19-day follow-up, TMS was found to provide greater pain relief than sham TMS.

Mixed Central and Peripheral Neuropathic Pain

VARIOUS MIXED NEUROPATHIES (TABLES 25.5 AND 25.10)

Two RCTs with 92 cases were uncovered for mixed central and peripheral neuropathic pain associated with various neuropathies.[47,48] A 1-week trial with a crossover design found that one session of high-frequency TMS and sham TMS resulted in greater pain relief than one session of low-frequency TMS, while there was no difference between high-frequency TMS and sham TMS.[48] A 6-day trial with a crossover design found greater improvements in global symptoms for high-frequency TMS compared with sham TMS but no difference in pain relief between the groups.[47]

HARMS

Data on harms were available in 25 RCTs[14,16, 18-25,27-32,34,35,37-40,46-48] and were not reported in 5 RCTs.[15,17,26,33,36]

Harms were noted in 12 of the 25 RCTs in which data on harms were available (Table 25.11). Harms were reported to be or appeared to be causally related to the experimental interventions in nine RCTs.[16,20,22,25,29,31,34,37,39] The relationship between harms and interventions was unclear in two RCTs.[14,21] One RCT reported harms in the oral placebo group only.[29]

Serious adverse events were noted in the experimental and control groups in one RCT on acupuncture for HIV-related peripheral neuropathy[14] and one RCT on ALA for diabetic peripheral neuropathy,[49] but the causal relationship between these adverse events and the interventions was not reported. No harms were noted in the three RCTs with TMS interventions for peripheral neuropathic pain.[40,47,48]

The harms deemed to be causally related to the experimental interventions were generally minor and self-limiting and included gastrointestinal symptoms following ALA for diabetic peripheral neuropathy[20,22] and use of B vitamins for diabetic peripheral neuropathy,[25] vertigo following ALA for diabetic peripheral neuropathy,[20] local cutaneous and muscular discomfort at the electrode site following TENS for peripheral neuropathy,[38,39,46] local pain, bruising, and paresthesia following acupuncture for CTS,[16] soreness and bruising in the treated upper extremity following manipulation for CTS,[31] and soreness in the neck following manipulation for CTS.[34]

DISCUSSION

This systematic review uncovered 30 RCTs assessing the efficacy of commonly used CAM therapies for the management of neuropathic pain. Overall, the quality of the included RCTs was poor to moderate, and the evidence base for many of these interventions was not strong. Numerous studies were carried out with small sample sizes and therefore were underpowered. Only a few studies assessed long-term clinical outcomes. Nevertheless, the currently available evidence allows certain conclusions to be drawn about the use of CAM approaches for the management of neuropathic pain. The evidence is summarized in this section and in Table 25.12.

Table 25-12. Summary of the Evidence for CAM Therapies for Short-Term Relief of Neuropathic Pain and Improvements in Global Symptoms (Including a Pain Component) for Various Neuropathies

	PAIN		GLOBAL SYMPTOMS	
INTERVENTION	EVIDENCE OF EFFECTIVENESS	EVIDENCE OF NO EFFECTIVENESS	EVIDENCE OF EFFECTIVENESS	EVIDENCE OF NO EFFECTIVENESS
Acupuncture	Lumbar radiculopathy/sciatica	HIV neuropathy	Diabetic neuropathy CTS	HIV neuropathy
ALA	Diabetic neuropathy		Lumbar radiculopathy/ sciatica	Diabetic neuropathy
B vitamins		Alcoholic neuropathy CTS Diabetic neuropathy		Alcoholic neuropathy CTS Diabetic neuropathy
Manipulation	CTS Lumbar radiculopathy/sciatica			
TENS	Diabetic neuropathy	Spinal cord injury Neuropathy	Diabetic neuropathy	
TMS	Trigeminal neuralgia Poststroke pain			

* Evidence of effectiveness: ≥1 RCT revealed statistically significant pain relief or improvement in global symptoms of intervention compared with control; evidence of no effectiveness: ≥1 RCT revealed no difference in pain relief or improvement in global symptoms of intervention compared with control. Blank cells or condition not listed in a given cell for particular intervention—no available evidence.

Abbreviations for Tables 25.1–25.12: AE, adverse event; ALA, alpha-lipoic acid; BMI, body mass index; BTCQ, Boston Carpal Tunnel Questionnaire; CNS, central nervous system; Con, control group; CT, computed tomography; CTOA-P, Carpal Tunnel Outcome Assessment—Physical; CTS, carpal tunnel syndrome; DC, doctor of chiropractic; DJD, degenerative joint disease; DOM, doctor of oriental medicine; DO, doctor of osteopathic medicine; DPM, doctor of podiatric medicine; EMG, electromyography; Exc, exclusion criteria; Exp, experimental group; GLA, gamma-linolenic acid; GSS, global symptom score; HPAL, Hamburg Pain Adjective List; HVLA, High-velocity, low-amplitude; IASP, International Association for the Study of Pain; Inc, inclusion criteria; LAC, licensed acupuncturist; LANSS, Leeds Assessment of Neuropathic Symptoms and Signs; LBP, low back pain; MD, doctor of medicine; MOB, mobilization; MPI-S, Multidimensional Pain Inventory—Swedish version, pain severity subscore; MPQ, McGill Pain Questionnaire; MRI, magnetic resonance imaging; NA, not applicable; NDS, neuropathy disability score; NIS, neuropathy impairment score; NIS-LL, neuropathy impairment score—lower limbs; NSS, neurological symptom score; NR, not reported; NRS, Numerical Rating Scale; NS, not significant ($p > .05$); NSAIDs, nonsteroidal anti-inflammatory drugs; NSC-LL, neuropathy symptoms and change—lower limbs; NSSS, neuropathy symptom and signs score; PNS, peripheral neurology score (somatic component); PT, physical therapist; RDQ, Roland Morris Disability Questionnaire; SCI, spinal cord injury; SF36-PF, Short Form 36 Physical Functioning Subscore; SLR, straight leg raise; SMT,: spinal manipulative therapy; TENS, transcutaneous electrical nerve stimulation; TMS, transcranial magnetic stimulation; TSS, total symptom score; VAS, Visual Analog Scale; VRS, Verbal Rating Scale.

Evidence Summary

PERIPHERAL NEUROPATHIC PAIN

Alcoholic Neuropathy B vitamins: There is some evidence to suggest that B vitamins are ineffective compared with placebo for short-term pain relief and improvements in global symptoms.

Carpal Tunnel Syndrome Acupuncture: There is some evidence to suggest that needle acupuncture is equivalent to oral corticosteroids in improving short-term global symptoms for CTS.

B vitamins: There is some evidence to suggest that B vitamins are ineffective compared with placebo for short-term pain relief and improvements in global symptoms and physical function for CTS. There is some evidence to suggest that B vitamins are less effective than a multisupplement containing ALA, GLA, B vitamins, and other dietary compounds for short-term pain relief and improvements in global symptoms and physical function.

Manipulation: There is some evidence to suggest that manipulation is equivalent to ibuprofen and wrist supports for short-term pain relief and improvements in physical function for CTS. There is also some evidence to suggest that two forms of manipulation may be effective for short-term pain relief and improvements in physical function.

Diabetic Neuropathy Acupuncture: There is some evidence to suggest that needle acupuncture is more effective than oral B vitamins for short-term improvements in global symptoms.

ALA: There is some evidence to suggest that intravenous and oral ALA are more effective than placebo in providing short-term pain relief. There is conflicting evidence on the relative efficacy of intravenous and oral ALA versus placebo in short-term functional improvements. There is some evidence to suggest that ALA is ineffective compared with placebo in providing long-term improvements in physical function and global symptoms.

B vitamins: There is some evidence to suggest that oral B vitamins are ineffective compared with placebo in terms of pain relief. There is some evidence to suggest that oral B vitamins are less effective than an oral multisupplement and needle acupuncture for pain relief and improvements in global symptoms.

TENS: There is some evidence to suggest that high-frequency TENS is more effective than sham TENS for short-term pain relief and improvements in global symptoms. There is some evidence to suggest that combining TENS with amitriptyline is superior to amitriptyline alone for short-term pain relief and improvements in global symptoms. There is some evidence to suggest that electrical muscle stimulation is more effective than TENS for short-term improvements in global symptoms.

HIV-Related neuropathy Acupuncture: There is some evidence to suggest that needle acupuncture is ineffective compared with placebo for pain relief and improvements in global symptoms.

Lumbar Radiculopathy and/or Sciatica Acupuncture: There is some evidence to suggest that electro-acupuncture is more effective than sham acupuncture and equivalent to physiotherapy for short-term pain relief for sciatica.

ALA: There is some evidence to suggest that oral ALA is more effective than acetyl-L-carnitine for improving global symptoms and physical function for symptomatic lumbar disc herniation.

Manipulation: There is some evidence to suggest that manipulation is more effective than chymopapain injections for short-term pain relief for symptomatic lumbar disc herniation, although these relative improvements are lost in the long term. There is some evidence to suggest that manipulation is more effective than sham manipulation for short-term and long-term pain relief for symptomatic lumbar disc herniation. There is some evidence to suggest that adding manipulation to physiotherapy is more effective than physiotherapy alone for short-term pain relief for sciatica.

Trigeminal Neuralgia TMS: There is some evidence to suggest that TMS is more effective than sham TMS for short-term pain relief.

Various Peripheral Neuropathies TENS: There is some evidence to suggest that high-frequency TENS is more effective than sham TENS for short-term pain relief.

CENTRAL NEUROPATHIES

Spinal Cord Injury-Related Neuropathy TENS: There is some evidence to suggest that high-frequency and low-frequency TENs are ineffective for short-term pain relief.

Poststroke Pain TMS: There is some evidence to suggest that TMS is more effective than sham TMS for short-term pain relief.

MIXED PERIPHERAL AND CENTRAL NEUROPATHIC PAIN

Various Neuropathies TMS: There is some evidence to suggest that TMS is ineffective compared with sham TMS for short-term pain relief. There is some evidence to suggest that TMS is more effective than sham TENS for short-term improvements in global symptoms.

HARMS

No serious complications have been reported in any of the RCTs to suggest that these treatment approaches have a high complication rate. No serious harms were reported in any of the trials that can be attributed to these treatments. As has been reported for other conditions, the therapies that involve insertion of needles (e.g., acupuncture) and the manipulative therapies can cause local discomfort or bruising, whereas the oral therapies have a number of commonly reported harms, such as gastrointestinal irritation or nausea, in a few patients.

CONCLUSIONS

As noted in the Introduction, a significant percentage (43%) of patients with peripheral neuropathy report that they had used CAM therapies. The reasons for this high percentage is that most of the commonly used treatments for neuropathic pain are prescription medications that, in these patients, either resulted in insufficient control of their symptoms, did not help their pain, or had unacceptable complication rates or harms. Considering that there is relatively little insurance coverage for most CAM treatment approaches, the observation that patients find it worthwhile to pay for CAM treatment approaches themselves should raise concern in all clinicians about current medical approaches to neuropathic pain and should result in an increased effort to search for alternative treatment options.

The major point that became apparent in searching the literature for this chapter was the paucity and relatively poor quality of the clinical trials available to assess the efficacy of the commonly used CAM treatment approaches utilized by patients to manage their neuropathic pain. Furthermore, the six treatment approaches discussed in this chapter have only been studied in a few of the different types of neuropathic pain conditions. These factors make it impossible to reach conclusions about the utility of these approaches in the management of the many neuropathic pain syndromes.

Despite these statements, a clinician can glean some information from the literature that should be helpful when discussing treatment options with patients. It is, for example, reasonable to state that no major harms appear to be reported from the use of these treatment approaches; this may be sufficient for some patients to ask for a brief trial of treatment. This stands in contrast with the well-documented harms reported with virtually all prescription medications that are currently used to treat neuropathic pain. It is also possible to state that none of the CAM treatment approaches have been proven to offer any long-term benefit to patients with neuropathic pain. It should be pointed out, however, that this is true for all medical and other treatments for neuropathic pain.

It can be reasonably stated that there is evidence that B vitamins are ineffective in the management of peripheral neuropathic pain and are not worth trying. On the other hand, there is some evidence that ALA may be of value in providing short-term relief of pain symptoms in patients with neuropathic pain associated with diabetic peripheral neuropathy and lumbar radiculopathy, although the evidence is very limited.

If asked, a clinician can reasonably inform patients that there is weak evidence that acupuncture and high-frequency TENS provide some short-term relief of pain in patients with neuropathic pain associated with various neuropathies, although the evidence is somewhat conflicting. Some clinicians may find the evidence sufficient to offer these treatments for a brief period to see if they are beneficial.

Similarly, there is weak evidence that spinal manipulation may be of some value in patients with neuropathic pain associated with CTS and lumbar radiculopathy. In the case of lumbar radiculopathy, there may be a long-term beneficial effect of manipulation. To date, there are no trials on the effectiveness of any non-invasive treatment, CAM, or classical medicine approaches for the management of cervical radiculopathy. This should be made clear to any patient who presents with neuropathic pain associated with cervical radiculopathy before a treatment is offered or recommended.

Considering that there is too little available information to guide treatment decisions regarding CAM therapies for neuropathic pain, a greater effort should be made to conduct well-designed clinical trials. The focus should initially be on whether the treatment approach offers any benefit when compared with some form of placebo or a known ineffective treatment that could be used as a control. The research, however, should not stop here. There is a need to know whether the CAM treatment approaches that appear to have some benefit are as effective as standard prescription medications. If so, the lower risk of harms and side effects of CAM therapies may make them the preferable choice. There is also a possibility that combining one or more CAM treatment approaches with prescription medication could enhance pain relief or result in reduced medication doses. Finally, it is important to begin to look at the relative cost effectiveness of the different treatment approaches for neuropathic pain. Treatment of patients with these conditions tends to require long-term pain management that can be very expensive, especially if some of the newer medications are used on a daily basis. It is possible that the utilization of the relatively less expensive CAM therapies may prove to be worth considering, assuming that future studies confirm their effectiveness.

In the final analysis, however, it is clear that the medical community cannot ignore the fact that patients are seeking better care than is currently being offered by their medical physicians and are using personal funds to try CAM treatments. It is incumbent on the scientific and health care communities to determine whether these funds are being appropriately spent and to guide patients as they seek alternative and complementary care options for the neuropathic pain.

ACKNOWLEDGEMENTS

We thank the following individuals for their contributions to this project: Allison Howard, MLIS, Kristen Morda, MA, and John Orriola, MA, MEd for assistance with designing and conducting the literature searches.

REFERENCES

1. National Center for Complementary and Alternative Medicine, National Institutes of Health. What is CAM? http://www.nccam.nih.gov. Accessed April 20, 2010. 2010.
2. Brunelli B, Gorson K. The use of complementary and alternative medicines by patients with peripheral neuropathy. *J Neurol Sci.* 2004; 218(1–2):59–66.
3. Ammendolia C, Furlan A, Imamura M, Irvin E, van Tulder M. Evidence-informed management of chronic low back pain with needle acupuncture. *Spine J.* 2008;8(1):160–172.
4. Audette J, Ryan A. The role of acupuncture in pain management. *Phys Med Rehabil Clin North Am.* 2004;15(4):749–772.
5. Foster T. Efficacy and safety of alpha-lipoic acid supplementation in the treatment of symptomatic diabetic neuropathy. *Diabetes Educ.* 2007;33(1):111–117.
6. Ang C, Alviar M, Dans A, et al. Vitamin B for treating peripheral neuropathy. *Cochrane Database Syst Rev.* 2008(3):1–39.
7. Anderson R. Spinal manipulation before chiropractic. In: Haldeman S, ed. *Principles and Practice of Chiropractic.* 2nd ed. Norwalk CT: Appleton Lange; 1992:3–14.
8. Lomax E. An historical perspective from ancient times to the modern era. In: Goldstein M, ed. *The Research Status of Spinal Manipulative Therapy.* Bethesda, MD: U.S. Department of Health Education and Welfare; 1975:11-A. NIH publication 76–998.
9. Shekelle P, Adams A, Chassin M, Hurwitz E, Phillips R, Brook R. *The Appropriateness of Spinal Manipulation for Low Back Pain: Indications and Ratings by a Multi-Disciplinary Expert Panel* (document no. R-4025/2-CCR). Santa Monica, CA: RAND Corporation; 1991.
10. Cherkin D, Mootz R, eds. *Chiropractic in the United States: Training, Practice, and Research.* Rockville, MA: U.S. Agency for Health Care Policy and Research; 1997. AHCPR Publication No. 98-N002.
11. Bronfort G, Haas M, Evans R, Kawchuk G, Dagenais S. Evidence-informed management of

chronic low back pain with spinal manipulation and mobilization. *Spine J.* 2008;8(1):213–225.

12. Poitras S, Brosseau L. Evidence-informed management of chronic low back pain with transcutaneous electrical nerve stimulation, interferential current, electrical muscle stimulation, ultrasound, and thermotherapy. *Spine J.* 2008;8(1):226–233.

13. Leo R, Latif T. Repetitive transcranial magnetic stimulation (rTMS) in experimentally induced and chronic neuropathic pain: a review. *J Pain.* 2007;8(6):453–459.

14. Shlay J, Chaloner K, Max M, et al. Acupuncture and amitriptyline for pain due to HIV-related peripheral neuropathy: a randomized controlled trial. *JAMA.* 1998;280(18):1590–1595.

15. Hollisaz M. Use of electroacupuncture for treatment of chronic sciatic pain. *Internet J Pain Symptom Control Palliative Care.* 2007;5(1):1–7.

16. Yang C, Hsieh C, Wang N, et al. Acupuncture in patients with carpal tunnel syndrome: a randomized controlled trial. *Clin J Pain.* 2009;25(4):327–333.

17. Jiang H, Shi K, Li X, Zhou W, Cao Y. Clinical study on the wrist-ankle acupuncture treatment for 30 cases of diabetic peripheral neuritis. *J Tradit Chin Med.* 2006;26(1):8–12.

18. Ametov A, Barinov A, Dyck P, et al. The sensory symptoms of diabetic polyneuropathy are improved with alpha-lipoic acid: the SYDNEY trial. *Diabetes Care.* 2003;26(3):770–776.

19. Ruhnau K, Meissner H, Finn J, et al. Effects of 3-week oral treatment with the antioxidant thioctic acid (alpha-lipoic acid) in symptomatic diabetic polyneuropathy. *Diabet Med.* 1999;16(12):1040–1043.

20. Ziegler D, Ametov A, Barinov A, et al. Oral treatment with alpha-lipoic acid improves symptomatic diabetic polyneuropathy: the SYDNEY 2 trial. *Diabetes Care.* 2006;29(11):2365–2370.

21. Ziegler D, Hanefeld M, Ruhnau K, et al. Treatment of symptomatic diabetic polyneuropathy with the antioxidant alpha-lipoic acid: a 7-month multicenter randomized controlled trial (ALADIN III Study). ALADIN III Study Group. Alpha-Lipoic Acid in Diabetic Neuropathy. *Diabetes Care.* 1999;22(8):1296–1301.

22. Ziegler D, Hanefeld M, Ruhnau K, et al. Treatment of symptomatic diabetic peripheral neuropathy with the anti-oxidant alpha-lipoic acid. A 3-week multicentre randomized controlled trial (ALADIN Study). *Diabetologia.* 1995;38(12):1425–1433.

23. Memeo A, Loiero M. Thioctic acid and acetyl-L-carnitine in the treatment of sciatic pain caused by a herniated disc: a randomized, double-blind, comparative study. *Clin Drug Investig.* 2008;28(8):495–500.

24. Di Geronimo G, Caccese A, Caruso L, Soldati A, Passaretti U. Treatment of carpal tunnel syndrome with alpha-lipoic acid. *Eur Rev Med Pharmacol Sci.* 2009;13(2):133–139.

25. Abbas Z, Swai A. Evaluation of the efficacy of thiamine and pyridoxine in the treatment of symptomatic diabetic peripheral neuropathy. *East Afr Med J.* 1997;74(12):803–808.

26. Levin E, Hanscom T, Fischer M, Lauvstad W, Lui A, Ryan A. The influence of pyridoxine in diabetic peripheral neuropathy. *Diabetes Care.* 1981;4(6):606–609.

27. Winkler G, Pal B, Nagybeganyi E, Ory I, Porochnavec M, Kempler P. Effectiveness of different benfotiamine dosage regimens in the treatment of painful diabetic neuropathy. *Arzneimittelforschung.* 1999;49(3):220–224.

28. Woelk H, Lehrl S, Bitsch R, Kopcke W. Benfotiamine in treatment of alcoholic polyneuropathy: an 8-week randomized controlled study (BAP I Study). *Alcohol Alcoholism.* 1998;33(6):631–638.

29. Yaqub B, Siddique A, Sulimani R. Effects of methylcobalamin on diabetic neuropathy. *Clin Neurol Neurosurg.* 1992;94(2):105–111.

30. Spooner G, Desai H, Angel J, Reeder B, Donat J. Using pyridoxine to treat carpal tunnel syndrome. Randomized control trial. *Can Fam Physician.* 1993;39:2122–2127.

31. Burke J, Buchberger D, Carey-Loghmani M, Dougherty P, Greco D, Dishman J. A pilot study comparing two manual therapy interventions for carpal tunnel syndrome. *J Manipulative Physiol Ther.* 2007;30(1):50–61.

32. Burton A, Tillotson K, Cleary J. Single-blind randomised controlled trial of chemonucleolysis and manipulation in the treatment of symptomatic lumbar disc herniation. *Eur Spine J.* 2000;9(3):202–207.

33. Coxhead C, Inskip H, Meade T, North W, Troup J. Multicentre trial of physiotherapy in the management of sciatic symptoms. *Lancet.* 1981;1(8229):1065–1068.

34. Davis P, Hulbert J, Kassak K, Meyer J. Comparative efficacy of conservative medical and chiropractic treatments for carpal tunnel syndrome: a randomized clinical trail. *J Manipulative Physiol Ther.* 1998;21(5):317–326.

35. Santilli V, Beghi E, Finucci S. Chiropractic manipulation in the treatment of acute back pain and sciatica with disc protrusion: a randomized double-blind clinical trial of active and simulated spinal manipulations. *Spine J.* 2006;6(2):131–137.

36. Cheing G, Luk M. Transcutaneous electrical nerve stimulation for neuropathic pain. *J Hand Surg Br.* 2005;30(1):50–55.

37. Kumar D, Alvaro M, Julka I, Marshall H. Diabetic peripheral neuropathy. Effectiveness of electrotherapy and amitriptyline for symptomatic relief. *Diabetes Care.* 1998;21(8):1322–1325.

38. Kumar D, Marshall H. Diabetic peripheral neuropathy: amelioration of pain with transcutaneous electrostimulation. *Diabetes Care.* 1997;20(11):1702–1705.

39. Reichstein L, Labrenz S, Ziegler D, Martin S. Effective treatment of symptomatic diabetic polyneuropathy by high-frequency external muscle stimulation. *Diabetologia.* 2005;48(5):824–828.

40. Khedr E, Kotb H, Kamel N, Ahmed M, Sadek R, Rothwell J. Longlasting antalgic effects of daily sessions of repetitive transcranial magnetic stimulation in central and peripheral neuropathic pain. *J Neurol Neurosurg Psychiatry.* 2005;76(6):833–838.

41. Piazzini D, Aprile I, Ferrara P, et al. A systematic review of conservative treatment of carpal tunnel syndrome. *Clin Rehabil.* 2007;21(4):299–314.

42. Luijsterburg P, Verhagen A, Ostelo R, van Os T, Peul W, Koes B. Effectiveness of conservative treatments for the lumbosacral radicular syndrome: a systematic review. *Eur Spine J.* 2007;16(7):881–899.

43. Carragee E, Hurwitz E, Cheng I, et al. Treatment of neck pain: injections and surgical interventions: results of the Bone and Joint Decade 2000–2010 Task Force on Neck Pain and Its Associated Disorders. *Spine.* 2008;33 (4 suppl):S153–S169.

44. Haldeman S, Carroll L, Cassidy J, Schubert J, Nygren A. The Bone and Joint Decade 2000–2010 Task Force on Neck Pain and Its Associated Disorders: executive summary. *Spine.* 2008;33 (4 suppl):S5–S7.

45. Hurwitz E, Carragee E, van der Velde G, et al. Treatment of neck pain: noninvasive interventions: results of the Bone and Joint Decade 2000–2010 Task Force on Neck Pain and Its Associated Disorders. *Spine.* 2008;33(4 Suppl):S123–S152.

46. Norrbrink C. Transcutaneous electrical nerve stimulation for treatment of spinal cord injury neuropathic pain. *J Rehabil Res Dev.* 2009;46(1):85–93.

47. Andre-Obadia N, Mertens P, Gueguen A, Peyron R, Garcia-Larrea L. Pain relief by rTMS: differential effect of current flow but no specific action on pain subtypes. *Neurology.* 2008;71(11):833–840.

48. Andre-Obadia N, Peyron R, Mertens P, Mauguiere F, Laurent B, Garcia-Larrea L. Transcranial magnetic stimulation for pain control. Double-blind study of different frequencies against placebo, and correlation with motor cortex stimulation efficacy. *Clin Neurophysiol.* 2006;117(7):1536–1544.

49. Reljanovic M, Reichel G, Rett K, et al. Treatment of diabetic polyneuropathy with the antioxidant thioctic acid (alpha-lipoic acid): a two year multicenter randomized double-blind placebo-controlled trial (ALADIN II). Alpha Lipoic Acid in Diabetic Neuropathy. *Free Radic Res.* 1999;31(3):171–179.

26

Neuropathic Pain

An Interdisciplinary Rehabilitation Approach

R. NORMAN HARDEN, KATHRYN RICHARDSON, MICHELLE SHUFELT, AND GADI REVIVO

INTRODUCTION

THE ESTIMATED NEARLY 4 million cases of chronic neuropathic pain in the United States include conditions as diverse as cancer-associated pain, stroke pain, spinal cord injury pain, low back pain (e.g., radiculopathy), and phantom pain.[1] Most nerve damage does not lead to clinically important neuropathic pain; however, in some cases, even small degrees of nerve injury can precipitate severe pain.[2] Neuropathic pain associated with disorders such as postherpetic neuralgia (PHN) and diabetes mellitus are the best characterized and studied, due primarily to the development of drugs using these models,[3] but they are certainly not the exclusive or even the most prevalent causes of pain due to nerve lesions. There are also a few other neuropathic pain research models in which there is increasing interest (e.g., human immune deficiency virus neuropathy and radiculopathy).

Clinically, neuropathic pain is a challenging problem that lacks a coherent treatment paradigm.[4] The best-executed treatment trials, using these models, are drug trials. In these trials, there is a recurring pattern: only one-fourth to one-third of subjects obtain significantly greater relief from drugs than from placebo,[5,6] which suggests that often clinicians will have to try more than one drug, and often will have to combine drugs; yet, there is very limited evidence for drug combination therapy. For neuropathic pain diagnoses other than PHN and diabetes mellitus, pharmacotheraputic decisions must rely on extrapolation,at best and on "empiricism" at worst.

The cumulative side effects and toxicity of drugs, and the risk and high cost of most technical nondrug treatments (e.g., surgery), provide the strongest arguments for trying the relatively low-cost, relatively safe nondrug, nonsurgical, and low-technical-rehabilitation approaches. In the spirit of "doing no harm," it is incumbent on physicians to use accessible, empowering, self-management therapeutic approaches, even in the absence of Western medicine-type "evidence."[7] On the risk side of the risk-benefit ratio, rehabilitation-based interventions have a strong advantage. If the clinician accepts *primum non nocere* as the first tenet of any therapeutic interaction, then there is certainly an overwhelming responsibility to understand and use rehabilitation principles to treat chronic neuropathic pain (or consult those who will). Unfortunately, concerning benefit, there is very little rigorous evidence. Most of the information discussed in this chapter is anecdotal or, at best, supported by case series. While it is clear that we immediately need better evidence for any treatment of neuropathic pain, it is also clear that we cannot postpone the necessity of making daily clinical decisions while awaiting that evidence. Hence the rationale for a chapter based primarily on anecdote.

At present, treatment approaches target "diagnoses" based on disease etiology rather than the best thinking about pathophysiology.[1,8–10] This is less than ideal for several reasons. First, most neuropathic pain disease states are associated with more than one mechanism of pain—and that mechanism usually changes over time. Second, different etiologies may produce mechanistically similar neuropathic pain syndromes. And finally, presenting symptoms, signs, and tests are often diverse within a single type of neuropathic pain syndrome.[11] Postherpetic neuralgia can be used to illustrate the pitfalls in treating neuropathic pain according to a simplistic view of "etiology." In PHN, at least three different pathophysiological mechanisms for pain have been identified, all of which are associated with direct neuronal damage to both the peripheral and central nervous systems (resulting from infectious, inflammatory, and ischemic processes).[12,13] Each of these mechanisms may be associated with different symptomatology. For instance, some patients present with profound sensory loss in an area of pain. Others have pronounced allodynia and hyperalgesia with minimal or no sensory loss. Still others present with sensory loss *and* allodynia.[10]

Studies have demonstrated that neuropathic pain, like all chronic pain, is prominently associated with psychosocial diagnoses; and comorbid conditions such as depression are common complications of chronic pain and further contribute to heterogeneous etiologies.[14,15] This diversity of potential mechanisms and symptoms results in complicated and ill-defined pathophysiological treatment targets; consequently, the response is unpredictable.[6] Thus, two seemingly similar patients with PHN may respond differently to the same treatment.[13] These limitations in our understanding of target mechanisms[8,9] often make the current and rather haphazard treatment approaches cumbersome and ineffective; and this diagnostic vagueness specifically corroborates the need to select simple, low-cost, and safe treatments early rather than to rush reflexively to relatively risky drug or other technical remedies.

THE RATIONALE FOR INTERDISCIPLINARY TREATMENT

Neuropathic pain syndromes can be very difficult to manage successfully.[4] Not only are the syndromes biomedically multifaceted, comprised of both central and peripheral pathophysiologies, but they also frequently encompass psychosocial components that are additional pivotal diagnostic features (and, thus, treatment targets[16]). The array of possible patient presentations and the fact that the presentation often changes over time complicate successful identification and treatment.[17] Given these obstacles to diagnosis, treatment, and research, how is a specialist to embark on a path toward the successful treatment of such complicated syndromes? The only treatment methodology that can possibly successfully span these gaps in medical science is a systematic and orderly interdisciplinary approach.[18,19] Interdisciplinary treatment is defined (here) as treatment provided by a dedicated, coherent, coordinated, specially trained group of relevant professionals who meet regularly to plan, coordinate care, and adapt to treatment eventualities.[16,18]

The integrated application of the holistic principles of rehabilitation in neuropathic pain often determines the success or failure of pain management. Because these rehabilitation techniques comprise nonsurgical, noninvasive, nontoxic, low-tech and self-management interventions, their use should always be an early consideration for every complicated case. The goals of rehabilitation treatment are decreased pain, increased functioning, decreased long-term health care utilization, and decreased use of medications. The rehabilitation methods discussed here are labor and thought intensive on the part of both patient and staff, yet they can yield significant long-term increases in health and in quality of life. Interdisciplinary programs are designed to help patients learn to cope more effectively with pain and help them maintain the highest possible functional level while optimally managing pain with empowering techniques. In the 1950s, Bonica was one of the first specialists to recognize that physical therapy and psychotherapy greatly enhanced outcomes in patients whom he would have previously treated with nerve blocks alone.[20]

It is critical to identify and aggressively treat all relevant spheres of the pain experience. Focusing exclusively on the biomedical sphere (and drug therapy) often dooms the approach to failure, especially in chronic neuropathic pain. The psychological targets of the pain experience can be identified with many validated psychometric measures with proven sensitivity and specificity.[21] These psychological features are critically important diagnostic components to identify, and the treatments (e.g., cognitive behavioral treatments and psychopharmacology) can be significantly effective.[16] Pain intensity and the psychological sequelae/comorbidities of pain are recognized fundamental elements in understanding and treating the whole patient, yet the subjective character of these elements and of their measurement render them problematic for interpreting clinical outcomes. Thus, more objective clinical benchmarks and outcomes should be identified—standards on which clinical decisions may be based and success measured. These types of benchmarks and outcomes are part of interdisciplinary care (e.g., physical and biometric measurements[18]).

It is important to note that meta-analyses have shown that an interdisciplinary approach improves symptoms in patients with general chronic pain,[22,23] although no level one data exist specifically for neuropathic pain.[3,19] Hard data concerning which particular components of an interdisciplinary program yield positive outcomes, as well as which modalities should be delivered, when, and for how long, are currently unavailable.[16] Thus, the interdisciplinary/holistic method is currently empirical, yet the highly favorable risk-benefit ratios of these tactics justify the trials.

THE ROLE OF PHYSICAL THERAPY IN NEUROPATHIC PAIN

Physical therapists (PTs) apply a wide range of physical and behavioral treatments to reduce pain, prevent dysfunction, and optimize outcomes in patients with neuropathic pain. Some of the diagnoses in which there is evidence for the role and effectiveness of PT include diabetic peripheral neuropathy, phantom limb pain, HIV sensory neuropathy, PHN, central poststroke pain, low back and neck pain with a neuropathic origin, complex regional pain syndrome (CRPS), carpel tunnel syndrome, and multiple sclerosis pain.[24,25] Neuropathic pain can be the underlying cause of many secondary orthopedic problems as well, such as adhesive capsulitis, lateral epicondylitis, or even low back pain.

The general role and responsibilities of a PT, as cited in the International Association for the Study of Pain's ad hoc Subcommittee for Occupational Therapy and Physical Therapy Curriculum, are "Assessment of the primary and secondary chemical (infection/inflammation), biomechanical (stress/strain), and behavioral factors that contribute to pain, the pain-activity cycle, and overall function. In collaboration with the patient, development of a physical therapy exercise program directed at modifying the effect of primary and secondary contributors to pain, promotion of tissue healing, and reduction of the factors that may lead to the recurrence of pain and dysfunction. Intervention may include education, exercise, manual therapy, movement facilitation techniques, and application of electro/physical agents based on thermal/mechanical/electrical phototherapeutic modalities. Education is focused on understanding pain and on improved posture, body mechanics, and gait. Exercise is directed toward the strengthening of specific muscle groups as well as counteracting the effects of generalized deconditioning. Movement is used as a mechanism to control and decrease pain and to increase mobility."[26]

Patients with neuropathic pain may often be deconditioned, have postural imbalances, have decreased strength, have decreased energy to perform activities of daily living (ADLs) or meet work responsibilities, decreased range of motion, and decreased balance/proprioception from lack of activity; all these deficits represent therapeutic targets for the PT. A wide array of treatments is used to address neuropathic pain: cardiovascular training, strengthening, stretching, proprioceptive/balance, McKenzie self-treatment, Gary Gray functional training, Feldenkrais, aquatic therapy, and mirror therapy for phantom limb pain. Passive modalities such as transcutaneous electrical nerve stimulation (TENS), electrical stimulation, ultrasound, heat, ice, and manual therapy are used in the beginning stages of pain, but they are often replaced with more active treatment. The PT may focus on correcting or modulating the factors that may be contributing to neuropathic pain, such as poor posture, spasm, contractures, or bony ankylosis. For instance, in a compressive neuropathy, the goals of PT are to teach the patient stretching and strengthening exercises that enhance flexibility in those muscle groups that would tend to compress the nerve and to simultaneously strengthen the muscle groups that would tend to relieve the compression. Clinical studies[27] suggest that patients with neuropathic pain experience kinesiophobia (fear of movement/[re]injury). A slow, graded PT program aimed at practicing movements and reducing fear can directly help overcome kinesiophobia.[28] Cognitive-behavioral strategies and supportive educational approaches for pain management are appropriately implemented *during* PT to motivate patients and reduce kinesiophobia.

Endurance Training, Strengthening/ Stabilization, Stretching, and Balance/ Proprioception

Cardiovascular conditioning is a vital component in the treatment of patients with chronic neuropathic pain. Patients are instructed on how to achieve and sustain their target heart rate (60%–80% of the maximum heart rate) and are encouraged to incorporate these principles into a daily aerobic conditioning regimen. Exercising at 60%–80% of the maximum heart rate for 30 minutes facilitates improvements in endurance, metabolic stimulation, maintenance of muscle bulk, immunological modulation, improved sleep, endorphin release, and various positive psychological effects.[29]

Isometric and isotonic strengthening exercises serve to minimize disuse atrophy, increase circulation, and maintain muscle condition. Strengthening typically consists of a regimen of active and passive range-of-motion exercises, eventually progressing to isometric exercises. Later, isotonic exercise and, ideally, supervised weight training may be useful, provided that they do not aggravate the compression.

Stabilization exercises are also utilized in the treatment of radiculopathy. Rasmussen-Barr has shown that stabilizing training is more effective than manual treatment in reducing pain, decreasing functional disability levels, and improving general health.[30]

Flexibility exercises are used to help restore normal joint motion and prevent reinjury. Stretching exercises are rarely used in isolation and are typically coupled with strengthening exercises to promote long-term progress. Proprioception/balance exercises are used to affect ligament, tendon, and joints that may have been injured and accompany impairments of body awareness or position sense, which may persist after the acute stage of an injury. One very useful approach is proprioceptive neuromuscular facilitation exercises. These exercises are designed to promote a sustained stretch reflex through increased elongation of related muscle groups. They involve a pattern of spiral and diagonal movements that mirror functional movement patterns in order to encourage stimulation of proprioceptors and the neuromuscular mechanism as a whole.[31]

Movement Therapies

Movement therapies can include such methods as Feldenkrais, t'ai chi, Gary Gray therapy, and yoga. Feldenkrais therapy, an empirical invention of the disabled physicist Moshe Feldenkrais, is a way of retraining the body. It is defined as "awareness through movement and functional integration." The Feldenkrais method teaches patients how to improve their ability to function in daily life. A study by Lundblad[32] shows a decrease in complaints of pain in the neck and shoulders and in disability during leisure time after Feldenkrais therapy.

T'ai chi has been practiced in China for centuries as a relaxation techinque and for exercise. It is unique in its slow, smooth movements with low impact, low velocity, and minimal orthopedic complications.[33] The various benefits of t'ai chi include balance improvement, fall prevention, cardiovascular enhancement, and stress reduction.[34] Yoga, philosophically related to t'ai chi, is intended to help bring about a natural balance of body and mind[33] while facilitating flexibility and relieving "tightness" over compressed or inflamed nerves. Gary Gray therapy includes functional training exercises to strengthen the entire kinetic chain. Simulated environmental testing and effective team communication facilitate a progressive return to physical activity after the achievement of full range of motion and adequate strength and control.

Aquatic Therapy

Patients with limitations (including pain) that do not allow them to move or exercise on land can often participate in exercises in the water. Exercises performed in warm water have shown that the buoyancy of water may block nociception by acting on thermal receptors and mechanoreceptors, and the warmth of the water may enhance blood flow and facilitate flexibility and muscle relaxation. The ease of movement many patients report in a water environment may activate supraspinal pathways, resulting in decreased pain intensity.[35]

Self-treatment Using McKenzie Techniques

Neuropathic pain (e.g., radiculopathy) is prevalent in patients with low back pain. McKenzie treatment for low back pain emphasizes education and active involvement of patients in the management of their treatment in order to increase the perception of self-efficacy, decrease pain quickly, and restore function and independence, minimizing the number of visits to the clinic.[36] The crux of the McKenzie technique is to build strength and flexibility directionally toward the positions of most comfort. A clinician who uses McKenzie philosophies allow patients to progress efficiently and provide additional advanced hands-on techniques until the patients can successfully perform the prescribed skills on their own. Self-treatment may not be possible right away if a problem is complex. An individualized self-treatment program tailored to the patient's lifestyle puts the patient in control safely and effectively and provides an experiential education in self-treating the problem. The management of these skills and behaviors will minimize the risk of symptom recurrence and empower patients to rapidly manage themselves when symptoms occur.

Modalities

Passive modalities, such as thermotherapies and ultrasound, have demonstrated limited usefulness in neuropathic pain treatment. Neuromuscular facilitation and other manipulation therapies can be particularly valuable, primarily in relieving pressure on a compressed nerve. Physical therapists should be consulted in decision making when orthotics are indicated. Although bracing may be indicated in the initial stages of rehabilitation, it is not commonly useful as a long-term modality, because it creates dependency and causes atrophy of supporting muscles.

Even though they are commonly used in the management of painful neuropathies, electrostimulation methods have not been sufficiently investigated. It remains to be seen whether recent techniques (burst technologies, strength duration variation modalities, or high-frequency, low-amplitude stimulation) improve upon traditional square-wave TENS. Optimal electrode placement (e.g., over a motor point, along the course of nerves, at acupuncture points) remains similarly unresolved. Until the results of more comprehensive studies are available, a patient, flexible, and pragmatic methodology developed by an experienced PT will provide the best outcome. The PT enhances stretching programs by training the patient to apply heat before sustained stretching and ice afterwards.

OCCUPATIONAL THERAPY FOR NEUROPATHIC PAIN

Occupational therapists (OTs) collaborate with patients to identify and optimize areas of everyday life that are adversely affected by disability. As such, OTs are often considered the ideal therapeutic leaders in the functional restoration process, as they are trained in the biopsychosocial principles of disease and are primary in functional assessment and treatment.[37] Patients with neuropathic pain may exhibit a loss of function in ADLs, work, leisure, or school. Mullersdorf[38] outlined a set of selection criteria that were strong predictive variables for the need of OT in neuropathic pain. These include the (rather nebulous) presence of "irresolute feelings" about pain, a "gnawing and searing" pain, gender, use of compensatory strategies, and an inability to perform tasks/work partially or fully.[38] The OT will assess and identify the specific components of pain that are impacting all relevant areas of function and occupation. The treatment plan should be centered on effective use of the body during these tasks, modifying the tasks to eliminate steps, and modifying the environment to support the patient in the most biomechanically advantageous position to decrease pain and maximize performance. Specifically, the patient may participate in posture exercises, body mechanics, ergonomic training, energy conservation, joint protection techniques, work simulation or work hardening, occasional splinting, edema management, and/or a rigorously structured home program in desensitization and stress loading.

Posture Retraining

Posture retraining is central to managing pain diagnoses during everyday activities. Neuropathic pain is often accompanied by a significant increase in pain with prolonged static positioning. In a recent randomized, controlled trial by Bernaards et al.,[39] it was found that the use of work-style intervention (changes in body posture, workplace adjustments, breaks, and coping strategies) was more effective in reducing pain outcomes than physical activity or no intervention at all. Through OT, the patient learns about maladaptive posturing and its effect on persistent pain—specifically, how to self-adjust in order to decrease overall pain during daily activities that require extended periods of sitting, standing, or lying down (sleep). Often, environmental modification is necessary to support the patient in an ideal posture during these activities. This can be accomplished by adjusting the workstation to encourage neutral positioning of the spine or an affected extremity, such as using lumbar supports or available office chair adjustments for height, seat depth, and seat angle or using footstools for prolonged standing. The importance of posture principles cannot be overemphasized to patients because these concepts are then carried over to more dynamic functional activities in the form of body mechanics training and the relief of stress or compression on neurological structures.

Body Mechanics

Body mechanics can be described as the application of kinesiology during dynamic activities such as bending, lifting, carrying, and reaching. Instruction in proper body mechanics, especially repetitive lifting, has demonstrated effectiveness in improving dynamic endurance for patients undergoing intensive work conditioning.[40] However, adapting the traditional principles of body mechanics to fit the workplace or work duties is essential to encourage carryover outside of treatment. The OT will assist the patient in identifying safe ways to use the body during activities that place increased demand on the body. The therapist will train the patient in proper use of larger muscle groups during heavy tasks and in minimizing overall energy expenditure during lighter but more repetitive tasks. It may be necessary to implement environmental modification (e.g., changing the level at which items are stored) or use adaptive equipment (e.g., reachers) when the patient's physical abilities are not sufficient to complete the task without increasing pain. Body mechanics training may also be used as part of an overall work hardening or work conditioning program.

Occupational therapy is becoming more widely recognized as an integral part of interdisciplinary care for neuropathic pain because of its emphasis on meaningful activity to increase independence in daily activities. In fact, the use of occupation-embedded/functional activities versus rote exercise to promote motor performance has been widely studied and supported by a high level of evidence.[41] Occupational therapy has also been shown to improve skill acquisition, retention, and transfer to everyday activities because of the emphasis on purpose and meaning during treatment activities.[42] Each of these findings has strengthened the empirical basis for the inclusion of OT as a component of the conservative management of multiple neurological conditions, translating into better outcomes and improved self-efficacy for the patient. The OT will work closely with PT, psychologists, medical doctors, and vocational counselors as needed to ensure that all areas of function affected by neuropathic pain are being addressed. Physical therapists may also employ some of the above treatments, depending on the size of the interdisciplinary team, the global treatment plan, and the availability of OTs at a particular site.

Work Hardening and Work Conditioning

Work hardening and work conditioning are therapeutic programs to build tolerance and maximize performance for return to work. While the terms *work hardening* and *work conditioning* are often used interchangeably, there is a difference in duration and scope of treatment between the two programs (see Table 26.1). In order to be eligible for either work hardening or work conditioning, the patient must have a target job, motivation to return to work, and no preexisting medical condition that would contraindicate such intensive therapy. The OT will design a work circuit tailored to the type of job to which the patient will return, which may include aerobic conditioning, simulated lifting, carrying, crawling, ladder climbing, and overhead activities. Work hardening and work conditioning programs can range from 2 to 8 hours a day, depending on the patient's tolerance for activity and the job requirements (and are optimally designed to mimic the patient's normal day). These programs are also designed to be upgraded as the patient builds tolerance to the work demands. The programs are terminated once the patient has plateaued or the

Table 26-1. Program Comparison

WORK CONDITIONING		
Focuses on physical and functional needs, may be provided by one discipline (single discipline model)	Utilizes physical conditioning and functional activities related to work	Provided in multi-hour sessions up to: −4 hours/day −5 days/week −8 weeks
WORK HARDENING		
Focuses on physical, functional, behavioral, and vocational needs within a multidisciplinary model	Utilizes real or simulated work activities	Provided in multi-hour sessions up to: −8 hours/day −5 days/week −8 weeks

Source: http://www.apta.org.

job demands are met; additionally, work place adaptation/modification may be necessary if the patient does not meet the physical requirements for the job. In returning patients to employment tasks that require physical activity, contact with the employer is helpful to determine which job roles can be safely undertaken. The decision to return to full activity should be made by the whole treatment team (which includes the patient).

Ergonomics

Ergonomics literally means "the laws of work," but for the management of neuropathic pain it can be considered the science of adapting the task or environment to optimize productivity and safety while minimizing pain. Ergonomic assessment and modification of the workplace have demonstrated a positive effect on pain levels when coupled with patient education. In a study by Amick et al.,[43] workers who received training in office ergonomics and the use of ergonomic equipment had a reduced increase in pain and discomfort over the course of a typical work day. Those study participants who received only training or no intervention at all demonstrated no significant reduction in progressive symptoms over the work day.[43] The OT will consider the patient's current abilities with respect to work tolerances for sitting, standing, and the use of bilateral extremities when making specific recommendations for job site modification. A work site visit may be necessary to evaluate job tasks, to devise a work simulation regimen, and to ensure that all modifications and devices are properly applied; however, the patient should be trained in the assessment process so that he or she can generalize these principles to other activities (e.g., household or leisure activities).

Splinting and Physical Agent Modalities

Splinting may be used to maintain tissue length and increase circulation to the affected area during the treatment of the early stages of neuropathic pain syndromes (e.g., carpal tunnel or CRPS). The OT may issue a customized or prefabricated splint and educate the patient on an appropriate wearing schedule to prevent tissue shortening and to decrease pain with functional activities. Splinting is most often used in the acute stages of neuropathic pain to help improve the functional use of the extremity; however, prolonged use of these adaptive devices may encourage disuse of the affected extremity and contribute to deconditioning of the underlying/supporting muscles. Physical agent modalities (e.g., fluidotherapy, TENS, iontophoresis) may be used as adjuncts to the above therapies, but typically they are discontinued after the subacute stages of neuropathic pain. Passive treatments, such as modalities and manual therapy, can encourage the patient's reliance on the therapist rather than the self-management of pain.

ENERGY CONSERVATION

Energy conservation is a therapeutic intervention focused on educating the patient to maximize the available energy in order to maintain stable levels of pain and endurance during daily activities. Energy conservation can include work simplification, activity pacing, and joint protection techniques. Neuropathic pain is often accompanied by a decrease in energy and a subsequent decrease in functional activities, in many cases making energy conservation the cornerstone of functional rehabilitation across disciplines. Mathiowetz et al.[44] demonstrated the importance of energy conservation education for persons with multiple sclerosis with respect to decreasing fatigue, increasing self-efficacy, and improving the quality of life. Additionally, these authors followed participants of their 2005 randomized clinical trial 1 year post-treatment and found that 70% continued to use the energy conservation techniques learned during the energy conservation course.[45] The OT (as well as the PT and the psychologist) will assist the patient in identifying the most appropriate techniques to integrate into specific functional activities.

MIRROR THERAPY

Most often used and studied in phantom limb pain and CRPS type II, pain relief associated with mirror therapy may be due to the activation of contralateral inhibitory (analgesic) cerebral systems to a painful (deafferented or lesioned) limb by normalized visual input from the unaffected "mirror" limb.[46] Visual input of what appears to be movement of the amputated limb may act to inhibit or modulate the activity of afferent pain systems through *gating*.[47] Although the underlying mechanism accounting for the success of this therapy remains to be elucidated, these results suggest that mirror therapy may be helpful in alleviating phantom pain[46] and CRPS.[48] In a case report study by Selles et al.,[49] the patient was able to perform exercises that were previously too painful before the mirror therapy treatment.

COMPLEX REGIONAL PAIN SYNDROME

Some of the strongest evidence for the inclusion of OT and PT in the rehabilitation process for neuropathic pain comes from the study of CRPS. In fact, interdisciplinary care is now generally accepted as a critical step toward rehabilitating persons with CRPS, and the treatment recommendations in this syndrome provide a useful template for the treatment of other neuropathic conditions. Oerlemans et al.[50] concluded that OT (and PT) produced increased improvement in functional use of the affected limb for patients diagnosed with CRPS. "In general, OT of CRPS should aim to normalize sensation, promote normal positioning, decrease muscle guarding, minimize edema, and increase functional use of the extremity in order to increase independence in all areas of occupation."[51] Harden et al.[7] have outlined a specific clinical pathway for conservative treatment of CRPS (see Figure 26.1). This algorithm presents a framework or guide for the progression of therapy that begins with reactivation/desensitization and moves toward more functional use of the affected extremity with range-of-motion exercises, stress loading, strengthening, and eventual normalization of use.

Desensitization

Of the characteristics of neuropathic pain in general and those of CRPS in particular, allodynia

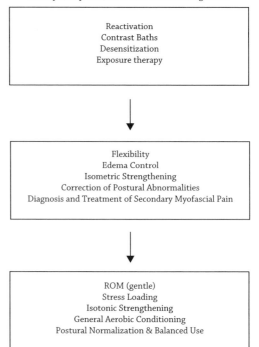

A sample, step-wise, functional restoration algorithm

Reactivation
Contrast Baths
Desensitization
Exposure therapy

Flexibility
Edema Control
Isometric Strengthening
Correction of Postural Abnormalities
Diagnosis and Treatment of Secondary Myofascial Pain

ROM (gentle)
Stress Loading
Isotonic Strengthening
General Aerobic Conditioning
Postural Normalization & Balanced Use

Ergonomics
Movement Therapies
Normalization of Use
Vocational/Functional Rehabilitation

FIGURE 26.1 Functional restoration algorithm for CRPS. From the outset, in appropriate cases, the patient should have access to medications and/or psychotherapy and/or injections. If the patient cannot begin, or fails to progress at any step or in any regard, the clinical team should consider starting (or adding) more or stronger medications and/or more intensive psychotherapies and/or different interventions.

Source: Reprinted with permission from Harden RN, Swan M, King A, et al. Treatment of complex regional pain syndrome: functional restoration. *Clin J Pain*. 2006;22(5):420–424.

or hyperalgesia can have a considerable impact on function. Desensitization is used to normalize the body's response to nonnoxious stimuli (e.g., light touch, temperature, and pressure). There are two commonly used protocols for desensitization. Hardy et al.[52] described a structured methodology for desensitizing the traumatized hand using paraffin, massage, vibration, constant touch-pressure activities, texture, and object identification. The Downey Hand Center Sensitivity Test, which later became the Three Phase Hand Sensitivity Test and the Three Phase Desensitization program, consists of 10 textured dowels, 10 contact particles, and vibration. Each component of the system is introduced in a systematic, structured, and function-oriented manner.[53] Textures can range from those of silk to Velcro, and contact particles can include cotton, rice, beans, pebbles, and plastic tubes. Vibration is useful in the early stages of focal desensitization, but it is less often incorporated into the patient's long-term home program.[54] Following a thorough assessment, the OT will determine the functional impact of these sensitivities and construct an individualized desensitization program according to the patient's needs.

Edema Management

Edema, or swelling of the extremity, must be addressed immediately once it has been identified in treatment. Edema is an accumulation of protein-rich fluid that can limit range of motion and tissue mobility by serving as an interstitial adhesive for fascia, skin, muscle tissue, and tendons. Edema prevents the smooth gliding of tissue during functional movement of the joint, contributing to increased pain. There are four main stages of edema, starting with soft and fluid and progressing toward a more fibrotic presentation. The first stages respond best to retrograde massage and elevation. However, once the edema has become more gelatinous or fibrotic and starts to adhere to underlying structures, compression bandaging or manual lymph drainage may be necessary to reverse the process and break up the edema into areas of softness.[55] Upon evaluation, the OT will use circumferential or volumetric measurement of the affected and unaffected limbs in order to determine the baseline presence of edema and the necessary therapeutic intervention to decrease swelling (e.g., retrograde massage, manual lymph drainage, bandaging, or compression garments). Once the

swelling is managed, treatment can progress toward more active use of the extremity.

Stress Loading

Watson and Carlson[56] introduced a structured regimen to treat CRPS that includes active traction and compression exercises to provide normal proprioceptive input with minimal joint motion to the affected limb. A *stress loading* protocol consists of two stages: scrubbing and carrying. The *scrubbing* portion of the program places the patient in a quadruped position with a scrub brush in the affected extremity. The patient is instructed to scrub a board with a back-and-forth motion, applying as much pressure as can be tolerated. The hand should be directly below the shoulder to ensure maximum pressure through the joint. This position may be modified for patients with decreased weight bearing by performing the task standing, with a table as the scrubbing surface. Some therapists may use a Dystrophile® in treatment to encourage maximal pressure through the upper extremity during scrubbing. The Dystrophile® is a handheld device that gauges the pressure applied during scrubbing by using a light-emitting diode light to indicate when the patient has applied and sustained the required amount of force.

Carrying (loading) requires the patient to carry a weighted bag (purse or briefcase) during the day whenever walking or standing, with the arm fully extended. The typical weight of the bag will range from 1 to 5 pounds, depending on the patient's tolerance. Watson and Carlson found that CRPS patients using a stress loading protocol had a significant increasein range of motion and a decrease in pain from an average of 7.7 to 2.7 on a 10-point scale.[56] While this seminal study introduced a treatment technique for CRPS that is clinically useful and anecdotally beneficial for many patients, further research is needed to substantiate its use in the clinical setting.

SUMMARY

Because the pathophysiology of neuropathic pain encompasses all the biopsychosocial complexities of chronic pain, the best way to help our patients is to adopt a systematic, stable, empathetic, and, above all, interdisciplinary approach that addresses all of these putative mechanisms.[16,19] A consideration of nondrug and noninterventional treatments should be foremost, as they demonstrate a very favorable cost-benefit ratio, and not an afterthought after drug failure. High-level evidence supporting the rationale for interdisciplinary treatment of neuropathic pain is fairly sparse (as it is for the treatment of chronic pain in general), and the anecdotal and empirical impression that rehabilitation-based treatments can and should be the pivotal intervention is a theory that must be tested.[19] Until then, the interdisciplinary approach for treating patients with neuropathic pain remains the most pragmatic, helpful, and cost-effective regimen available.

REFERENCES

1. Bennett G. Neuropathic pain: an overview. In: Borsook D, ed. *Molecular Neurobiology of Pain.* Seattle: IASP Press; 1997:109–113.
2. Farrar JT, Portenoy RK. Neuropathic cancer pain: the role of adjuvant analgesics. *Oncology (Williston Park).* 2001;15(11):1435–1442, 1445; discussion 1445, 1450–1433.
3. Dworkin RH. An overview of neuropathic pain: syndromes, symptoms, signs, and several mechanisms. *Clin J Pain.* 2002;18(6):343–349.
4. Jensen TS, Gottrup H, Sindrup SH, Bach FW. The clinical picture of neuropathic pain. *Eur J Pharmacol.* 2001;429(1–3):1–11.
5. Rowbotham M, Harden N, Stacey B, Bernstein P, Mangus-Miller L. Gabapentin for the treatment of postherpetic neuralgia: a randomized controlled trial. *JAMA.* 1998;280(21):1837–1842.
6. Orza F, Boswell MV, Rosenberg SK. Neuropathic pain: review of mechanisms and pharmacologic management. *NeuroRehabilitation.* 2000;14(1): 15–23.
7. Harden RN, Swan M, King A, Costa B, Barthel J. Treatment of complex regional pain syndrome: functional restoration. *Clin J Pain.* 2006;22(5): 420–424.
8. Woolf CJ, Bennett GJ, Doherty M, et al. Towards a mechanism-based classification of pain? *Pain.* 1998;77(3):227–229.
9. Attal N, Bouhassira D. Mechanisms of pain in peripheral neuropathy. *Acta Neurol Scand Suppl.* 1999;173:12–24; discussion 48–52.
10. Baron R. Peripheral neuropathic pain: from mechanisms to symptoms. *Clin J Pain.* 2000;16 (2 suppl):S12–S20.
11. Fields HL, Rowbotham MC. Multiple mechanisms of neuropathic pain: a clinical perspective. In: Gebhart GF, Hammond DL, Jensen TS, eds. *Proceedings of the 7th World Congress on Pain.* Seattle: IASP Press; 1994:437–454.
12. Fields HL, Rowbotham M, Baron R. Postherpetic neuralgia: irritable nociceptors and deafferentation. *Neurobiol Dis.* 1998;5(4):209–227.
13. Bonezzi C, Demartini L. Treatment options in postherpetic neuralgia. *Acta Neurol Scand Suppl.* 1999;173:25–35; discussion 48–52.
14. Gallagher RM, Verma S. Managing pain and comorbid depression: a public health challenge. *Semin Clin Neuropsychiatry.* 1999;4(3): 203–220.
15. Clark MR, Heinberg LJ, Haythornthwaite JA, Quatrano-Piacentini AL, Pappagallo M, Raja SN. Psychiatric symptoms and distress differ between patients with postherpetic neuralgia and peripheral vestibular disease. *J Psychosom Res.* 2000;48(1):51–57.
16. Harden RN. Neuropathic pain. In: Von Roenn JH, Paice JA, Preodor M, eds. *Current Diagnosis and Treatment of Pain.* New York: Lange Medical Books/McGraw-Hill Medical Publication. Division; 2006:122–135.
17. Bruehl S, Harden RN, Galer BS, Saltz S, Backonja M, Stanton-Hicks M. Complex regional pain syndrome: are there distinct subtypes and sequential stages of the syndrome? *Pain.* 2002;95(1–2): 119–124.
18. Harden RN. The rationale for integrated functional restoration. In: Wilson PR, Stanton-Hicks MDA, Harden RN, eds. *CRPS: Current Diagnosis and Therapy.* Vol. 32. Seattle: IASP Press; 2005:163–172.
19. Gilron I, Watson CP, Cahill CM, Moulin DE. Neuropathic pain: a practical guide for the clinician. *CMAJ.* 2006;175(3):265–275.
20. Bonica JJ. *The Management of Pain.* Philadelphia: Lea and Feibiger; 1953.
21. Turk D, Melzack R. The measurement of pain and the assessment of people experiencing pain. In: Turk D, Melzack R, eds. *Handbook of Pain Assessment.* New York: Guilford Press; 2001:3–14.
22. Flor H, Fydrich T, Turk DC. Efficacy of multidisciplinary pain treatment centers: a meta-analytic review. *Pain.* 1992;49(2):221–230.
23. Guzmán J, Esmail R, Karjalainen K, Malmivaara A, Irvin E, Bombadier C. Multidisciplinary rehabilitation for chronic low back pain: systematic review. *BMJ.* 2001;322(7301):1511–1516.

24. Lee MHM, Itoh M, Yang G-FW, Eason AL. Physical therapy and rehabilitation medicine. In: Bonica JJ, ed. *The Management of Pain*. Vol. 2. 2nd ed. Philadelphia: Lea & Febiger; 1990:1769–1788.

25. APTA. Guidelines: Occupational Health Physical Therapy: Work Conditioning and Work Hardening Programs BOD G03-01-17-58 [Retitled: Occupational Health Guidelines: Work Conditioning and Work Hardening Programs, Amended BOD 03-00-25-62; BOD 03-99-16-49; BOD 11-94-33-109; Initial BOD 11-92-29-134] www.apta.org/ . . . /APTAorg/ . . . /OccupationalHealth-WorkConditioningHardening.pdf - Accessed April 14, 2009

26. IASP. Ad hoc Subcommittee for Occupational Therapy and Physical Therapy Curriculum. Pain curriculum for students in occupational therapy or physical therapy. IASP Newsletter. November-December; 1994:3–8.

27. Picavet HS, Vlaeyen JW, Schouten JS. Pain catastrophizing and kinesiophobia: predictors of chronic low back pain. *Am J Epidemiol.* 2002;156(11):1028–1034.

28. Trost Z, France CR, Thomas JS. Exposure to movement in chronic back pain: evidence of successful generalization across a reaching task. *Pain.* 2008;137(1):26–33.

29. Farrell PA, Gustafson AB, Morgan WP, Pert CB. Enkephalins, catecholamines, and psychological mood alterations: effects of prolonged exercise. *Med Sci Sports Exerc.* 1987;19(4):347–353.

30. Rasmussen-Barr E, Nilsson-Wikmar L, Arvidsson I. Stabilizing training compared with manual treatment in sub-acute and chronic low-back pain. *Man Ther.* 2003;8(4):233–241.

31. Voss DE, Ionta MK, Myers BJ, Knott M. *Proprioceptive Neuromuscular Facilitation: Patterns and Techniques*. 3rd ed. Philadelphia: Harper & Row; 1985.

32. Lundblad I, Elert J, Gerdle B. Randomized controlled trial of physiotherapy and Feldenkrais interventions in female workers with neck-shoulder complaints. *J Occup Rehabil.* 1999;9(3):179–194.

33. Galantino ML, Lucci SL. Living with chronic pain: exploration of complementary therapies and impact on quality of life. In: Wittink H, Hoskins Michel T, eds. *Chronic Pain Management for Physical Therapists*. 2nd ed. Boston: Butterworth-Heinemann; 2002:279–291.

34. Chen KM, Snyder M. A research-based use of Tai Chi/movement therapy as a nursing intervention. *J Holist Nurs.* 1999;17(3):267–279.

35. Hall J, Swinkels A, Briddon J, McCabe CS. Does aquatic exercise relieve pain in adults with neurologic or musculoskeletal disease? A systematic review and meta-analysis of randomized controlled trials. *Arch Phys Med Rehabil.* 2008;89(5):873–883.

36. Clare HA, Adams R, Maher CG. A systematic review of efficacy of McKenzie therapy for spinal pain. *Aust J Physiother.* 2004;50(4):209–216.

37. Severens JL, Oerlemans HM, Weegels AJ, van't Hof MA, Oostendorp RA, Goris RJ. Cost-effectiveness analysis of adjuvant physical or occupational therapy for patients with reflex sympathetic dystrophy. *Arch Phys Med Rehabil.* 1999;80(9):1038–1043.

38. Mullersdorf M. Factors indicating need of rehabilitation—occupational therapy among persons with long-term and/or recurrent pain. *Int J Rehabil Res.* 2000;23(4):281–294.

39. Bernaards CM, Ariens GA, Knol DL, Hildebrandt VH. The effectiveness of a work style intervention and a lifestyle physical activity intervention on the recovery from neck and upper limb symptoms in computer workers. *Pain.* 2007;132(1–2): 142–153.

40. Lieber SJ, Rudy TE, Boston JR. Effects of body mechanics training on performance of repetitive lifting. *Am J Occup Ther.* 2000;54(2):166–175.

41. Lin K, Wu C, Tickle-Degnen L, Coster W. Enhancing occupational performance through occupationally embedded exercise: a meta-analytic review. *Occup Ther J Res.* 1997;17(1):25–47.

42. Ferguson JM, Trombly CA. The effect of added-purpose and meaningful occupation on motor learning. *Am J Occup Ther.* 1997;51(7):508–515.

43. Amick BC 3rd, Robertson MM, DeRango K, et al. Effect of office ergonomics intervention on reducing musculoskeletal symptoms. *Spine (Phila Pa 1976).* 2003;28(24):2706–2711.

44. Mathiowetz VG, Finlayson ML, Matuska KM, Chen HY, Luo P. Randomized controlled trial of an energy conservation course for persons with multiple sclerosis. *Mult Scler.* 2005;11(5): 592–601.

45. Mathiowetz VG, Matuska KM, Finlayson ML, Luo P, Chen HY. One-year follow-up to a randomized controlled trial of an energy conservation course for persons with multiple sclerosis. *Int J Rehabil Res.* 2007;30(4):305–313.

46. Rossi S, Tecchio F, Pasqualetti P, et al. Somatosensory processing during movement observation in humans. *Clin Neurophysiol.* 2002;113(1):16–24.

47. Henson RA. Henry Head: his influence on the development of ideas on sensation. *Br Med Bull.* 1977;33(2):91–96.

48. McCabe C, Haigh R, Ring E, Halligan P, Wall P, Blake D. A controlled pilot study of the

utility of mirror visual feedback in the treatment of complex regional pain syndrome (type 1). *Rheumatology (Oxford)*. 2003;42(1): 97–101.

49. Selles RW, Schreuders TA, Stam HJ. Mirror therapy in patients with causalgia (complex regional pain syndrome type II) following peripheral nerve injury: two cases. *J Rehabil Med*. 2008;40(4):312–314.

50. Oerlemans HM, Oostendorp RA, de Boo T, Goris RJ. Pain and reduced mobility in complex regional pain syndrome I: outcome of a prospective randomised controlled clinical trial of adjuvant physical therapy versus occupational therapy. *Pain*. 1999;83(1):77–83.

51. Swan M. *Treating CRPS: A Guide for Therapy*. Milford, CT: RSDSA Press; 2004.

52. Hardy MA, Moran CA, Merritt WH. Desensitization of the traumatized hand. *Va Med*. 1982;109(2):134–137.

53. Rendell JW. Desensitization of the traumatized hand. In: Hunter JM, Mackin E, Callahan AD, eds. *Rehabilitation of the Hand: Surgery and Therapy*. 4th ed. St. Louis: Mosby; 1995:693–700.

54. Hochreiter NW, Jewell MJ, Barber L, Browne P. Effect of vibration on tactile sensitivity. *Phys Ther*. 1983;63(6):934–937.

55. Ryerson SD. Hemiplegia. In: Umphred DA, ed. *Neurological Rehabilitation*. 4th ed. St. Louis: Mosby; 2001:741–786.

56. Watson HK, Carlson L. Treatment of reflex sympathetic dystrophy of the hand with an active "stress loading" program. *J Hand Surg Am*. 1987;12(5 pt 1):779–785.

27

Preventing Neuropathic Pain in Experimental Models and Predictable Clinical Settings

J. ROBINSON SINGLETON AND A. GORDON SMITH

INTRODUCTION

PAIN IS NOT a condition that either patients or physicians typically contemplate in advance. As a result, the literature on neuropathic pain prevention is sparse. However, some clinical conditions cause neuropathic pain with such regularity that prophylaxis can be contemplated. These include treatment of cancer patients with potentially neurotoxic chemotherapy, surgery, diabetic neuropathy, and the development of postherpetic neuralgia after shingles. This chapter explores pain prophylaxis with a focus on human studies and clinical utility. Peripheral nerve causes of neuropathic pain are emphasized because they are generally much more predictable, though rare diseases such as thalamic stroke can also lead to neuropathic pain. Experience with treatment to prevent neuropathic pain can be considered in three broad categories: (1) experimental settings in which normal animals or humans are treated to prevent or lessen intentionally induced neuropathic pain; often these studies are not important in validating a particular medication, but rather as a way of understanding neuropathic pain pathogenesis; (2) trials of prophylaxis in diseases in which neuropathic pain is a predictable consequence of treatment, including cancer chemotherapy and postsurgical pain; and (3) diseases commonly associated with neuropathic pain (e.g., diabetic neuropathy) in which treatment reduces the disease incidence and thereby the associated neuropathic pain.

EXPERIMENTAL MODELS OF NEUROPATHIC PAIN

Animal Models

Experimental animal models in which nerve injury results in pain are important for exploring the pathogenesis of acute and chronic neuropathic pain and in preclinical screening for new drug development. Several different paradigms for neuropathic pain generation have been validated, including ligation of the sciatic nerve and spinal cord, injection of directly neurolytic or neurotoxic chemicals, and treatment with medications known to cause neuropathic pain in humans. Some paradigms, such as paclitaxel injection, are derived directly from clinical applications, while others are essentially irrelevant to human disease. A representative list of animal pain prophylaxis studies, grouped by neuropathic pain paradigm, is provided in Table 27-1. Most of these studies have clinical relevance in localizing and elucidating the mechanisms of pain pathogenesis, covered in greater detail in Chapter 2. A few examples illustrate the power of these studies to localize pain mechanisms to specific sites and neurotransmitters.

The development of chronic neuropathic pain requires molecular remodeling at the spinal level. Studies requiring manipulation or histological evaluation of spinal neurons are not feasible in humans and thus are typically a focus of rodent research. Partial sciatic nerve ligation predictably decreases withdrawal latencies to thermal and mechanical pain stimuli in rats or mice and has been used as an experimental model of neuropathic pain in response

Table 27-1. Experimental Paradigms for Neuropathic Pain

PAIN MODEL	TESTED MECHANISM	AGENT	SITE OF ACTION
Sciatic ligation	$GABA_B$ overexpression	Amitriptyline	Spinal neurons[1]
Sciatic ligation	Inflammatory cytokine interleukin-6	Minocycline i.p.	Peripheral axons[59]
Sciatic ligation	PPAR gamma agonism	Pioglitazone p.o.	Spinal glia[60]
Sciatic ligation	Immune cell-expressed opioids	Corticotropin releasing hormone	Peripheral axons[4]
Sciatic ligation, formalin paw injection	Nav 1.8 Na^+ channel	Ambroxol (Nav 1.8 inhibitor)	Peripheral small fibers[3]
Sciatic branch transection	PPAR gamma agonism	Rosiglitazone, i.t.	Spinal neurons, glia[61]
Spinal nerve injury	Glucocorticoid receptor	GCC antagonists RU-486, dexamethasone 21 mesylate	Spinal neurons[2]
Spinal nerve ligation	Voltage-gated Ca^{2+} channel inhibition	Gabapentin, pregabalin, other α-2δ binders	Spinal neurons[62]
Streptozotocin diabetic neuropathy	TNF-α and nitric oxide release	Curcumin	Peripheral small fibers[63]
Paclitaxel injection, i.p.	Unknown	Intrathecal interleukin-10	Dorsal root ganglia[64]
Paclitaxel injection, i.p.	Unknown	Acetyl-L-carnitine	C-fiber axonal mitochondria[65]
Paclitaxel injection, i.p.	Sodium channel activation	Tetrodotoxin	Peripheral axons[66]
Cisplatin i.p.	Prevent neuronal apoptosis	Growth hormone secretagogue gherelin	Peripheral axons[67]
Vincristine	Cannabinoid receptor activation	Cannabinoid CB1/CB2 receptor agonist	Spinal neurons[68]

PPAR, peroxisome proliferator-activated receptor; TNF-α, tumor necrosis factor-α.

to peripheral nerve injury. Ligation is associated with increased $GABA_B$ receptor subunit expression in lumbar spinal cord. Amitriptyline given as an intraperitoneal infusion prior to ligation prevents this increase in $GABA_B$ subunit expression and blunts reduction in pain thresholds to thermal and mechanical stimuli.[1] These results suggest that amitriptyline may act in part by maintaining spinal cord $GABA_B$ receptor activity.

Similarly, spinal nerve injury causes mechanical allodynia and thermal hyperalgesia associated with central overexpression of glucocorticoid receptor mRNA. Intrathecal or intraperitoneal prophylactic treatment with the glucocorticoid receptor antagonists RU-486 or dexamethasone 21-mesylate potently suppressed pain.[2] Interestingly, glucocorticoid antagonists given by intracerebroventricular injection were not effective, suggesting that glucocorticoid receptor overexpression in spinal neurons is particularly important for neuropathic pain generation. Similar peripheral and central injury models have been used to demonstrate the prophylactic efficacy of the voltage-gated sodium channel inhibitor Ambroxol.[3]

A novel mechanism for neuropathic regulation is demonstrated by work examining the release of opioid substances from peripheral leukocytes. Up to 40% of reactive white blood cells recruited to the site of acute peripheral nerve injury produce counterregulatory and anti-inflammatory endogenous opioids, including B-endorphin, met-enkephalin, and dynorphin A.[4] Release of these opioids from leukocytes in response to corticotropin releasing factor significantly reduces tactile allodynia in mice subjected to neuropathic pain by sciatic nerve ligation. These results both confirm an important role for the inflammatory response in peripheral neuropathic pain pathogenesis and recognize a novel potential site for pain prophylaxis.

Human Experimental Models of Neuropathic Pain

Trials of neuropathic pain medication in patients with existing pain are often inefficient, burdened by high dropout rates and a powerful placebo effect. As a result, screening of potential pain agents in human subjects is expensive, and historically has often failed to replicate the favorable results of animal testing. Human models of induced neuropathic pain have been developed as a platform for rapid preclinical screening of potential pain treatments. Use of human subjects has obvious advantages for measurement of an intrinsically subjective experience: unlike rodents, whose behavior must be observed, human subjects can directly report pain severity.[5] Moreover, because neuropathic pain is reproducibly evoked, testing of true pain prophylaxis is possible. Studies of evoked pain in human volunteers raise obvious potential ethical concerns. Institutional review board approval, careful oversight to ensure that monetary or other inducements are not coercive, and close monitoring by ombudsmen are necessary.

Simple paradigms for quantitative sensory testing of cutaneous heat-pain thresholds have been used to examine pain prophylaxis induced by drugs and other modalities. A metal disc applied to the skin is gradually heated (typically using circulating hot water) until the patient reports that the sensation has become painful. This system does not itself induce neuropathic pain, since there is no element of central sensitization unless the test is performed repeatedly. However, it allows recognition of the threshold for heat hyperalgesia. Serial measurement of thermal hyperalgesia has been suggested as a predictive measure of early neurotoxicity in patients receiving oxaliplatin therapy for colorectal cancer.[6]

The perception threshold for thermal hyperalgesia has also been deliberately manipulated using transcranial magnetic stimulation (TMS). The left prefrontal cortex, through its connections with the nucleus cuneiformis and periaqueductal grey matter, has been proposed as a region for the central regulation of pain perception.[7] Transcranial magnetic stimulation of either the dominant motor cortex or the premotor cortex has been shown to ameliorate chronic neuropathic pain associated with diverse injuries, including cervical root avulsions and stroke. In controlled trials, repetitive motor cortex TMS results in suppression of pain associated with trigeminal neuralgia or poststroke pain for up to 2 weeks.[8] Transcranial magnetic stimulation has been used prophylactically to reduce neuropathic pain perception in experimental models. In healthy adult volunteers, 15 minutes of prefrontal TMS significantly increased thermal pain thresholds compared to sham treatment.[9] After undergoing a standardized assessment of their individual resting motor threshold, subjects received a magnetic stimulus sufficient to stimulate thumb movement 50% of the time, at 20-second intervals for 15 minutes. These studies demonstrate that thermal hyperalgesia can be prospectively manipulated.

Development and maintenance of chronic peripheral neuropathic pain requires reinforcement of nociceptive signaling at the level of spinal interneurons and central projections through repeated painful stimuli.[10] This central sensitization (see Chapter 1 of this volume) is recognized as critical to chronic pain behavior in animal models. Human models of central sensitization have been developed using either intradermal injection of capsaicin[11,12] or painful subdermal electrical stimulation.[13] Subdermal capsaicin-induced neuropathic pain has been validated with placebo-controlled trials of gabapentin.[12] However, repeated painful electrical stimulation to produce central sensitization in the skin of the volar forearm is probably the best-validated technique. For each subject, 2 Hz pulses of electrical current are delivered via two intradermal wire electrodes at gradually increasing intensities over 15 minutes to achieve a subjective pain rating of 6 on an 11-point numeric rating scale, then maintained at constant current for the 180-minute testing session. Subjects develop hyperalgesia to pin sensation over the stimulated skin, as well as allodynia to pressure from a 256 mN von Frey filament or light touch with a cotton ball. The area of skin affected by these neuropathic pain responses is measured at 20- minute intervals. Subjects serve as their own controls across multiple treatment sessions.

Comparison of capsaicin and electrical stimulation in human volunteers shows that both methods induce primary hyperalgesia to heat and pinprick with good test-retest reproducibility.[5] Clinically, central sensitization can be quantitated by examining the area of skin

with resultant hyperalgesia or allodynia for reproducible sensory stimuli. Stimulation of small unmyelinated nociceptive fibers results in reflex activation of adjacent axonal branches leading to release of calcitonin gene-related peptide, histamine, and other inflammatory mediators and a vascular *flare* response that may be used as a measure of peripheral C-fiber activation.[14] Electrical stimulation produces a more robust vasogenic flare. The temporal profiles of the two techniques differ. Electrical stimulation produces central stimulation that increases with the duration and intensity of the stimulus, while capsaicin causes rapid onset of pain with diminution over time despite continued capsaicin stimulation, a less favorable and less controllable profile.

Chizh et al. validated the subdermal electrical stimulus model by comparing the pain prophylactic effects of the neuropathic agent pregabalin and the centrally acting tachykinin (substance P) NK1 receptor antagonist aprepitant in a prospective, double-blind, placebo-controlled two-period crossover design.[15] Thirty-two healthy control subjects were given baseline stimulus testing, then randomized to pretreatment for 6 days with either oral pregabalin (titrated to 300 mg), aprepitant (titrated to 320 mg/day), or placebo, prior to repeat electrical stimulus testing. In a subsequent session, subjects who had received active medication crossed over to placebo and vice versa. Even in this small group, pregabalin demonstrated very significant reduction in skin areas of punctate mechanical allodynia and pin hyperalgesia compared to the placebo prophylaxis trial ($p < .0001$). In contrast, aprepitant showed no significant prophylaxis for hyperalgesia or allodynia, demonstrating the specificity of the model for neuropathic pain agents. As an added nuance, intravenous injection of the nonsteroidal agent parecoxib, but not intravenous saline, produced an additive antinociceptive effect when given 120 minutes into the experimental electrical stimulus period. Prophylactic intravenous parecoxib has been previously shown to reduce central hyperalgesia in the electrical stimulation model.[16] Measurement of the flare response by laser Doppler flowmetry together with areas of heat or pin hyperalgesia allow determination of whether the study drug has a component of peripheral nerve activity.

These studies illustrate the sophistication with which human neuropathic pain models can compare the acute prophylactic effects of drugs alone or in combination. Use of such models may reduce costs and shorten the time necessary to provide validation for novel neuropathic pain agents translated from animal studies. However, human models are necessarily limited by ethical considerations, and will never be able to fully recapitulate the complex process of altered nociceptive signaling, and cellular remodeling of spinal and central afferent neurons and support cells, that contribute to chronic neuropathic pain emergence and maintenance.

DISEASE TREATMENTS ASSOCIATED WITH PREDICTABLE NEUROPATHIC PAIN

Chemotherapy-Induced Peripheral Neuropathy

A sensory-predominant peripheral polyneuropathy develops in 30%–40% of cancer patients receiving a broad spectrum of chemotherapeutic agents[17,18] (Figure 27.1). Not surprisingly, the presence of chemotherapy-induced peripheral neuropathy (CIPN) is a predictor of subsequent neuropathic pain.[19] Uncomfortable paresthesias often segue into chronic distal neuropathic pain in proportion to the severity of the sensory deficits. The platinum-derived compounds, vinca alkaloids, and paclitaxel are particularly likely to cause neuropathic pain (see also Chapters 14 and 24). Despite their common use in clinical practice, traditional neuropathic pain medications have generally not been shown to be effective once CIPN is established. A retrospective comparison of cancer patients with neuropathic pain following chemotherapy found that the 75 patients receiving gabapentin were significantly more likely to report a "complete" neuropathic pain reduction than the 33 patients receiving fixed-dose naproxen/codeine/paracetemol.[20] However, randomized, placebo-controlled trials of sufficient size in established CIPN patients have failed to demonstrate efficacy for nortriptyline,[21] amitriptyline,[22] gabapentin,[23] or lamotrigine.[24]

These discouraging results suggest that, as with shingles, prophylactic therapy to prevent CIPN may be the only effective strategy. In fact, a variety of agents have shown efficacy in reducing the incidence of CIPN and limiting the severity of associated neuropathic pain. Vitamin E (alpha-tocopherol) has been examined in two small prospective but unblinded, randomized trials. Patients were randomized to receive vitamin E or no additional therapy during and for 3 months following the completion of cisplatin

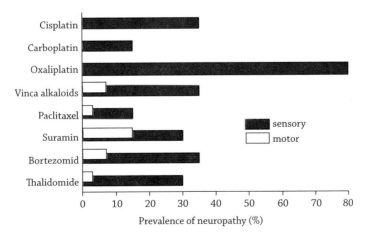

FIGURE 27.1 Common chemotherapeutic agents associated with peripheral neuropathy.

Source: Windebank AJ, Grisold W. Chemotherapy-induced neuropathy. *J Peripher Nerv Syst*. 2008;13(1):27–46.

therapy. Chemotherapy-induced peripheral neuropathy developed in only 4 of 13 vitamin E patients but in 12 of 13 controls. Similarly, of 40 patients receiving combination chemotherapy including cisplatin and paclitaxel, 25% of those randomized to vitamin E (alpha tocopherol 300 mg BID) developed CIPN, while 73% of controls did so. The results for both small trials were statistically significant. A large placebo-controlled study has been initiated in response to these promising results. A barrier to adoption of vitamin E therapy has been concern that it might diminish the effectiveness of chemotherapy. Vitamin E treatment (along with the antioxidant beta-carotene) has been linked to a higher recurrence rate in head and neck cancer patients receiving radiation therapy.[25] However, animal studies[17] and at least one randomized trial of multiple oral antioxidants (vitamin E, beta carotene, and vitamin C) in patients receiving carboplatin and paclitaxel[26] found no evidence of altered in vitro cancer cell lethality, clinical treatment response rates, or median patient survival times in association with vitamin E administration.

Calcium and magnesium infused at the time of chemotherapy have been proposed as treatment to prevent CIPN because of the cations' inhibitory effect on excitatory sodium channel activation by chemotherapeutic agents, particularly oxaliplatin. A prospective, double-blinded study randomized colon cancer patients receiving oxaliplatin to receive either calcium/magnesium or saline infusion. Although the study was stopped early due to the (ultimately unfounded) concern that calcium/magnesium infusion might reduce oxaliplatin efficacy, a post hoc analysis demonstrated that the calcium/magnesium infusion was associated with reduced CIPN cumulative incidence rates (28% vs. 51%) and with reduced overall neurotoxicity compared to placebo treatment.[17] The amino acid glutamine, the antioxidants n-acetylcysteine and glutathione, and the neurotrophic agent xaliproden have demonstrated reduced CIPN incidence compared to placebo or no treatment in small randomized studies,[17] but additional data from more rigorously designed trials are necessary.

Interestingly, few trials have addressed the prophylactic effects of common neuropathic pain agents on the incidence of CIPN or associated pain. An open-label prospective study randomized 32 patients undergoing oxaliplatin therapy for colon cancer to receive either oxcarbazepine (titrated to 600 mg BID) or no additional treatment.[27] Thirty-one percent of oxcarbazepine-treated subjects developed peripheral neuropathy (judged by the clinical features on exam) compared to 75% of controls, a statistically significant difference. In a separate study, patients with advanced colorectal cancer receiving oxaliplatin therapy were assigned to receive either the antiepileptic medication carbamazepine, titrated to achieve a plasma level of 4–6 mg/L, or no treatment. The study was underrecruited, and no significant difference in the severity of neurotoxicity was observed between the groups.[28] Large, carefully designed studies of neuropathic pain agents focused specifically on prevention of neuropathic pain due to chemotherapy have not been performed.

Postoperative Pain

Major surgery reliably causes postoperative pain, which results from a combination of superficial tissue and visceral injury, positioning, a diffuse inflammatory response, and peripheral nerve damage. Visceral nociception may be enhanced in the immediate postoperative period by acetic acid-driven inflammatory release of aspartate, glutamate, serine, and glycine from spinal neurons or support cells.[29] The presence of postoperative allodynia and hyperalgesia experienced by many patients points to a component of secondary neuropathic pain.[30] Repetitive TMS has been used to temporarily reduce pain perception in surgical settings. In two similar prospective studies, 20 patients undergoing elective gastric bypass surgery were randomized to receive either repetitive transcranial magnetic stimulation (TMS; 10 Hz, 10 seconds on, 20 seconds off) or sham TMS for 20 minutes in the immediate postoperative period.[31,32] Patients receiving real TMS used less self-administered morphine in the postoperative period and reported less pain on the Visual Analogue Scale (VAS) scales than sham- treated control patients ($p < .05$ for both groups). Several caveats limit the potential significance of these findings. All of the described studies were performed by a single investigative group, and TMS has not been validated for pain prophylaxis by other groups or in other clinical settings. True blinding is difficult since rTMS intensity was calibrated to produce a hand or thumb twitch that could be noticed by the subject. Postoperative pain is probably not primarily neuropathic. Finally, TMS has been posited to affect mood and has been proposed for the treatment of depression. Postoperatively, patients who received brief repetitive TMS reported fewer depressive symptoms, as measured by the Beck Depression Index, than did sham-treated controls. Thus, reduced pain or need for medications might, in part, reflect a better mood rather than pain prophylaxis.

Among potential prophylactic agents, the α2-δ subunit inhibitors of voltage-gated Ca^{2+} channel activation, gabapentin and pregabalin, have attracted interest because of their benign side effect profiles and relative lack of interaction with other drugs. Unlike opiates, neither drug affects ventilatory drive, heart rate, or blood pressure directly, making them suitable for prophylactic use immediately before surgery. Several prospective, randomized, placebo-controlled trials have evaluated the efficacy of presurgical gabapentin or pregabalin for postsurgical pain. In a typical study, 80 patients scheduled to undergo elective decompressive lumbar laminectomy and one- or two-level spinal fusion were randomized to receive preoperative placebo, pregabalin, celecoxib, or these drugs in combination.[33] Patients reported pain using a VAS, and used a patient-controlled analgesia (PCA) device to self-administer postoperative opiates. Preoperative dosing with either pregabalin or celecoxib reduced postoperative VAS scores and PCA use compared to placebo. The greatest benefit was seen with combination therapy. Meta-analysis of eight placebo-controlled, randomized trials of preoperative gabapentin for postoperative pain found significantly lower VAS pain scores and opiate consumption in the first 24 hours after surgery among those receiving gabapentin.[34] A single preoperative dose of gabapentin was estimated to reduce the average postoperative morphine requirement by 30 mg.[35] As an exception to this markedly positive prophylactic effect, preoperative gabapentin showed no significant pain reduction compared to placebo

in women scheduled for minor gynecological surgery (cervical dilation and curettage, uterine hysteroscopy) that did not require tissue incision.[36] The authors speculated that this might reflect the sparing of peripheral nerves in this surgical paradigm. Overall, prospective studies support the concept that postsurgical pain is a predictable cause of neuropathic pain for which prophylaxis can be effective. These results have begun to influence surgical practice; a single dose of gabapentin is now often given prior to orthopedic procedures in some practices.

TREATMENT TO PREVENT DISEASES ASSOCIATED WITH NEUROPATHIC PAIN

Postherpetic Neuralgia

Successful and economical treatment to prevent neuropathic pain requires identification of a population at high risk. Herpes zoster reactivation from dorsal root ganglion or trigeminal neurons results in a painful shingles rash in one or several dermatomes. Postherpetic neuralgia (PHN) is a feared but predictable consequence of acute herpes zoster reemergence that becomes increasingly common with age. Once established, dermatomal PHN neuropathic pain persists for up to 3 months in 20% of patients and for more than 6 months in 12%–15%. The prevalence of PHN corresponds to the severity of acute pain, and the extent and severity of the herpetic rash, and increases with age.[37] In a prospective evaluation of 280 patients with herpes zoster, age over 50 years and significant pain during the acute zoster flare with a VAS score above 50 mm were the features most predictive of progression to PHN.[38]

Primary prevention of shingles with vaccine was proposed in the early 1990s,[39] and has been shown to unequivocally reduce the incidence of both herpes zoster eruption and subsequent PHN. Among 38,456 patients older than age 60 randomized to receive an injection of either placebo or live attenuated vaccine delivered in a double-blinded manner, 957 developed herpes zoster over an average 3-year follow-up period, and 277 went on to develop PHN lasting for at least 30 days.[40] Vaccination significantly reduced the incidence of herpes zoster

(5.42 cases/1000 patient-years versus 11.22) and PHN (1.39 cases/1000 patient-years versus 3.39 for placebo) and also the duration and intensity of associated neuropathic pain, as measured by the area under the pain severity-duration curve. Patients receiving vaccine were more likely to experience adverse events, most of them related to irritation at the injection site. Primary vaccination of children to prevent varicella infection may eventually reduce incidence of PHN, but it has been estimated that over the next 20 years these vaccines will actually increase the number of PHN cases, since older adults will less commonly experience the exogenous immune stimulus associated with exposure to children with varicella. In the United States, the licensed vaccine used currently is Zostavax®, which is a live attenuated virus vaccine indicated for prevention of herpes zoster (shingles) in individuals 60 years of age and older. Like most live vaccines, it should not be used in pregnant women or in people with immunosuppression.

Prophylactic treatment at the time of shingles development has met with only limited success in preventing subsequent PHN. Prompt recognition and treatment of herpes zoster with antiviral medication has been shown to reduce progression to PHN. Among 419 patients with acute zoster randomized to receive famciclovir or placebo within 72 hours of rash eruption, famciclovir recipients were less likely to experience PHN (hazard ratio 1.9) and had a PHN course that was 2 months shorter on average than that of placebo recipients.[41] A more recent randomized trial in 2027 zoster patients found that famciclovir and the newer once-daily agent bromovinyl deoxyuridine (Brivudin) yielded equivalent reductions in PHN incidence and duration.[37]

Oral corticosteroids do not appear to prevent future attacks or to reduce the risk of developing PHN, so they are not routinely used. Treatment designed explicitly to prevent or limit neuropathic pain has shown mixed results. The PINE (Prevention by epidural Injection of posttherpetic Neuralgia in the Elderly) study randomized 598 active zoster patients, 50 years or older, to receive standardized treatment with oral antivirals alone or with the addition of a single epidural injection of methylprednisolone acetate (80 mg) plus bupivocaine (10 mg). All patients had dermatomal involvement below C6, and patients were recognized and treated less than 7 days after developing a rash. There was no sham or placebo injection, and investigators were not blinded to the treatment assignment. Epidural steroid treatment was associated with a modest decrease in reports of neuropathic pain that was statistically significant at 30 days (137 [48%] vs. 164 [58%]) but not at 3 or 6 months. A far more intensive model of this anti-inflammatory treatment randomized active zoster patients to standard care or repeated administration of methylprednisolone/bupivocaine using an image-guided indwelling epidural catheter. Treatment was continued for at least 7 days, then until the patient reported being pain free or for up to 21 days. This study achieved a highly significant relative risk for PHN of 0.19, but it does not represent a very practical or cost-effective model.

In summary, herpes zoster has been a successful clinical model for exploration of treatments for prophylaxis of neuropathic pain because of its predictable characteristics. Zoster onset is abrupt, easily recognized, and transitions to PHN within weeks in more than 20% of sufferers. Statistically, primary prevention of zoster reactivation has proven to be the most effective means of pain prophylaxis, while later and more pain-specific treatments have proven to be less efficacious. In this regard, zoster is likely to serve as a model for more common conditions, such as painful diabetic neuropathy, in which the treatment of established neuropathy typically provides only limited benefit.

Diabetic Peripheral Neuropathy

Neuropathy is a predictable consequence of diabetes, ultimately affecting half of diabetic patients over their lifetimes. A majority of diabetic peripheral neuropathy (DPN) patients complain of neuropathic pain, making diabetes the single most common cause of neuropathy and neuropathic pain in industrialized countries worldwide. A cross-sectional study comparing 350 people with diabetes to 344 age- and sex-matched controls in Liverpool, England, found chronic painful neuropathy in 16% of diabetic patients but in only 4% of controls.[42] Evaluation of the same cohorts 5 years later found that neuropathic pain had continued for 77% of the diabetic subjects.[43] One-third had not received specific treatment despite requests for pain medication from their physician. For those with persistent pain, there was no significant improvement in neuropathic pain intensity as measured by VAS despite multimodal pain treatment. This result mirrors the frustrating experience of many patients and physicians in treating established neuropathic pain in DPN.[44,45] Although a wide variety of antidepressants, antiepileptic drugs, opiates, and mixed serotonin/norepinephrine reuptake inhibitors have been shown to significantly reduce neuropathic pain compared to placebo in randomized controlled trials[45] (see Chapter 11), pain relief is incomplete for most patients. Diabetic peripheral neuropathy should be an attractive target for treatment to preemptively prevent neuropathic pain. However, no studies have prospectively treated patients with diabetes or DPN with the explicit goal of preventing pain. No basis for identification of patients at particularly high risk for neuropathic pain has been developed.

The duration and intensity of hyperglycemia increase the incidence of neuropathy in patients with diabetes. However, features of metabolic syndrome appear to confer an additional independent neuropathy risk and may play a particularly important role in the development of neuropathic pain. In a cross-sectional study of 548 type 2 diabetic subjects, those with metabolic syndrome were twice as likely to have neuropathy.[46] The EuroDiab study followed 3000 type 1 diabetic subjects for up to 7 years. Among the 1200 subjects without neuropathy at baseline, hypertension, serum lipids and triglyceride levels, body mass index, and smoking were each independently associated with an increased risk of developing neuropathy at follow-up.[47] Elevated triglyceride levels have recently been linked to faster progression of diabetic neuropathy.[48] These epidemiological data linking metabolic syndrome and neuropathy are supported by experimental models of early neuropathy in obese mice[49] and reflect an evolving understanding of the neurotoxic effects of free fatty acid excess and adipokine secretion in central obesity.[50] Adipokines may

have complex and perhaps conflicting pathogenic influences on neuropathy and neuropathic pain. For instance, the adipokine leptin is released from enlarged adipocytes and limits appetite, but it also stimulates an inflammatory response from macrophages. Mice made obese by genetic silencing of leptin production (ob/ob) develop an early peripheral neuropathy.[51] However, these mice do not develop tactile allodynia evoked by partial sciatic nerve ligation,[52] suggesting inhibition of chronic neuropathic pain.

Recognition of the independent contribution of obesity, dyslipidemia, and hypertension to the risk of macrovascular disease has prompted controlled trials designed to directly or indirectly remediate these metabolic syndrome components. While the incidence of neuropathy has not typically been the primary endpoint, these studies support the concept that intervention can prevent progression to DPN and the inevitable accompanying neuropathic pain. The Steno-2 trial demonstrated that aggressive therapy to normalize hypertension and lipid abnormalities, together with smoking cessation, was superior to conventional therapy in reducing the risk of developing large and small vessel diabetic outcomes. Those in the multifactorial treatment arm were significantly less likely to develop coronary, cerebral, or peripheral vascular occlusive disease, but also nephropathy, retinopathy, and autonomic neuropathy.[53] Somatic neuropathy and associated pain were not evaluated.

Balducci and colleagues prospectively examined the effect of long-term aerobic exercise on the incidence of diabetic neuropathy. They randomized 78 type 2 diabetes patients without neuropathy at baseline to receive either nondescript exercise counseling or to perform supervised treadmill walking 4 hours weekly.[54] Measures of fitness, metabolic function, and peripheral nerve integrity were evaluated annually. No dietary counseling was provided, and no direct attempt was made to influence glucose control; The adult hemoglobin level did not improve significantly for either cohort. However, the exercise subjects improved their fitness, increasing their maximum oxygen consumption from 25 to 41 mL/kg/min, and lost waist circumference, while the nonexercisers experienced a worsening over 4 years. Over the 4-year follow-up period, 30% of nonexercisers progressed to clinical sensory neuropathy, while only 7% of exercisers did so ($p < .05$). More than half of the subjects who developed neuropathy in either group complained of new neuropathic pain. These results suggest that regular exercise reduced the risk for DPN and the accompanying neuropathic pain through a mechanism other than improvement in glucose control. Direct neurotrophic effects of exercise may result from vasodilation, increased oxygen delivery, and neovascularization driven by upregulation of vascular endothelial growth factor and other vasogenic growth factors. Smaller studies have shown that exercise can improve electrodiagnostic metrics of nerve function in diabetic patients with neuropathy[55] and measures of epidermal innervation on skin biopsy.[55a]

FUTURE DIRECTIONS

As the causes of neuropathic pain become better understood and more predictable, the prophylactic therapy of patients at high risk for neuropathic pain will use agents that have previously been shown to reduce neuropathic pain or improve peripheral nerve function. Two likely candidates are alpha-lipoic acid (ALA) and acetyl-L-carnitine (ALC). Oxidative stress has been identified as a key component of neuropathy pathogenesis. In diabetes, excess lipids and glucose both produce oxidative free radicals that directly damage axonal mitochondria and divert nitric oxide from its normal vasodilatory role, resulting in impaired vasoregulation and ischemia of nutritive arterioles.[50] Alpha-lipoic acid is an orally bioavailable antioxidant that has been shown to reduce neuropathic pain in the Symptomatic Diabetic Neuropathy (SYDNEY) study, which randomized diabetic neuropathy patients to double-blinded treatment with either placebo or one of three doses of oral ALA (600, 1200, or 1800 mg; 43–45 subjects per group). Over the 5-week treatment course, subjects treated with any of the ALA doses reported a significantly greater reduction in neuropathic pain, as measured by the validated Total Symptom Score, than did the placebo-treated controls.[56] Most clinical measures of neuropathy severity did not

significantly improve; the 600 mg cohort showed a just significant improvement in the Neuropathy Impairment Score (Lower Leg) compared to placebo, an effect not achieved by the larger doses. Previous studies had reported modest improvement in neuropathy measures following intravenous ALA injection.[57]

Diabetes is associated with reduced serum levels and cellular concentrations of ALC, another antioxidant that has been shown to inhibit lipid peroxidation and increase nitric oxide synthase and nitric oxide in experimental models. Two parallel randomized, blinded, controlled trials used pain VAS, various nerve conduction measures, the vibration perception threshold, and, most remarkably, morphometric analysis of sural nerves to assess neuropathy severity at baseline and after 52 weeks of treatment. A total of 1257 diabetic neuropathy patients were randomized to receive either placebo or one of two ALC doses (500 mg or 1000 mg daily).[58] Acetyl-L-carnitine significantly improved sural morphology, but not nerve conduction study measures at 52 weeks. Pain, as measured by VAS, also improved significantly with the larger ALC dose. Responsiveness of pain to ALC treatment diminished with the duration of diabetes, suggesting that early treatment with ALC would be more effective. Alpha-lipoic acid or ALC has been proposed as prophylactic treatment to prevent the onset of neuropathy and the accompanying neuropathic pain in patients with diabetes and those with multiple myeloma undergoing chemotherapy.

The prophylactic effects of recognized neuropathic pain agents have been demonstrated in experimental animal models and in settings such as surgery, where pain is an expected consequence of therapy. However, prospective treatment in other settings where neuropathic pain is predictable would be welcome. Pain associated with chemotherapy-induced peripheral neuropathy is a ready example. Future studies will need to evaluate neuropathic pain specifically, rather than simply measuring peripheral nerve injury. This will require the use of clinical pain scales, but it could also employ quantitative measures of hyperalgesia such as those developed for the heat pain threshold in human experimental settings. Greater use of human experimental models in preclinical testing, and development of combination treatments exploiting synergistic mechanisms, can be expected to provide more effective prophylaxis for patients at high risk for neuropathic pain.

REFERENCES

1. McCarson KE, Ralya A, Reisman SA, Enna SJ. Amitriptyline prevents thermal hyperalgesia and modifications in rat spinal cord GABA(B) receptor expression and function in an animal model of neuropathic pain. *Biochem Pharmacol.* 2005;71(1–2):196–202.
2. Takasaki I, Kurihara T, Saegusa H, et al. Effects of glucocorticoid receptor antagonists on allodynia and hyperalgesia in mouse model of neuropathic pain. *Eur J Pharmacol.* 2005;524(1–3):80–83.
3. Gaida W, Klinder K, Arndt K, Weiser T. Ambroxol, a Nav1.8-preferring Na(+) channel blocker, effectively suppresses pain symptoms in animal models of chronic, neuropathic and inflammatory pain. *Neuropharmacology.* 2005;49(8):1220–1227.
4. Labuz D, Schmidt Y, Schreiter A, et al. Immune cell-derived opioids protect against neuropathic pain in mice. *J Clin Invest.* 2009;119(2):278–286.
5. Geber C, Fondel R, Kramer HH, et al. Psychophysics, flare, and neurosecretory function in human pain models: capsaicin versus electrically evoked pain. *J Pain.* 2007;8(6):503–514.
6. Attal N, Bouhassira D, Gautron M, et al. Thermal hyperalgesia as a marker of oxaliplatin neurotoxicity: a prospective quantified sensory assessment study. *Pain.* 2009;144(3):245–252.
7. Hadjipavlou G, Dunckley P, Behrens TE, Tracey I. Determining anatomical connectivities between cortical and brainstem pain processing regions in humans: a diffusion tensor imaging study in healthy controls. *Pain.* 2006;123(1–2):169–178.
8. Khedr EM, Kotb H, Kamel NF, et al. Longlasting antalgic effects of daily sessions of repetitive transcranial magnetic stimulation in central and peripheral neuropathic pain. *J Neurol Neurosurg Psychiatry.* 2005;76(6):833–838.
9. Borckardt JJ, Smith AR, Reeves ST, et al. Fifteen minutes of left prefrontal repetitive transcranial magnetic stimulation acutely increases thermal pain thresholds in healthy adults. *Pain Res Manage.* 2007;12(4):287–290.
10. Zimmermann M. Pathobiology of neuropathic pain. *Eur J Pharmacol.* 2001:429(1–3):23–37.
11. Simone DA, Ngeow JY, Putterman GJ, LaMotte RH. Hyperalgesia to heat after intradermal injection of capsaicin. *Brain Res.* 1987;418(1):201–203.
12. Gottrup H, Juhl G, Kristensen AD, et al. Chronic oral gabapentin reduces elements of central sensitization in human experimental hyperalgesia. *Anesthesiology.* 2004;101(6):1400–1408.
13. Koppert W, Dern SK, Sittl R, et al. A new model of electrically evoked pain and hyperalgesia in human skin: the effects of intravenous alfentanil, S(+)-ketamine, and lidocaine. *Anesthesiology.* 2001;95(2):395–402.
14. Schmelz M, Michael K, Weidner C, et al. Which nerve fibers mediate the axon reflex flare in human skin? *Neuroreport.* 2000;11(3):645–648.
15. Chizh BA, Gohring M, Troster A, et al. Effects of oral pregabalin and aprepitant on pain and central sensitization in the electrical hyperalgesia model in human volunteers. *Br J Anaesth.* 2007;98(2):246–254.
16. Koppert W, Wehrfritz A, Korber N, et al. The cyclooxygenase isozyme inhibitors parecoxib and paracetamol reduce central hyperalgesia in humans. *Pain.* 2004;108(1–2):148–153.
17. Wolf S, Barton D, Kottschade L, et al. Chemotherapy-induced peripheral neuropathy: prevention and treatment strategies. *Eur J Cancer.* 2008;44(11):1507–1515.
18. Windebank AJ, Grisold W. Chemotherapy-induced neuropathy. *J Peripher Nerv Syst.* 2008;13(1):27–46.
19. Reyes-Gibby CC, Morrow PK, Buzdar A, Shete S. Chemotherapy-induced peripheral neuropathy as a predictor of neuropathic pain in breast cancer patients previously treated with paclitaxel. *J Pain.* 2009;10(11):1146–1150.
20. Tsavaris N, Kopterides P, Kosmas C, et al. Gabapentin monotherapy for the treatment of chemotherapy-induced neuropathic pain: a pilot study. *Pain Med.* 2008;9(8):1209–1216.
21. Hammack JE, Michalak JC, Loprinzi CL, et al. Phase III evaluation of nortriptyline for alleviation of symptoms of cis-platinum-induced peripheral neuropathy. *Pain.* 2002;98(1–2):195–203.
22. Kautio AL, Haanpaa M, Saarto T, Kalso E. Amitriptyline in the treatment of chemotherapy-induced neuropathic symptoms. *J Pain Symptom Manage.* 2008;35(1):31–39.
23. Rao RD, Michalak JC, Sloan JA, et al. Efficacy of gabapentin in the management of chemotherapy-induced peripheral neuropathy: a phase 3 randomized, double-blind, placebo-controlled, crossover trial (N00C3). *Cancer.* 2007;110(9):2110–2118.

24. Rao RD, Flynn PJ, Sloan JA, et al. Efficacy of lamotrigine in the management of chemotherapy-induced peripheral neuropathy: a phase 3 randomized, double-blind, placebo-controlled trial, N01C3. *Cancer.* 2008;112(12):2802–2808.

25. Bairati I, Meyer F, Gelinas M, et al. A randomized trial of antioxidant vitamins to prevent second primary cancers in head and neck cancer patients. *J Natl Cancer Inst.* 2005;97(7): 481–488.

26. Pathak AK, Bhutani M, Guleria R, et al. Chemotherapy alone vs. chemotherapy plus high dose multiple antioxidants in patients with advanced non small cell lung cancer. *J Am Coll Nutr.* 2005;24(1):16–21.

27. Argyriou AA, Chroni E, Polychronopoulos P, et al. Efficacy of oxcarbazepine for prophylaxis against cumulative oxaliplatin-induced neuropathy. *Neurology.* 2006;67(12):2253–2255.

28. von Delius S, Eckel F, Wagenpfeil S, et al. Carbamazepine for prevention of oxaliplatin-related neurotoxicity in patients with advanced colorectal cancer: final results of a randomised, controlled, multicenter phase II study. *Invest New Drugs.* 2007;25(2):173–180.

29. Feng Y, Cui M, Willis WD. Gabapentin markedly reduces acetic acid-induced visceral nociception. *Anesthesiology.* 2003;98(3):729–733.

30. Dahl JB, Mathiesen O, Moiniche S. "Protective premedication": an option with gabapentin and related drugs? A review of gabapentin and pregabalin in the treatment of post-operative pain. *Acta Anaesthesiol Scand.* 2004;48(9):1130–1136.

31. Borckardt JJ, Weinstein M, Reeves ST, et al. Postoperative left prefrontal repetitive transcranial magnetic stimulation reduces patient-controlled analgesia use. *Anesthesiology.* 2006;105(3): 557–562.

32. Borckardt JJ, Reeves ST, Weinstein M, et al. Significant analgesic effects of one session of postoperative left prefrontal cortex repetitive transcranial magnetic stimulation: a replication study. *Brain Stimulat.* 2008;1(2):122–127.

33. Reuben SS, Buvanendran A, Kroin JS, Raghunathan K. The analgesic efficacy of celecoxib, pregabalin, and their combination for spinal fusion surgery. *Anesth Analg.* 2006;103(5):1271–2717.

34. Seib RK, Paul JE. Preoperative gabapentin for postoperative analgesia: a meta-analysis. *Can J Anaesth.* 2006;53(5):461–469.

35. Tiippana EM, Hamunen K, Kontinen VK, Kalso E. Do surgical patients benefit from perioperative gabapentin/pregabalin? A systematic review of efficacy and safety. *Anesth Analg.* 2007;104(6):1545–1556, table of contents.

36. Paech MJ, Goy R, Chua S, et al. A randomized, placebo-controlled trial of preoperative oral pregabalin for postoperative pain relief after minor gynecological surgery. *Anesth Analg.* 2007;105(5):1449–1453, table of contents.

37. Wassilew S. Brivudin compared with famciclovir in the treatment of herpes zoster: effects in acute disease and chronic pain in immunocompetent patients. A randomized, double-blind, multinational study. *J Eur Acad Dermatol Venereol.* 2005;19(1):47–55.

38. Coen PG, Scott F, Leedham-Green M, et al. Predicting and preventing post-herpetic neuralgia: are current risk factors useful in clinical practice? *Eur J Pain.* 2006;10(8):695–700.

39. Oxman MN. Immunization to reduce the frequency and severity of herpes zoster and its complications. *Neurology.* 1995;45(12 suppl 8):S41–S46.

40. Oxman MN, Levin MJ, Johnson GR, et al. A vaccine to prevent herpes zoster and postherpetic neuralgia in older adults. *N Engl J Med.* 2005;352(22):2271–2284.

41. Tyring S, Barbarash RA, Nahlik JE, et al. Famciclovir for the treatment of acute herpes zoster: effects on acute disease and postherpetic neuralgia. A randomized, double-blind, placebo-controlled trial. Collaborative Famciclovir Herpes Zoster Study Group. *Ann Intern Med.* 1995;123(2):89–96.

42. Daousi C, MacFarlane IA, Woodward A, et al. Chronic painful peripheral neuropathy in an urban community: a controlled comparison of people with and without diabetes. *Diabet Med.* 2004;21(9):976–982.

43. Daousi C, Benbow SJ, Woodward A, MacFarlane IA. The natural history of chronic painful peripheral neuropathy in a community diabetes population. *Diabet Med.* 2006;23(9):1021–1024.

44. Davies HT, Crombie IK, Lonsdale M, Macrae WA. Consensus and contention in the treatment of chronic nerve-damage pain. *Pain.* 1991;47(2): 191–196.

45. Ziegler D. Treatment of diabetic neuropathy and neuropathic pain: how far have we come? *Diabetes Care.* 2008;31(Suppl 2):S255–S261.

46. Costa LA, Canani LH, Lisboa HR, et al. Aggregation of features of the metabolic syndrome is associated with increased prevalence of chronic complications in type 2 diabetes. *Diabet Med.* 2004;21(3):252–255.

47. Tesfaye S, Chaturvedi N, Eaton SE, et al. Vascular risk factors and diabetic neuropathy. *N Engl J Med.* 2005;352(4):341–350.

48. Wiggin TD, Sullivan KA, Pop-Busui R, et al. Elevated triglycerides correlate with progression

of diabetic neuropathy. *Diabetes*. 2009;58(7): 1634–1640.

49. Vareniuk I, Pavlov IA, Drel VR, et al. Nitrosative stress and peripheral diabetic neuropathy in leptin-deficient (ob/ob) mice. *Exp Neurol*. 2007;205(2):425–436.

50. Singleton JR, Smith AG, Russell JW, Feldman EL. Microvascular complications of impaired glucose tolerance. *Diabetes*. 2003;52(12): 2867–2873.

51. Drel VR, Mashtalir N, Ilnytska O, et al. The leptin-deficient (ob/ob) mouse: a new animal model of peripheral neuropathy of type 2 diabetes and obesity. *Diabetes*. 2006;55(12):3335–3343.

52. Maeda T, Kiguchi N, Kobayashi Y, et al. Leptin derived from adipocytes in injured peripheral nerves facilitates development of neuropathic pain via macrophage stimulation. *Proc Natl Acad Sci USA*. 2009;106(31):13076–13081.

53. Gaede P, Vedel P, Larsen N, et al. Multifactorial intervention and cardiovascular disease in patients with type 2 diabetes. *N Engl J Med*. 2003;348(5):383–393.

54. Balducci S, Iacobellis G, Parisi L, et al. Exercise training can modify the natural history of diabetic peripheral neuropathy. *J Diabetes Complications*. 2006;20(4):216–223.

55. Fisher MA, Langbein WE, Collins EG, et al. Physiological improvement with moderate exercise in type II diabetic neuropathy. *Electromyogr Clin Neurophysiol*. 2007;47(1):23–28.

55a Smith AG, Russell J, Feldman EL, et al. Lifestyle intervention for pre-diabetic neuropathy. Diabetes Care. 2006; 29 (6):1294-1299.

56. Ziegler D, Ametov A, Barinov A, et al. Oral treatment with alpha-lipoic acid improves symptomatic diabetic polyneuropathy: the SYDNEY 2 trial. *Diabetes Care*. 2006;29(11):2365–2370.

57. Ziegler D, Nowak H, Kempler P, et al. Treatment of symptomatic diabetic polyneuropathy with the antioxidant alpha-lipoic acid: a meta-analysis. *Diabet Med*. 2004;21(2):114–121.

58. Sima AA, Calvani M, Mehra M, Amato A. Acetyl-L-carnitine improves pain, nerve regeneration, and vibratory perception in patients with chronic diabetic neuropathy: an analysis of two randomized placebo-controlled trials. *Diabetes Care*. 2005;28(1):89–94.

59. Zanjani TM, Sabetkasaei M, Mosaffa N, et al. Suppression of interleukin-6 by minocycline in a rat model of neuropathic pain. *Eur J Pharmacol*. 2006;538(1–3):66–72.

60. Maeda T, Kiguchi N, Kobayashi Y, et al. Pioglitazone attenuates tactile allodynia and thermal hyperalgesia in mice subjected to peripheral nerve injury. *J Pharmacol Sci*. 2008;108(3): 341–347.

61. Churi SB, Abdel-Aleem OS, Tumber KK, et al. Intrathecal rosiglitazone acts at peroxisome proliferator-activated receptor-gamma to rapidly inhibit neuropathic pain in rats. *J Pain*. 2008;9(7):639–649.

62. Lynch JJ 3rd, Honore P, Anderson DJ, et al. (L)-Phenylglycine, but not necessarily other alpha2delta subunit voltage-gated calcium channel ligands, attenuates neuropathic pain in rats. *Pain*. 2006;125(1–2):136–142.

63. Sharma S, Kulkarni SK, Agrewala JN, Chopra K. Curcumin attenuates thermal hyperalgesia in a diabetic mouse model of neuropathic pain. *Eur J Pharmacol*. 2006;536(3):256–261.

64. Ledeboer A, Jekich BM, Sloane EM, et al. Intrathecal interleukin-10 gene therapy attenuates paclitaxel-induced mechanical allodynia and proinflammatory cytokine expression in dorsal root ganglia in rats. *Brain Behav Immun*. 2007;21(5):686–698.

65. Jin HW, Flatters SJ, Xiao WH, et al. Prevention of paclitaxel-evoked painful peripheral neuropathy by acetyl-L-carnitine: effects on axonal mitochondria, sensory nerve fiber terminal arbors, and cutaneous Langerhans cells. *Exp Neurol*. 2008;210(1):229–237.

66. Nieto FR, Entrena JM, Cendan CM, et al. Tetrodotoxin inhibits the development and expression of neuropathic pain induced by paclitaxel in mice. *Pain*. 2008;137(3):520–531.

67. Garcia JM, Cata JP, Dougherty PM, Smith RG. Ghrelin prevents cisplatin-induced mechanical hyperalgesia and cachexia. *Endocrinology*. 2008;149(2):455–460.

68. Rahman M, Griffin SJ, Rathmann W, Wareham NJ. How should peripheral neuropathy be assessed in people with diabetes in primary care? A population-based comparison of four measures. *Diabet Med*. 2003;20(5):368–374.

28

Peripheral Neuropathy

Educating Patients and Providers

TAMARA S. RITSEMA AND BETH B. MURINSON

THIS CHAPTER DESCRIBES the education of patients and physicians with regard to peripheral neuropathy. The first section focuses on patient education and the latter portion of the chapter discusses the advances and challenges in educating providers about peripheral neuropathy.

PATIENT EDUCATION IN PERIPHERAL NEUROPATHY

Peripheral neuropathy has important effects on quality of life, perception of self, and the emotional state[1]. It is typically characterized by impairment in motor and sensory function and secondarily coordination; pain is a frequent part of peripheral neuropathy. Beyond this, patients can experience a deep sense of isolation from those around them. This arises in part because neuropathy is not well recognized by the general public despite having a prevalence approaching 10% in older adults.

A feeling of stigma can develop as progressive deterioration of gait and agility can prompt patients to worry that others suspect alcoholism or senescence. Relatively few studies have examined patients' cognitive understanding of, and emotional experiences related to, diabetic neuropathy. One study found moderate levels of knowledge in British and American patients and noted that patients' misperceptions about diabetic foot ulcers were related to pragmatic experience with ulcers.[1a] The study did not elucidate whether patients had received neuropathy or foot care education. A recent Veterans Administration study found that patient education, as a specific intervention, had an important impact on foot care practices related to peripheral neuropathy, observing that basic and advanced patient education was associated with patient practices such as checking the feet daily and keeping them clean.[2] The potential importance of patient education has been known for some time, but patient education practices vary widely and best practices are not uniformly adopted.[3,4, 4a]

PERIPHERAL NEUROPATHY AND THE ROLE OF SELF-CARE

Patients with peripheral neuropathy are expected to perform considerable self-care. The quality of the care these patients can provide themselves is improved when patients have a better understanding of the disease process, treatment options, self-care routines, and available resources. At the end of the day, however, self-care requires a commitment to change on the part of the patient and others close by. Advances in the area of behavior modification indicate that the patient's willingness to make the changes necessary is not enough.[5] Support from healthcare providers is needed. Specifically, the benefits that result from engaging in positive health behaviors and the consequences of failing to adopt appropriate changes need to be explored with the patient in order to establish the momentum needed for implementation of new regimens and routines. Although nursing staff and patient educators can be extremely helpful in educating patients about neuropathy, there is evidence from behavior modification studies in other areas of medicine that physician inquiry and counseling has an important role in generating positive outcomes.[6,7]

Taken as a whole, the studies indicate that more work is needed to find the most effective ways of educating patients about neuropathy. There may be a role for formal foot-care classes, which have been shown to have a positive impact on patient practices. Nonetheless, reinforcement of key messages by physicians (e.g., "Do you check your feet daily?") will continue to be needed. There is increasing awareness that certain physician behaviors can influence the likelihood of a patient's following recommendations. Daily foot exams are one example of a patient behavior that can prevent more severe problems. If you are trying to increase the frequency of the patient's daily foot exams, make sure to ask about these exams at the next visit; this helps to let the patient know that this practice is important. Motivational interviewing techniques utilize the concerns and questions that patients have.

If a patient asks, "Will I wind up in a wheelchair?" this represents an opportunity to explore a patient's fears about neuropathy and hopes for the future. By understanding what motivates a patient, the physician is better prepared to discuss behavior change in terms that are most meaningful to the patient. Continuing with the example, the physician could reply, "It sounds like you're worried about winding up in a wheelchair. What if checking your feet every day could help prevent this?" and "What are the barriers that prevent you from checking your feet every day?" Using the approach of motivational interviewing, the patient's concerns become the fuel that drives discussions about changing important patient behaviors.

Patient Education About Disease Processes

Peripheral neuropathy has many known causes. Patients whose neuropathy has an identified etiology require pathology-specific education. They may need advice on glucose control, alcohol cessation, or avoidance of neurotoxic agents. A significant percentage of patients have idiopathic peripheral neuropathy. These patients need to know that idiopathic neuropathy is common and that they are not alone. They also need to be reassured that their physician will continue to reevaluate them over time to potentially identify an etiology for the neuropathy.

Patients are often confused about the clinical course of peripheral neuropathy. After a few visits, they may be frustrated to discover that they still have neuropathy, having expected to be cured. It is helpful for clinicians to provide an opening for patients to ask questions about neuropathy and to provide a "safe space" for feelings of discouragement or disappointment.

The use of patient-friendly analogies has been described as especially appropriate when discussing neurological problems.[8] One analogy that seems to work fairly well in describing peripheral nerves is the "wires in the house" analogy. By describing this familiar arrangement, it is possible to explain the differences between large-fiber neuropathies (wires to air conditioners and large appliances), mid-caliber neuropathies (wires to small appliances and lights), and small-fiber neuropathies (the little cobundled wires that supply landline telephones). Patients often need explanations about these technical aspects to better understand why both nerve conduction studies and skin biopsies are needed to assess neuropathy.

Patient Education About Treatments

Patients often fail to understand the nature of treatments for peripheral neuropathy. They may need additional counseling to accept the fact that anticonvulsants or antidepressants need to be taken on a regular basis to prevent neuropathic symptoms. As one indicator of this misconception, they may complain that taking these medications intermittently is not effective for the treatment of acute pain.

Providers can anticipate this problem and address it with basic anticipatory guidance. Explain to the patient that these medications are "pain prevention pills," not "pain treatment pills." It may help to compare neuropathy medications to other medications taken for preventive reasons, such as antihypertensive agents or statins. Providing some anticipatory guidance can spare the patient from neuropathic pain and can spare physicians from having to respond to a patient who is upset when his or her gabapentin does not work when taken twice per week. Written reminders or patient instructional materials can help reinforce these messages.

Patients who are treated with disease-modifying medications such as azathioprine or prednisone need to be given guidance about the specific issues concerning these medications. In general, these patients need to be cautioned to avoid abrupt cessation of these medications without consultation with their physician. They may need encouragement to persist in taking medications that have unpleasant side effects that are evident long before the potential benefits are perceived. Providers should tell these patients that the goal of using these medications is both to promote healing and to prevent further neurological degeneration.

Patients who are taking opiates need special instructions and oversight. First, if the physician anticipates long-term treatment with opiates, the physician should initiate a pain contract with the patient advising the patient that certain behaviors or test results will be met with a predetermined series of responses, which may include treatment termination. Behaviors that indicate active addiction, diversion, or abuse of the health care system (doctor-shopping, frequent emergency room visits, etc.) should be extensively documented and responded to with consistency. At the same time, the patient should be advised that sometimes increasing doses of the medication are needed to achieve the same degrees of pain relief. Both staff and patients should be told that this phenomenon represents physiological tolerance, not opioid addiction. Patients should be instructed on how to properly use long-acting opiates— for example, not to crush the pills and to take medications regularly instead of only as needed. Finally, patients who are taking opiates need to be counseled to prevent constipation. Patients should be advised to combine fiber supplements, stool softeners, increased dietary fiber, and significantly increased water intake to avoid debilitating and potentially hazardous constipation.

Regardless of treatment methodology, all patients should be counseled about effective and ineffective adjunct therapies. No single adjunct therapy is effective for every patient. Patients can be advised to try several noninvasive approaches, such as soaking the feet in cool water, using over-the-counter topical analgesics such as capsaicin or menthol gel, or performing foot massage. They should be cautioned against taking high doses of vitamin B_6 (often promoted by health food stores as a treatment for neuropathy), as these can worsen neuropathic pain. The physician should inquire at each visit about adjunctive therapies the patient is using, as patients often fall victim to unscrupulous people who sell ineffective and even harmful "therapies" or "cures" to desperate patients.

Early integration of physical therapy into the regimen of care for peripheral neuropathy can be instrumental for long-term success. As many patients with peripheral neuropathy continue to slowly worsen, the input of a skilled physical therapist whom the patient trusts is especially valuable. Early in the course of disease, the physical therapist can teach strengthening and balance exercises that will enhance the patient's ability to compensate for the limitations imposed by peripheral neuropathy.[9] Physical therapists often infuse their advice with a positive life-affirming attitude that can be helpful to patients coping with pain and lifestyle changes. Later in the course of disease, as it becomes necessary to add assistive devices, patients may be more receptive to this guidance if the neurologist's opinion is supported by the perspectives of the physical therapist.

Self-Care for Peripheral Neuropathy

Like all patients with a chronic illness, patients with peripheral neuropathy need to perform significant self-care. Specific instruction from the medical team can help patients to avoid painless injuries, falls, and amputations.

Patients should be advised to perform daily foot inspection. If the patient inspects the feet daily, painless injuries can be identified before they cause infection or ulceration. We advise our patients to inspect their feet when they are getting out of the shower each day. We demonstrate the technique to them in the clinic and always include specific instructions for inspecting the soles of the feet and the spaces between the toes. Patients who are not flexible enough to examine their own feet can either have their feet examined by a family member who lives with them or can be taught to use a mirror to complete the daily inspection. The physician should specifically ask each neuropathy patient about daily foot inspection at each visit.

At each visit, the physician should also query each patient about falls. Asking about falls is essential if the patient has proprioceptive loss or gait abnormalities on examination. Patients may need to be encouraged to consider using a cane or advancing to a walker. Many patients resist the idea of using these devices. We have found it helpful to remind patients that using an assistive device that allows them to safely work, attend social events, or continue their hobbies is much better than either sitting at home or sustaining a fall with life-changing consequences. All patients must be warned about the dangers they face in the bathroom. Patients with neuropathy should have solid grab bars installed in the shower/bathtub. Some patients may need to be advised to use a shower chair. These are particularly important safety features for patients who live alone and may not have anyone to help them should they fall in the bathroom. Finally, patients should be counseled against the use of throw rugs, the dangers of uneven floors, and other tripping hazards. Occupational therapists can provide an invaluable in-home assessment with practical recommendations for improving the safety of the home for neuropathy patients.

All patients should be encouraged to establish a relationship with a qualified podiatrist. Most insurance companies, including Medicare, will pay for a podiatrist to trim the toenails of neuropathy patients four times per year. Many patients have difficulty trimming their own nails due to arthritis and/or vision problems. Well-trimmed nails can prevent painless injuries and serious infections. Podiatrists can also provide excellent guidance to the patients about shoe choice and advise modifications to shoes to make them safer for patients who have lost protective sensation. In addition, podiatrists can treat those foot ulcers that do occur despite the use of preventive measures.

Family Education and the Patient with Peripheral Neuropathy

As mysterious as peripheral neuropathies can be to patients, they are often even more mysterious to patients' family members. Family members may think that the patient is simply a complainer because nothing appears to be wrong with the patient's feet or hands. It can be hard for children to understand why their formerly active father now feels the need to sit down after 10 minutes of walking or why their mother believes that she can no longer babysit for her grandchildren. The physician can ask the patient to bring family members with them to clinic. Sometimes a simple explanation about neuropathy from a physician will enable family members to believe the patient and to provide more effective assistance to the patient.

PATIENT EDUCATION RESOURCES

Many useful patient-centered resources are available. The Neuropathy Association hosts a Web site and in many larger cities provides support groups. Patients may benefit from disease-specific resources offered by organizations such as the American Diabetes Association and the American Cancer Society. Table 28-1 lists some of the Internet addresses for helpful organizations.

PERIPHERAL NEUROPATHY AND MEDICAL TRAINEES

Introduction

Peripheral neuropathy is a diagnostic term applied to a prevalent medication condition, the most common cause of which is diabetes. Other causes are important especially in patients without known abnormalities of glucose metabolism, including autoimmune processes, infection, repetitive trauma, genetic factors, metabolic conditions, toxicities, and deficiencies. In short, peripheral neuropathyarises from a diverse number of medical conditions. The study of peripheral neuropathy should be deeply challenging to medical trainees, as it essentially compels integrative clinical reasoning; for unknown reasons, peripheral neuropathy continues to suffer from a pervasive lack of interest among medical students.[10] This attitude may relate to the nonacute nature of most neuropathies, in contrast to the more dramatic presentations of other neurological conditions such as stroke and seizure. Nonetheless, peripheral neuropathy leads to dramatic reductions in quality of life and thousands of amputations yearly, many related to the complications of peripheral neuropathy. In this respect,

peripheral neuropathy is a serious disease that is often suboptimally managed; improved education of medical trainees is needed.

Recently, substantial advances have been made with regard to understanding and improving the process of trainee education[10a]. There are pragmatic lessons to be learned from advances in the area of medical education process, that is, how learners learn well and how teachers can deliver their lessons more effectively.[11] The application of conceptual insights about trainee development may enhance medical training in peripheral neuropathy; however, persisting challenges face those seeking to strengthen education about neuropathy.

Despite the high to moderate prevalence of peripheral neuropathy, medical trainees as a group receive only limited training about the pathophysiology, assessment, and treatment of peripheral nervous system (PNS) disorders. And although academicians of previous generations viewed medical teaching as a series of practices acquired through apprenticeship, reflecting an inchoate understanding of how trainees develop, the process of clinical learning has attracted the attention of educational psychologists.[11,12] Research in this area has challenged several closely held beliefs about teaching and learning, but in other areas it has supported conventional wisdom.

Peripheral Neuropathy and the Multiple Dimensions of Trainee Education

The clinical tasks associated with delivering care for neuropathy include not only diagnosis, where possible, and symptomatic relief but also anticipation of patients' needs in the areas of physical rehabilitation, accommodations for mobility restrictions, addressing the inevitable questions about dietary impacts on neuropathy, and education of the patient and relevant others about clinical trials in peripheral neuropathy as appropriate. In the event that neuropathy is painful, it is necessary to ascertain and address the impact of neuropathic pain on sleep, cognition, mood, and role functioning. Depending on the circumstances, patients may require counseling with regard to participation in clinical trials, the risks and benefits associated with particular medical therapies, and their interest in attempting complementary and alternative therapies. Some patients with neuropathy will pursue unproven therapies out of desperation. Maintaining the therapeutic relationship with patients is essential, but this may be difficult if abruptly dismissive skepticism or overt ridicule is evident when responding to these queries. Because of the distressing nature of neuropathy, the care of patients with peripheral neuropathy requires not only knowledge but also a degree of emotional development on the part of medical providers.[13]

There are several ways in which recently identified best practices in medical education can be applied in everyday clinical teaching encounters. First and foremost, every moment counts. Never underestimate the influence of personal and professional commitment in working with others who are learning. The identification of exceptional role models is by far the most important event in medical school and subsequent training for most trainees.[14,15] Part of becoming an exceptional clinical educator in the modern era is to recognize that particular behaviors are especially effective in promoting rapid and meaningful learning. Stu-

dents and trainees need to acquire new information in a way that allows them to build on existing knowledge. For this reason, most brief clinical educational experiences need to begin with a rapid but nonjudgmental assessment of the existing knowledge base (Table 28-2). A few quick questions at the start of a clinic session will usually suffice to generally gauge trainees' clinical knowledge about peripheral neuropathy. This allows a limited clinical education experience to make strong associations with established cognitive elements. The clinical encounter presents great opportunities to engage students in immediately applying new knowledge; communicating with patients will lead nascent providers to reinforce their own understanding of a clinical problem. It is important to provide feedback that is timely and specific and focused on encouraging the positive aspects of care already present while providing direction for incremental change. Flippant or inappropriate conduct by students should be responded to with immediate and exceptionally detailed comments, as generic expressions of disapproval are not correctly interpreted by trainees.[16] Finally, a "learning prescription" is

Table 28-2. Recommended Steps for Successful Teaching in a Clinical Setting

1. Begin with non-threatening inquiry to determine learner readiness for specific material:
   a. Ask learners if they have seen or taken care of patients with peripheral neuropathy.
   b. Ask if they have previously observed a nerve conduction study.
   c. Ask if they would be comfortable choosing a medication for relief of neuropathic pain.
2. Assign tasks that require a learner to apply new knowledge.
   a. Have a medical student explain "small versus large neuropathy" to a patient.
   b. Ask a resident to explain his or her interpretation of the electromyography/nerve conduction study.
   c. Formulate the plan with the fellow and have the fellow communicate it to the patient with observation and later feedback
3. Provide a learning prescription: "I'd like you to read about autoimmune neuropathies this evening and send me a revised differential diagnosis for this patient with an explanation. Include your recommendations for further workup."
4. When providing feedback use recommended techniques
   a. Provide feedback that is timely and specific; don't delay until the details of the experience have faded.
   b. When possible, provide formative feedback at the midpoint of a teaching encounter and summative feedback at the end.
   c. Make sure to give feedback that includes both positive and negative points. The "feedback sandwich" approach uses a negative comment sandwiched between two positive observations.

a tailored recommendation for the learner to engage in a specific task relating to the clinical encounter. The learning prescription may identify a specific area of medical knowledge that needs additional study. Increasingly, students are being asked to cultivate the habit of lifelong learning by actively reflecting on challenges specific to a clinical experience and verbalizing or writing about their own formulation of a learning prescription.[17]

Conceptual Organization of Clinical Development and Applications to Peripheral Neuropathy

There has been increasing awareness that the traditional models of professional competence are insufficient to describe the broad range of skills required for the full expression of medical excellence. One formulation of the multiple dimensions of professional competence is widely used and includes domains of knowledge, technical skill, clinical reasoning, communication, emotions, values, and reflection.[18] This model is helpful in addressing those domains of clinical care that extend beyond the database of medicine.

The relationship of the various domains to each other is overlapping (Figure 28.1), and medical practitioners will have varying degrees of strength in each domain. Interestingly, the seven-domain model is a gateway to considering further how each of the domains is structured. Clearly, broad terms like *knowledge* and *emotions* need further elaboration.[19] To date, selected domains have been expanded to varying degrees but, for example, it is clear that the cognitive aspects of clinical medicine, incorporating knowledge and clinical reasoning and to some degree each of the other domains, have a particular structure that may be especially familiar to neurologists as semantic knowledge, explicit knowledge, and so on. Recognition that multiple domains of accomplishment are necessary to fully attain clinical excellence has direct relevance in educational settings. Application of the multidimensional model of professional competence to training in peripheral neuropathy is illustrated for trainees at various stages in Table 28-3. As an example of this, medical students can be viewed as having developmentally appropriate learning tasks germane to each of the dimensions in the Epstein model.

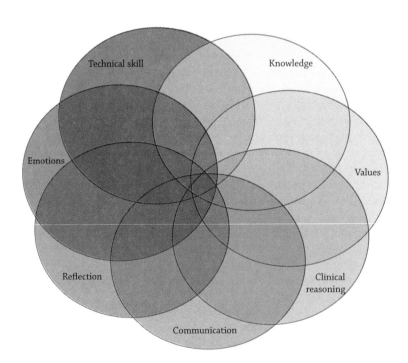

FIGURE 28.1   Multiple domains of clinical development as described by Epstein and Hundert.[18] The domains interact but are required in combination for full attainment of clinical excellence.

Table 28-3. Basic Learning Tasks for Major Skill Areas in Medicine, Classified by Stage of Training

STAGE OF TRAINING	KNOWLEDGE	TECHNICAL SKILL	CLINICAL REASONING	EMOTIONAL DEVELOPMENT	VALUES FORMATION	REFLECTIVE CAPACITY	COMMUNICATION
Medical student	Neuropathy as classified by modality and fiber size; diabetes is a major cause	Basic reflexes, sensory testing, explaining testing maneuvers to the patient as appropriate	Description of syndrome in terms of motor, sensory, and autonomic involvement	Neuropathy is painful and/or disabling; this has emotional effects on patients	Neuropathy is prevalent and potentially serious	Role models are profoundly important	Practice explaining basics of nerve structure and the neuropathy process
Resident	Neuropathy due to many causes: repetitive injury, metabolic, genetic	Reflexes with reinforcement Sensory: dermatomal vs. gradient	Sensory exam is essential for neuropathy assessment	Resisting compassion fatigue for those with pain or disability	Neuropathy, while not as dramatic as stroke or epilepsy, needs neurologicalcare	Modeling respectful conduct and concern for patient well-being	Foster open dialogue and shared decision making, assess risks for adverse effects of medications
Fellow	Genetic variants and acquired variants	Reflexes: consonant with other modalities Sensory: mono-neuropathy vs. other patterns	Integration of modalities from exam, history, and laboratory information	Instilling hope and managing expectation for care outcomes	Neuropathy has profound impacts on quality of life; active intervention mitigates negative effects	How best to manage impacts of neuropathy on ADLs and other functions	Dialogue concerning lifestyle impacts on/ of neuropathy
Peer review	Essential screening strategies and when to refer	Major mono-neuropathies	Assessment of neuropathy for progression	Avoiding therapeutic nihilism	Neuropathy merits expert assessment and care	Advocate for impacts of neuropathy	Impact of neuropathy on other conditions

Because neuropathy, and especially small-fiber neuropathy has very subtle physical findings concomitant with profound impacts on the patient's affective state, it may be important to actively shape the emotional responses of medical students and interns who may exhibit undue skepticism toward patients with many somatic complaints. Students, many of whom will be unfamiliar with the details of peripheral neuropathy, need to become comfortable with acknowledging limitations and avoid hiding the limits of their knowledge through the use of medical jargon. It is important to encourage students to calibrate their use of language to the patient's understanding.

Challenges to Teaching About Peripheral Neuropathy

Clinical conditions related to diseases of the PNS, such as sciatica and peripheral neuropathy, have high to moderate prevalence. Despite this, medical students receive scant training about the pathophysiology, assessment, and treatment of PNS disorders. In addition, because of limited preclinical preparation during medical school, students often have substantial deficits in general knowledge about nociception (pain processing) and lack professional development in the diagnosis, assessment, and treatment of pain-associated medical conditions. We have found that junior medical students who affirm multiple negative emotions in response to clinical pain vignettes are more likely to underestimate pain than students who endorse two or fewer negative emotions.[20] We believe that this compels a careful examination of how medical students both understand and feel about pain. In order to better understand the educational challenges particular to neuropathy, we conducted a survey to gauge students' reactions to peripheral neuropathy and sciatica and to determine if they have a specific tendency to underestimate the pain of these conditions.[10]

In the context of the 4-year neurosciences curriculum at Johns Hopkins, we asked 190 students from all 4 years of medical school training about their knowledge of neuropathy, their interest in neuropathy, and their expectation of needing knowledge about neuropathy in the future. Surprisingly, many students had relative difficulty

Table 28-4. Second-Year Medical Students' Knowledge About Peripheral Neurology

CORE KNOWLEDGE TESTED	% CORRECT
Identifies pain system components	68
Locates primary afferent neuron in the Dorsal Root Ganglion	82
Knows that glutamate is the major neurotransmitter of primary afferents	82
Recognizes that nonsteroidal anti-inflammatory drugs are the least likely of various medications to relieve neuropathic pain	78
Chooses an appropriate differential diagnosis for a case of radicular pain	83

answering basic questions about neuropathy and pain pathophysiology (Table 28-4). The students' responses to clinical vignettes depicting radiculopathy and peripheral neuropathy turned up a surprising discrepancy: students asked to assess the case with peripheral neuropathy slightly underestimated the amount of pain, but those assigned to assess the amount of pain associated with radiculopathy demonstrated markedly underestimated it; as a group, the students estimated pain to be 2 full points below that reported by the patient (Figure 28.2). Given our previous finding that pain underestimation by medical students was related to their emotional responses, we wanted to explore student empathy and interest. As shown in Figure 28.3, the students self-identified as having strong empathy for patients with pain in general but expressed relatively less interest in patients' neuropathy and radiculopathy specifically. It seems that students may be unaware of the prevalence and importance of these conditions in clinical practice. We conclude from these data that making peripheral neuropathy and radiculopathy interesting for medical students represents a significant educational challenge.

Synopsis and Goals for the Future

Peripheral neuropathy is a prevalent disorder in the older patient population. More broadly

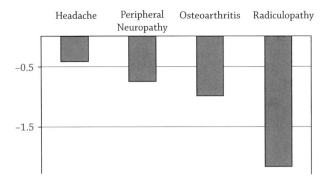

FIGURE 28.2   Underestimation of pain by second-year medical students varies with the medical condition. Students estimated the intensity of pain described by a patient in a clinical vignette. Using a 0–10 scale to make this estimate, students assigned to the peripheral neuropathy group demonstrated intermediate pain ratings compared to students in the headache and osteoarthritis groups. Pain associated with radiculopathy was underestimated by all students. Radiculopathy pain was assessed prior to the start of a 1-hour training session on nonpharmacological approaches to pain management; other conditions were assessed at the end of this session. Significant improvements were seen; radiculopathy vs. headache, peripheral neuropathy and osteoarthritis, $p < .05$).

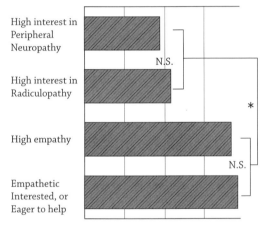

FIGURE 28.3   Percentage of students expressing interest or empathy. Students were asked to endorse levels of interest and empathy for patients with peripheral neuropathy, radiculopathy, or pain in general (empathy measures). Students who expressed more than moderate levels of interest or empathy were identified as expressing high levels of these qualities, and percentages were derived from the whole. N.S. indicates no significant differences in the proportions of students with high interest in neuropathy or radiculopathy. Measures of empathy were not different (N.S.). The proportions of students endorsing high interest in peripheral neuropathy and radiculopathy were significantly lower than the proportion of students expressing empathy more generally; $p < .05$.

speaking, peripheral nerve disease, including disease of the peripheral nerves, ganglia, and roots, is even more prevalent. Sciatica, due to disease of the lumbosacral roots, ganglia, or sciatic nerve, is common. Spinal disorders are among the 10 most common primary diagnoses in the United States and the second most common primary diagnosis in the population aged 44–64.[21] Sciatica can present as radiating low back pain, also a very common diagnosis.

Given the prevalence of pain and pain-associated medical conditions, most medical graduates lack sufficient preparation to competently to distinguish among osteoarthritis, peripheral neuropathy, and radiculopathy, each requiring specialized treatment. Fewer still are prepared to counsel patients with regard to the care and self-care of these conditions.

Do physicians committed to the study and clinical care of peripheral neuropathy need a nationally recommended curriculum for medical students and medical trainees? This question remains unanswered. It would appear from the foregoing discussion that the challenges associated with educating patients and providers about peripheral neuropathy are substantial. It stands to reason that a coordinated effort to understand the process of learning and the optimization of knowledge transfer is this area is needed.

REFERENCES

1. Torpy JM, Kincaid JL, Glass RM. JAMA patient page. Peripheral neuropathy. *JAMA*. 2010; 303(15):1556.

1a. Vileikyte L, Gonzalez JS, Leventhal H, Peyrot MF, Rubin RR, Garrow A, Ulbrecht JS, Cavanagh PR, Boulton AJ. Patient Interpretation of Neuropathy (PIN) questionnaire: an instrument for assessment of cognitive and emotional factors associated with foot self-care. *Diabetes Care*. 2006;29(12):2617–2624.

2. Johnston MV, Pogach L, Rajan M, Mitchinson A, Krein SL, Bonacker K, Reiber G. Personal and treatment factors associated with foot self-care among veterans with diabetes. *J Rehabil Res Dev*. 2006;43(2):227–238.

3. el-Shazly M, Abdel-Fattah M, Scorpiglione N, Benedetti MM, Capani F, Carinci F, Carta Q, Cavaliere D, De Feo EM, Taboga C, Tognoni G, Nicolucci A. Risk factors for lower limb complications in diabetic patients. The Italian Study Group for the Implementation of the St. Vincent Declaration. *J Diabetes Complications*. 1998;12(1): 10–17.

4. Oguejiofor OC, Oli JM, Odenigbo CU. Evaluation of "care of the foot" as a risk factor for diabetic foot ulceration: the role of internal physicians. *Niger J Clin Pract*. 2009;12(1):42–46.

4a. Collins J. Education techniques for lifelong learning: making a PowerPoint presentation. *Radiographics*. 2004;24(4):1177–1183.

5. Chobanian AV, Bakris GL, Black HR, Cushman WC, Green LA, Izzo JL Jr, Jones DW, Materson BJ, Oparil S, Wright JT and Roccella EJ. The Seventh Report of the Joint National Committee on Prevention, Detection, Evaluation, and Treatment of High Blood Pressure: The JNC 7 Report. *JAMA*. 2003;289(19):2560–2572.

6. Lemmens V, Oenema A, Knut IK, Brug J. Effectiveness of smoking cessation interventions among adults: a systematic review of reviews. *Eur J Cancer Prev*. 2008;17(6):535–544.

7. Law M, Tang JL. An analysis of the effectiveness of interventions intended to help people stop smoking. *Arch Intern Med*. 1995;155(18): 1933–1941.

8. Gregory RJ. Neuro-talk: an intervention to enhance communication. *J Psychosoc Nurs Ment Health Serv*. 1998;36(10):28–31.

9. Yentes JM, Perell KL. Diabetic peripheral neuropathy and exercise. 2006 *Clin Kinesiol*. 2006:60(3):25–32.

10. Murinson BB, Agarwal A, Haythornthwaite JA. Medical students report high levels of empathy for sciatica but only moderate interest in learning about peripheral neuropathy. Paper presented at: Biennial Meeting of the Peripheral Nerve Society; July 2007; Snowbird, UT.

10a. Woods NN, Brooks LR, Norman GR. It all makes sense: biomedical knowledge, causal connections and memory in the novice diagnostician. *Adv Health Sci Educ Theory Pract*. 2007;12(4): 405–415.

11. Norman G. Teaching basic science to optimize transfer. *Med Teach*. 2009;31(9):807–811.

12. Nendaz MR, Bordage G. Promoting diagnostic problem representation. *Med Educ*.2002;36: 760–766.

13. Paqueta C, Kergoat M-J, Dube L.The role of everyday emotion regulation on pain in hospitalized elderly: insights from a prospective within-day assessment. *Pain*. 2005;115: 355–363.

14. Murinson BB, Klick B, Haythornthwaite JA, Shochet R, Levine RB, Wright SM. Formative experiences of emerging physicians: gauging the impact of events that occur during medical school. *Acad Med*. 2010;85(8):1331–1337.

15. Wright SM, Kern DE, Kolodner K, Howard DM, Brancati FL. Attributes of excellent attending-physician role models. *N Engl J Med*. 1998; 339(27):1986–1993.

16. Burack JH, Irby DM, Carline JD, Root RK, Larsen EB. Teaching compassion and respect: attending physicians' responses to problematic behaviors. *J Gen Intern Med*. 1999;14:49–55.

17. Knowles MS. Facilitating learner-centered learning through learning contracts. *Med Encounter*. 1992;8(3):4–5.

18. Epstein RM, Hundert EM. Defining and assessing professional competence. *JAMA*. 2002;287(2):226–235.

19. Roter DL, Frankel RM, Hall JA, Sluyter D. The expression of emotion through nonverbal behavior in medical visits. Mechanisms and outcomes. *J Gen Intern Med*. 2006;21(suppl 1): S28–S34.

20. Klick B, Agarwal AK, Haythornthwaite JA, Murinson BB. Negative emotional responses impair pain assessment by medical Ssudents. Presented at: IASP Triennial World Congress of the IASP; August 2008; Glasgow, Scotland.

21. Konstantinou K, Dunn KM. Sciatica: review of epidemiological studies and prevalence estimates. *Spine*. 2008;33(22):2464–2472.

Index

McGill Pain Questionnaire (MPQ), 89–90. *See also* Short-Form
    McGill Pain Questionnaire
    for DNP, 173
McKenzie techniques, 476
mechanical hyperalgesia, 25
Melville, Herman, 3
memantine, 320–321
Mendell, Lorne, 9
meningitis. *See* aseptic meningitis
metabolic disorders, 416
methadone, 122
    cardiac risks with, 159–160, 160
methotrexate, 27
N-methyl-D-aspartate (NMDA) receptors, 171–172
    in DNP therapy, 179
    SCDH event signaling, 171
    in TPNI therapy, 320–321
mexiletine, 119
MFS. *See* Miller Fish syndrome
microcompression. *See* balloon microcompression, for TN
microglia, in HIV-DSP, 194
microvascular decompression (MVD), 406–407
midazolam, 27
Miller Fish syndrome (MFS), 264
minocycline, 28
MIRE. *See* monochromatic infrared photo energy
mirror visual feedback therapy, 335, 479–480
Mitchell, John, 374
Mitchell, S. Weir, 1, 3–4, 5, 307
    CRPS for, 372
MMN. *See* multifocal motor neuropathy
Moby Dick (Melville), 3
monoamines, 119–122
    bupropion, 122
    dosage guidelines for, 121
    receptor activation in, 120
    SSRIs, 120–122
        duloxetine, 27, 120–121
        venlafaxine, 30, 31, 121–122
    tricyclic agents, 120
        amitriptyline, 27, 29, 120
        clinical risks with, 120
monochromatic infrared photo energy (MIRE), 182
monoclonal gammopathy of undetermined significance.
        See chronic sensory-motor neuropathy
morphine, 29, 123
movement exercises, 475–476
MPQ. *See* McGill Pain Questionnaire
MS. *See* multiple sclerosis
multifocal acquired demyelinating sensory and motor neu-
    ropathy (MADSAM), 271
multifocal motor neuropathy (MMN), 271
multiple sclerosis (MS), 60
    CNeP with, 343–345
        clinical characteristics, 343–344
        diagnosis of, 344
        treatment therapies for, 344–345
    TN and, 399
MVD. *See* microvascular decompression
myelin, during Wallerian degeneration, 310
myelinated low threshold mechanoreceptors, 10

NA. *See* neuralgic amyotrophy
Namenda. *See* memantine
nerve biopsies. *See* skin and nerve biopsies
nerve conduction studies, 76–77
    CMAP in, 76
    diagnostic utility of, 76

limitations of, 77
principles of, 76
SNAP in, 76
for SSN, 233
strengths of, 76–77
nerve growth factor (NGF), 170–171
nerve system
    afferent fibers
        overtrophed, 17
        undertrophed, 17
    anatomy of, 307
    peripheral nerves
        neuropathic pain and, 4
        segregation of function in, 6–7
nerve toxicity, neuropathy from. *See* toxic nerve neuropathy
neuralgic amyotrophy (NA), 260–264
    clinical features of, 260–262
    diagnosis of, 262–263
        through electrodiagnostic findings, 263
    discovery of, 260
    HNA and, 262, 263
    treatment for, 263–264
neurapraxia injuries, 307
neurogenic claudication, 361
    animal models for, 361
neuromyotonia, 238
    clinical features of, 238
    laboratory findings for, 238
    treatment for, 238
neuropathic pain. *See also* allodynia; animal models; can-
        cer, neuropathic pain from; cognitive-behavior
        therapy; complementary and alternative medicine;
        drug development; entrapment syndromes; experi-
        mental models, for neuropathic pain; hyperalgesia;
        pain management; peripheral neuropathic pain;
        psychosocial factors, for neuropathic pain
    action potential and, 5–7
        in peripheral sensory axons, 5
    anatomic localization of, 59–60
        in CNS, 59–60
        peripheral nerves, 59
    assessment for, 64–72
        in animal research models, 67
        bedside, 63, 61–63, 63, 71
        for classifications, 71–72
        through interviews, 71
        with NPS, 64
        with NPSI, 65
        phenotype heterogeneity in, 67
        with PQAS, 64–65
        with QST, 65–67, 65–67, 72
        through questionnaires, 68–71
        with SF-MPQ 2, 65, 89–90
        standardized protocols for, 65–67
        subgroup definition in, 67–71
    causalgia and, 3–4, 5, 5
    central sensitization in, 18–19, 19
        cortical field reorganization and, 21, 20–21
        drug development for, 50
        signal transduction cascades in, 19
        spinal neurons and, 18, 19
        synaptic plasticity in, 18–19
        tactile somatotopy in, 21
    from chronic liver disease, 424
    chronic nonmalignant
        definition of, 151
        prevalence rates for, 151
    classifications of, 14–16, 71–72